Chronic Lymphocytic Leukemia

CONTEMPORARY HEMATOLOGY

Gary J. Schiller, MD, Series Editor

Chronic Lymphocytic Leukemia

Molecular Genetics, Biology,

Diagnosis, and Management

Edited by

Guy B. Faguet, MD

Veterans Affairs Medical Center, Augusta, GA

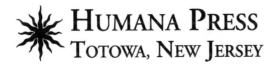

HUMANA PRESS
TOTOWA, NEW JERSEY

Library of Congress Cataloging-in-Publication Data

Chronic lymphocytic leukemia ; molecular genetics, biology, diagnosis, and management / edited by Guy B. Faguet.
p. ; cm. -- (Contemporary hematology)
Includes bibliographical references and index.
ISBN 1-58829-099-9 (alk. paper)
1. Lymphocytic leukemia. I. Faguet, Guy B. II. Series.
[DNLM: 1. Leukemia, Lymphocytic, Chronic. WH 250 C556505 2003]
RC643.C4846 2003
616.99'419--dc21

2003041670

PREFACE

Chronic lymphocytic leukemia (CLL) is usually described as the most common leukemia in the United States, Canada, and Western Europe, whereas it is rare in Japan *(1)* and infrequent in other Asian societies *(2)*. In the United States, CLL remained the most common leukemia between 1973 and 1991 with a mean age- and population-adjusted incidence of 4.4/100,000, whereas it was 3.2/100,000 for acute myelocytic leukemia (AML), the second most frequent leukemia during that time. However, the incidence of CLL began declining in the mid-1990s as AML's rose, resulting in reversed positions after 1997, with rates of 3.4 for CLL and 3.9 for AML in 2000, the last year of available Surveillance, Epidemiology, and End Results (SEER) data *(3)* (Fig. 1). Likewise, according to American Cancer Society projections for the 2000–2002 period, CLL accounted for 22.7–26.3% of all leukemias in the United States, whereas AML represented 31.5–34.4% *(4)*, and in 2003 approximately 7300 new cases of CLL and 10,500 new cases of AML are expected in the United States *(5)*. On the other hand, these data probably underestimate the true incidence and prevalence of CLL *(6)*. Indeed, the ease of suspecting the disease based on blood lymphocytosis revealed by ubiquitous CBCs, coupled with the highly specific and sensitive diagnostic power of immunophenotyping, makes a cytologic diagnosis of CLL possible in many asymptomatic individuals with emerging clones that are likely to remain indolent and untreated for many years *(7)*. This, and the fact that many of these individuals are likely to die of unrelated deaths, suggest that their leukemia might be considered incidental by their physicians and not be reported to tumor registries nor listed in death certificates.

Yet, whether it is the most common or the second most common leukemia in the Western world, it is noteworthy that CLL attracts a disproportionate amount of interest in the scientific community despite accounting for less than 1% of all new cancers and all cancer deaths in the United States in any given year *(3,5)*, after a frequently benign course compatible with a multiyear survival (Table 1). This interest is illustrated by a recent Medline survey that yielded 4002 articles on CLL in the last 10 years (January 1993 through December 2002), compared

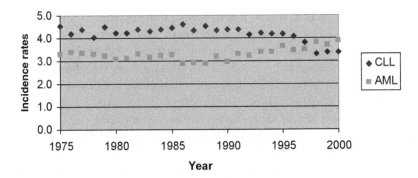

Age- and population-adjusted incidence rates for CLL and AML between 1975 and 2000. (Data from ref. *3*, SEER Cancer Statistics Review, 1975–2000)

Table 1
CLL vs Lung Cancer in the US: Incidence, Mortality, and Survival Rates *(3,4,6)*

	CLL	Lung Cancer
New cases (2003 estimates)	7300	171,900
New cases as percentage of total cancers (2003)	0.55	12.9
Age-adjusted incidence rate (1999)	3	68
Mortality (total deaths in 1999)	4300	152,480
Mortality as percentage of total cancer deaths (1999)	0.79	28.2
Age-adjusted mortality rate (1995–1999)	1.6	58
Percentage of patients surviving 5 years (1992–1998)	73	15

to 38,222 on lung cancer, the most lethal cancer accounting for 12.9% of all cancer deaths expected in the United States in 2003 *(5)*, after a relentless progression and an average survival that barely exceeds 6 months *(8)*. Several factors render CLL an interesting subject for study by scientists and clinical researchers. They include marked progress in understanding the molecular biology of normal and neoplastic lymphocytes and recent advances in molecular genetic techniques culminating in microarray technology. The former, facilitated by highly sophisticated and versatile flow cytometry instruments, powerful analytical software *(9)*, and a rapidly evolving hybridoma technology with its myriad of monoclonal antibodies targeted to lymphoid antigens, enable the discriminant analysis of complex and heterogeneous cellular components within tissues and fluids, their differentiation, activation, and proliferative potential. The latter enables the study of thousands of genes, their expression and interactions, simultaneously *(10)*. These tools together with the ease of procuring blood and bone marrow samples repeatedly with little discomfort or risk to patients, whose prolonged survival enables long-term follow-up studies, are largely responsible for the fascination of CLL. This fascination at the molecular level extends to human trials. Indeed, as of December, 2002, there were 69 ongoing National Cancer Institute (NCI)-sponsored clinical trials on CLL and 185 on lung cancer *(11)*, a ratio of 1:2.7 despite the relative age-adjusted incidence and death ratios in the 1995–1999 period of 1:23 and 1:36, respectively (Table 1). Not surprisingly, the pharmaceutical industry has also participated in and financially benefited from these heightened bench and clinical research activities, launching new agents with activity in CLL, such as Fludarabine®, Rituxan®, and Campath®.

Because the aim of medical research is to generate the scientific database as a foundation for ultimately improving health care, a pertinent and timely question is whether this extraordinary focus on CLL has improved patient outcomes and where it is leading. Thus, the purpose of *Chronic Lymphocytic Leukemia: Molecular Genetics, Biology, Diagnosis, and Management*, is to review recent advances in molecular genetics and biology of CLL, to assess the impact on the diagnosis and management of this disease, and to suggest future directions. To do so, a panel of senior experts was assembled from the United States and Europe, and each was assigned the task of updating the status of his or her area of expertise in a comprehensive yet concise chapter. This effort yielded 23 chapters, carefully prepared by 43 scientists and clinical researchers from 24 medical centers or research institutions. Chapters were organized into five sectional themes beginning with Dr. Marti's enlightening historical perspective that sets the stage for sequentially reviewing recent progress in the molecular genetics and biology of CLL and the extent to which these

CONTENTS

CONTRIBUTORS

JULIA ALMEIDA, MD, PhD • *Service of Cytometry, Department of Medicine and Cancer Research Center, University of Salamanca, Salamanca, Spain*

GERALD P. BODEY, MD • *Department of Infectious Diseases, The University of Texas M.D. Anderson Cancer Center, Houston, TX*

FRANCESC BOSCH, MD • *Department of Hematology, Hospital Clinic, University of Barcelona, Barcelona, Spain*

RAUL C. BRAYLAN, MD • *Department of Pathology, Immunology, and Laboratory Medicine, University of Florida College of Medicine, Gainesville, FL*

JOHN C. BYRD, MD • *Division of Hematology and Oncology, The Ohio State University, Columbus, OH*

JANUARIO E. CASTRO, MD • *Division of Hematology and Oncology, University of California, San Diego, School of Medicine, La Jolla, CA*

DANIEL CATOVSKY, MD, DSc • *Academic Department of Haematology and Cytogenetics, Institute of Cancer Research, Royal Marsden Hospital, London, UK*

GUILLAUME DIGHIERO, MD, PhD • *Unité d'Immuno-Hematologie et d'Immunopathologie, Institut Pasteur, Paris, France*

HARTMUT DÖHNER, MD • *Department of Internal Medicine III, University of Ulm, Ulm, Germany*

VONDA K. DOUGLAS, MD • *Department of Pathology, Immunology, and Laboratory Medicine, University of Florida College of Medicine, Gainesville, FL*

GUY B. FAGUET, MD • *Section of Hematology/Oncology, Veterans Affairs Medical Center, Augusta, GA*

ALESSANDRA FERRAJOLI, MD • *Department of Leukemia, The University of Texas M.D. Anderson Cancer Center, Houston, TX*

ROBIN FOA, MD, PhD • *Dipartimento di Biotecnologie Cellulari ed Ematologia, Università degli Studi di Roma "La Sapienza," Rome, Italy*

ARTHUR E. FRANKEL, MD • *Wake Forest University School of Medicine, Winston-Salem, NC*

NIRAJ GUPTA, MD • *Division of Hematology-Oncology, Long Island Jewish Medical Center, New Hyde Park, NY*

TERRY HAMBLIN, MB, DM • *Department of Haematology, Royal Bournemouth Hospital, Bournemouth, UK*

UPENDRA P. HEGDE, MD • *Division of Hematology/Oncology, University of Connecticut Health Center, Farmington CT*

RICHARD S. HOULSTON, MD, PhD • *Section of Cancer Genetics, Institute of Cancer Research, Sutton, Surrey, UK*

PATRICK B. JOHNSTON, MD • *Department of Internal Medicine, Division of Hematology, Mayo Clinic, Rochester, MN*

GUNNAR JULIUSSON, MD • *Department of Biomedicine and Surgery, Faculty of Health Sciences, Department of Hematology, University Hospital, Linkoping, Sweden*

NEIL E. KAY, MD • *Department of Internal Medicine, Division of Hematology, Mayo Clinic, Rochester, MN*

MICHAEL J. KEATING, MB, BS • *Department of Leukemia, The University of Texas M.D. Anderson Cancer Center, Houston, TX*

THOMAS J. KIPPS, MD, PhD • *Division of Hematology and Oncology, University of California-San Diego, School of Medicine, La Jolla, CA*

DIMITRIOS KONTOYIANNIS, MD • *Department of Infectious Diseases, The University of Texas M.D. Anderson Cancer Center, Houston, TX*

ROBERT J. KREITMAN, MD • *Laboratory of Molecular Biology, National Cancer Institute, Bethesda, MD*

PETER LICHTER, PhD • *DKIZ, Heidelberg, Germany*

THOMAS S. LIN, MD, PhD • *Division of Hematology and Oncology, The Ohio State University, Columbus, OH*

MARGARET S. LUCAS, PA • *Division of Hematology and Oncology, The Ohio State University, Columbus, OH*

GERALD E. MARTI, MD, PhD • *Division of Cell and Gene Therapies, Laboratory of Stem Cell Biology, CBER FDA NIH, Bethesda, MD*

FRANCESCA R. MAURO, MD • *Dipartimento di Biotecnologie Cellulari ed Ematologia, Università degli Studi di Roma "La Sapienza," Rome, Italy*

MAURICETTE MICHALLET, MD, PhD • *Chief, Department of Hematology, Hôpital Edouard Herriot, Lyon, France*

EMILI MONTSERRAT, MD • *Department of Hematology, Hospital Clinic, University of Barcelona, Barcelona, Spain*

SUSAN M. O'BRIEN, MD • *Department of Leukemia, The University of Texas M.D. Anderson Cancer Center, Houston, TX*

ALBERTO ORFAO, MD, PhD • *Service of Cytometry, Department of Medicine and Cancer Research Center, University of Salamanca. Salamanca, Spain*

ENRICA ORSINI, MD • *Dipartimento di Biotecnologie Cellulari ed Ematologia, Università degli Studi di Roma "La Sapienza," Rome, Italy*

KANTI R. RAI, MD • *Division of Hematology-Oncology, Long Island Jewish Medical Center, New Hyde Park, NY; Albert Einstein College of Medicine, Bronx, NY*

MARIA LUZ SANCHEZ, PhD • *Service of Cytometry, Department of Medicine and Cancer Research Center, University of Salamanca, Salamanca, Spain*

JESUS F. SAN MIGUEL, MD, PhD • *Hematology Service, University Hospital, Department of Medicine, Cancer Research Center, Salamanca, Spain*

STEPHAN STILGENBAUER, MD • *Department of Internal Medicine III, University of Ulm, Ulm, Germany*

WILLIAM G. WIERDA, MD, PhD • *Department of Leukemia, The University of Texas M.D. Anderson Cancer Center, Houston, TX*

WYNDHAM H. WILSON, MD, PhD • *Medical Oncology Research Unit, Center for Cancer Research NCI, NIH, Bethesda, MD*

MARTIN R. YUILLE, PhD • *Academic Department of Haematology and Cytogenetics, MRC UK Genome Mapping Project Resource Centre, Babraham, Cambridge, UK*

VINCENT ZENGER, PhD • *Division of Cell and Gene Therapies, Center for Biologics Research FDA, Bethesda, MD*

I INTRODUCTION

1

The Natural History of CLL

Historical Perspective

Gerald E. Marti, MD, PhD and Vincent Zenger, PhD

1. INTRODUCTION

By convention, the history of chronic lymphocytic leukemia (CLL) begins in 1845, but it could be said to have started when the first white cells, "the globuli albicanates," were noted by Joseph Lieutaud in 1749 *(1)*. During the intervening years, many events have aided in our understanding of the etiology and treatment of CLL. In his discussion of the history of CLL, Rai *(2)* found it informative to define three eras: (1) the recognition of CLL as a clinical entity, 1845–1924; (2) initial clinical investigations, 1924–1973; and (3) the modern era, 1973–2002. We too have found this division informative and have grouped the events into those three periods.

In evaluating the recent history of CLL, Rai *(2)* also recognized four major scientific advances that have contributed greatly to our understanding of CLL and lymphoid neoplasms. They are: (1) immunological classification; (2) molecular cytogenetics; (3) systematic studies of natural history and prognostic factors; and (4) development of new therapeutic agents offering hope for long-term control of these diseases. To this we would add genomic-scale cDNA microarray expression profiling and a better understanding of normal B-cell differentiation and development as it relates to B-cell neoplasia.

2. HISTORICAL EVOLUTION

2.1. First Era, 1845–1924: Recognition of CLL As a Distinct Entity

The reports of Rai *(2)*, Galton *(3)*, Gunz *(4)*, Hamblin *(5)*, Piller *(6)*, and Videbaek *(7)* are useful in reconstructing this early historical period.

Gunz *(4)* attributes the first accurate description of a case of leukemia to Dr. Velpeau, who in 1827 *(8)* described a 63-yr-old florist and lemonade seller Monsieur Vernis, who had abandoned himself to the abuse of spirituous liquor and women *(8)*. Hamblin *(5)* shed further light on this subject by noting that in this profession and in his former job as a florist, Vernis had been a happy, carefree individual with an eye for the ladies, yet he managed to avoid the ravages of syphilis. This florist-lemonade seller fell ill in the summer of 1825 with pronounced swelling of the abdomen, fever, weakness, and symptoms caused by urinary stones. He died soon after admission to the hospital and at autopsy was found to have an enormous liver and spleen, the latter weighing 10 pounds. The blood was thick like gruel, and Velpeau wondered if it was laudable pus mixed with a blackish colored matter. Gunz *(4)* notes that it was this peculiar character of the blood, as seen

From: *Contemporary Hematology*
Chronic Lymphocytic Leukemia: Molecular Genetics, Biology, Diagnosis, and Management
Edited by: G. B. Faguet © Humana Press Inc., Totowa, NJ

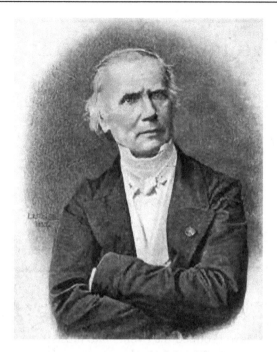

Fig. 1. Dr. A. Velpeau. Courtesy of the National Library of Medicine (http://www.nlm.nih.gov/).

at postmortem, which first attracted the attention of all the early observers. Despite Dr. Velpeau's eminence, no one else seemed interested in the disease. In 1839, Barth submitted the blood of one such postmortem examination to Donne, who performed a microscopic examination and stated that he could not distinguish the mucous globules from pus. Later, he examined the blood of a leukemic patient during life and thought that the blood was so full of colorless corpuscles that at first he thought it was pus.

In his 1963 dissertation, Galton *(3)* begins the history of CLL with Craigie's two recorded cases of leukemia. Rather than publishing the first case, Craigie waited to confirm his observations when another patient appeared 4 yr later in 1845. Craigie *(9)* then published both cases in 1845. On the following pages of the same journal, Bennett *(10)* presented a complete autopsy report of the last case including microscopy of the cadaver blood. Both noted the purulent matter in the blood and thought it was unrelated to infection. Based on the abnormal appearance of the blood at postmortem examinations in 37 cases with 17 followed during life, Bennett called this suppuration of the blood "leucocythemia" (reported in four papers and a monograph). In the same year, 1845, Virchow *(11)* described two further cases and suggested a distinction between the splenic and a lymphatic type. In the lymphatic case, besides lymph node enlargement, Virchow found large and small single "rundzellen" in the bone marrow. Using the term "veisses Blut," Virchow argued that there was no evidence of local suppuration with diffuse spread and coined the term "leukemia," of which he said there were two forms: splenic and lymphatic. Virchow was able to differentiate a leukocytosis from lymphatic leukemia again permitting him to classify leukemia, into splenic and lymphatic forms. He recognized that splenic leukemias had granular leukocytes with trefoil-like nuclei, in contrast to the agranular leukocytes with smooth round nuclei of lymphatic leukemias. He also recognized a group of conditions in which lymph nodes and spleens were enlarged without alteration of the blood picture, which he termed "lymphosarcoma" and

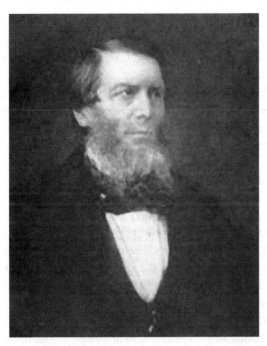

Fig. 2. John Hughes Bennett. Courtesy of the National Library of Medicine (http://www.nlm.nih.gov/).

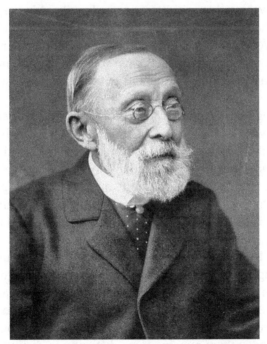

Fig. 3. Rudolf Virchow. Courtesy of the National Library of Medicine (http://www.nlm.nih.gov/).

considered not essentially different from lymphocytic leukemia. He also noted very aggressive tumors, frequently of the neck and sometimes in the mediastinum, that metastasized to other organs. These metastases, although nodular, could easily be distinguished from other malignant tumors by their less circumscribed character and their tendency to merge with the surrounding tissues. The concepts of absolute and relative lymphocytosis were introduced rather early.

Most historical reviewers consider that the history of leukemia and therefore of CLL begins with these descriptions by John Hughes Bennett (1812–1875) and Rudolph Virchow (1821–1902). After both men performing autopsies on their respective patients, are credited with having virtually simultaneously and entirely independently of each other discovered the pathology in 1845 that is now readily recognized as leukemia *(10,11)*. Thus, in 1845, independent publications from Bennett, a physiologist in Scotland, and Virchow, a pathologist in Germany, made leukemia a recognized clinical entity. Much has been made of the supposed rivalry between Bennett and Virchow, but Hamblin *(5)* supplies details about this nonexistent rivalry and concludes that since many of the colorless corpuscles were described as cells, each containing one large nucleus, the case described by Bennett might indeed represent a case of CLL. However, Galton *(3)* attributes the first description of CLL to Virchow: gradual, painless enlargement of cervical, axillary, and inguinal nodes over a 2-yr period. At death the spleen was firmer than normal but not enlarged. The blood in the heart and great vessels was leukemic, with the proportions of white to red corpuscles roughly estimated as 2–3:1.

The term "pseudoleukemia" was used to describe those conditions in which enlargement of spleen, lymph nodes, and other organs was found at autopsy. The macroscopic and microscopic findings resemble the lymphatic leukemia without involvement of the blood. Because the word "pseudoleukemia" was gradually understood to refer to several unrelated conditions, the term "true pseudoleukemia" was used to indicate primary lymphoid hyperplasia, which resembled leukemia but lacked the characteristic blood picture. The term "pseudoleukemia" also took another turn in which organ involvement was consistent with a lymphoid neoplasm, but a relative lymphocytosis was present. Fortunately, the terms "pseudoleukemia and true pseudoleukemia" were gradually dropped and became synonymous with aleukemic or subleukemic lymphocytic leukemia.

Paul Ehrlich, publishing in 1877, 1880, 1887, and 1891 *(12–14)* developed the triacid staining method to study red and white corpuscles in thin dried films of blood. His method allowed a clear distinction among the nucleus, the cytoplasm, and other details of blood cells. The stains allowed three types of granulocytes to be distinguished: the eosinophil, the basophil, and the neutrophil *(13)*. His work allowed leukemias to be classified into two types: myeloid (granulocytes) of the bone marrow and lymphoid (lymphocytes) from nongranular cells. By 1881, Einhorn *(16)* had named the lymphocyte and made a distinction without staining between small and large lymphocytes.

Kundrat, in 1893 *(17)*, followed by Turk, in 1903 *(18)* provided case summaries and other clinical data to separate CLL from lymphoma systematically. Kundrat used the same term, "lymphosarcoma," recognizing that the disease spreads between different groups of lymph nodes but spares the blood and bone marrow, thus distinguishing it from leukemia. However, Turk pointed out that transitions between lymphosarcoma and CLL did occur, and he regarded them as part of a family of diseases. A lively debate between these two extreme positions continued well into the 20th century, and even today there remains some difficulty in distinguishing CLL from some forms of lymphoma.

Turk *(18)* also devised a classification scheme for hyperplastic conditions of lymphoid tissue (lymphomatosis), based on clinical behavior, the mode of growth and spread, and hematological features. He described three chronic benign lymphomatoses, which were indistinguishable clinically and histologically but could be divided hematologically. They are: (1) alymphatic or

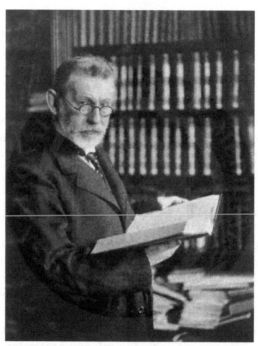

Fig. 4. Paul Ehrlich. Courtesy of the National Library of Medicine (http://www.nlm.nih.gov/).

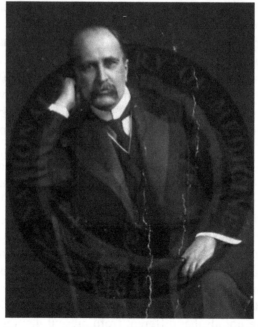

Fig. 5. Sir William Osler. Courtesy of the National Library of Medicine (http://www.nlm.nih.gov/).

alymphemic with a normal lymphocyte count throughout the course of the disease; (2) sublymphatic, in which there was a relative lymphocytosis; and (3) lymphocytic, in which there was an absolute lymphocytosis. Chronic lymphocytic leukemia was thus termed "chronic benign lymphemic lymphomatosis."

The chronic malignant lymphomatoses of Turk were referred to as chronic malignant lympho-sarcoma forms. Turk also notes that large cells were more often found in the blood and associated with more rapidly advancing disease. He cited cases of leukemia with both large and small cell and transitional forms present. In other cases in which the change was from a small cell to a large cell type, they were without any change in clinical behavior or evidence of locally aggressive growth. Thus, the chronic malignant lymphomatoses were considered to be true malignant tumors that began as local tumors, and although benign for long periods eventually became locally aggressive and spread rapidly by lymphatic pathways from one group of lymph nodes to the next regional lymph node. It should be noted that a plasma cell on the blood film is often referred to as a Turk cell.

Also during this time, patients were observed for long periods with just lymphadenopathy alone. After local radiation, a rapid increase in lymphocyte count could be noted with subsequent death of the patient. Although the cells in the blood were described as being small lymphocytes, microscopic examination of lymphoid tissue at autopsy revealed both large and small lympho-cytes with varying degrees of massive infiltration. Galton *(3)* believes that many of these have been examples of generalized follicular lymphoma. Eventually the term "lymphosarcoma cell leukemia" was added. The term "terminal blast cell leukemia of lymphosarcoma" preceded the term "lymphosarcoma cell leukemia."

Galton *(13)* points out that the merit of Turk's classification was that the name of each condition was a concise definition of its clinical, pathological, and hematological characteristics. Lym-phomatosis was a family of conditions ranging from benign to highly malignant. Galton further points out that such confusion has arisen because the leukemia associated with lymphosarcoma has not always been differentiated from chronic lymphocytic leukemia. Galton concluded that the term "leukosarcoma" had been used in a variety of circumstances as follows: (1) infiltrating tumors developing during the course of acute lymphoblastic leukemia and perhaps chronic lym-phocytic leukemia; (2) lymphosarcoma with terminal leukemia; and (3) follicular lymphoma with sarcomatous features and terminal leukemia. Thus, this term may have led to the confusion of possibly distinct conditions, and, in addition, its use appears to have been partially responsible for the confusion, whereby the terminal blast cell leukemia of lymphosarcoma has not been differentiated from CLL. With regards to the pathogenesis of CLL, Galton returns to Turk's concept of a systemic diffuse hyperplasia of the lymphoid system, in contradistinction to a focally arising lymphosarcoma. After a long discussion regarding the bone marrow as a source of lym-phocytic leukemias, Galton concludes that it seems reasonable to conclude that the bone marrow is rarely if ever the site of origin of CLL.

In his review, Rai *(2)* notes that in the first edition of Sir William Osler's monumental book *The Principles and Practice of Medicine* in 1892 until the 7th edition in 1909, there was little change in the description of CLL *(19)*. In Osler's experience at Johns Hopkins Hospital, CLL constituted 20% of all leukemias and was associated with a generalized enlargement of lymph nodes. The confusion that arose historically between the terms "chronic lymphocytic leukemia" and "lymphosarcoma" are not all that different from present day terms: chronic lymphocytic leukemia vs a well-differentiated lymphocytic lymphoma vs small lymphocytic leukemia. Cli-nicians, hematologists, oncologists, surgeons, and pathologists all contribute their observations to this disease. The difficulty lies in the different clinical behavior of lesions that appear morpho-logically similar: a lymphadenopathy without lymphocytosis and a lymphocytosis without lym-phadenopathy. The clinical course in either case cannot be predicted without observation. It will only be by the continued observation of these two extremes that the heterogeneity of the CLL

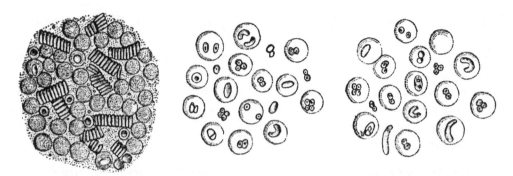

—Appearance of a drop of blood, magnified 250 diameters, taken from Tinlay's finger.
—The same, after the addition of acetic acid.
—A drop of blood, treated by acetic acid 24 hours after being taken from the arm by venesection.

Fig. 6. (From ref. *20*, Bennett, 1852, Figs. 6, 7, and 8). With permission from Sutherland and Knox, Edinburg, UK.

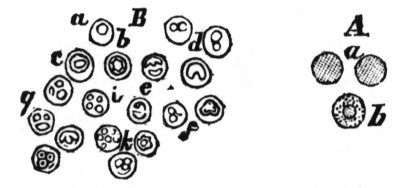

Fig. 7. Colorless blood corpuscles from a vein of the pia mater of a lunatic. **(A)** Examined when fresh: *a,* in their natural fluid; *b,* in water. **(B)** After the addition of acetic acid: *a–c,* cells with a singular, granular nucleus, which becomes progressively larger and is finally provided with a nucleolus; *d,* simple division of the nuclei; *e,* a more advanced stage of the division; *f–h,* gradual division of the nuclei into three parts; *i–k,* four or more nuclei. 280 diameters. (From ref. *21*, Virchow, 1863, Fig. 56.)

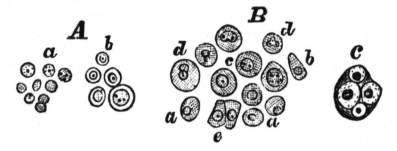

Fig. 8. Lymph corpuscles from the interior of the follicles of a lymph gland. **(A)** As usually seen: *a,* free nuclei, with and without nucleoli, simple and divided; *b,* cells with smaller and larger nuclei, which are closely invested by the cell wall. **(B)** Enlarged cells from a hyperplastic bronchial gland in a case of variolous pneumonia: *a,* largish cells with granules, and single nuclei; *b,* club-shaped cells; *c,* larger cells with larger nuclei and nucleoli; *d,* division of nuclei; *e,* club-shaped cells in close apposition (cell division?) **(C)** Cells with an endogenous brood. 300 diameters. (From ref. *21*, Virchow, 1863, Fig. 62.)

population can be discerned not only for etiological purposes but also for the prognosis and care of these patients.

In ending our discussion of this first era, we wish to draw attention to the early microscopic illustrations provided by Virchow and Bennett, as shown in Figs. 6, 7, and 8. Regardless of the type of construction of microscope used to make these observations and recordings, the drawings that remain are remarkable for their similarity. It would be of historical interest to follow the progression from these earliest microscopic observations of the CLL lymphocyte morphology up to and including modern day image analysis.

2.2. Second Era, 1924–1973: Initial Clinical Investigations Into CLL

2.2.1. MAJOR CONTRIBUTORS

2.2.1.1. Ward: 1917. In the first era, CLL was separated from leukemia, and its separation from lymphomas was initiated. The second era, between 1924 and 1973, was marked by significant contributions to our understanding of the natural history of the disease, the diagnosis, and (as poor as they were) the various treatments for this disease. It should be noted that chronic leukemia was often the subject of a given report and that both forms (myelogenous and lymphocytic) were studied.

Just before the start of the second era in 1917, Ward *(22)*, a military officer, analyzed 1457 cases of leukemia of all varieties. He compared the age and sex incidences of 398 cases of acute leukemia, 247 cases of chronic myelemia, and 84 cases of chronic lymphemia (CLL). Most of the CLL pateints were between 45 and 60 yr of age, and 73–80% were males (Figs. 9 and 10). He concluded that the marked preferences for a particular sex and age of onset argued for a noninfectious etiology of leukemia, resembling metabolic diseases and cancer.

2.2.1.2. Minot and Isaacs: 1924. In the first comprehensive report on CLL in 1924, Minot (Fig. 11) and Isaacs *(23)* compared their series of 92 CLL patients with 84 CLL patients reported by Ward. Figures 12 and 13 are extracted from their report. They showed that most cases of CLL occurred at 45–54 yr of age. The male/female ratio was 3:1, symptoms were usually present 9 mo before the patient presented, and another 6 mo more was required to confirm the diagnosis. Minot and Isaacs *(23)* further report on 50 patients who received irradiation and 30 patients who did not and who served as controls. The source of irradiation was radium, administered over the lymph nodes and spleen. They noted that there was no difference in the duration of life span for the two groups: 3.45 yr (40 mo). We have taken the liberty of using their data to draw Fig. 14. However, they did note that individual patients did benefit if the irradiation was given at 1 or more years prior to death. Although there seemed to be an improvement in the patients' efficiency and/or a decrease in metabolic rate, improvement in formed blood elements was not the rule. Lymph nodes and spleen size showed the greatest effect. Irradiation usually had no effect if the hemoglobin level was below 50%, if thrombocytopenia and purpura were present, or if the blood contained immature and atypical lymphocytes. In Rai's opinion *(2)*, the formal beginnings of CLL as a recognized and well-described clinical entity should be considered to have occurred in 1924 with this report by Minot and Isaacs.

In 1938, Leavell *(24)* reported the incidence and factors influencing survival times for 128 CLL patients seen in three large city clinics between 1917 and 1936 and reported similar findings. The greatest number of cases occurred between ages 45 and 55 yr, with 60% being male and an average duration of life of 3.6 yr. Patients with marked anemia had a shorter course, and the duration of life was slightly longer in patients with lower white counts. The number of patients with a history of bleeding was too small to be significant. Skin involvement in CLL

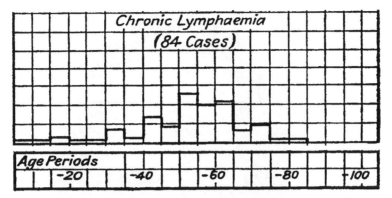

Fig. 9. Age incidence of CLL arranged in 5-yr periods. (From ref. *22*, Ward, 1917; The "Chronic Lymphaemia" chart was extracted from Fig. 1.)

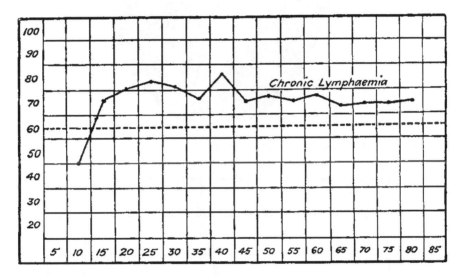

Fig. 10. Proportions of males with CLL at each age period. (From ref. *22*, Ward, 1917; The "Chronic Lymphaemia" curve was extracted for clarity from Fig. 3.)

seemed to have no effect on the duration of disease compared with those CLL patients without specific skin lesions.

2.2.1.3. Wintrobe and Hasenbush: 1939. The early phase of the disease was emphasized in a report published in 1939 by Wintrobe and Hasenbush *(25)* containing clinical data on 86 cases of chronic (myeloid and lymphoid) leukemia from the Department of Medicine, John Hopkins University. They studied 47 CLL patients of whom 39 were men (83%) seen between 1926 and 1938. The age of disease onset was 60–65 yr for 61.7% of the CLL patients. A representative figure from this work is shown in Fig. 16. Examples of patient presentation included three men with prostatic hypertrophy, one patient with sugar in the urine, one patient with a psychoneurotic disorder, and one patient with indigestion. One-third of their patients presented with an unexplained leukocytosis, and one-third had glandular enlargement. A distinct absolute lymphocytosis with a normal or low-normal white blood count (WBC) was frequently seen. Only one patient had splenomegaly. They observed an average life span of 2.33 yr but noted great variation in their patients and in the literature. Infections were common in CLL and did not correlate with spon-

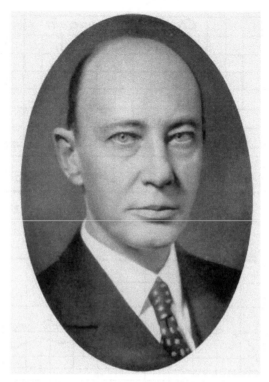

Fig. 11. George R. Minot. Courtesy of the National Library of Medicine (http://wwwihm.nlm.nih.gov/).

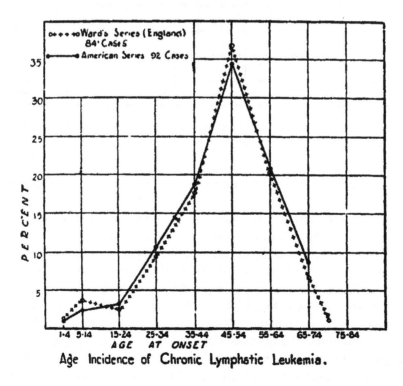

Fig. 12. Age incidence of CLL in the American and English population. (From ref. *23*, Minot and Issacs, 1924; the curves were extracted for clarity from Fig. 1. Copyright © 1924, Massachusetts Medical Society.)

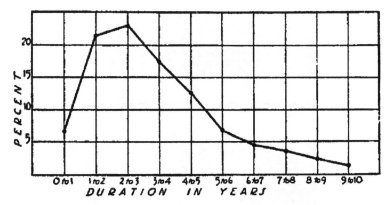

Fig. 13. Frequency of duration of CLL (87 cases). (From ref. *23*, Minot and Isaacs, 1924, Fig. 5. Copyright © 1924, Massachusetts Medical Society.)

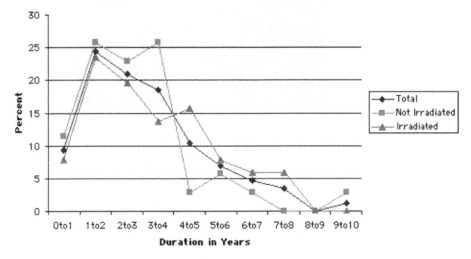

Fig. 14. Frequency of duration of CLL. (Redrawn from the data of ref. *23*, Minot and Isaacs, 1924. Copyright © 1924, Massachusetts Medical Society.)

taneous remissions. These investigators also found no benefit from irradiation or the use of potassium arsenite solutions with CLL.

2.2.1.4. Boggs et al.: 1966. Boggs et al. *(26)* followed 130 CLL patients from 1945 to 1964 in the Hematology Clinic, University of Utah and reported their findings in 1966. Patients with "aleukemic" CLL and lymphosarcoma were excluded. Seventy-four had died, 46 were alive, and 10 were lost to follow-up. Death owing to CLL was caused by infection (23 patients), thrombocytopenic hemorrhage (2 patients), meningeal leukemic infiltrates (1 patient), and congestive heart failure (CHF) with acute myocardial infarction (AMI) and autoimmune hemolytic anemia (AIHA; 1 patient). Deaths unrelated to CLL consisted of AMI and CHF (five patients), pulmonary embolus (PE; two patients), cancer [three patients: prostate cancer, bile duct carcinoma, and Hodgkin's disease (HD)], and diabetes and uremia (two patients), as well as perforated ulcer, cerebral vascular thrombosis, and automobile accident in one patient each. Treatment-related deaths occurred in eight patients (*see* Table 1 of their report for a summary of deaths). The mean age of this CLL group was 59.5 yr, and 74% were male. Most patients were symptomatic,

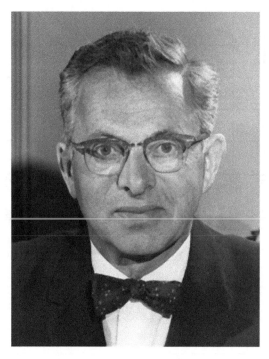

Fig. 15. Maxwell M. Wintrobe.

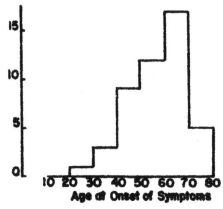

Fig. 16. Age at onset of symptoms in 47 cases of chronic lymphogenous leukemia. (From ref. *25*, Wintrobe and Hasenbush, 1939; extracted from Chart 1. Copyrighted 1939, American Medical Association.)

complaining of fatigue (76%), enlarged lymph nodes (39%), recent infection (25%), and easy bruising or minor bleeding (6%). In 25% there were no symptoms referable to CLL, and the patient was being seen either for a routine visit or for complaints unrelated to CLL. The duration of symptoms was 12.9 mo. Physical findings consisted of lymphadenopathy and splenomegaly in more than 75% of patients, with hepatomegaly and sternal tenderness in 45% and 27%, respectively. Palpable retroperitoneal (mesenteric or pelvic?) lymph nodes (three patients) and skin infiltrates (two patients) were also seen. An absolute lymphocytosis (7000–978,000), was noted in 100% of patients, with 32% showing greater than 100,000; anemia, thrombocytopenia, and neutropenia, were seen in 55%, 39%, and 23 % respectively. Triethylenemelamine, chlorambucil,

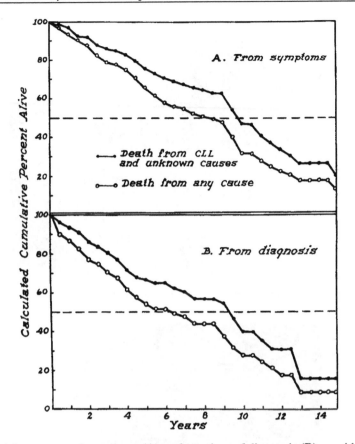

Fig. 17. Survival from onset of symptoms (**A**) or from time of diagnosis (**B**) considering deaths from all causes and deaths related to CLL. Calculations from which this figure was derived are listed in Tables IV and V of ref. *26*. (From ref. *26*, Boggs et al.,1966, Fig. 1. Copyright 1966, with permission frtom Excerpta Medica Inc.)

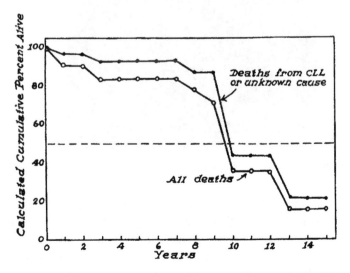

Fig. 18. Survival of 31 patients in whom the diagnosis was made before symptoms attributable to CLL developed. Calculations from which this figure was derived are listed in Table VI of ref. *26*. (From ref. *26*, Boggs et al., 1966, Fig. 4. Copyright 1966, with permission from Excerpta Medica Inc.)

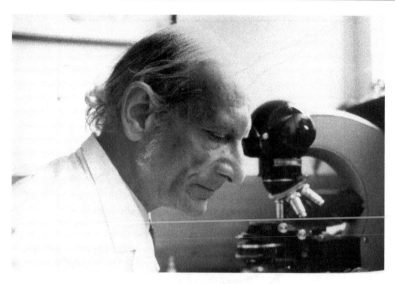

Fig. 19. Professor D. A. G. Galton. (Digital image kindly provided by Professor Daniel Catovsky.)

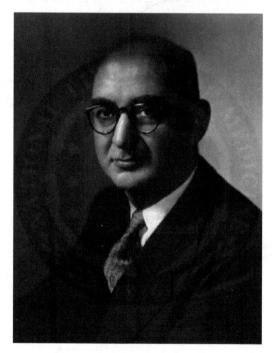

Fig. 20. William Dameshek. Courtesy of the National Library of Medicine (http://www.nlm.nih.gov/).

and prednisone were used in the treatment of these patients. Treatment was associated with a reduction in lymphoid tissue, but often there was no improvement or there was a worsening of anemia, thrombocytopenia, and neutropenia. In addition, prednisone was associated with compression fractures, diabetes, and severe infections. Their analysis of survival (Fig. 18) suggests a median survival of 6 yr from time of diagnosis to death, 9 yr if non-CLL causes of death are excluded, and 10 yr for asymptomatic CLL. In their series, untreated patients lived as long or longer than treated patients.

2.2.1.5. Galton: 1960s. In his 1963 thesis on "The natural history of chronic lymphocytic leukemia" and in a later (1966) paper, Galton *(27)* summarized much of his experience and understanding of CLL. In his description of the natural history of CLL lay the beginning of a staging system that would later be used by Rai and Binet. His attention to the rediscovered patterns of lymphocytosis would also lead to a valuable prognostic indicator, i.e., the lymphocyte doubling time (LDT). Later, he also made seminal observations not only of the differential diagnosis of CLL but also the subclassification of CLL. In his observations of 88 cases over 15 yr, he starts by noting the need to evaluate and intergrate the presence or absence of symptoms, and physical and laboratory findings. Most importantly, he stressed the desirability of evaluating the hematological and blood film findings in conjunction with the histopathology of *both* the lymph node and bone marrow biopsies. An increase in symptoms and physical findings tends to be associated with a higher absolute lymphocyte count (ALC) and decreased normal marrow function. Marked marrow infiltration with normal function was often noted with isolated splenomegaly, i.e., so-called splenomegalic CLL.

In addition, he defined three patterns (trends) of ALC evolution in CLL. In the type I trend, the ALC continued to increase constantly during the period of observation. In the type IIa trend, the ALC rose to a certain level, reached a plateau, and remained relatively constant during the period of observation. Today CLL patients with type I and IIa patterns would be thought to have LDTs of less than 6–12 mo and more than 12 mo, respectively. A third pattern, type IIb, showed a fluctuation around a mean, which Galton interpreted to mean the stationary phase of type IIa. However, it could just as well be that the type IIb pattern could precede the type IIa pattern, as seen in early CLL. Regardless of these subtleties in the etiology of the type IIb pattern, Galton appropriately noted that the type II pattern favored superior survival and the type II trend was thus associated with slowly progressive disease. Parenthetically, Galton further notes: "The patterns shown by the lymphocyte counts in these cases were clearly seen when they were plotted on a semilogarithmic scale, on which the amplitude of fluctuations about the mean values does not increase as the mean counts rise." Thus he was able to define two groups of patients on the basis of their ALC: one whose absolute lymphocyte counts rose throughout the observation period and another in which the absolute lymphocyte count stabilized around a mean value and was associated with a more benign form of the disease. How strikingly similar these observations are to the recent correlation of Ig gene mutational status and CD38 expression correlating with two variants of CLL! Galton's speculations on the pathogenesis of CLL begin with his observations on the evolution of CLL: the gradual accumulation of aged, small, mature, well-differentiated lymphocytes as seen on blood films that are fragile (smudge cells) in the blood, lymph nodes, spleen, and bone marrow. This lymphocytosis is further characterized as having a low mitotic index and being poorly responsive to several mitogenic stimuli.

2.2.1.6. Dameshek: 1960s. In 1967, William Dameshek, attending hematologist at The Mount Sinai Hospital and Medical School, published a special article in *Blood* entitled: "Chronic Lymphocytic Leukemia—an Accumulative Disease of Immunologically Incompetent Lymphocytes" *(28)*. Dameshek drew attention to several features of CLL. First he proposed a clinical stratification of CLL into four stages similar to those of Galton as follows: stage I, the patient is entirely asymptomatic, with a blood and marrow lymphocytosis; stage II, a year or decade later, the patient would develop night sweats, generalized lymphadenopathy, and variable splenomegaly (here recognized isolated splenomegalic CLL); stage III, the patient was increasingly symptomatic, with palpable intra-abdominal lymph nodes and frequent bouts of infection; and stage IV, "bouts of fever, frequent infections, disturbances referable to various organs such as nasal sinuses, the lung, the skin, various autoimmune disorders and increasing anemia take place often in rapid succession." Anemia was increasingly marked and associated with stages III and IV, as was a packed non-aspiratable marrow. Hypogammaglobulinemia was already recognized at that time, and the findings of autoimmunity (AIHA and idiopathic thrombocytopenia [ITP]) were beginning to emerge. The manifestations of autoimmunity and a reduced or absent response to common bacterial antigens led to the second concept of immune incompetence. The lack of skin graft rejection, fatal viral infections, the dissemination of live vaccines, and allergic reactions to insect bites suggested that there were defects in both the humoral and cellular immune systems. Although better understood today, the lack of a response to the plant mitogen phytohemagglutinin (PHA) led to the concept of a "block in differentiation" in this lymphoproliferative disorder of the CLL lymphocyte. He was also aware of familial CLL. In addition, Dameshek drew attention to the use of large-dose corticosteroids (prednisone 50–150 mg daily) and the pattern of response. Thus he defined CLL as an abnormal, generalized, self-perpetuating proliferation of small lymphocytes with a variety of immunological aberrations resulting in immunoincompetency.

2.2.1.7. Hansen: 1973. In 1973 Hansen *(29)* presented detailed clinical data on 189 patients with CLL followed for a long time in his department in Copenhagen. This report, along with Galton's thesis should be required reading for all students of CLL. This stand-alone report, a single issue of the *Scandinavian Journal of Haematology* devoted to CLL, is not unlike the early editions of *Dameshek and Gunz's Leukemia (30)*. Because of the wealth of clinical material in this publication, a brief summary follows.

In Hansen's historical review *(29)*, he notes that Hayhoe *(31)* assigns the first reported case of CLL to Craigie. The spleen of Craigie's 30-yr-old patient weighed 7 pounds, 3.5 ounces. He also notes the early recognition of splenic and lymphatic leukemia that was subsequently corrected by Neumann *(32)*, who described bone marrow changes in leukemia as " 'pyoid' hyperplasia, predominated by highly granulated cells and 'lymphadenoid' hyperplasia, predominated by cells having pale homogeneous cytoplasm." Hansen aptly notes that difficulties in diagnosis led to a profusion of such terms as lymphosarcoma and leukosarcoma leukemia, to be differentiated from CLL. Hansen defined CLL as an increasing accumulation and infiltration of small lymphocytes with the characteristic presence of "smudge cells" or Gumprecht shadows. If the typical presentation of lymphadenopathy or splenomegaly with a leukemic blood picture is lacking, then either a lymph node and or bone marrow biopsy is required to document the typical lymphoid infiltrate. Generalized lymph node enlargement was defined as clinical or radiological evidence of enlarged lymph nodes in at least three regions. The WBC was required to be more than 10,000 cells/μL, with at least 60% lymphocytes (mostly mature forms) and a hypercellular marrow with more than 40% mature lymphocytes.

The 189 cases reported by Hansen came from three institutions in Denmark during the time period 1954–1963. When the analysis was completed in 1966/1967, 28 patients were still alive and had been followed for at least 3 yr. Autopsy reports were available on 109 of 161 deceased CLL patients (68%). It was felt that these cases represented 15% of all cases of CLL in Denmark during the period 1954–1963. The sex and age distribution is shown in Fig. 21; the mean age at diagnosis was 63.3 yr, and the overall male/female ratio was 1.8:1. Initial symptoms are shown in Table 1, and causes of death are listed in Table 2. Lymph node enlargement was present in 91%, splenomegaly in 47%, hepatomegaly in 30%, leukemic skin infiltrates in 6–7%, and herpes zoster in 13%. Mediastinal and or hilar lymphadenopathy was 27%, rising to 38% during the course of disease, whereas plural effusions were unusual, seen in only 2% at presentation but during the course of the disease in 17%. Microscopic pulmonary leukemia infiltrates were seen in 52% of

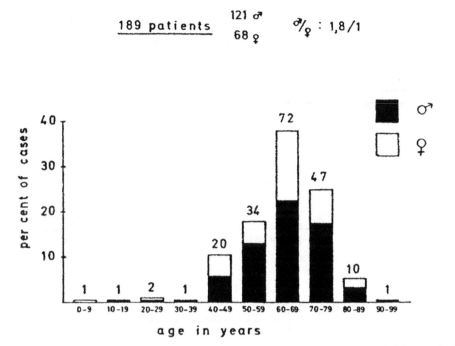

Fig. 21. Sex and age distribution at diagnosis. (From ref. *29*, Hansen, 1973, Fig. 1. With permission from the *European Journal of Hematology.*)

autopsy samples—gross leukemic gastrointestinal infiltrates were seen in 9% of patients and were generally clinically silent. Gross renal leukemic infiltrates were seen in 18%, with 70% microscopic involvement. Fatal uremia was seen in 2%, with urolithiasis in 7–8%. Skeletal changes consisted primarily of osteoporosis and vertebral body collapse. Osteosclerosis was seen less frequently, and lytic lesions were not seen. At presentation, 45% of the patients had a normal hemoglobin level, but 21% were Coombs test positive, and 47% had a normal platelet count. Normal marrow function persisted even though more than 80% of the marrow was involved with a leukemic infiltrate. Median survival was estimated at 3 yr and the single survival curve from this study is shown in Fig. 22. This extensive clinical review is followed by individual case reports and graphic presentations of each patient.

Rai *(2)* and Hamblin *(5)* both note in their reviews that Galton and Dameshek, virtually simultaneously but independently of each other, concluded that the primary pathology in CLL was the progressive accumulation (rather than an abnormally rapid proliferation) of lymphocytes. It is further noted that both of these leaders in hematology recognized that CLL lymphocytes were functionally incompetent and did so before the era of immunotyping and the classification of lymphoid neoplasms according to their T- and B-cell origin. Although Hansen did not propose a staging system, he seems to be the first to have laid down extensive criteria for the diagnosis of CLL. Hansen's extensive clinical description confirmed the patterns that Galton described. These observations, combined with Dameshek's symptomatic stages, set the stage for Rai and later Binet to develop clinical staging systems.

In his book *Leukemia: Research and Clinical Practice* published in 1960, Hayhoe *(31)* provided a comprehensive description of the clinical aspects of CLL prior to Hansen's report. Hamblin in his review *(5)* felt that Hayhoe's description remained the most up-to-date summary of knowledge of CLL nearly 35 yr later. Hayhoe's description of the latent autoimmune sensitization of

Table 1
Initial Symptoms of Chronic Lymphocytic Leukemia in 188 Patients

	Patients
	No. (%)
Symptom	
Lymph node enlargement	84 (45)
Symptoms of anemia	48 (26)
Sweating	38 (20)
Fever	22 (12)
Complaints owing to an enlarged liver or spleen	20 (11)
Cutaneous or mucosal hemorrhages	11 (6)
Itching	11 (6)
Accidental finding	30 (16)

From ref. *29*, 1973, Table 4. With permission from the *European Journal of Hematology.*

Table 2
Causes of Death in 161 Patients
With Chronic Lymphocytic Leukemia

	Patients
	No. (%)
Cause	
Infection	101 (63)
Other disease	31 (19)
Cachexia	22 (14)
Anemia	14 (9)
Hemorrhage	5 (3)
Uncertain	21 (13)

From ref. *29*, 1973, Table 5. With permission from the *European Journal of Hematology.*

red cells (macrocytosis, anisocytosis, and sometimes spherocytosis with polychromatophilia) is particularly apt in the absence of a slight rise in the serum bilirubin and when reticulocytes are not noticeably increased. For reviews of the etiology of anemia in CLL, which is beyond the scope of this report, see Dameshek and Schwartz, 1938 *(33)*, Berlin, 1951 *(34)*, Coons et al., 1955 *(35)*, Wasserman et al., 1955 *(36)*, Troup et al., 1960 *(37)*, Videbaek, 1962 *(38)*, Myint et al., 1995 *(39)*, and Casadevall et al., 2002 *(40)*. His distinction between "amegakaryocytic thrombocytopenia" and "megakaryocytic thrombocytopenia" remains relevant today. In his chapter on CLL, Hayhoe references the early work (1957) of Scott *(41)*. Three figures have been selected from that report and are shown here (Figs. 23, 24, and 25). Our summary of this second era in the history of CLL might best be closed with a discussion of the discovery and use of chlorambucil and steroids in the treatment of CLL.

2.2.2. Therapies of the Second Era

2.2.2.1. Chlorambucil (CB1348). In 1955, a landmark paper in the history of CLL, "Clinical Trials of p(DI-2-Chloroethylamino)-phenylbutyric Acid (CB 1348) in Malignant Lymphoma," Galton et al. *(42)* gave the first report of the treatment of patients with CLL with chlorambucil.

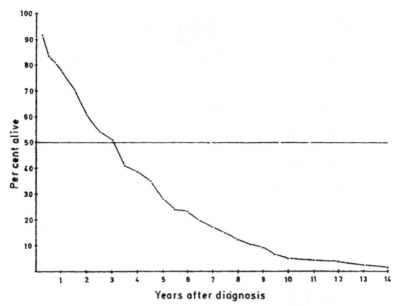

Fig. 22. Single survival curve from Hansen's study. (From ref. *29*, Hansen, 1973, Fig. 6. With permission from the *European Journal of Hematology*.)

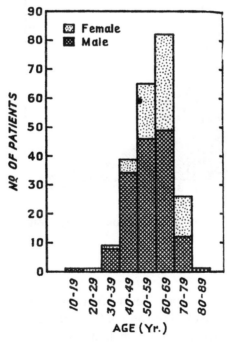

Fig. 23. Age at onset of symptoms in CLL. (From ref. *41*, Scott, 1957, Fig. 9. Reprinted with permission from Elsevier, *The Lancet*.)

Ironically, the use of chlorambucil, a water-soluble aromatic nitrogen mustard, followed a fairly intensive study of mustard gas as a result of World War II. This drug was found to be a powerful inhibitor of the transplanted Walker rat tumor 256 and was therefore submitted to clinical trials.

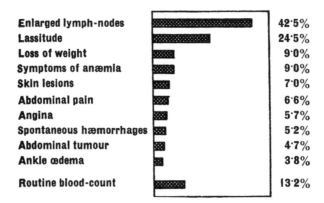

Enlarged lymph-nodes	42·5%
Lassitude	24·5%
Loss of weight	9·0%
Symptoms of anæmia	9·0%
Skin lesions	7·0%
Abdominal pain	6·6%
Angina	5·7%
Spontaneous hæmorrhages	5·2%
Abdominal tumour	4·7%
Ankle œdema	3·8%
Routine blood-count	13·2%

Fig. 24. Presenting symptoms in 212 patients with CLL. (From ref. *41*, Scott, 1957, Fig. 10. Reprinted with permission from Elsevier, *The Lancet.*)

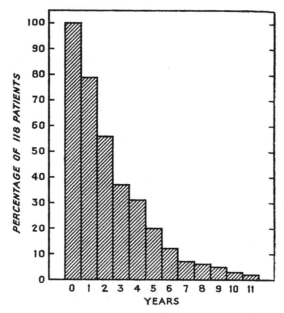

Fig. 25. Survival from onset of symptoms in CLL. (From ref. *41*, Scott, 1957, Fig. 12. Reprinted with permission from Elsevier, *The Lancet.*)

We quote liberally from this report as it provides the first description of how the drug chlorambucil was used for over 40 yr, before the discovery of fludarabine. In this first study, 93 patients suffering from advanced carcinoma and from lymphoma were treated with chlorambucil. The report was restricted to those patients with malignant lymphoma of which there were 62 including 23 with HD, 20 with lymphocytic lymphoma (including 8 patients with CLL), 11 with reticulum cell sarcoma, and 6 with follicular lymphoma. The oral dose ranged from 2 to 20 mg/d (0.03–0.34 mg/kg/body weight), and in most cases it was either 0.1 or 0.2 mg/kg daily or 6 or 12 mg for a patient weighing approx 10 stone (63.5 kg). The course of treatment usually lasted for 3–6 wk.

Results were summarized by the presence of "benefit," "some effect," or "no effect." The CLL cases are summarized in Table 2 of that report; 4 of the 8 CLL patients had a benefit, and 7 of 12

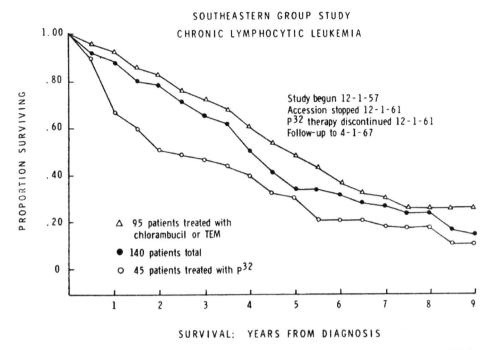

Fig. 26. Overall survival of patients treated with chlorambucil, triethylenemelamine (TEM), and radioactive phosphorus (P³²). It is to be noted that the administration of P³² ended at yr 4. (For an early study on the use of P³² in CLL, *see* ref. *45*, Lawrence et al., 1949). (From ref. *43*, Huguley, 1970, Fig. 4, as cited in ref. *44* by Rundles in Williams et al. [eds.] *Hematology*, 2nd and 3rd editions. With permission from Elsevier.)

patients with a lymphocytic lymphoma (subleukemic), also had a benefit. These benefits were associated with increases in hemoglobin and platelet counts and decreases in size of splenomegaly and degree of lymphadenopathy. The toxic effects of chlorambucil on blood elements included lymphopenia, which was slowly progressive and continued as long as the drug was given. Most patients showed some neutropenia after the third week of treatment. Severe neutropenia was closely related to the dosage of chlorambucil. All but one patient received a total dose of 6.5 mg/kg or more (450–550 mg) in one course. About one-fourth of all patients receiving 6.5 mg/kg may be expected to develop severe neutropenia, and if this dose is taken in 8 wk or less, the proportion approaches one-third. It may be significant that 16 of the 20 patients who derived most benefit from treatment received comparatively small doses suggesting that administration of chlorambucil need not be pushed to its limits of tolerance to achieve the best therapeutic results. In the lymphoma group, most patients who developed severe neutropenia and thrombocytopenia had infiltration of the bone marrow, but others who tolerated the drug well had similar infiltrations. The administration need not be discontinued as soon as the neutrophil count begins to fall, but it should be remembered that the fall may continue for 10 d after the last dose and that as the total dose is approached (6.5 mg/kg), there is a real risk of causing irreversible bone marrow damage. With regards to platelets, platelet depression was rarely serious in patients treated with chlorambucil.

In summary, 62 patients suffering from malignant lymphoma were treated with chlorambucil. Striking remissions were obtained in four cases of HD, seven of lymphocytic lymphoma, four of CLL, and of five follicular lymphoma. Chlorambucil therapy is relatively free from gastrointes-

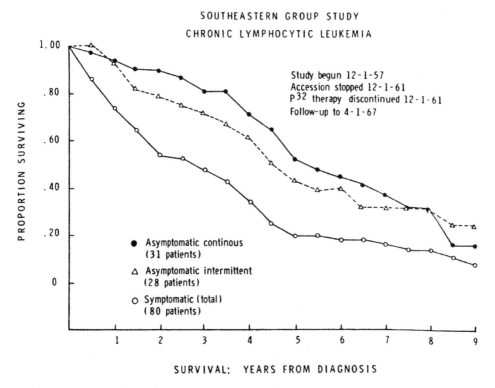

SOUTHEASTERN GROUP STUDY
CHRONIC LYMPHOCYTIC LEUKEMIA

Study begun 12-1-57
Accession stopped 12-1-61
P^{32} therapy discontinued 12-1-61
Follow-up to 4-1-67

● Asymptomatic continous
(31 patients)

△ Asymptomatic intermittent
(28 patients)

○ Symptomatic (total)
(80 patients)

PROPORTION SURVIVING

SURVIVAL: YEARS FROM DIAGNOSIS

Fig. 27. Overall survival of asymptomatic and symptomatic patients comparing continuous and intermittent regimens. (From ref. *43*, Huguley, 1970, Fig. 4, as cited in ref. *44* by Rundles in Williams et al. [eds.] *Hematology*, 2nd and 3rd editions. With permission from Elsevier.)

tinal side effects and has proved to be less damaging to hemopoietic tissue than the cytotoxic agents heretofore available for the treatment of malignant lymphoma.

The introduction of chlorambucil led to clinical trials evaluating continuous vs intermittent therapy and a single large oral vs the same dose divided over 4 d. The addition of prednisone was also evaluated. Clorambucil became the mainstay of treatment in CLL. More importantly, clinical trials led to the discontinuation of the use of radioactive P^{32} owing to increased deaths compared with chlorambucil. This development is illustrated in Figs. 26 and 27.

2.2.2.2. Steroids. In 1961 Shaw et al. *(46)* reported on a National Cancer Institute (NCI) sponsored study of prednisone therapy to define its antileukemic effect and ascertain its effect on the frequency and/or character of infections in CLL. Eighteen patients were randomized to (1) prednisone for 12 wk followed by a 12-wk control period or (2) a control period of 12 wk followed by prednisone for 12 wk. Prednisone was given at 1 mg/kg for 4 wk. At the end of 4 wk, it was reduced to 0.5 mg/kg for 4 wk, and after 8 wk it was reduced to 0.25 mg/kg. At the end of 12 wk, prednisone was discontinued. No other anti-eukemic therapy was given and antacids were not routinely administered.

This study showed an improved sense of well-being and increased strength and appetite in all subjects. There was a dramatic reduction in splenomegaly, with a comparable decrease in lymphadenopathy and hepatomegaly in most of patients. (Figure 28 shows the reduction in spleen size.) There was an initial increase in the WBC ("paradoxical lymphocytosis") with a subsequent decrease. Improvements in hemoglobin, platelet, and absolute granulocyte counts were also

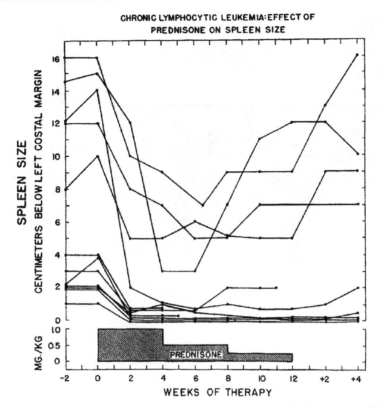

Fig. 28. Effect of prednisone on spleen size in CLL. (From ref. *46*, Shaw et al., 1961, Fig. 1. Copyright American Society of Hematology, used with permission.)

noted. All these changes were transient. Although there was no statistically significant increase in fever and infections during the prednisone period compared with the control period, infections in the prednisone-treated subjects were more severe and more difficult to treat.

3. THIRD ERA, 1973–2000: CLINICAL STAGING SYSTEMS FOR CLL

The third era begins with the emergence of the Rai staging system and we will end our discussion of it with Rai et al.'s 2000 comparison of chlorambucil with a new drug for CLL called fludarabine *(47)*. In this modern era, two major areas for investigation became evident. First, because extremely wide range of survival time in this disease, clinicians were frustrated by the difficulty of making therapeutic decisions in patients newly diagnosed with CLL. Second, we needed a better understanding of the abnormalities of the leukemic cell in CLL and how it might predict prognosis; such an understanding would help us to understand normal B-cell differentiation.

3.1. Clinical Staging

3.1.1. RAI

Rai *(2)* notes that the roots of the Rai staging system for CLL can be traced back to the work of Galton presented in a Burroughs Wellcome Lecture in 1965 and subsequently published by the Canadian Medical Association in 1966 *(27)*. Galton presented data on 88 CLL patients followed for 15 yr classifying them into four groups:

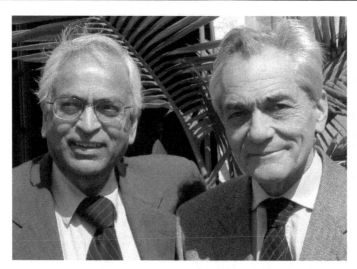

Fig. 29. Kanti Rai (left) and Jacque Louis Binet (right). This digital image was taken with permission at the IWCLL March 2002 meeting in San Diego outside the poster display pavilion.

   i. Neither lymph node nor spleen enlargement
  ii. Only lymph node enlargement
 iii. Only spleen enlargement
 iv. Both lymph node and spleen enlargement.

The distributions of these four groups (i–iv) were 19, 27, 8, and 56, respectively. Galton further noted that patients with high ALC tended to be group iv and that 71% of patients in group iv had evidence of bone marrow compromise. On the other hand, only 56% of patients with splenomegaly and 24% of patients with lymphadenopathy had symptoms related to their CLL. As already noted, Galton also described two patterns in the rise in ALC: type I (aggressive) and type II (indolent). Rai further notes that Wintrobe and colleagues *(26)* reported that all the physical and laboratory evidence of disease tended to be more severe in CLL patients surviving for less than 5 yr. However, he credits Dameshek *(28)* with proposing the first formal staging system in 1967: stage 1, asymptomatic blood and marrow lymphocytosis; stage 2, symptomatic generalized lymphadenopathy with variable splenomegaly; stage 3, symptomatic bulky disease with frequent infections; and stage 4, fevers, infections, pneumonias, and increasing anemia.

On the basis of these observations, in 1975 Rai et al. *(48)* proposed the following five stages:

Stage 0   blood and marrow lymphocytosis
Stage I   lymphocytosis with lymphadenopathy
Stage II   lymphocytosis with splenomegaly and/or hepatomegaly with or without lymphadenopathy
Stage III lymphocytosis with anemia (Hgb < 11 g/dL); nodes, spleen, or liver may or may not be enlarged
Stage IV lymphocytosis with thrombocytopenia (platelet count < 100,000/μL); anemia and organomegaly may or may not be present.

Several observations can be made from this progression of events, but first it should be noted that the Rai staging system has been proved to have prognostic value. When this system was tested on their own data and confirmed on the data of Boggs et al. *(26)* and Hansen et al. *(29)*, the following median values were found: 150, 101, 71, 19, and 19 mo for Rai stages 0–IV, respectively. It would appear that the Rai stage 0, Galton's group (i), and Dameshek's asymptomatic stage 1 are identical. Galton's group (ii), Dameshek's stage 2, and Rai stage I are likewise nearly identical. Isolated splenomegaly, Galton's group (iii), and Rai stage II are also identical. Galton's group (iv), and Dameshek's stage 3 are identical. With regard to Rai stages III and IV, Galton does not specify these two groups, and Dameshek's stage 4 would be equivalent to the Rai stage III. Thus the physical examination and clinical laboratory findings of CLL are recognized in the Rai Staging System. The lymphocytosis is systemic and progressive, involving the blood and bone marrow, and there is a progressive, generalized, symmetrical lymphadenopathy involving the spleen and the liver and resulting in anemia, thromboyctopenia, and death.

3.1.2. BINET

After publication of the Rai staging system and the general realization that patients with anemia and thrombocytopenia defined high-risk CLL, the question arose as how to define the nonanemic, nonthrombocytopenic patients who constitute 75% of CLL patients. It was felt that the large variability in this group was not well explained. The French CLL group, under the leadership of Binet, proposed in 1977, revised in 1981, and presented in 1981 a new classification based on three prognostic groups: C, B, and A *(49–51)*. Group C was defined as anemia (Hgb < 10 g/dL) and/or thrombocytopenia (platelets < 100,000 µL); group B as no anemia, no thrombocytopenia, three or more involved areas (counting as one each of the following: cervical, axillary, inguinal lymph nodes, whether unilateral or bilateral, spleen, and liver); and group A as no anemia, no thrombocytopenia, and less than three involved areas. In the study group that they used, the distributions of patients were 15% in group C, 35% in group B, and 50% in group A. The median survivals were 2 yr in group C, 7 yr in group B, and in group A survival did not seem to differ at the time from that of the French population of the same age and sex as noted by Binet in 1988 *(52)*.

After the emergence of the Rai system, Montserrat and Rozman *(53)*, in an analysis of prognostic factors in CLL, noted in 1988 that the widely used Rai staging system had been confirmed in more than seven or eight studies. They classified their 269 patients according to both the Rai and Binet systems, and their figures are shown for the sake of comparison (Figs. 30 and 31). They note the problems that still exist regarding the limitations of these staging systems: too many clinical stages in the Rai system; [it should be noted that in 1987 Rai *(54)* also revised the original five groups down to three groups]; lack of an explanation for median survival of Rai stage II patients being the same as the whole population of CLL patients; failure to separate out the causes of anemia and thrombocytopenia on the basis of marrow failure or autoimmune destruction as separate prognostic groups; and failure to identify progressive and quiescent clinical forms in either Rai stage 0/I or Binet stage A. In 1988 Binet *(52)* made an extensive comparative analysis of the Binet and Rai systems: the low-risk stages A (0), A (I), A (II); the intermediate-risk stages B (I), B (II); and the high-risk stages C (III) and C (IV). As would be expected, Binet stage A contains more better outcome patients (66%) than Rai stage 0 (31%); both Rai stage I and II patients can be further subdivided in into Rai stage IA and IB and Rai stage IIA and IIB, with prognostic significance. Rai stage IA contains two-thirds of the patients, and Rai stage IB contains one-third of the patients, with 5-yr survivals of 78% and 52%, respectively. Rai stage IIA contains one-third of the patients, and Rai stage IIB contains two-thirds of the patients, with 5-yr survivals of 68% and 38%, respectively. *See* Figs. 32 and 33 for a comparison of the Rai and Binet systems, and *see* Fig. 34 for the overall survival of Rai stage IA and IB, Rai stage IIA and IIB, and Rai stage IIIA, IIIB, and IIIC. Of course the Binet system confirms the poor prognostic outcome of the anemic and thrombocytopenic patient *(52)*.

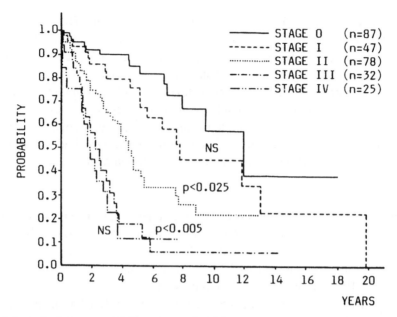

Fig. 30. Actuarial survival curves of 269 patients classified according to the Rai et al. staging system. Median survivals are as follows: stage 0, 126 mo; stage I, 92 mo; stage II, 53 mo; stage III, 23 mo; stage IV, 20 mo. (From ref. 53, Montserrat and Rozman, 1988, Fig. 1. With permission from Harwood Academic Publishers, Inc.)

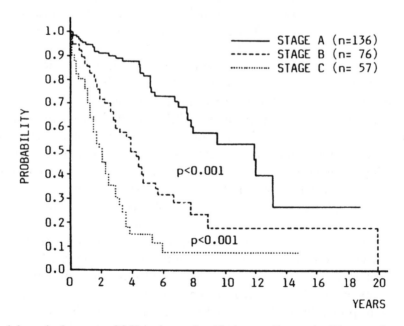

Fig. 31. Actuarial survival curves of 269 patients classified according to the Binet et al. staging system. Median survivals are as follows: stage A, 128 mo; stage B, 47 mo; stage C, 24 mo. (From ref. 53, Montserrat and Rozman, 1988, Fig. 2. With permission from Harwood Academic Publishers, Inc.)

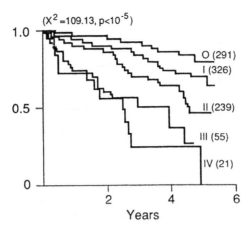

Fig. 32. Stages A, B, and C-COP cases. Overall survival according to Rai's staging (second interim analysis). (From ref. *52*, Binet, 1988, Fig. 6. With permission from Harwood Academic Publishers, Inc.)

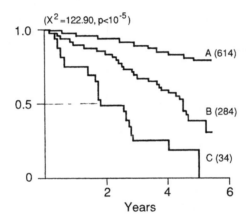

Fig. 33. Overall survival according to the (A, B, C) staging (second interim analysis); group C includes only COP treated patients. (From ref. *52*, Binet, 1988, Fig. 5. With permission from Harwood Academic Publishers, Inc.)

3.2. Prognostic Indicators

In 1981 and in 1989, the International Workshop on CLL (IWCLL) recommended the combined use of the Rai and Binet systems *(51,55)*. This recommendation has not been widely implemented, and clinicians use one or the other in their practice, as the combination is too cumbersome. In reality, the Americans continue to use the Rai system and the Europeans the Binet system. As noted above, in 1987, the five stages in the original Rai system were reduced to three in recognition of the three survival curves, which were different from each other *(54)*. The high-risk group, which combines Rai stages III and IV, is similar to Binet's worst prognosis group, stage C. Binet's stage A and Rai's lowest group 0 are, however, not as similar. In 1988, Rai and Sawitsky *(56)* described the staging system of Jaksic and Vitale proposed in 1981 *(57)*, which attempts to estimate the total tumor mass (TTM) of leukemic cells in CLL. The TTM score was further reviewed in 1999 by Rai and Han *(59)*. The TTM is the sum of the square root of the ALC plus the diameter in centimeters of the largest lymph node plus the number of centimeters the spleen is below the left costal margin. Scores below and above 9.0 were associated with median

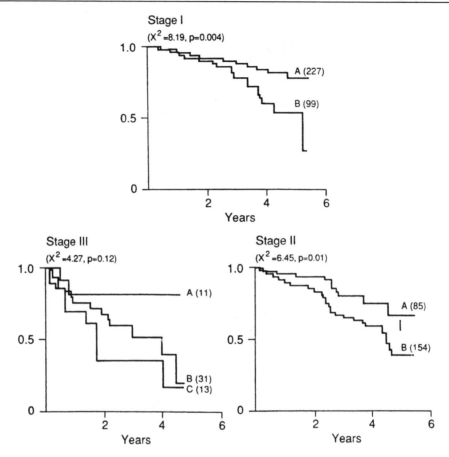

Fig. 34. Overall survival according to the A, B, C staging within Rai's staging system (second interim analysis). Stage III excludes C-CHOP cases. (From ref. *52*, Binet, 1988, Fig. 8. With permission from Harwood Academic Publishers, Inc.)

survivals of 101 and 39 mo, respectively. In 1973 Zippin et al. *(59)* performed a statistical analysis of 839 CLL patients diagnosed between 1955 and 1964 in 24 hospitals participating in the End Results Program of the NCI. They reported that the overall 5-yr survival was 44%, and the relative 5-yr survival decreased with increasing age. Five-year survival was greater in women (50%) than in men (41%). They also noted an unusual plateau or peak in the WBC, with increasing survival peaking in the WBC interval 25,000–49,000 cells/μL and then decreasing.

In an attempt to improve on these clinical staging systems, a host of prognostic factors have been studied. In 1982 Rozman et al. *(60)* showed the prognostic value of the ALC in Rai stage I and II and in Binet stage A and B. Survival is shortened in both clinical stages when the ALC is greater than 50×10^9 cells/L. In 1987 Lee et al. *(61)*, using a regression model as well as uric acid and lactate dehydrogenase (LDH) levels, were able to separate risk groups within a given clinical Rai stage, but this approach does not appear to have been widely used *(61)*. In 1987 Mandelli et al. *(62)* drew attention to the ALC ($> 60 \times 10^9$ cells/L) and the size of a given lymph node and spleen and likewise were able to improve on the present staging systems. It is of interest that they defined their first stage as a benign monoclonal lymphocytosis. Using plastic embedding methods, in 1974 Gray et al. *(63)* were one of the first groups to investigate bone marrow pattern and cellularity using the ratio of percent lymphocytes in the marrow over the ALC. As predicted, patients with marked marrow infiltration had a shortened survival. Notably, these investigators also described the large cell in CLL as "having a large nucleus, an increased quantity of cytoplasm, increased nuclear indentation, and most notably a single, prominent nucleolus with a dense nucleolar chromatin ring."

A long list of prognostic indicators were reviewed by Molica in 2001 *(64)* and Montserrat and Rozman in 1988 *(53)*. Some of these indicators are clinical stage, lymphocyte count (ALC), lymphocyte morphology, size, immunophenotype, molecular cytogenetics, lymphocyte doubling time, bone marrow histology, response to chemotherapy, autoimmune disease, other medical problems, and a number of serum factors. In addition to cytogenetics, CD38 expression and Ig gene sequence have emerged as potential prognostic indicators that will be clinically useful. Immunophenotyping has for the most part played a role in both establishing B-cell monoclonality and contributing significantly to the differential diagnosis of CLL. Zwiebel and Cheson in 1998 *(65)* noted that the usefulness of many prognostic factors remains uncertain unless they are evaluated in prospective randomized studies.

3.3. Immunological Classification

Flow cytometry (FCM) has played a crucial role in CLL and B-cell identification. We *(66)* have recently reviewed the technology, its quantitative aspects, the application of FCM to BCLL, and its potential for the detection of early disease in familial CLL. With regard to the identification of the B-cell in CLL, the original work of Aisenberg and Block in 1972 *(67)* and that of Preud'homme and Seligmann also in 1972 *(68)*, are usually cited. In the ensuing years, the work by Geisler et al. in 1991 *(69)*, Freedman et al. in 1987 *(70)*, and Freedman and Nadler in 1987 and 1993 *(71,72)* has led to a comprehensive description of the surface markers in CLL.

Hamblin *(5)* reviewed the history of B-cell identification in CLL and noted that Wilson and Nossell in 1971 *(73)* and Papamichael et al. in 1971 *(74)* reported in the Lancet that B-cells were found in human peripheral blood. Both papers included CLL patients among their study subjects and found a much larger percentage of lymphocytes, expressing IgM in CLL subjects vs normal subjects. Grey et al. also in 1971 *(75,76)* demonstrated the presence of surface immunoglobulin on cells of 20 CLL patients. Preud'homme et al. *(77)* and Pernis et al. *(78)* also published reports in 1971. Although Hamblin *(5)* believed that any of a dozen labs could have made the discovery, he seems to give the prize to Eva Klein, who published a single case report in 1970 *(79)*.

Hamblin's review *(5)* notes the useful discovery of the ability of CLL lymphocytes to form rosettes with mouse red cells by Stathopoulos and Elliot in 1974 *(80)*. The IgM immunophenotype of CLL was quickly defined, and most cells also carried IgD *(81,82)*. Surface immunoglobulin density was much lower than for normal B-cells *(83–86)*. In this same vein, the reduction in CD20 expression on CLL lymphocytes should also be noted *(87)*. Paradoxically, an antigen initially regarded as T-cell specific and later designated as CD5, was recognized on the surface of CLL cells by the monoclonal antibodies RFT-1, Leu-1, and OKT-1 *(88)*. In fact, CD5 expression is now thought to be necessary for the diagnosis of CLL and CD5-negative CLL is considered another disease such as marginal cell lymphoma or immunocytoma.

Concerning the differential diagnosis of BCLL, we find it best to start with the advice of Galton *(89)*. Thirty years ago, a blood and marrow lymphocytosis, if confirmed by a bone marrow aspirate, was not pursued further. The routine use of a bone marrow biopsy did not come about until it was widely used in lymphoma staging. And then it was a bilateral procedure! When this was done, the distinctions between nodular and interstitial and paratrabecular and non-

Table 3
WHO Histological Classification of Mature B-Cell Neoplasms

B-cell neoplasms
    Precursor B-cell neoplasm
    Precursor B lymphoblastic leukemia/lymphoma
Mature B-cell neoplasms
    Chronic lymphocytic leukemia/small lymphocytic lymphoma
    B-cell prolymphocytic leukemia
    Lymphoplasmacytic lymphoma
    Splenic marginal zone lymphoma
    Hairy cell leukemia
    Plasma cell myeloma
    Monoclonal gammopathy of undetermined significance (MGUS)
    Solitary plasmacytoma of bone
    Extraosseous plasmacytoma
    Primary amyloidosis
    Heavy chain diseases
    Extranodal marginal zone B-cell lymphoma of mucosa-associated lymphoid tissue (MALT lymphoma)
    Nodal marginal zone B-cell lymphoma
    Follicular lymphoma
    Mantle cell lymphoma
    Diffuse large B-cell lymphoma
    Mediastinal (thymic) large B-cell lymphoma
    Intravascular large B-cell lymphoma
    Primary effusion lymphoma
    Burkitt's lymphoma/leukemia
B-cell proliferations of uncertain malignant potential
    Lymphomatoid granulomatosis
    Post-transplant lymphoproliferative disorder, polymorphic

From ref. *92*, IARC, 2001, p. 120.

paratrabecular growth patterns and the composition of neoplastic lymphoid aggregates (small cells and large cells) were recognized. Of course, even prior to the advent of T- and B-cell immunophenotyping, as Galton points out, confusing conditions such as hairy cell leukemia, Waldenstrom's macroglobulinemia, and Sézary syndrome should have been resolved. In retrospect, exclusion of T-cell disease was not a major problem as T-cell neoplasms are uncommon and most of the morphological heterogeneity could be and still is attributed to the leukemic phase of non-Hodgkin's lymphomas. The evolution of the lymphoma classification systems was presented by Dr. Jaffe *(90)* in a recent highly informative lecture given by her at the NIH (Hematological Malignancies Series 2001–2002). For the purposes of this review, it is useful to keep in mind the most recent REAL/WHO classification list of B-cell neoplasms available for the differential diagnosis of CLL (Table 3) *(91,92)*.

More specifically, the differential diagnosis of low-grade indolent lymphoma is aided or prompted by the use of flow cytometric immunophenotyping. In general, CLL is a CD5-positive, CD19/CD20/CD23-positive, CD10/C79b/CD103-negative monoclonal (light chain restricted) B-cell lymphocytosis. In particular, the absence of CD5 expression should raise the index of suspicion for another closely related chronic B-cell lymphoid neoplasm. Likewise, the absence of CD23 should initiate the same thought process. The role of the lymph node biopsy should not be overlooked, and serum immunoglobulins levels along with serum protein electrophoresis and immunofixation electrophoresis should be evaluated for evidence of a paraprotein or gammopathy. We need not mention the role of immunohistochemical (IHC) evaluation of lymph nodes in the clinical setting of lymphoid neoplasm because it is both a standard and routine. However, it is unfortunate that the IHC evaluation of trephine bone morrow biopsies is not more common. Although there are fewer reliable reagents for fixed and acid-decalcified bone marrow biopsies, the few that are available are quite useful. This is of particular importance when the blood lymphocytosis is minimal and the marrow is unaspirable. Unless it is done routinely, the normal admixture of T-, B-, and NK cells will not be appreciated, and, more importantly, insight into the early events of a polyclonal B-cell hyperplasia coexisting with a slight B-cell monoclonal interstitial infiltrate will not be seen. The routine application of polymerase chain reaction (PCR)-based molecular techniques is still hampered by the nonjudicious and/or suboptimal use of present day fixatives for bone marrow biopsies.

Given that immunophenotyping has improved the differential diagnosis of CLL, what can be said about the subclassification of CLL? This implies that CLL should first be carefully differentiated from other closely related, low-grade malignant lymphoproliferative disorders such as prolymphocytic leukemia (PLL), hairy cell leukemia and its variants, splenic lymphoma with villous lymphocytes, Waldenstrom's disease (immunocytoma) and the leukemic phase of small cell lymphocytic, centrocytic, or follicular lymphoma, and other non-Hodgkin's lymphomas by a combination of cytomorphology and immunophenotyping. Then one can use further subclassification. To date, in addition to conventional CLL/SLL (small lymphocytic lymphoma), two further subtypes have been recognized: CLL/PL (the prolymphocyte fraction, which varies from 10 to 55%) and CLL/mixed (in patients who have a component of larger cells that are not prolymphocytes) *(93)*. It is important to point out that much of this subclassification has been based on careful review of the routine blood films from untreated patients and does not involve the use of a standardized albumin blood preparation *(94)*.

In the absence of a standardized blood film preparation *(94)*, we do not believe that there is a reliable correlation between the blood film and certain cytogenetic abnormalities reported in BCLL *(95,96)*. In a previous review *(66)*, we noted that Criel et al. *(97)* have attempted to bring some order into the subclassification of BCLL. In their morphological review of 390 cases of CLL selected from a total of 418 cases, they concluded that typical and atypical BCLL are two distinct but closely related clinical entities. Atypical CLL, regardless of clinical stage, is thought to be a biologically more aggressive disease. Of further interest, these investigators have correlated typical and atypical CLL with nodal patterns characterized by the presence or absence of paraimmunoblasts, prolymphocytes, pseudofollicles, and nuclear irregularities *(98)*. Criel et al. *(97)* provide two types of survival curves: the effects of typical and atypical morphology (Fig. 35) and the effects of cytogenetics upon typical and atypical morphology (Fig. 36).

3.4. Molecular Genetics

In 1987 and 1989, Shen et al. *(99)* and Kipps et al. *(100)* made a major contribution to the molecular analysis of Ig genes in CLL. Their initial observation was that the B-cell antibody repertoire in CLL was limited. This was based on the finding that certain variable (V) region heavy chain (H) Ig genes were expressed more frequently and in fact that certain genes within a given family were expressed at an even higher frequency. Further analysis by Fais et al. *(101)* in 1998 of the B-cell receptor (BCR) showed that it can be either mutated or unmutated. Continued

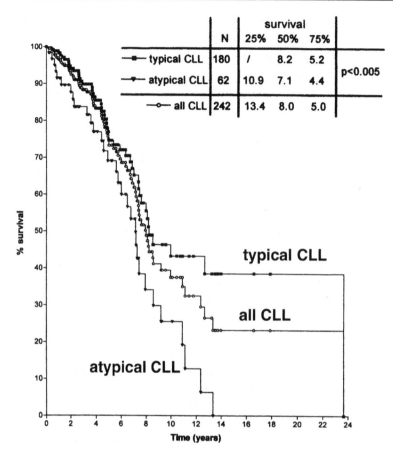

The following table appears within the figure:

	N	survival			
		25%	50%	75%	
typical CLL	180	/	8.2	5.2	p<0.005
atypical CLL	62	10.9	7.1	4.4	
all CLL	242	13.4	8.0	5.0	

Fig. 35. Overall survival of all CLL cases with typical and atypical morphology. (From ref. *97*, Criel et al., 1999, Fig. 2.)

analysis of the Ig genes in CLL led to a further finding that some patients had their Ig gene nucleic acid sequence in a germline configuration *(102)*. This meant that the Ig gene in a given CLL clone varied less than 1.5% from known germline Ig gene sequences. On the other hand, some patients had an Ig gene sequence that demonstrated multiple somatic mutations *(102)*. Clones bearing germline, unmutated Ig genes were thought to arise from pregerminal center lymphocytes. Clones bearing somatically mutated Ig genes were thought to arise from postgerminal center lympho-cytes. These two types of lymphocytes are also referred to as naïve (virgin) and memory cells. Recently the naïve cells were termed "naïve, experienced" *(103)*. Independent memory cells were also postulated to have developed via an alternative or germinal center pathway. Patients with germline naïve cell CLL had a shorter life span, required more regimens of chemotherapy, and were treated sooner. Just the opposite was seen for patients with mutated, memory cell CLL; they had a longer survival, required treatment later, and had fewer courses of chemotherapy. What is remarkable is that the initial findings of the clinical correlation of Ig gene sequences reported by Damle et al. *(104,105)* have been confirmed in two subsequent independent reports *(106,107)*. Of interest is an identical finding by Sakai and colleagues *(108)* in familial CLL. Naylor and Capra *(109)* in their editorial point out that the reports of Damle et al. *(104)* and Hamblin et al. *(106)* put to rest two previous questions concerning Ig gene analysis: the existence of unmutated and mutated IgV_H genes and restricted use.

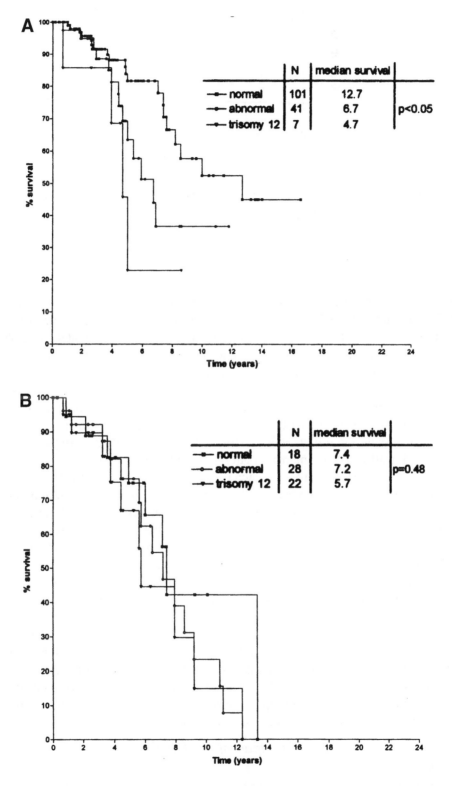

Fig. 36. Survival of typical CLL (**A**) and atypical CLL (**B**) with a normal karyotype vs abnormal karyotype and trisomy 12. (From ref. *97*, Criel et al., 1999, Fig. 3.)

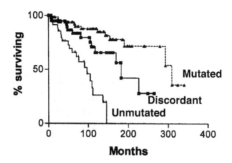

Fig. 37. Survival curves for 145 patients with B-CLL from date of diagnosis, comparing patients whose cells are CD38+ and who have unmutated IgV_H genes ($n = 34$), with those whose cells are CD38– and who have mutated IgV_H genes ($n = 70$) and those whose cells gave discordant results for the two assays ($n = 41$). (From ref. *110*, Hamblin et al., 2002, Fig. 5. Copyright American Society of Hematology, used with permission.)

In the initial report by Damle et al. *(104,105)*, a correlation was shown with Ig gene sequence and CD38 expression. Those CLL patients with 30% or more lymphocytes positive for CD38 expression were also found to have the germline configuration. Unfortunately, this observation of the correlation between CD38 expression and Ig gene status has not been confirmed *(111)*. However, a recent paper has appeared showing a striking correlation between CD38 expression and survival in CLL *(112)*. In this report, 20% or more of the cells positive for CD38 cells were associated with a worse prognosis. This was an excellent three-color flow cytometric study. It also showed further subgroups within early Rai or Binet stage disease. D'Arena et al. *(113)* showed that patients expressing more than 30% CD19/CD38-positive cells had atypical morphology, trisomy 12, and a diffuse bone marrow pattern. An interstitial bone marrow pattern, 13q14 deletion, and early Binet stage were associated with CD38-negative BCLL. Median survival was 90 mo in the CD38-positive group, and median survival had not reached 180 mo in the CD38-negative group. Heintel et al. *(114)* found a strong positive correlation with β2-microglobulin levels of 3 mg/L or more ($p < 0.0001$) and interpreted this to mean that CD38 is a marker of tumor mass as well as disease progression. They also showed that a borderline association was found with LDT of less than 12 mo ($p = 0.05$). They too noted discordance between the two groups.

In conclusion, Ig gene mutational status and CD38 expression stand as newly defined independent prognostic indicators. Other recent publications tend to support the relationship between CD38 expression with Ig gene configuration, with rare exceptions *(115–119)*. This is where things stood until 2002, when Hamblin et al. *(110)* re-examined the relationship between Ig gene mutation status and CD38 expression as independent prognostic variables for survival. Their major contribution was to confirm the relationship between unmutated IgV_H genes and CD38 positivity and mutated IgV_H genes and CD38 negativity and to unravel the effects of discordant values. Survival of the discordant group is intermediate to the CD38-positive unmutated and CD38-negative mutated patients. These results are shown in Fig. 37.

3.5. *Therapies of the Third Era*

3.5.1. FLUDARABINE

The modern era of CLL also saw the introduction of a new drug into the treatment armamentarium. In the post-chlorambucil period, numerous studies has searched for multidrug regimens

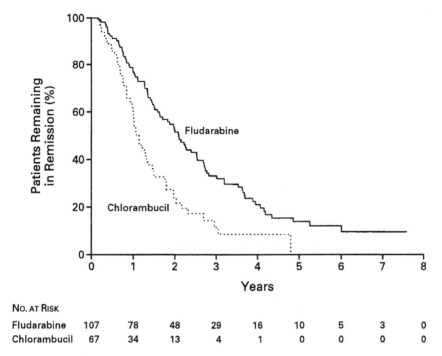

Fig. 38. Proportion of patients with an initial response to fludarabine or chlorambucil who continued in remission. Shown are the proportions of the 107 patients assigned to fludarabine and the 67 assigned to chlorambucil who had a response to treatment and remained in complete or partial remission. In both groups combined, 78% of patients (135 of 174) had relapses. The median duration of the response was significantly longer in the fludarabine group than in the chlorambucil group (25 vs. 14 mo, $p < 0.001$). (From ref. *47*, Rai et al., 2000, Fig. 1. Copyright © 2000 Massachusetts Medical Society. All rights reserved.)

that would be more effective in CLL. Unfortunately, the toxicity associated with multiple drug regimens did not result in increased survival. Then, a new class of drugs emerged, the nucleoside analogs: fludarabine, 2-chlorodeoxyadenosine (CdA), and 2'-deoxycoformycin (pentostatin, or DCF). The definitive fludarabine study by Rai et al. in 2000 *(47)* is of importance for several reasons. First clinical responsiveness was based upon published NCI guidelines *(120)*. Second, there was a comparative control arm for chlorambucil treatment by itself, and third, there was a third arm that compared the combination of fludarabine and chlorambucil. The findings of this study were striking. First of all, the combined arm of fludarabine and chlorambucil was terminated early owing to excessive toxicity. Second the overall response rate was superior for fludarabine vs chlorambucil with complete response (CR) and partial response (PR) of 20 and 43% for fludarabine and 4 and 33% for chlorambucil. Toxicity was greater for the fludarabine-treated patients and consisted of infections, neutropenia, and thromboyctopenia. However, there was no survival difference when fludarabine was compared with chlorambucil, yet because of its superior CR rate, overall response rate, and duration of response, fludarabine is now considered the first-line choice for untreated CLL. Figure 38 shows the initial response for fludarabine- and chlorambucil-treated patients who continued in remission (25 vs 14 mo). Figure 39 compares patients without disease progression (20 vs 14 mo). Figure 40 compares overall survival (66 vs 56 mo).

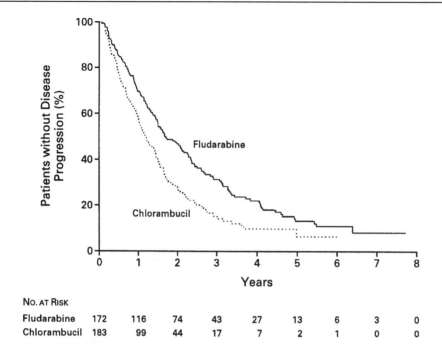

No. at Risk

Fludarabine	172	116	74	43	27	13	6	3	0
Chlorambucil	183	99	44	17	7	2	1	0	0

Fig. 39. Proportion of patients without disease progression, according to treatment group. Shown are the proportions of the 172 patients assigned to fludarabine and the 183 assigned to chlorambucil in whom disease progression could be evaluated who did not have progression of disease from the time of entry into the study. The disease progressed in 79 and 81% of the patients in the two groups, respectively. The median time to progression was significantly longer in the fludarabine group than in the chlorambucil group (20 vs. 14 mo, $p < 0.001$). (From ref. *47*, Rai et al., 2000, Fig. 2. Copyright © 2000 Massachusetts Medical Society. All rights reserved.)

3.5.2. Monoclonal Antibody Therapy

Recently the chimeric monoclonal antibody to CD20, rituximab or rituxan, has been approved for use in the treatment of CLL (FDA Approval Letter Nov. 26, 1997). Although initial responses were low and consisted only of PRs and no CR, interest has continued in its use in CLL *(121–123)*. The original studies used 375 mg/m^2 once a week for 4 wk. Subsequent studies have suggested that this same dose three times a week for 4 wk for a total of 12 doses instead of 4 doses has resulted in better overall responses *(124,125)*. Also, early data suggest that the CR is increased by the addition of Rituxan to fludarabine, but survival data are not yet available. Campath (anti-CD52) has also been recently approved for use in CLL patients refractory to alkylating agents and fludarabine (FDA Approval Letter of May 7, 2001). The FDA approved a novel treatment regime for one type of non-Hodgkin's lymphoma that for the first time includes a monoclonal antibody combined with a radioactive chemical (FDA Approval Letter of Feb. 20, 2002). The product, zevalin, must be used along with rituxan.

3.5.3. Growth Factors

In 1995 Pangalis et al. *(126)* reported that 8/9 CLL patients responded to recombinant human erythropoietin (r-HuEPO) treatment regardless of the pretreatment serum EPO level. A slower response was attributed to a "packed marrow." In 1988 Casadevall *(127)* reviewed a multicenter study of 146 patients by Cazzaola et al. *(128)* and 121 patients reported by Osterborg et al. *(129)*.

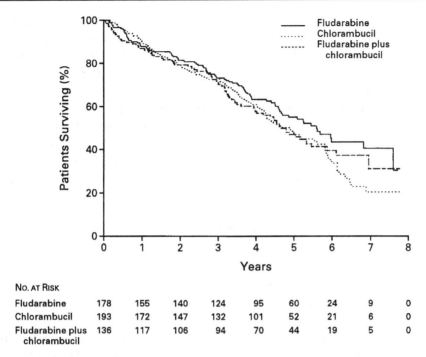

Fig. 40. Overall survival according to treatment group. Shown are the proportions of 178 patients assigned to fludarabine, the 193 assigned to chlorambucil, and the 136 assigned to fludarabine plus chlorambucil who were still alive during follow-up. Forty-seven percent, 57%, and 56% of the patients in the three groups, respectively, died. There was no statistically significant difference in overall survival among the three groups (median, 66, 56, and 55 mo, respectively; $p = 0.21$). (From ref. *47*, Rai et al., 2000, Fig. 3. Copyright © 2000 Massachusetts Medical Society. All rights reserved.)

Both reports concerned patients with non-Hodgkin's lymphoma and multiple myeloma. The probability of a response in the first study (increase > 2 g Hgb) reached 62% in the group treated with 10,000 IU daily after 8 wk. In the second study a cumulative response frequency of 60% for the fixed dose and variable stepwise dose was seen. In both of these studies, Hgb levels could be corrected without obvious side effects.

Casadevall *(127)* also reviewed two reports evaluating the effects of epoetin-α therapy in anemic CLL patients. The first report is unfortunately only an abstract from Rose et al. *(130)*, who treated 221 anemic CLL patients and evaluated them for hematologic parameters and health status. They reported that 47% of treated patients had an increase of at least six points in the Hct over baseline values unrelated to transfusions, compared with 15% in the placebo group ($p > 0.001$). The second article on the treatment of anemic CLL patients with EPO reviewed by Casadevall is the aforementioned report of Pangalis et al. *(126)*.

Russo et al. *(131)* make a cogent argument for the combined use of granulocyte/macrophage colony stimulating factor (GM-CSF) and EPO in the refractory, chemotherapy nonresponsive patient. The antileukemic and antitumor effect is of interest in these four patients.

The most interesting paper is by Siakantaris et al. *(132)* and represents an expansion of the earlier 1995 study by Pangalis et al. *(126)*. For this study, 22 patients with CLL, 5 patients with SLL, and 6 patients with lymphoplasmocytic lymphoma (LPL)—all with anemia (Hct < 32%)—

were treated three times weekly with 50 U/kg for 3 mo. After 1.5 mo, the dose was incrementally increased to a maximum of 300 U/kg if the response was unsatisfactory. Of these patients, 50% had a complete response (Hct > 38%) and an overall response rate of 80% (PR = Hct increase of 6% over baseline). All patients on maintenance therapy have a continuous response. There was no correlation with low or high pretreatment EPO serum levels, ongoing chemotherapy, presence or absence of B-cell symptoms, diffuse or nondiffuse bone marrow pattern, or the presence or absence of splenomegaly. Of further interest, 14 CLL Rai stage III patients were downstaged after treatment with r-HuEPO: 11 became Rai stage II, 2 became Rai stage I, and 1 became Rai stage 0 (*see* Table III of that report). They apparently did not see any reduction in absolute lymphocyte count, as noted by Russo et al. *(131)*, suggesting that the combined use of cytokine growth factors may be required for the antileukemic effect.

3.6. Cytogenetics

In 1914, Boveri *(133)* described chromosomal changes in tumor cells. In 1960, Nowell and Hungerford *(134)* identified the first tumor-specific chromosomal abnormality, the Philadelphia (Ph) chromosome, a minute chromosome in chronic myeloid leukemia. After the development of chromosome banding Caspersson et al. *(135,136)* identified the Ph chromosome as an abbreviated chromosome 22.

When chromosome banding became available, the chromosomes were enumerated from 1 (the largest) to 22 (the shortest). The sex chromosomes were designated X and Y. The shortest arm of the chromosome is designated p (shown above the centromere in figures), and the long arm is termed q.

Differences in the number of copies were presented with a minus sign for monosomy and a plus for trisomy. Other abnormalities are indicated by letters. The chromosomes involved in the abnormality are placed in parentheses in numerical order separated by a semicolon (;). Following in a second parentheses are the specific breakpoint bands for each chromosome, also separated by a semicolon. Translocations are designated with a "t" before the first parentheses, deletions with a "del," interstitial deletions, with "int del," duplications with "dup," and inversions with "inv." Abnormal chromosomes with the same arm on both sides of the centromere, isochromosomes, are designated as "iso." To be defined as a clonal change, two metaphases with the same abnormality or extra chromosome, or three metaphases with the loss of the same chromosome, are required.

Cytogenetic techniques require metaphase cells of good quality. Rapidly proliferating tumors, such as those in acute leukemia, usually present spontaneous mitosis. Cells from indolent disease such as CLL have a very low mitotic index, and in vivo activation with mitogens is required to induce mitosis in tumor cells from these diseases. To evaluate constitutional abnormalities, the established technique is to culture blood cells with phytohemagglutinin (PHA), which is a T-cell activator. Thus, when this was done in the early 1970s, the conclusion was that there were no chromosomal abnormalities in CLL. As late as 1975, Crossen *(137)*, in viewing 100 metaphases from 20 CLL patients concluded that 97 of them had a normal banding pattern. The remaining three, all from one patient, had a pattern similar to those seen in aging.

As noted just above, CLL have a very low mitotic index, and activation with mitogens is required to induce mitosis. When PHA, a potent T-cell activator, is used on bone marrow cultures, or when peripheral blood samples from patients with CLL have been analyzed, only normal cells were available for analysis. As late as 1975, the conclusion was that there were no chromosomal abnormalities in CLL. Most cells from patients had a normal chromosome number and chromosome morphology. A slight increase in aneuploid cells was seen, but none were considered cell lines because they were isolated occurrences. The finding of normal banding patterns in CLL suggested that chromosomal changes were not a feature of this leukemia. Crossen *(137)* did recognize that there might be a problem with PHA not stimulating B-cells. Using dextran sulfate, lipopolysaccharide from *E. coli*, purified protein derivative (PPD) from tuberculin, and rabbit IgG antihuman B_2-microglobulin, Robert et al. *(138)* documented the first successful activation of B-cells in 1978. In addition to these early B-cell-activating agents, pokeweed mitogen (PWM), concanavalin A, tetradecanoyl phorbol acetate (TPA), cytochalasin B, antihuman IgM, B-cell growth factor, calcium ionophore, and anti-CD40 antibody have been used in an attempt to generate mitotic figures from CLL samples. After stimulation with Epstein-Barr virus, Gahrton et al. *(139)* first reported trisomy 12 in a CLL patient in 1979 and subsequently in a fairly large proportion (15%) of cases examined *(140,141)*.

The use of newer molecular genetics techniques has contributed greatly to advances in the understanding of CLL. Fluorescence *in situ* hybridization (FISH) can detect changes in interphase as well as metaphase cells. PCR analysis allows chromosomal breakpoints to be identified. Comparative genomic hybridization, developed in 1992 *(142)*, has the ability to survey the whole genome in a single hybridization and can detect and map relative DNA sequence copy number between genomes. It can distinguish changes as low as several kilobases up to as many as a few megabases. These techniques have identified a number of new chromosomal aberrations as well as previously known aberrations in previously normal-seeming cases.

While it is still not quantified, the fraction of CLL patients with identifiable genetic aberrations has increased with the use of molecular genetic techniques. Using conventional cytogenetic techniques, Jarosova et al. *(143)* found that 17% of nonstimulated bone marrow samples of 88 CLL patients had abnormalities. Comparative genomic hybridization and FISH revealed chromosomal changes in an additional 33 individuals, bringing the total with abnormalities to 57%. In 2000, Dohner et al. *(144)* detected genomic aberrations using FISH in 82% of 325 patients with CLL.

Juliusson and Gahrton *(145–147)*, Juliusson et al. *(148)*, and Dohner et al. *(144)* summarize the status of cytogenetics in CLL. First discovered in the 1980s, the most frequent genetic aberration in CLL now appears to be a deletion in 13q14 *(149–151)*. A 13q14 deletion may confer protection. Another frequent genetic aberration is a deletion in 11q *(152–155)*. It is associated with disease progression and reduced survival *(156,157)*. The area may contain the neural cell adhesion molecule, or the ataxia telangiectasia (AT) gene may be mutated (ATM). Dohner et al. *(158)* notes that these patients tend to have massive lymphadenopathy and do not do well clinically. Trisomy 12 appears in between 7 and 25% of the CLL cases, and is said to be associated with atypical CLL *(159)*. Another common aberration is a 17p deletion. The short arm of chromosome 17 is the site of the TP53 tumor suppressor gene. G-banding analysis demonstrated abnormalities of chromosome 17 in 13 of these 17 patients, leading to the loss of band 17p13. These 17 patients exhibited a monoallelic p53 gene deletion, as demonstrated by FISH *(160)*. The median survival time from the date of diagnosis of patients with a p53 gene deletion was 2.1 yr compared with 10.3 yr in the patients without the deletion ($p < 0.001$). None of 12 patients with a deletion responded to therapy with either fludarabine ($n = 7$) or pentostatin ($n = 5$), whereas 20 of 36 (56%) patients without a deletion achieved a remission ($p < 0.001$). A 6q deletion may be found in approx 6% of CLL cases *(161–163)*. The pathogenic significance has not yet been identified. Figure 41 is a convenient summary of the distribution of known cytogenetic abnormalities in CLL, and Figs. 42 and 43 show survival and disease progression data in CLL patients as a function of their cytogenetic abnormality.

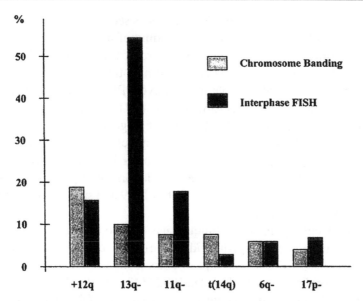

Fig. 41. This is a frequency distribution of the common cytogenetic lesions in CLL. Approximately one-third of the patients will have more than one abnormality, and approx 15% will have a normal karyotype. Given the frequency of the 13q14 deletion in CLL, a more detailed summary of this deletion is shown in Fig. 44. FISH, fluorescence *in situ* hybridization. (From ref. *164*, p. 353, Stilgenbauer et al., 2001 by courtesy of Dekker, Inc.)

3.7. cDNA Microarray and Comparative Genomic Hybridization

Other new molecular techniques also hold promise for the future. Expression profiling, both DNA microarray *(167)* and protein expression profiles (proteomics) *(168)* has yielded some interesting results for a limited number of CLL patients. In a pilot study, Voss et al. *(168)* determined that a patient population with a decreased survival time showed changed levels of redox enzymes, heat shock protein 27, and protein disulfide isomerase. Stratowa et al. *(167)* showed that low expression levels of IL-1β and IL-8 correlated with poor survival, higher Rai clinical stage, and 11q deletions.

Comparative genomic hybridization studies of CLL have been reported from three laboratories. Bentz et al. *(169)* note that 13q14 deletions in CLL can sometimes be too small to be detected with present diagnostic thresholds. Karhu et al. *(170)* confirmed the consistent loss of the 11q14-24 region in a subset of CLL patients. Odero et al. *(171)* compared comparative genomic hybridization with amplotyping using arbitrarily primed PCR (AP-PCR) and found that AP-PCR was more sensitive in the detection of small 13q14 deletions.

Using genomic-scale gene expression profiling, Rosenwald et al. *(172)* have shown that CLL patients share a characteristic gene expression signature in their leukemic cells. Although they were unable to find two separate and distinct subgroups, they did confirm the relationship between unmutated and mutated Ig genes and clinical course. They were able to show that patients with germline, unmutated Ig genes compared with patients with mutated Ig genes, had a median time to treatment of 28 and 95 mo, respectively (Fig. 45). They interpret this to mean that CLL consists of a single disorder rather than two distinct diseases and suggest that their data support a common cell of origin and or a common mechanism of neoplastic transformation. Interestingly, they were able to show that the unmutated subtype genes were associated with B-cell activation

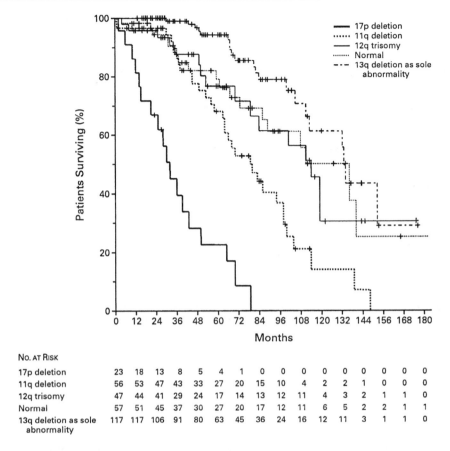

No. at Risk

17p deletion	23	18	13	8	5	4	1	0	0	0	0	0	0	0	0	0
11q deletion	56	53	47	43	33	27	20	15	10	4	2	2	1	0	0	0
12q trisomy	47	44	41	29	24	17	14	13	12	11	4	3	2	1	1	0
Normal	57	51	45	37	30	27	20	17	12	11	6	5	2	2	1	1
13q deletion as sole abnormality	117	117	106	91	80	63	45	36	24	16	12	11	3	1	1	0

Fig. 42. Probability of survival from the date of diagnosis among the patients in the five genetic categories. The median survival times for the groups with 17p deletion, 11q deletion, 12q trisomy, normal karyotype, and 13q deletion as the sole abnormality were 32, 79, 114, 111, and 133 mo, respectively. Twenty-five patients with various other chromosomal abnormalities were not included in the analysis. (From ref. *144*, Dohner et al., 2000, Fig. 1. Copyright © 2000 Massachusetts Medical Society. All rights reserved.)

(Fig. 46). They interpret this finding to suggest that Ig-unmutated CLL cells may be continuously stimulated in vivo via antigen through the BCR. Alternatively, the malignant transformation activates the same B-cell activation signaling process independently in the absence of antigen stimulation. Finally, for the molecular differential diagnosis of CLL, i.e., the two Ig gene variants of unmutated and mutated CLL, they offer a simpler diagnostic test (PT-PCR) for one to three genes rather than the DNA sequence analysis of Ig gene variable regions. One of these genes, ZAP70, is being tested.

4. CHANGING NATURAL HISTORY OF CLL

Molica and Levato *(173)* analyzed 518 CLL patients diagnosed between 1970 and 1998 by forming three groups. Group I consisted of 75 patients, group II consisted of 149 patients, and group III consisted of 293 patients diagnosed with CLL in the time periods 1970–1979, 1980–1989, and 1990–1998, respectively. As expected, there was no difference between age and sex in these three time periods. The median survival values were 38, 54, and 93 mo for the time periods 1970–1979, 1980–1989, and 1990–1998, respectively. This was associated with an increase in stage A patients:

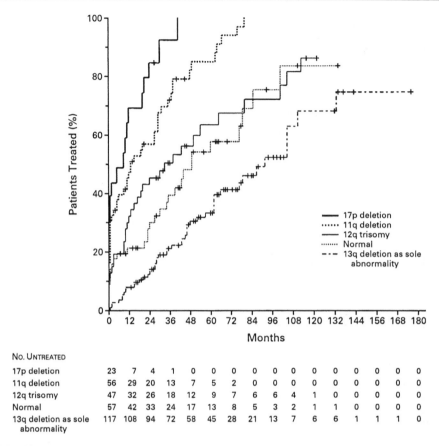

No. Untreated

17p deletion	23	7	4	1	0	0	0	0	0	0	0	0	0	0	0	0
11q deletion	56	29	20	13	7	5	2	0	0	0	0	0	0	0	0	0
12q trisomy	47	32	26	18	12	9	7	6	6	4	1	0	0	0	0	0
Normal	57	42	33	24	17	13	8	5	3	2	1	1	0	0	0	0
13q deletion as sole abnormality	117	108	94	72	58	45	28	21	13	7	6	6	1	1	1	0

Fig. 43. Probability of disease progression, as indicated by the treatment-free interval in the patients in five genetic categories. The median treatment-free intervals for the groups with 17p deletion, 11q deletion, 12q trisomy, normal karyotype, and 13q deletion as the sole abnormality were 9, 13, 33, 49, and 92 mo, respectively. The differences between the curves were significant ($p < 0.001$). Twenty-five patients with various other chromosomal abnormalities were not included in the analysis. (From ref. *144*, Dohner et al., 2000, Fig. 2. Copyright © 2000 Massachusetts Medical Society. All rights reserved.)

Fig. 44. *(opposite page)* Chromosome 13. (Modification or combination of Figs. 5 and 6 in ref. *165*, Bullrick and Croce, 2001 and ref. *166*, Tyazhelova et al., 2001. The figure legend is taken from refs. *165*, Bullrick and Croce and *164*, Stilgenbauer et al., 2001.) Chromosome banding and recently FISH and CGH have confirmed 13q14 deletions in CLL. Although RB1, a prominent tumor suppressor gene, is located in this region, biallelic deletions in CLL are rare. Homozygous deletions at the D13S25 locus suggested a CLL gene located telomeric to RB1/D13S273 and centromeric to D13S31 and D13S294. LOH and YAC cloning led to the definition of a minimum region of loss, and BAC, PAC and cosmid contigs have further defined two core regions of loss. The smaller of the two core regions is bounded by D13S273 and D13S272 and contains three genes: Leu1, Leu2, and Leu5. This is contrary to the findings of Tyazhelova et al. *(166)*, who find at least 10 genes (DLeu through DLeu10, where D signifies "deletion"). R. Dalla-Favera says that based on work from his laboratory and in agreement with several others reports, there are no critical genes in this area and that the assignment of genes in this region on the basis of sequences is arbitrary (IWCLL Meeting, San Diego, CA, March, 2002, personal communication). Absence of mutational inactivation of these 3genes or 10 genes suggests that they are not critical genes in B-CLL leukemogenesis.

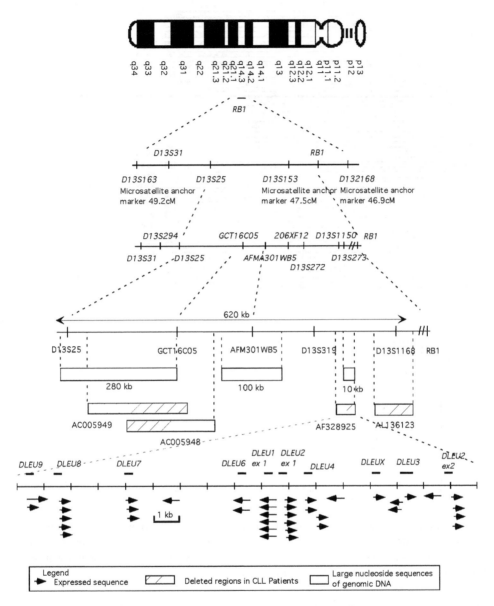

Fig. 44. *(continued from previous page)* The larger core region of loss is bounded by D13S272 and D13S25. Tyazhelova et al. *(166)* have investigated large nucleotide sequences in the q14 region of chromosome 13. They suggest an arbitrary division of two intervals: D13S1168 to D13S319 and GCT16C05 to D13S25. The D13S1168 to D13S319 interval is rich in Alu repeats, whereas the GCT16C05 to D13S25 interval is rich in LINE repeats. In addition, they define a new human gene, C13orf1 (chromosome 13 open reading frame 1), that is conserved in the nematode *C. elegans*, the fruit fly *D. melanogaster*, and the mouse. Another potential tumor suppressor gene has been designated PLCC (putative large CLL candidate, EST AA431979). Stilgenbauer et al. *(164)* pointed out that these 13q14 deletion clusters in CLL are also seen in 50% of patients with mantle cell lymphoma (MCL), and Bullrick and Croce *(165)* state that 13q14 deletions are associated with the transition of MGUS to multiple myeloma. One can imagine one gene (number of Alu repeats) controlling the level of the absolute lymphocytosis and the other genes controlling the transition from a benign B-cell monoclonal lymphocytosis to CLL or MCL or MGUS to MM. (With permission from MAIK "Nauka/Interperiodica," Moscow, Russia and by courtesy of Marcel Dekker, Inc.)

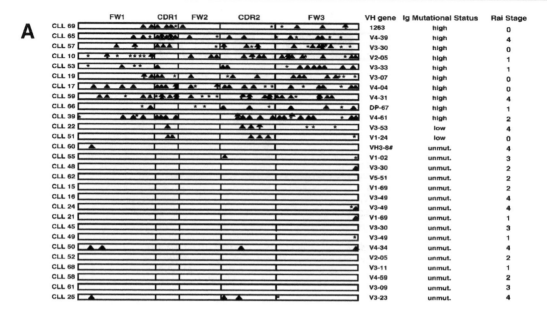

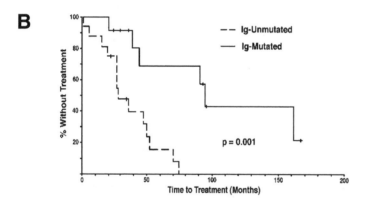

Fig. 45. Distribution of Ig gene sequences as either unmutated (**A**, bottom) or mutated (**A**, top). (**B**) Difference in the time to treatment in these two groups: median time to treatment in Ig-mutated CLL patients 95 mo; median time to treatment in Ig-unmutated CLL patients 28 mo. (From ref. *172*, Rosenwald et al., 2001, by copyright permission of the Rockefeller University Press.)

26.3% in group I, 50.3% in group II, and 72% in group III. Despite this increasing early stage distribution, survival values did not change when they were analyzed according to individual stages. Even when controlled for early smoldering CLL (so-called stage A) and compared with age- and sex-matched controls, CLL remains an incurable disease with a decreased overall survival. Earlier diagnosis and better health care for the elderly contribute to some of the observed changes. Molica and Levato *(173)* further note that an increase in survival has occurred mainly in the high-risk category patient. However, given that the introduction of purine analogs has not increased overall survival, they consider the improvement in overall survival to be a function of time to the prevention and treatment of both disease- and treatment-related complications. This has probably led to or accounted for the observed gain in overall survival of stage C patients in the last decade. It should be noted that Rozman et al. *(174)* have noted a shift in the age of onset of CLL in Spain, and this is thought to be partially related to the increase in longevity in Spain over the last 50 yr.

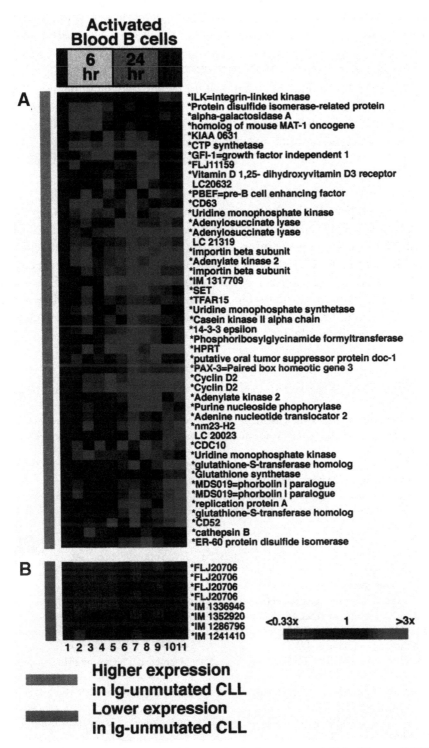

Fig. 46. Higher **(A)** and lower **(B)** B-cell gene expression in Ig-unmutated CLL. (From ref. *172*, Rosenwald et al., 2001, by copyright permission of the Rockefeller University Press.)

5. CLL RESEARCH CONSORTIUM AND CLL LIST SERVE

Two developments in the recent history of CLL bear further mention. The first is the evolution of the CLL Research Consortium (CRC) under the direction of Thomas Kipps. As Cheson *(175)* notes in the preface of his new book, *Chronic Lymphoid Leukemias,* the CRC is a "highly interactive collaboration among some of the foremost basic and clinical researchers in the United States" and "this new integrated research model is likely to result in major progress." At the time of this writing, the CRC had submitted an application for supplemental funding. There is also a bill before Congress called the Hematological Cancer Research Investment and Education Act of 2001, to amend the Public Health Service Act to provide for research, information, and education with respect to blood cancer. This bill is to contain special language referring to CLL. At a recent IWCLL meeting (San Diego, March, 2002), an NCI Familial CLL Consortium was formed under the leadership of Neil Caporaso.

In November of 1996, the CLL E-mail Listserv Digest was formed. The CLL List represents a group of CLL patients founded by Barbara Lackritz, Tony Bradford, Paul Copper, and Loren Buhle. It began with 25 people and has now grown to over 2000 members. The CLL List performs several functions. First, it is a source of information on the Internet for newly diagnosed patients. Second, it provides a forum for CLL patients to communicate with one another at any time. It has developed a CLL questionnaire and has a list of frequently asked questions. It has also worked with Healthtalk.com, a source of several audiocasts that can be downloaded. More recently, some of its members have piloted the development of a CLL Registry and Database to chart individual patient blood values and to calculate the lymphocyte doubling time.

REFERENCES

1. Lieutaud J. Elementa Physiologiae, Amsterdam, 1749, pp. 82–84. Translated by Dreyfus C. Milestones in the History of Haematology, New York, 1957, pp. 11–12.
2. Rai K. Progress in chronic lymphocytic leukemia: a historical perspective. Bailliere's Clin Hematol 1993;6:757–765.
3. Galton DAG. The natural history of chronic lymphocytic leukemia. M.D. thesis, Cambridge University, Cambridge, 1963.
4. Gunz FW. The dread leukemias and the lymphomas: their nature and their prospects. In: Wintrobe MM, ed. Blood, Pure and Eloquent. McGraw Hill, New York, 1980, pp. 511–546.
5. Hamblin T. Historical review: historical aspects of chronic lymphocytic leukemia. Br J Hematol 2000;111:1023–1024.
6. Piller GJ. Historical review: leukemia—a brief historical review from ancient times to 1950. Br J Haematol 2001;112:282–292.
7. Videbaek A. Chronic lymphocytic leukemia: historical aspects. In: Polliack A, Catovsky D, eds. Chronic Lymphocytic Leukemia. Harwood Academic Publishers, New York, 1988, pp. 1–9.
8. Velpeau A. Sur la resorption du pusuaet sur l'alteration du sang dans les maladies clinique de persection nenemant. Premier observation. Rev Med Fr Etrang 1827;2:216–240.
9. Craigie D. Case of disease and enlargement of the spleen in which death took place from the presence of purulent matter in the blood. Edinb Med Surg J 1845;64:400–412.
10. Bennett JH. Case of hypertrophy of the spleen and liver, in which death took place from suppuration of the blood. Edinb Med Surg J 1845;64:413–423.
11. Virchow R. (1943) Weisses Blut. In: Neue Notizen aus dem Gebiete der Natur- und Heilkunde, vol 36. Berlin, 1845, pp. 151–156.
12. Ehrlich P. Beitrag zur Kenntnis der Anilinfarbungen under ihrer Verwendung in der Microskopischen Technik. Arch Mikrochir Anat 1877;13:263–277.
13. Ehrlich P. Methodologische Beitrage zur Physiologie und Pathologie der verschisdenen Formen der Leukocyten. Z Klin Med 1880;1:553–558.
14. Ehrlich P. Uber die Bedeutung der neutrophilen Kornung. Charite Annales 1887;12:288–295.
15. Ehrlich P. Farbenanalytische Untersuchungen Zur Histologie und Klinik Des Blutes. Hirschwald, Berlin, 1891.

16. Einhorn M. Uber das Verhalten der Lymphocyten zu den weissen Blutkorperschen Inaugural-Dissertat., Berlin, 1881.
17. Kundrat H. Ueber Lympho-Sarkomatosis. Wien Klin Wochenschr 1893;6:211–213.
18. Turk W. Ein System der Lymphomatosen. Wein. Klin Wochenschr 1903;16:1073–1085.
19. Osler W. Leukaemia. In: Appleton D, ed. Principles and Practice of Medicine, 7th ed. New York, 1909, pp. 731–738.
20. Bennett JH. Leucocythemia or White Cell Blood, in Relation to the Physiology and Pathology of the Lymphatic Glandular System. Edinburgh: Sutherland and Knox, 1852.
21. Virchow R. Cellular Pathology as Based upon Physiological and Pathological Histology, Twenty Lectures translated from the second edition by F. Chance. JB Lippincott, Philadelphia, 1863.
22. Ward G. The infective theory of acute leukaemia. Br J Child Dis 1917;14:10–20.
23. Minot GR, Isaacs R. Lymphatic leukemia: age incidence, duration, and benefit derived from irradiation. Boston Med Surg J 1924;191:1–10.
24. Leavell BS. Chronic leukemia: a study of incidence and factors influencing the duration of life. Am J Med Sci 1938;196:329–340.
25. Wintrobe MM, Hasenbush LL. Chronic leukemia: the early phase of chronic leukemia, the results of treatment and the effects of complicating infections; a study of 86 adults. Arch Int Med 1939;64:701–718.
26. Boggs DR, Sofferman SA, Wintrobe MM, Cartwright GE. Factors influencing the duration of survival of patients with chronic lymphocytic leukemia. Am J Med 1966;40:243–254.
27. Galton DAG. The pathogenesis of chronic lymphocytic leukaemia. Can Med Assoc J 1966;94:1005–1010.
28. Dameshek W. Chronic lymphocytic leukemia-an accumulative disease of immunologically incompetent lymphocytes. Blood 1967;29:566–584.
29. Hansen MM. Chronic lymphocytic leukemia. Clinical studies based on 189 cases followed for a long time. Scand J Haematol 1973;18(suppl):1–286.
30. Henderson E, Lister T, eds. Dameshek and Gunz's Leukemia, 5th ed. WB Saunders, Philadelphia, 1990.
31. Hayhoe FGJ. Chronic lymphocytic leukemia: clinical aspects. In: Leukemia: Research and Clinical Practice. Little Brown, Boston, 1960, pp. 262–287.
32. Neumann E. Ueber myelognie Leukamie. Berl Klin Wochenschr 1878;15:69.
33. Dameshek W, Schwartz SO. Hemolysins as the cause of clinical and experimental hemolytic anemias. With particular reference to the nature of spherocytosis and increased fragility. Am J Med Sci 1938;196:769–792.
34. Berlin R. Red cell survival studies in normal and leukaemic subjects: latent haemolytic syndrome in leukaemia with splenomegaly—nature of anaemia in leukaemia-effect of splenomegaly. Acta Med Scand Suppl 1951;252:1–141.
35. Coons AH, Leduc EH, Connolly JM. Studies on antibody production. I. A method for the histochemical demonstration of specific antibody and its application to a study of the hyperimmune rabbit. J Exp Med 1955 102:49–72.
36. Wasserman LR, Stats D, Schwartz L, Fudenberg H. Symptomatic and hemopathic hemolytic anemia. Am J Med 1955;18:961–989.
37. Troup SB, Swisher SN, Young LE. The anemia of leukemia. Am J Med 1960;28:751–763.
38. Videbaek A. Auto-immune haemolytic anaemia in some malignant systemic diseases. Acta Med Scand 1962;171:463–476.
39. Myint H, Copplestone JA, Orchard J, et al. Fludarabine-related autoimmune haemolytic anaemia in patients with chronic lymphocytic leukaemia. Br J Haematol 1995;91:341–344.
40. Casadevall N, Nataf J, Viron B, et al. Pure red-cell aplasia and antierythropoietin antibodies in patients treated with recombinant erythroppietin. N Engl J Med 2002;346:469–475.
41. Scott RB. Leukaemia: chronic lymphatic leukaemia. Lancet 1957;1:1162–1167.
42. Galton DAG, Israels LG, Nabarro JDN, Till M. Clinical trials of p-(DI-2-chloroethylamino)-phenylbutyric acid (CB 1348) in malignant lymphoma. BMJ 1955;12:1172–1176.
43. Huguley CM. Survey of current therapy and of problems in chronic leukemia, In: Leukemia-Lymphoma. Year Book Medical Publishers, Chicago, 1970, p. 317.
44. Rundles RW. Chapter 114 Chronic lymphocytic leukemia. In: Williams WJ, Beutler E, Erslev AJ, Rundles RW, eds. Hematology, 2nd ed. McGraw-Hill , New York, 1977.
45. Lawrence JH, Low-Beer BVA, Carpenter JWJ. Chronic lymphatic leukemia. JAMA 1949;140:585.
46. Shaw RK, Boggs DR, Silberman HR, Frei E. A study of prednisone therapy in chronic lymphocytic leukemia. Blood 1961;17:182–189.
47. Rai KR, Peterson BL, Applebaum FR, Kolitz J, Elias L, Shepherd L, et al. Fludarabine compared with chlorambucil as primary therapy for chronic lymphocytic leukemia. N Engl J Med 2000;343:1750–1757.
48. Rai KR, Sawitsky A, Cronkite EP, et al. Clinical staging of chronic lymphocytic leukemia. Blood 1975;46:219–234.

104. Damle RN, Wasil T, Fais T, et al. Ig V gene mutation status and CD38 expression as novel prognostic indicators in chronic lymphocytic leukemia. Blood 1999;94:1840–1847.

105. Damle R, Wasil T, Allen S, et al. Updated data on V gene mutation status and CD38 expression in B-CLL. Blood 2000;95:2456–2457.

106. Hamblin TJ, Davis Z, Gardiner A, Oscier DG, Stevenson FK. Unmutated Ig V (H) genes are associated with a more aggressive form of chronic lymphocytic leukemia. Blood 1999;94:1848–1854.

107. Maloum K, Davi F, Merle-Beral H, et al. Expression of unrealted VH genes is a detrimental prognostic factor in chronic lymphocytic leukemia (editorial). Blood 2000;96:377–379.

108. Sakai A, Marti GM, Caporaso N, et al. Analysis of expressed immunoglobulin heavy chain genes in familial B-CLL. Blood 2000;95:1413–1419

109. Naylor M, Capra JD. Mutational status of Ig V(H) genes provides clinically valuable information in B-cell chronic lymphocytic leukemia. Blood 1994;94:1837–1839.

110. Hamblin TJ, Orchard JA, Ibbotson RE, et al. CD38 expression and immunoglobulin variable region mutations are independent prognostic variables in chronic lymphocytic leukemia, but CD38 expression may vary during the course of the disease. Blood 2002;99:1023–1029.

111. Hamblin TJ, Orchard JA, Gardiner A, Oscier DG, Davis Z, Stevenson FK. Immunoglobulin V genes and CD38 expression in CLL. Blood 2000;95:2455–2457.

112. Ibrahim S, Keating M, Do KA, et al. CD38 expression as an important prognostic factor in B-cell chronic lymphocytic leukemia. Blood 2001;98:181–186.

113. D'Arena G, Musto P, Cascavilla N, et al. CD38 expression correlates with adverse biological features and predicts poor clinical outcome in B-cell chronic lymphocytic leukemia. Leuk Lymph 2001;42:109–114.

114. Heintel D, Schwarzinger I, Chizzali-Bonfadin C, et al. Association of CD38 antigen expression with other prognostic parameters in early stages of chronic lymphocytic leukemia. Leuk Lymph 2001;42:1315–1321.

115. Chevallier P, Penther D, Avet-Loiseau H, et al. CD38 expression and secondary 17p deletion are important prognostic factors in chronic lymphocytic leukemia. Br J Haematol 2002;116:142–150.

116. Del Poeta G, Maurill L, Venditti A, et al. Clinical significance of CD38 expression in chronic lymphocytic leukemia. Blood 2001;98:2633–2639.

117. Matrai Z, Lin K, Dennis M, et al. CD38 expression and Ig VH gene mutation in B-cell chronic lymphocytic leukemia. Blood 2001;97:1902–1903.

118. Morabito F, Mangiola M, Oliva B, et al. Peripheral blood CD38 expression predicts survival in B-cell chronic lymphocytic leukemia. Leuk Res 2001;25:927–932.

119. Thunberg U, Johnson A, Roos G, et al. CD38 expression is a poor predictor for VH gene mutational status and prognosis in chronic lymphocytic leukemia. Blood 2001;97:1892–1893.

120. Cheson BD, Bennett JM, Grever M, et al. National Cancer Institute–sponsored working group guidelines for chronic lymphocytic leukemia: revised guidelines for diagnosis and treatment. Blood 1996;87:4990–4997.

121. Maloney DG, Liles TM, Czerwinski DK, et al. Phase I clinical trial using escalating single-dose infusion of chimeric anti-CD20 monoclonal antibody (IDEC-C2B8) in patients with recurrent B-cell lymphoma. Blood 1994;84:2457–2466.

122. Maloney DC, Grillo-Lopez AJ, White CA, et al. IDEC-C2B8 (rituximab) anti-CD20 monoclonal antibody therapy in patients with relapsed low-grade non-Hodgkin's lymphoma. Blood 1997;90:2188–2195.

123. McLaughlin P, Grillo-Lopez AJ, Link BK, et al. Rituximab chimeric anti-CD20 monoclonal antibody therapy for relapsed indolent lymphoma: half of patients respond to a four-dose treatment program. J Clin Oncology 1998;16:2825–2533.

124. Byrd JC, Murphy T, Howard RS, et al. Rituximab using a thrice weekly dose schedule in B-cell chronic lymphocytic leukemia and small lymphocytic lymphoma demonstrates clinical activity and acceptable toxicity. J Clin Oncol 2001;19:2153–2164.

125. O'Brien SM, Kantarjian H, Cortes J, et al. Rituximab dose escalation trial in chronic lymphocytic leukemia. J Clin Oncol 2001;19:2165–2170.

126. Pangalis GA, Poziopoulos C, Angelopoulou MK, Siakantaris MP, Panayiotidis P. Effective treatment of disease – related anaemia in B-chronic lymphocytic leukemia patients with recombinant human erythropoietin. Br J Haematol 1995;89:627–629.

127. Casadevall N. Update on the role of epoetin in hematologic malignancies and myelodysplastic syndromes. Semin Oncol 1998;25(suppl 7):12–18.

128. Cazzola M, Messinger D, Battistel V, et al. Recombinant human erythropoietin in anemia associated with multiple myeloma or non-Hodgkin's lymphoma: dose finding and identification of predictors of response. Blood 1995;86:4446–4453.

129. Osterborg A, Boogaerts MA, Cimino R, et al. Recombinant human erythropoietin in transfusion dependent anemic patients with multiple myeloma and non-Hodgkin's lymphoma—a randomized multicenter study. Blood 1996;87:2675–2682.

130. Rose E, Rai K, Revicki D, Brown R, Reblando J. Clinical and health status assessments in anemic chronic lymphocytic leukemia (CLL) patients treated with epoetin alfa (EPO). Blood 1994;80(Suppl 1):526a.

131. Russo F, Guadagni S, Mattera G, Esposito G, Abate G. Combination of granulocyte-macrophage colony-stimulating factor (GM-CSF) and erythropoietin (EPO) for the treatment of advanced non-responsive chronic lymphocytic leukemia. Eur J Haematol 1999;63:325–331.

132. Siakantaris MP, Angelopoulou MK, Vassilakopoulos TP, Dimopoulou MN, Kontopidou FN, Pangalis GA. Correction of disease related anaemia of B-chronic lymphoproliferative disorders by recombinant human erythropoietin: maintenance is necessary to maintain response. Leuk Lymph 2000;40:141–147.

133. Boveri T. Zur Frage der Enstehung maligner Tumoren. Fischer, Jena, 1914.

134. Nowell PC, Hungerford DA. A minute chromosome in human chronic granulocytic leukemia. Science 1960;132:1497.

135. Caspersson T, Gahrton G, Lindsten J, Zech L. Identification of the Philadelphia chromosome as a number 22 by quinacrine mustard fluorescence analysis. Exp Cell Res 1970;63:238–249.

136. Caspersson T, Lomakka G, Zech L. The 24 fluorescence patterns of the human metaphase chromosomes-distinguishing characters and variability. Hereditas 1971;67:89–102.

137. Crossen PE. Giemsa banding patterns in chronic lymphocytic leukaemia. Humangenetick 1975;27:151–156.

138. Robert KH, Moller E, Gahrton G, et al. B-cell activation of peripheral blood lymphocytes from patients with chronic lymphatic leukemia. Clin Exp Immunol 1978;33:302–308.

139. Gahrton G, Zech L, Robert KH, Bird AG. Mitogenic stimulation of leukemic cells by Epstein-Barr virus. N Engl J Med 1979;301:438.

140. Gahrton G, Robert KH, Friberg K, et al. Extra chromosome 12 in chronic lymphocytic leukemia. Lancet 1980;i:146.

141. Gahrton G, Robert KH, Friberg K, et al. Nonrandom chromosomal aberrations in chronic lymphocytic leukemia revealed by polyclonal B-cell mitogen stimulation. Blood 1980;56:640–647.

142. Kallioniemi A, Kallioniemi OP, Sudar D, et al. Comparative genomic hybridization for molecular cytogenetic analysis of solid tumors. Science 1992;258:818–821.

143. Jarosova M, Jedlickova K, Holzerova M, et al. Contribution of comparative genomic hybridization and fluorescence in situ hybridization to the detection of chromosomal abnormalities in B-cell chronic lymphocytic leukemia. Onkologie 2001;24:60–65.

144. Dohner H, Stilgenbauer S, Benner A, et al. Genomic aberrations and survival in chronic lymphocytic leukemia. N Engl J Med 2000;343:1910–1916.

145. Juliusson G, Gahrton G. Chromosome aberrations in B cell chronic lymphocytic leukemia. Pathogenetic and clinical implications. Cancer Genet Cytogenet 1990;45:143–160.

146. Juliusson G, Gahrton G. Chromosome abnormalities in B-cell chronic lymphocytic leukemia. In: Cheson BD, ed. Chronic Lymphocytic Leukemia: Scientific Advances and Clinical Developments. Marcel Dekker, New York, 1993, pp. 83–103.

147. Juliusson G, Gahrton G. Cytogenetics in CLL and related disorders. Bailliere's Clin Haematol 1993;6:821–848.

148. Juliusson G, Oscier DG, Fitchett M, et al. Prognostic subgroups in B-cell chronic lymphocytic leukemia defined by specific chromosomal abnormalities. N Engl J Med 1990;323:720–724.

149. Ross FM, Stockdill G. Clonal chromosome abnormalities in chronic lymphocytic leukemia patients revealed by TPA stimulation of whole blood cultures. Can Genetic Cytogenet 1987;25:109–121.

150. Fitchett M, Griffiths MJ, Oscier DG, et al. Chromosome abnormalities involving band 13q14 in hematologic malignancies. Cancer Genet Cytogenet 1987;24:143–150.

151. Zech L, Mellstedt H. Chromosome 13-a new marker for B-cell chronic lymphocytic leukemia. Heriditas 1988;108:77–84.

152. Pittman S, Catovsky D. Prognostic significance of chromosome abnormalities in chronic lymphocytic leukaemia. Br J Haematol 1984;58:649–660.

153. Juliusson G, Robert KH, Ost A, et al. Prognostic information from cytogenetic analysis in chronic B-lymphocytic leukemia and leukemic immunocytoma. Blood 1985;65:134–141.

154. Callen DF, Ford JH. Chromosome abnormalities in chronic lymphocytic leukemia revealed by TPA as a mitogen. Cancer Genet Cytogent 1983;10:87–93.

155. Dohner H, Stilgenbauer S, James MR, et al. 11q deletions identify a new subset of B-cell chronic lymphocytic leukemia characterized by extensive nodal involvement and inferior prognosis. Blood 1997;89:2516–2522.

156. Fegan C, Robinson H, Thompson P, et al. Karyotypic evolution in CLL. Identification of a new subgroup of patients with deletions of 11q and advanced or progressive disease. Leukemia 1995;9:2003–2008.

157. Neilson JR, Auer R, White D, et al. Deletions at 11q identify a subset of patients with typical CLL who show consistent disease progression and reduced survival. Leukemia 1997;11:1929–1932.

158. Dohner H, Pohl S, Bulgay-Morschel M, et al. Detection of trisomy 12 in chronic lymphoid leukemias using fluorescence in situ hybridization. Leukemia 1993;7:516–520.

159. Gahrton G, Robert KH, Friberg K, et al. Cytogenetic mapping of the duplicated segment of chromosome 12 in lymphoproliferative disorders. Nature 1982;297:513–514.

160. Dohner H, Fischer K, Bentz M, et al. p53 gene deletion predicts for poor survival and non-response to therapy with purine analogs in chronic B-cell leukemias. Blood 1995;85:1580–1589.

161. Juliusson G, Oscier D, Gahrton G, for the International Working Party on Chromosomes in CLL (IWCCLL). Cytogenetic findings and survival in B-cell chronic lymphocytic leukemia. Second IWCCLL compilation of data on 662 patients. Leuk Lymph 1991;5:21–25.

162. Gaidano G, Newcomb EW, Gong JZ, et al. Analysis of alterations of oncogenes and tumor suppressor genes in chronic lymphocytic leukemia. Am J Path 1994;144:1312–1319.

163. Stilgenbauer S, Bullinger L, Schroder M, et al. Deletions of chromosome regions 6q21 and 6q27 in B-CLL detected by FISH: incidence and correlation with clinical parameters in 208 patients. Blood 1996;88(suppl 1):238a.

164. Stilgenbauer S, Lichter P, Dohner H. Genomic aberrations in B-CLL chronic lymphocytic leukemia. In: Cheson BD, ed. Chronic Lymphoid Leukemias, 2nd ed. Marcel Dekker, New York, 2001, pp. 353–376.

165. Bullrich F, Croce CM. Molecular biology of chronic lymphocytic leukemia. In: Cheson BD, ed. Chronic Lymphoid Leukemias, 2nd ed. Marcel Dekker, New York, 2001, pp. 9–32.

166. Tyazhelova TV, Ivanov DV, Makeeva NV, et al. The transcription map of the 13q14 region frequently deleted in B-cell chronic lymphocytic leukemia. Russian J Genet 2001;37:1286–1292.

167. Stratowa C, Loffler G, Lichter P, et al. cDNA microarray gene expression analysis of B-cell chronic lymphocytic leukemia proposes potential new prognostic markers involved in lymphocyte trafficking. Int Jo Cancer 2001;91:474–480.

168. Voss T, Ahorn H, Haberl, P, et al. Correlation of clinical data with proteomics profiles in 24 patients with B-cell chronic lymphcyticleukemia. Int J Cancer 2001;91:180–186.

169. Bentz M, Huck K, du Manoir S, et al. Comparative genomic hybridization in chronic B-cell leukemias shows a high incidence of chromosomal gains and losses. Blood 1995;85:3610–3618.

170. Karhu R, Knuutila S, Kallioniemi OP, et al. Frequent loss of the 11q14-24 region in chronic lymphocytic leukemia: a study by comparative genomic hybridization. Tampere CLL Group. Genes Chromosom Cancer 1997;19:286–290.

171. Odero MD, Soto JL, Matutes E, et al. Comparative genomic hybridization and amplotyping by arbitrarily primed PCR in a Stage A B-CLL. Cancer Genet Cytogenet 2001;130:8–13.

172. Rosenwald A, Alizadeh AA, Widhopf G, et al. Relation of gene expression phenotype to immunoglobulin mutation genotype in B cell chronic lymphocytic leukemia. J Exp Med 2001;194:1639–1647.

173. Molica S, Levato D. What is changing in the natural history of chronic lymphocytic leukemia? Haematologica 2001;86:8–12.

174. Rozman, C, Bosch, F, Montserrat E. Review: state of the art of chronic lymphocytic leukemia: a changing natural history. Leukemia 1997;11:775–778.

175. Cheson BD, ed. Chronic Lymphoid Leukemias, 2nd ed. Marcel Dekker, New York, 2001.

II BIOLOGY AND GENETICS

2

Genetics of B-Cell Chronic Lymphocytic Leukemia

Stephan Stilgenbauer, MD, Peter Lichter, PhD, and Hartmut Döhner, MD

1. INTRODUCTION

B-cell chronic lymphocytic leukemia (B-CLL) is the most frequent type of leukemia among adults in the Western world, with an incidence of about 5 cases per 100,000 residents annually *(1,2)*. The disease affects mainly people of advanced age, but about 20% of patients are younger than 55 *(3)*. B-CLL is characterized by the accumulation of lymphocytes that appear morphologically mature but are functionally incompetent in bone marrow, blood, lymph nodes, and other organs, primarily of the lymphatic system (Fig. 1). During the course of the disease, there is increasing suppression of normal hematopoiesis and impairment of organ functions, resulting in B-symptoms, susceptibility to infection, and hemorrhage (Fig. 1). Currently available conventional therapeutic procedures are aimed at palliation. In younger patients, potentially curative approaches like autologous or allogeneic stem cell transplantation and antibody therapies are currently being investigated. The prognosis is influenced by the degree of dissemination of the disease at the time of diagnosis. This is reflected in the prognostic importance of the clinical staging systems defined by Rai and Binet *(4,5)*. Both systems differentiate among early (Rai 0, Binet A), intermediate (Rai I, II; Binet B) and advanced (Rai III, IV; Binet C) stages, which are characterized by different survival times (Fig. 2) *(6)*. However, the prognostic value of clinical staging is limited, especially in early stages, and there is marked heterogeneity in the speed of disease progression within the individual stages. For this reason, there has been intensive work in recent years on the identification of other clinical and biological factors with potential prognostic relevance. Genetic characteristics of the B-CLL cells have attained considerable importance among these factors *(7–10)*.

2. GENOMIC ABERRATIONS IN B-CLL

Two major subjects can be differentiated with respect to the genetic analysis of B-CLL: on the one hand, genomic aberrations, which, as acquired changes, may be involved in the initiation and progression of the disease, and, on the other hand, the mutation status of the variable segments of immunoglobulin heavy chain genes (V_H), which may reflect the cellular origin of B-CLL.

Since the early 1980s, chromosome banding analyses of malignant B-cells have been performed using B-cell mitogens *(11–18)*. Up to the early 1990s, clonal aberrations could be dem-

From: *Contemporary Hematology*
Chronic Lymphocytic Leukemia: Molecular Genetics, Biology, Diagnosis, and Management
Edited by: G. B. Faguet © Humana Press Inc., Totowa, NJ

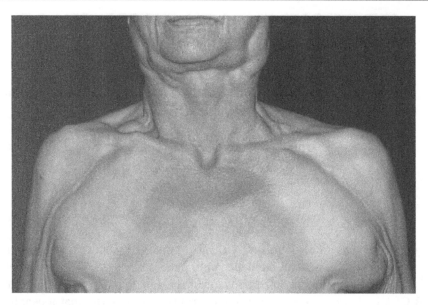

Fig. 1. Marked cervical and axillary lymphadenopathy in a B-CLL patient with deletion 11q. (From ref. *9*, with permission.)

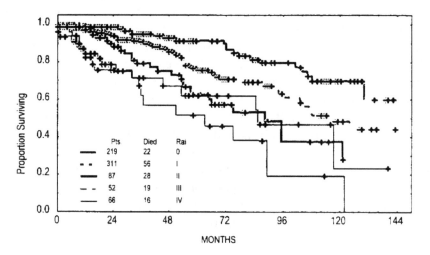

Fig. 2. Estimated survival times of B-CLL subgroups according to Rai stage (from ref. *6*, with permission).

onstrated in only 40–50% of B-CLL cases using chromosome banding *(19–21)*. Frequently, and despite the use of B-cell mitogens, nonclonal T-cells without chromosomal aberration were analyzed *(22)*. More recently, the development of molecular cytogenetic techniques like fluorescence *in situ* hybridization (FISH) has led to considerable improvement in the diagnostics of genetic aberrations in tumor cells *(23,24)*. FISH allows sensitive detection of specific sequences in the genome using cloned DNA fragments as probes. Signal number and location reflect numerical and structural changes of the corresponding chromosomal regions. The ability to detect aberrations not only on metaphase chromosomes but also in interphase cell nuclei is of great importance, especially in B-CLL (interphase cytogenetics; Fig. 3) *(25)*. Interphase cytogenetic studies using FISH showed that the incidence of genomic aberrations in B-CLL was markedly

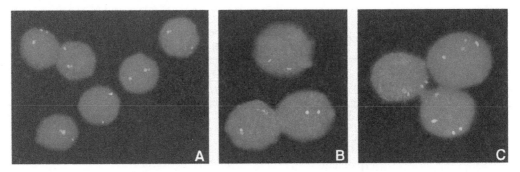

Fig. 3. Interphase FISH in B-CLL. **(A)** 11q deletion as demonstrated by the single red signal in five of the six nuclei shown. Two green signals of an internal control probe prove a high hybridization efficiency. The single cell with two red signals probably represents a nonleukemic cell from the specimen. **(B)** Biallelic deletion at 13q. Two of the three nuclei show no red hybridization signal of a probe containing marker D13S272, demonstrating biallelic loss of this region, whereas an adjacent probe containing marker D13S273 is retained in a disomic fashion. The single cell with two red and two green signals probably represents a nonleukemic cell. **(C)** Trisomy 12q (three green hybridization signals) and monoallelic deletion 13q14 (single red signal) in two of three nuclei in a B-CLL specimen. A single cell reflecting the normal disomic status of the two regions is shown for comparison. (From ref. *27*, with permission.)

underestimated in banding studies *(9)*. In B-CLL cases with abnormal karyotype by banding analysis but clonal aberrations by interphase FISH, the metaphase cells are derived from nonclonal T-cells and therefore do not reflect the karyotype of the malignant B-CLL cells.

Among the genomic aberrations whose incidence has been underestimated in B-CLL in banding studies are particularly the deletions of bands 13q14 and 11q22-q23, *(9)*; while trisomy 12, which was originally described as the most frequent aberration of B-CLL in studies using chromosome banding, has been rated the third most frequent aberration by interphase FISH *(9,26,27)*. In a study on 325 B-CLL patients, a comprehensive disease-specific probe set was used to detect the most important genomic gains, like partial trisomies 12q13, 3q27, and 8q24 and the most frequent genomic losses in bands 13q14, 11q22-q23, 6q21, 6q27, and 17p13 and translocations in band 14q32 using FISH *(9)* (Table 1). Overall genomic aberrations were found in more than 80% of all cases. The most frequent aberration by far was deletion of band 13q14, which was found in 55% of the cases. Other frequent aberrations were deletion 11q22-q23 (18%), trisomy 12q13 (16%), deletion 17p13 (7%), deletion 6q21 (6%), trisomy 8q24 (5%), translocation 14q32 (4%), and trisomy 3q27 (3%). Somewhat more than half of the cases showed only a single aberration; one-fifth of the cases showed two and nearly one-tenth showed more than two aberrations.

This precise determination of the incidence of chromosomal aberrations provides the basis for further studies of the role of these changes in the pathogenesis and progression of the disease. Thus, genes assumed to be involved in the pathogenesis of B-CLL could be identified by physical mapping of the minimal affected regions and by the strategy of positional cloning as well as the analysis of candidate genes (for review, see ref. *27*).

2.1. Deletions Within Band 13q14 and Identification of Candidate Genes

The structural chromosome aberration most frequently found in cytogenetic studies of B-CLL is deletion of band 13q14 *(18,28–31)*. Recurrent deletion of a chromosomal region indicates the existence of a tumor suppressor gene, whose inactivation is caused by the loss of an allele and the mutation in the remaining allele (two-hit hypothesis). The retinoblastoma tumor suppressor

Table 1
Incidence of Genomic Aberrations
in 325 Patients With B-CLL

| | Patients | |
Aberration	No.	%
13q deletion	178	55
11q deletion	58	18
12q trisomy	53	16
17p deletion	23	7
6q deletion	21	7
8q trisomy	16	5
t(14q32)	12	4
3q trisomy	9	3
Clonal abnormalities	268	82

From ref. *9*, with permission.

gene (*RB1*) is a candidate gene localized in band 13q14 that codes for a nuclear phosphoprotein involved in cell cycle regulation and transcription control. Its inactivation is involved in the pathogenesis of numerous tumors *(32)*. The deletion of an allele of *RB1* was detected using molecular cytogenetic techniques in about one-fourth of all B-CLL cases *(33–36)*. However, the inactivation of both *RB1* gene copies by deletion and/or mutation could only be extremely rarely detected, which raises questions about the pathogenetic role of *RB1* in B-CLL.

Various groups have constructed high-resolution genomic maps of the critical region in 13q14 to identify a new B-CLL-tumor suppressor gene *(37–47)*. By means of positional cloning, several groups identified fragments of several new genes from these subregions in parallel. Based on their localization in the minimal deleted 13q14 region, BCMS (ep272-3-t5, LEU1) and BCMSUN (ep272-3-t4, LEU2) are currently considered the most promising candidate tumor suppressor genes in B-CLL *(41–43,45,47)*. However, in mutation analyses to date, no inactivation of these candidate genes could be demonstrated in B-CLL in the sense of the two-hit hypothesis. BCMS inhibits a complex genomic organization. The gene extends over at least 560 kb genomic DNA and is transcribed in a number of heterogeneous mRNA transcripts *(48)*. Expression analyses are currently being performed to clarify the pathogenetic importance of the candidate genes in the 13q14 region *(49,50)*.

2.2. Deletions of Bands 11q22-q23 With ATM As the Candidate Gene

In a study using FISH, a critical region was identified around the neural cell adhesion molecule (NCAM) gene in band 11q23.1 in 15 hematological tumors *(51)*. In another study, the extent of 11q deletions among 40 B-CLL cases was determined using a FISH probe set of overlapping yeast artificial chromosome (YAC) clones spanning bands 11q14-q24 *(52,53)*. All aberrations affected a minimal consensus region of 2–3 Mb in size in bands 11q22.3-q23.1. In the minimal deleted region, the ataxia telangiectasia mutated (ATM) gene was localized, which, owing to its role in DNA repair and the frequent observation of lymphomas in *ATM* knockout mice, appeared to be a candidate tumor suppressor gene *(54,55)*. In fact, the changes in both *ATM* alleles by deletion and/or mutation in the sense of the two-hit hypothesis of tumor suppressor gene inactivation could be demonstrated for the first time in human tumors in T-prolymphocytic leukemia (T-PLL) *(56,57)*. Because of a lack of *ATM* protein expression, the involvement of *ATM* in B-CLL was also postulated, and inactivation of *ATM* by deletion and/or mutation could actually be demonstrated *(58–61)*. It was shown that *ATM* mutant B-CLL cases exhibited a deficient *ATM*-dependent response of p21 to γ-irradiation, failure to upregulate tumor necrosis factor-related apoptosis-inducing ligand receptor 2 (TRAIL-R2), and inability to repair induced chromosomal breaks *(62)*. An association of deletion 11q with a more aggressive clinical course of B-CLL was suggested in a chromosome banding study *(63)*. Interestingly, all *ATM* mutant cases showed absence of somatic V_H hypermutation (*see* also Subheading 2.8. below), indicating that *ATM* may play a role at the pregerminal center stage of B-cell maturation and may lead to the development of B-CLL derived from pregerminal center cells *(10,64)*. However, mutation of the remaining *ATM* allele was found only in 5 of 22 B-CLL cases with 11q22-q23 deletion of our series, which indicates a possible involvement of additional genes in this region in B-CLL *(59)*. By contrast, in mantle cell lymphoma, in which the 11q22-q23 deletion occurs in nearly half the cases *(65,66)*, mutation of the remaining allele could be demonstrated in all cases with deletion of an *ATM* allele *(67)*. Thus, *ATM* appears to be the tumor suppressor gene inactivated in connection with 11q22-q23 deletions in T-PLL, mantle cell lymphoma, and some cases of B-CLL. Elucidation of the situation in B-CLL cases with 11q deletion without mutation in the remaining *ATM* allele is currently in progress.

2.3. Trisomy 12 As Recurrent Aberration in B-CLL

Trisomy 12 was described in the early 1980s as the first recurrent aberration in B-CLL; with a prevalence between 10 and 25%, it was among the most frequent aberrations in nearly all subsequent studies using chromosome banding *(14,20,30,68–73)*. However, the identification of a critical region remained difficult, since usually a complete additional chromosome 12 was present and partial trisomy was observed only in very rare cases *(17,68,74)*.

Molecular cytogenetics by interphase FISH was used in numerous studies to detect trisomy 12 in B-CLL and revealed incidences of 10–20% in European studies and more than 30% in two US studies *(17,75–82)* (Table 1). The observation of one case of B-CLL with isolated over-representation of bands 12q13-q14 is interesting with respect to identification of a critical segment on chromosome 12 *(83)*. Merup et al. *(84)* examined a tumor with a complex 12q rearrangement and that found bands 12q13-q15 were most frequently amplified. Dierlamm et al. *(85)* observed partial trisomy 12 using FISH in 11 of more than 1000 lymphomas. Bands 12q13-q22 were the smallest mutually duplicated segment in four B-CLL cases in this series. Among others, genes of oncogenic potential, like CDK4, GLI, and MDM2, are localized in this genomic region, but no pathogenetic relevance for B-CLL has been shown to date for any of these genes. Currently the innovative approach of DNA microarray chip technology is being used, employing matrix comparative genomic hybridization (CGH) for identification of the smallest replicated genomic regions in bands 12q13-q21 in B-CLL *(86–89)* (Fig. 4).

2.4. Deletion 6q in Lymphatic Neoplasms

Among the most frequent aberrations in both acute lymphoblastic leukemia and aggressive as well as indolent lymphoma are deletions involving the long arm of chromosome 6 *(90)*. In B-CLL, 6q deletions were found in 6% of the evaluable cases by means of chromosome banding, whereby bands 6q15 and 6q23 were most often affected *(21)*. In an extensive analysis of various types of lymphoma, at least two independent deletion regions were identified, one in bands 6q21-q23 and

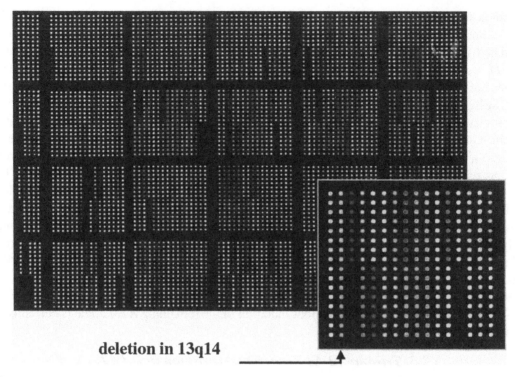

deletion in 13q14

Fig. 4. Matrix CGH in B-CLL. Hybridization of DNA derived from a patient with a 13q14 deletion (labeled in green) vs human control DNA (labeled in red). Inset: PAC clone localized in band 13q14 exhibits a dominant red fluorescence signal after hybridization, indicating the deletion of this region (arrow) *(89)*.

another in bands 6q25-q27 *(91)*. Deletion 6q21-q23 was associated with the subgroup of lymphomas with lymphocytic differentiation, which may be considered as nonleukemic correlates to B-CLL *(92)*.

Deletions in band 6q21 in B-CLL were also described in several more recent molecular genetic studies. Merup et al. *(93)* found 6q deletions in 6% of B-CLL cases, with a minimal deletion region in band 6q21. Gaidano et al. *(94)* observed 6q deletions in only 4 of 100 B-CLL cases in band 6q27. In another extensive series, 285 B-CLL cases were examined with probes from bands 6q21 and 6q27 *(95)*. The incidence of deletion 6q was 6%, and all deletions affected band 6q21, whereas band 6q27 was deleted in only one-third of the cases, and isolated 6q27 deletion was not observed in any case. In agreement with this, Zhang et al. *(96)* described a 4–5-Mb large minimal deleted region in band 6q21 in a series of various subtypes of lymphomas and leukemias. Although several candidate genes are located in the critical 6q21 region, it has not yet been possible to demonstrate a pathogenic role for one of these genes.

2.5. Deletion 17p13 and Mutation of the p53 Gene in B-CLL

Involvement of *p53* in band 17p13 in B-CLL was found in molecular genetic studies. Because of its role in nearly all kinds of tumors, *p53* was examined as a candidate gene in B-CLL. By means of single-strand conformational polymorphism analyses and direct DNA sequencing, *p53* mutations could be proved, with a prevalence between 10 and 15% in B-CLL *(94,97–100)*.

17p13 deletions were found in 4–9% in B-CLL *(9,101)*. To examine the relationship of 17p13 deletion and *p53* inactivation by mutation in the remaining allele, 110 B-CLL cases were analyzed *(102)*. Fifteen showed mutations in the *p53* gene, of which half were biallelic aberrations. Among the cases with deletion, most showed mutations in the remaining *p53* allele, whereas among the cases without 17p13 deletion, *p53* mutation occurred only rarely. The high rate of *p53* mutations in the B-CLL cases with 17p13 deletions suggests that, in the case of 17p13 deletion in B-CLL, *p53* is the tumor suppressor gene affected by the aberrations.

2.6. Rearrangement of the IgH Locus in Band 14q32

Translocation breakpoints in band 14q32, in which the heavy chain immunoglobulin genes (IgH) are located, were described as the most frequent aberration in B-CLL in early banding studies *(13,14,18,20,68,71,72,73,103–105)*. In the most extensive studies, aberrations of chromosome 14 could be demonstrated in 8% of evaluable cases *(21)*. The aberrations were often the result of translocation t(11;14)(q13;q32), which leads to deregulation of the cyclin-D1 gene (CCND1) in 11q13 by the Ig_H locus (14q32) *(106–110)*. The t(11;14)(q13;q32) and cyclin-D1 overexpression are now considered characteristic of mantle cell lymphoma and occur rarely in other lymphoproliferative diseases *(106,107,110,111)*. Many of the cases with t(11;14)(q13;q32) in early cytogenetic B-CLL studies were probably leukemic mantle cell lymphoma. Neither the t(11;14)(q13;q32) nor the deregulation of CCND1 was described as a frequent event in B-CLL in recent studies *(94,112–115)*. In our monocentric series of 325 B-CLL cases, there was no case of t(11;14)(q13;q32) *(9)*.

The situation is similar for translocations t(14;18)(q32;q21) and t(14;19)(q32;q13), which are rare but recurrent aberrations (<5%) in B-CLL. In today's view, 14q32 rearrangements are rare events in B-CLL, and the high incidence of these aberrations in early banding analyses was probably caused by the inclusion of other leukemic lymphomas in these series *(94,112–122)*.

2.7. Rare Aberrations in B-CLL: Trisomies 3q27 and 8q24

Additional genetic aberrations were discovered either by genome-wide screening methods like chromosome banding and CGH, or by analysis of prominent candidate genes. Banding and CGH identified several further aberrations that were rare but recurrent in B-CLL. Often, these were trisomies, like trisomy 3q, which was described in several studies *(30,71,73)*. CGH analyses point to the distal arm of 3q as the minimal duplicated region with possible pathogenetic relevance in B-CLL *(83)*. In addition to trisomy 3, which was also described in banding analyses, CGH analyses identified gains of 8q and 15q as new aberrations in B-CLL *(83)*. With C-MYC in 8q24 and BCL6 in 3q27, for example, candidate genes are known for some of these regions, but their role in the pathogenesis of B-CLL has not yet been confirmed.

2.8. Mutation Status of the V_H Genes

A novel genetic parameter of B-CLL is the mutation status of the V_H genes *(123–125)*. Although in the past, B-CLL was considered to be a lymphoma derived from pregerminal center B-cells, somatically mutated V_H genes could be demonstrated in about half of the cases in these studies. Accordingly, a separation was made into two different B-CLL groups: one with unmutated V_H genes, assumed to originate in pregerminal center cells, and another with mutated V_H genes, thought to stem from postgerminal center cells. Moreover, it could be demonstrated that the V_H mutation status is clinically relevant. Although B-CLL with unmutated V_H shows an unfavorable course, with rapid disease progression, B-CLL with mutated V_H often shows slow progression

(7,8). In addition, there was a correlation between V_H mutation status and CD38 expression of B-CLL cells as further evidence of the biological difference between the two forms (7). The relationship of the V_H mutation status to genomic aberrations and the differential influence of these factors in the pathogenesis and progression of B-CLL are currently undergoing intensive examination.

3. CLINICAL IMPACT OF GENOMIC ABERRATIONS IN B-CLL

The multicenter International Working Party on Chromosomes in CLL (IWCCLL) studies examined the correlation between clinical data and genomic aberrations based on chromosome banding (19,21). A longer estimated survival time (median 15 yr) was found in the group of patients with normal karyotype compared with the group with clonal aberrations (median 7.7 yr). Moreover, a relation was found between the complexity of the karyotype and unfavorable prognosis. In the subgroup analyses of patients with specific aberrations, a correlation was found between trisomy 12 and shorter survival time; in contrast, aberrations in chromosome 13 were associated with more favorable prognoses. In multivariate analysis, however, neither the presence nor the number of chromosomal aberrations showed independent prognostic relevance.

Precise detection of genomic aberrations using interphase FISH provided a more reliable basis for correlations between genomic aberrations and clinical parameters in B-CLL. In an extensive FISH analysis of 325 B-CLL cases with probes for regions 3q27, 6q21, 8q24, 11q22-q23, 12q13, 13q14, 14q32, and 17p13, multivariate analysis revealed an independent prognostic relevance of genomic aberrations (9) (Fig. 5). It was found that deletion 13q14 as a single aberration was associated with long median survival times (133 mo), whereas deletions 11q22-q23 and 17p13 were associated with poor prognoses (79 and 32 mo, respectively). Intermediate survival times were found for B-CLL cases without aberrations or with trisomy 12 (111 and 114 mo, respectively) (9).

3.1. Prognostic Relevance of Deletion 11q22-q23

B-CLL cases with deletion 11q show more rapid progression of the disease and shorter survival times. In interphase FISH, deletion 11q22-q23 is the second most frequent aberration in B-CLL, with an incidence of approx 20%, and identifies a patient group with a characteristic clinical picture (26). B-CLL patients with 11q deletion present with advanced stages of disease and pronounced lymphadenopathy, reflected by large palpable peripheral, thoracic, and abdominal lymph nodes (Fig. 1). Moreover, patients with 11q deletion have a more rapid progression of disease, as measured by shorter therapy-free intervals (9 mo vs 43 mo; $p < 0.001$). In the survival time analysis, 11q deletion was associated with a poor prognosis, and the effect of this aberration on the course of the disease was age-dependent. In B-CLL patients younger than 55 yr, the survival time was significantly shorter in the group with 11q deletion than in the group without 11q deletion, whereas in patients 55 yr or older, there was only a trend to shorter survival times. Another, likewise age-dependent prognostic relevance was found in an examination of ATM protein expression in B-CLL (61). The poor outcome of B-CLL with 11q deletion was confirmed in an independent series (126). In multivariate analysis, 11q deletion was found to be an independent adverse factor (26). Since the 11q deletion appears to be prognostically relevant, especially in younger B-CLL patients, this aberration could serve to identify a patient group that could benefit from modern experimental strategies, such as autologous or allogeneic blood stem cell transplantation.

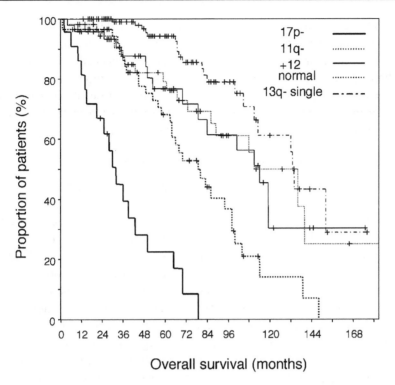

Fig. 5. Survival probability in B-CLL according to risk groups defined by genomic aberrations. The estimated median survival times were as follows: 17p deletion, 32 mo; 11q deletion, 79 mo; normal karyotype, 111 mo; 12q trisomy, 114 mo; and 13q deletion as single abnormality, 133 mo. (From ref.*9*, with permission.)

3.2. Clinical Characteristics of Trisomy 12

In a large comparison of individual chromosomal aberrations in banding analysis, B-CLL with trisomy 12 had the shortest survival time *(19,21)*. However, the negative prognostic relevance of trisomy 12 could not be confirmed in further studies *(18,68,69,73)*.

In interphase FISH studies, trisomy 12 was associated with atypical morphology and immunophenotype in B-CLL *(77,79,81)*. An effect of trisomy 12 on survival time was found in a series of 83 B-CLL patients *(78)*. Patients with trisomy 12 had a mean survival time of 7.9 yr compared with 14.4 yr in the group with normal karyotype. No significant difference was found in a comparison of trisomy 12 vs no trisomy 12 on the basis of the FISH results alone. Patients with trisomy 12 had undergone more intensive prior treatment and were in advanced stages of disease. The response rates to treatment with fludarabine did not differ *(78)*. In a series of 325 B-CLL patients, the prognosis in the group with trisomy 12 (median survival time 114 mo) was intermediate to that of 13q deletion as a single aberration and deletions 11q22-q23 or 17p13 (Fig. 5) *(9)*.

3.3. Clinical Relevance of Deletion 6q

In B-CLL patients with deletion 6q, shorter therapy-free intervals could be demonstrated, reflecting more rapid progression of the disease *(18)*. By contrast, however, no association of deletion 6q with shorter survival time was proved in the IWCCLL studies *(19,21)*. An interphase

FISH study on 285 B-CLL patients revealed a correlation between deletion 6q and greater tumor mass, measured by leukocyte count (median 49.3×10^9/L vs 31.7×10^9/L; $p = 0.036$) and lymphadenopathy *(95)*. The sum of the products of the largest cervical, axillary, and inguinal lymph nodes (median 7.3 cm^2 vs 3.0 cm^2; $p = 0.029$) and the longest lymph node diameter (median 4.0 cm vs 2.0 cm; $p = 0.008$) were greater in the group with 6q deletion. There was, however, no significant difference in survival time or therapy-free intervals between the two groups *(95)*. Thus, 6q deletion does not appear to be of prognostic relevance in B-CLL.

3.4. Prognostic Impact of 17p13 (p53) Aberrations

Early mutation analyses showed that *p53* mutations are of significant negative prognostic relevance and are associated with treatment failure in B-CLL *(98)*. In banding studies, the relevance of aberrations of band 17p13, where *p53* is localized, was only recently described in B-CLL. In a study of 480 B-CLL patients with no prior treatment, 17p aberrations were the only chromosomal aberration of prognostic relevance *(101)*. An interphase FISH study also showed that patients whose leukemia cells had a *p53* deletion had significantly shorter survival times than patients without this aberration *(100)*. Moreover, a relationship was found between the deletion and the response to treatment. Whereas 56% of patients without *p53* deletion went into remission on treatment with purine analogs, none of the patients with *p53* deletion responded *(100)*. In a multivariate analysis, *p53* deletion was the strongest prognostic factor, followed by established clinical prognosis factors like stage and age *(9)*. Prediction of the prognosis and therapeutic success in B-CLL thus appears possible with the parameter *p53* aberration/17p deletion. Despite the chemoresistance of B-CLL with 17p deletion, there is evidence that durable therapeutic success can be achieved with the monoclonal antibody campath-1H *(127)*.

3.5. Clinical Relevance of 14q32 (IgH) Translocations

The negative prognostic relevance of translocation breakpoints in band 14q32, often the result of a t(11;14) *(19,21)*, is probably explicable by the diagnostic ambiguity of these cases, since, for example, differentiation from leukemic mantle cell lymphomas often remains doubtful. Today, in a case with cytogenetic or molecular evidence of the t(11;14)(q13;q32) or *CCND1* over expression, a diagnosis of MCL should be considered until another diagnosis is proved otherwise *(94,106–115)*.

4. V$_H$ MUTATION, CD38, AND GENOMIC ABERRATIONS IN B-CLL

Several studies over the past few years have demonstrated that there is somatic hypermutation of the rearranged V$_H$ genes (mutated V$_H$) in about half of the B-CLL cases *(123–125)*. This was surprising since B-CLL had been considered a pregerminal center-derived lymphoma. Pivotal studies on a small number of patients showed an unfavorable prognosis in B-CLL with unmutated V$_H$ genes *(7,8)*. In some studies, there was a strong correlation between CD38 expression of the B-CLL cells and the V$_H$ mutation status *(7,128)*. Other authors could not confirm this, so it still remains unclear whether CD38 expression can be applied as a prognostic surrogate marker for the V$_H$ mutation status *(129–131)*.

4.1. Prognostic Impact of the V$_H$ Mutation Status

To examine the V$_H$ mutation status in a large series ($n = 300$) of B-CLL patients, the VDJ-rearrangement of the immunoglobulin genes was amplified by PCR from genomic DNA, and the

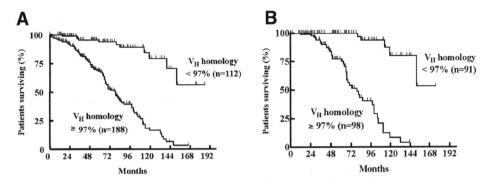

Fig. 6. Probability of survival in B-CLL patients with mutated and unmutated V_H genes according to the 97% cutoff values. **(A)** The estimated median survival time for the V_H homology $\geq$ 97% group was 79 mo. The last observed death in the V_H homology < 97% group was after 152 mo of follow-up time (survival probability 56%). **(B)** When only patients diagnosed at Binet stage A were evaluated the estimated median survival times for the V_H homology $\geq$ 97% and V_H homology < 97% groups were 79 mo vs not reached (last observed death after 152 mo of follow-up time; survival probability 53%). (From ref. *10*, with permission.)

mutation status of the V_H genes was determined by DNA sequencing *(10,132)*. Taking the classical cutoff value of 98% homology to the nearest related germline gene to differentiate between mutated and unmutated V_H genes, 132 cases (44%) showed mutated and 168 cases (56%) unmutated V_H genes. The method of maximally selected log rank statistics was applied to test the prognostic relevance of the V_H mutation status. A corrected p value (p_{cor}) for the best possible separation of two subgroups with different survival probabilities was found at a V_H homology to the nearest related germline gene of 97% ($p_{cor} < 0.001$; 95% confidence interval 96–98%) *(10)*. With a cutoff value of 97% homology to the nearest related germline gene, 112 cases (37%) showed mutated and 188 cases (63%) unmutated V_H. The Kaplan-Meier estimate of the median survival time in the two V_H subgroups differed both for the overall group ($n = 300$) and within the subgroup of patients in Binet stage A at the time of diagnosis ($n = 189$) (Fig. 6) *(10)*.

4.2. Structure of the VDJ Rearrangement

In addition to the V_H mutation status, the study of the structure of the VDJ rearrangement and the character of the mutations with respect to biological factors of disease etiology, like antigen selection, is of interest. Until recently, there were only studies available on small numbers of cases *(123,125,133,134,* and references therein). In a large B-CLL series, at least one clonal VDJ rearrangement of genomic DNA could be amplified in all 300 cases *(132)*. Cases with mutated V_H showed a different VDJ rearrangement structure than cases with unmutated V_H. Genes of the V_H3 and V_H4 families were over-represented in the mutated V_H subgroup, whereas the V_H1 family was found more frequently in the V_H unmutated subgroup. Specific V_H genes were responsible for the differences, and these imbalances were in line with previous studies *(123,125,133,134,* and references therein). The mean length of the CDR3 region differed significantly between the V_H mutated and unmutated subgroups. The median mutation rates and ratios of replacement/silent (R/S) mutations were greater within the V_H subregions in the CDRs than in the FRs. Cases with less than 98% homology to the nearest related germline gene were examined by means of the algorithm of Chang and Casali *(135)* for evidence of an antigen selection in the mutation pattern of the V_H gene. In 43 cases, mutation patterns consistent with antigen selection were found, whereas no such patterns could be recognized in 41 cases *(132)*. The survival probabilities did not differ significantly between the two groups. Taking these data together, there are differences in the biological background of V_H mutated vs unmutated B-CLL; however, the pathogenetic role of external stimuli still needs to be confirmed.

4.3. CD38 Expression in Relationship to the V_H Mutation Status

The prognostic relevance of CD38 expression and particularly the question of whether CD38 might be used as a surrogate marker for the V_H mutation status in B-CLL is a topic of controversy *(7,128–131,136,137)*. The measurement of CD38 using fluorescence-activated cell sorting (FACS) would be technically less difficult and costly compared with V_H mutation analysis and thus would be an attractive procedure in estimating prognosis. CD38 expression was tested in 157 B-CLL cases of our series *(10)*. The group with expression of CD38 in more than 30% (56 cases, 36%) or less than 30% (101 cases, 64%) of B-CLL cells were compared, but no significant difference in estimated survival time was found. In this study, a high CD38 expression correlated with unmutated V_H status, but there was a discrepancy between CD38 expression and V_H mutation status in about one-third of the cases *(10)*. Thus, CD38 appears to be suitable for predicting the V_H mutation status only to a limited degree. Moreover, variability in CD38 expression is observed in some studies during the course of the disease *(10,130,136)*.

4.4. Distribution of Genomic Aberrations in the V_H Subgroups

Using interphase FISH, genomic aberrations were demonstrable in 246 of 300 (82%) B-CLL cases with known V_H mutation status in our series *(10)*. The incidences of the individual genomic aberrations in the total group and in dependence on the V_H mutation status are shown in Table 2. The incidences of genomic aberrations overall and of trisomy 12 in the two V_H subgroups were comparable; by contrast, prognostically unfavorable aberrations (11q-, 17p-) occurred almost exclusively in the V_H unmutated, and prognostically favorable aberrations (13q-, 13q- single) more frequently in the V_H mutated subgroup. This unbalanced distribution of genomic aberrations emphasizes the different biological backgrounds of the B-CLL subgroups with mutated or unmutated V_H and could in part explain their different clinical course. On the other hand, about two-thirds of the V_H unmutated B-CLL cases show no unfavorable genomic aberrations, which indicates a differential influence of these factors. Comprehensive studies of gene expression in B-CLL based on DNA chip technology indicate that the global gene expression "signature" of V_H mutated and unmutated B-CLL is very similar and that only the expression of a small number of genes discriminates between the two groups *(138,139)*.

4.5. Prognostic Relevance of Genomic Aberrations and V_H Mutation Status

To examine the individual prognostic value of genomic aberrations, the V_H mutation status, and other clinical and laboratory features, a multivariate analysis was made of the survival time by means of a Cox regression *(10)*. The V_H mutation status, 17p deletion, 11q deletion, age, leukocyte count and lactate dehydrogenase levels were identified as independent prognostic factors in this analysis. When the V_H mutation status, and 11q and 17p aberrations were included, the clinical stage of disease according to the systems of Rai or Binet was not identified as an independent prognostic factor. Similar results, demonstrating a very strong prognostic impact of the V_H mutation status and genomic aberrations, were independently found in two other B-CLL series *(140,141)*. Based on this model, four subgroups with widely differing survival probabilities can be defined by the V_H mutation status, 11q deletion and 17p deletion (Fig. 7).

Table 2
Relation of V_H Mutation Status and Genomic
Aberrations in 300 B-CLL Cases

| Aberration | V_H (%) | | p-value[a] |
	Mutated (homology < 98%) [n = 132 (44%)]	Unmutated (homology > 98%) [n = 168 (56%)]	
Clonal aberrations	80	84	0.37
13q deletion	65	48	0.004
13q deletion single	50	26	< 0.001
Trisomy 12	15	19	0.44
11q deletion	4	27	< 0.001
17p deletion	3	10	0.03
17p or 11q deletion	7	35	< 0.001

[a]Fisher's exact test.
From ref. 10, with permission.

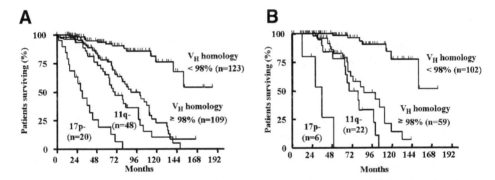

Fig. 7. Probability of survival among patients in the following genetic categories: 17p- (17p deletion irrespective of V_H mutation status), 11q- (11q deletion irrespective of V_H mutation status), unmutated V_H (V_H homology >98% and no 17p or 11q deletion), and mutated V_H (V_H homology <98% and no 17p or 11q deletion). **(A)** Among all stages (n = 300) the estimated median survival times for the respective genetic subgroups were as follows: 17p deletion, 30 mo; 11q deletion, 70 mo; V_H unmutated, 89 mo; and V_H mutated, not reached (54% survival at 152 mo). **(B)** Among Binet stage A patients (n = 189) the estimated median survival times for the respective genetic subgroups were as follows: 17p deletion, 36 mo; 11q deletion, 68 mo; V_H unmutated, 86 mo; and V_H mutated, not reached (52% survival at 152 mo). (From ref. 10, with permission.)

These studies show that genomic aberrations and V_H mutation status appear to have complementary relevance in estimating the prognosis in B-CLL. Unmutated V_H and genomic aberrations were among the strongest prognostic factors and gives us insight into the biological bases of the clinical heterogeneity of B-CLL. For this reason, genomic aberrations and V_H mutation status are currently being tested in relation to other clinical and laboratory factors in prospective multicenter studies of the German CLL Study Group (GCLLSG). If these factors allow us to predict the course of disease in individual patients at the time of diagnosis, independent of the stage, they could serve as the basis for future risk-adapted treatment strategies.

5. PERSPECTIVE: NEW DIAGNOSTIC TOOLS

As in other leukemias, genetic markers correlate with the clinical course, response to therapy, and survival time in B-CLL. To determine the relevance of such genetic markers for the stratification of patient groups to various treatments of different intensity, extensive clinical studies must be performed. As a rapid and robust diagnostic test matrix CGH (comparative genomic hybridization against a matrix of defined genomic DNA fragments) can be utilized *(86,89)*. In this procedure, total genomic tumor DNA is labeled with fluorescent dyes and hybridized on a DNA chip containing microarrays of defined genomic DNA fragments. After cohybridization with differently labeled normal control-DNA, the relative intensity of the two fluorescences is used to determine whether a certain DNA-sequence is over- or under-represented in the genome of the tumor cell population (Fig. 4). Since all relevant genomic aberrations in B-CLL are imbalances, a matrix CGH chip was constructed to test specific aberrations that might occur in B-CLL *(89)*. For this purpose, genomic DNA fragments of the chromosomal areas that are deleted or over represented in B-CLL were selected, isolated, and printed on a matrix CGH chip. This chip allows automated analysis of the genomic imbalances in B-CLL and will be evaluated in clinical studies aiming at risk stratification of individual patients.

ACKNOWLEDGMENTS

This work was supported by Wilhelm Sander-Stiftung (2001.004.1), Deutsche Krebshilfe (70-2434-DöI), and BMBF (01KW9934, 01KW9938).

REFERENCES

1. Rozman C, Montserrat E. Chronic lymphocytic leukemia. N Engl J Med 1995;1333:1052–1057.
2. Zwiebel JA, Cheson BD. Chronic lymphocytic leukemia: staging and prognostic factors. Semin Oncol 1998;25:42–59.
3. Mauro FR, Foa R, Giannarelli D, et al. Clinical characteristics and outcome of young chronic lymphocytic leukemia patients: a single institution study of 204 cases. Blood 1999;94:448–454.
4. Rai KR, Sawitsky A, Cronkite EP, Chanana AD, Levy RN, Paternack BS. Clinical staging of chronic lymphocytic leukemia. Blood 1975;46:219–234.
5. Binet JL, Auquier A, Dighiero G, et al. A new prognostic classification of chronic lymphocytic leukemia derived from a multivariate survival analysis. Cancer 1981;48:198-206.
6. Keating MJ Improving the complete remission rate in CLL. In: Hematology 1999. The American Society of Hematology Education Program Book, 1999, pp. 262–269.
7. Damle JN, Wasil T, Fais F, et al. Ig V gene mutation status and CD38 expression as novel prognostic indicators in chronic lymphocytic leukemia. Blood 1999;94:1840–1847.
8. Hamblin TJ, Davis Z, Gardiner A, Oscier DG, Stevenson FK. Unmutated Ig VH genes are associated with a more aggressive form of chronic lymphocytic leukemia. Blood 1999;94:1848-1854.
9. Döhner H, Stilgenbauer S, Benner A,. Genomic aberrations and survival in chronic lymphocytic leukemia. N Engl J Med 2000;343:1910-1918.
10. Kröber A, Seiler T, Benner A, et al. VH mutation status, CD38 expression level, genomic aberrations, and survival in chronic lymphocytic leukemia. Blood 2002;100:1410–1416.
11. Robèrt KH, Möller E, Gahrton G, Eriksson H, Nilsson B. B-cell activation of peripheral blood lymphocytes from patients with chronic lymphocytic leukaemia. Clin Exp Immunol 1978;33:302–308.
12. Mitelman F, Levan G. Clustering of aberrations to specific chromosomes in human neoplasms. Hereditas 1978;89:207–232.
13. Autio K, Turunen O, Penttilä O, Erämaa E, de la Chapelle A, Schröder J. Human chronic lymphocytic leukemia: Karyotypes in different lymphocyte populations. Cancer Genet Cytogenet 1979;1:147–155.
14. Gahrton G, Robèrt KH, Friberg K, Zech L, Bird AG. Nonrandom chromosomal aberrations in chronic lymphocytic leukemia revealed by polyclonal B-cell-mitogen stimulation. Blood 1980;56:640–647.

15. Hurley JN, Fu SM, Kunkel HG, Chaganti RSK, German J. Chromosome abnormalities of leukaemic B lymphocytes in chronic lymphocytic leukaemia. Nature 1980;283:76–78.

16. Crawford DH, Catovsky D. In vitro activation of leukaemia B cells by interleukin-4 and antibodies to CD40. Immunology 1993;80:40–44.

17. Döhner H, Pohl S, Bulgay-Mörschel M, Stilgenbauer S, Bentz M, Lichter P. Detection of trisomy 12 in chronic lymphoid leukemias using fluorescence in situ hybridization. Leukemia 1993;7:516–520.

18. Oscier DG, Stevens J, Hamblin TJ, Pickering RM, Lambert R, Fitchett M. Correlation of chromosome abnormalities with laboratory features and clinical course in B-cell chronic lymphocytic leukaemia. Br J Haematol 1990;76:352–358.

19. Juliusson G, Oscier DG, Fitchett M, et al. Prognostic subgroups in B-cell chronic lymphocytic leukemia defined by specific chromosomal abnormalities. N Engl J Med 1990;323:720–724.

20. Juliusson G, Gahrton G. Chromosome aberrations in B-cell chronic lymphocytic leukemia. Pathogenetic and clinical implications. Cancer Genet Cytogenet 1990;45:143–160.

21. Juliusson G, Oscier D, Gahrton G, for the International Working Party on Chromosomes in CLL (IWCCLL). Cytogenetic findings and survival in B-cell chronic lymphocytic leukemia. Second IWCCLL compilation of data on 662 patients. Leuk Lymphoma 1991;5:21–25.

22. Autio K, Elonen E, Teerenhovi L, Knuutila S. Cytogenetic and immunologic characterization of mitotic cells in chronic lymphocytic leukemia. Eur J Haematol 1986;39:289–298.

23. Lichter P, Ward DC. Is non-isotopic in situ hybridization finally coming of age? Nature 1990;345:93–95.

24. Lichter P, Bentz M, Joos S. Detection of chromosomal aberrations by means of molecular cytogenetics: Painting of chromosomes and chromosomal subregions and comparative genomic hybridization. Methods Enzym 1995;254:334–359.

25. Cremer T, Landegent J, Brückner A, et al. Detection of chromosome aberrations in the human interphase nucleus by visualization of specific target DNAs with radioactive and non-radioactive in situ hybridization techniques: diagnosis of trisomy 18 with probe L1.84. Hum Genet 1986;74:346–352.

26. Döhner H, Stilgenbauer S, James MR, et al. 11q deletions identify a new subset of B-cell chronic lymphocytic leukemia characterized by extensive nodal involvement and inferior prognosis. Blood 1997;89:2516–2522.

27. Stilgenbauer S, Bullinger L, Lichter P, Döhner H. Genetics of chronic lymphocytic leukemia: genomic aberrations and V(H) gene mutation status in pathogenesis and clinical course. Leukemia 2002;16:993–1007.

28. Fitchett M, Griffiths MJ, Oscier DG, Johnson S, Seabright M. Chromosome abnormalities involving band 13q14 in hematologic malignancies. Cancer Genet Cytogenet 1987;24:143–150.

29. Peterson LC, Lindquist LL, Church S, Kay NE. Frequent clonal abnormalities of chromosome band 13q14 in B-cell chronic lymphocytic leukemia: Multiple clones, subclones, and nonclonal alterations in 82 Midwestern patients. Genes Chromosom Cancer 1992;4:273–280.

30. Ross FM und Stockdill G. Clonal chromosome abnormalities in chronic lymphocytic leukemia patients revealed by TPA stimulation of whole blood cultures. Cancer Genet Cytogenet 1987;25:109–121.

31. Zech L, Mellstedt H. Chromosome 13—a new marker for B-cell chronic lymphocytic leukemia. Hereditas 1988;108:77–84.

32. Weinberg RA. The retinoblastoma protein and cell cycle control. Cell 1995;81:323–330.

33. Döhner H, Pilz T, Fischer K, et al. Molecular cytogenetic analysis of Rb-1 deletions in chronic B-cell leukemias. Leuk Lymph 1994;16:97–103.

34. Liu Y, Grandér D, Söderhäll S, Juliusson G, Gahrton G, Einhorn S. Retinoblastoma gene deletions in B-cell chronic lymphocytic leukemia. Genes Chrom Cancer 1992;4:250–256.

35. Liu Y, Szekely L, Grandér D, et al. Chronic lymphocytic leukemia cells with allelic deletions at 13q14 commonly have one intact RB1 gene: Evidence for a role of an adjacent locus. Proc Natl Acad Sci USA 1993;90:8697–8701.

36. Stilgenbauer S, Döhner H, Bulgay-Mörschel M, Weitz S, Bentz M, Lichter P. High frequency of monoallelic retinoblastoma gene deletion in B-cell chronic lymphoid leukemia shown by interphase cytogenetics. Blood 1993;81:2118–2124.

37. Bouyge-Moreau I, Rondeau G, Avet-Loiseau H, et al. Construction of a 780-kb PAC, BAC, and cosmid contig encompassing the minimal critical deletion involved in B cell chronic lymphocytic leukemia at 13q14.3. Genomics 1997;46:183–190.

38. Brown AG, Ross FM, Dunne EM, Steel CM, Weir-Thompson EM. Evidence for a new tumour suppressor locus (DBM) in human B-cell neoplasia telomeric to the retinoblastoma gene. Nat Genet 1993;3:67–72.

39. Bullrich F, Veronese ML, Kitada S, et al. Minimal region of loss at 13q14 in B-cell chronic lymphocytic leukemia. Blood 1996;88:3109–3115.

40. Chapman RM, Corcoran MM, Gardiner A, Hawthorn LA, Cowell JK, Oscier DG. Frequent homozygous deletions of the D13S25 locus in chromosome region 13q14 defines the location of a gene critical in leukaemogenesis in chronic B-cell lymphocytic leukaemia. Oncogene 1994;9:1289–1293.

41. Corcoran MM, Rasool O, Liu Y, et al. Detailed molecular delineation of 13q14.3 loss in B-cell chronic lymphocytic leukemia. Blood 1998;91:1382–1390.

42. Migliazza A, Bosch F, Komatsu H, et al. Nucleotide sequence, transcription map, and mutation analysis of the 13q14 chromosomal region deleted in B-cell chronic lymphocytic leukemia. Blood 2001;97:2098–2104.

43. Kalachikov S, Migliazza A, Cayanis E, et al. Cloning and gene mapping of the chromosome 13q14 region deleted in chronic lymphocytic leukemia. Genomics 1997;42:369–377.

44. Liu Y, Hermanson M, Grandér D, et al. 13q deletions in lymphoid malignancies. Blood 1995;86:1911–1915.

45. Liu Y, Corcoran M, Rasool O, et al. Cloning of two candidate tumor suppressor genes within a 10 kb region on chromosome 13q14, frequently deleted in chronic lymphocytic leukemia. Oncogene 1997;15:2463–2473.

46. Stilgenbauer S, Leupolt E, Ohl S, et al. Heterogeneity of deletions involving RB-1 and the D13S25 locus in B-cell chronic lymphocytic leukemia revealed by FISH. Cancer Res 1995;55:3475–3477.

47. Stilgenbauer S, Nickolenko J, Wilhelm J, et al. Expressed sequences as candidates for a novel tumor suppressor gene at band 13q14 in B-cell chronic lymphocytic leukemia and mantle cell lymphoma. Oncogene 1998;16:1891–1897.

48. Wolf S, Mertens D, Schaffner C, Korz C, Dohner H, Stilgenbauer S, Lichter P. B-cell neoplasia associated gene with multiple splicing (BCMS): the candidate B-CLL gene on 13q14 comprises more than 560 kb covering all critical regions. Hum Mol Genet 2001;10:1275–1285.

49. Korz C, Pscherer A, Benner A, et al. Evidence for distinct pathomechanisms in B-cell chronic lymphocytic leukemia and mantle cell lymphoma by quantitative expression analysis of cell-cycle and apoptosis associated genes. Blood 2002;99:4554–4461.

50. Mertens D, Wolf S, Schroeter P, et al. Downregulation of candidate tumor suppressor genes within chromosome band 13q14.3 is independent of the DNA methylation pattern in B-cell chronic lymphocytic leukemia. Blood 2002;99:4116-4121.

51. Kobayashi H, Espinosa R III, Fernald AA, et al. Analysis of deletions of the long arm of chromosome 11 in hematologic malignancies with fluorescence in situ hybridization. Genes Chrom Cancer 1993;8:246–252.

52. James MR, Richard III CW, Schott JJ, et al. A radiation hybrid map of 506 STS markers spanning human chromosome 11. Nat Genet 1994;6:70–76.

53. Stilgenbauer S, Liebisch P, James MR, et al. Molecular cytogenetic delineation of a novel critical genomic region in chromosome bands 11q22.2-q23.1 in lymphoproliferative disorders. Proc Natl Acad Sci USA 1996;93:11,837–11,841.

54. Barlow C, Hirotsune S, Paylor R, et al. Atm-deficient mice: a paradigm of ataxia telangiectasia. Cell 1996;86:159–171.

55. Rotman G, Shiloh Y. ATM: from gene to function. Hum Mol Genet 1998;7:1555–1563.

56. Stilgenbauer S, Schaffner C, Litterst A, et al. Biallelic mutations in the ATM gene in T-prolymphocytic leukemia. Nat Med 1997;3:1155–1159.

57. Vorechovsky I, Luo L, Dyer MJS, et al. Clustering of missense mutations in the ataxia-telangiectasia gene in a sporadic T-cell leukaemia Nat Genet 1997;17:96–99.

58. Bullrich F, Rasio D, Kitada S, et al. ATM mutations in B-cell chronic lymphocytic leukemia. Cancer Res 1999;59:24–27.

59. Schaffner C, Stilgenbauer S, Rappold G, Döhner H, Lichter P. Somatic ATM mutations indicate a pathogenic role of ATM in B-cell chronic lymphocytic leukemia. Blood 1999;94:748–753.

60. Stankovic T, Weber P, Stewart G, et al. Inactivation of ataxia telangiectasia mutated gene in B-cell chronic lymphocytic leukaemia. Lancet 1999;353:26–29.

61. Starostik P, Manshouri T, O'Brien S, et al. Deficiency of the ATM protein defines an aggressive subgroup of B-cell chronic lymphocytic leukemia. Cancer Res 1998;58:4552–4557.

62. Pettitt AR, Sherrington PD, Stewart G, Cawley JC, Taylor AM, Stankovic T. p53 dysfunction in B-cell chronic lymphocytic leukemia: inactivation of ATM as an alternative to TP53 mutation. Blood 2001;98:814–822.

63. Fegan C, Robinson H, Thompson P, Whittaker JA, White D. Karyotypic evolution in CLL. Identification of a new sub-group of patients with deletions of 11q and advanced or progressive disease. Leukemia 1995;9:2003–2008.

64. Stankovic T, Stewart GS, Fegan C, et al. Ataxia telangiectasia mutated-deficient B-cell chronic lymphocytic leukemia occurs in pregerminal center cells and results in defective damage response and unrepaired chromosome damage. Blood 2002;99:300–309.

65. Monni O, Zhu Y, Franssila K, et al. Molecular characterisation of deletion at 11q22.1-23.3 in mantle cell lymphoma. Br J Haematol 1999;104:665–671.

66. Stilgenbauer S, Winkler D, Ott G, et al. Molecular characterization of 11q deletions points to a pathogenic role of the ATM gene in mantle cell lymphoma. Blood 1999;94:3262–3264.

67. Schaffner C, Idler I, Stilgenbauer S, Döhner H, Lichter P. Mantle cell lymphoma is characterized by inactivation of the ATM gene. Proc Natl Acad Sci USA 2000;97:2773–2778.

68. Bird ML, Ueshima Y, Rowley JD, Haren JM, Vardiman JW. Chromosome abnormalities in B cell chronic lymphocytic leukemia and their clinical correlations. Leukemia 1989;3:182–191.

69. Han T, Ozer H, Sadamori N, et al. Prognostic importance of cytogenetic abnormalities in patients with chronic lymphocytic leukemia. N Engl J Med 1984;310:288–292.

70. Juliusson G, Robèrt KH, Öst A, et al. Prognostic information from cytogenetic analysis in chronic B-lympho-cytic leukemia and leukemic immunocytoma. Blood 1985;65:134–141.

71. Morita M, Minowada J, Sandberg AA. Chromosomes and causation of human cancer and leukemia. XLV. Chromosome patterns in stimulated lymphocytes of chronic lymphocytic leukemia. Cancer Genet Cytogenet 1981;3:293–306.

72. Nowell PC, Vonderheid EC, Besa E, Hoxie JA, Moreau L, Finan JB. The most common chromosome change in 86 chronic B cell or T cell tumors: a 14q32 translocation. Cancer Genet Cytogenet 1986;19:219–227.

73. Pittman S, Catovsky D. Prognostic significance of chromosome abnormalities in chronic lymphocytic leu-kaemia. Br J Haematol 1984;58:649–660.

74. Gahrton G, Robèrt KH, Friberg K, Juliusson G, Biberfeld P, Zech L. Cytogenetic mapping of the duplicated segment of chromosome 12 in lymphoproliferative disorders. Nature 1982;297:513–514.

75. Anastasi J, Le Beau MM, Vardiman JW, Fernald AA, Larson RA, Rowley JD. Detection of trisomy 12 in chronic lymphocytic leukemia by fluorescence in situ hybridization to interphase cells: a simple and sensitive method. Blood 1992;79:1796–1801.

76. Arif M, Tanaka K, Asou H, Ohno R, Kamada N. Independent clones of trisomy 12 and retinoblastoma gene deletion in Japanese B cell chronic lymphocytic leukemia, detected by fluorescence in situ hybridization. Leukemia 1995;9:1822–1827.

77. Criel A, Wlodarska I, Meeus P, et al. Trisomy 12 is uncommon in typical chronic lymphocytic leukaemias. Br J Haematol 1994;87:523–528.

78. Escudier SM, Pereira-Leahy JM, Drach JW, et al. Fluorescence in situ hybridization and cytogenetic studies of trisomy 12 in chronic lymphocytic leukemia. Blood 1993;81:2702–2707.

79. Matutes E, Oscier D, Garcia-Marco J, et al. Trisomy 12 defines a group of CLL with atypical morphology: correlation between cytogenetic, clinical and laboratory features in 544 patients. Br J Haematol 1996;92:382–388.

80. Perez Losada A, Wessman M, Tiainen M, et al. Trisomy 12 in chronic lymphocytic leukemia: an interphase cytogenetic study. Blood 1991;78:775–779.

81. Que TH, Garcia Marco J, Ellis J, et al. Trisomy 12 in chronic lymphocytic leukemia detected by fluorescence in situ hybridization: Analysis by stage, immunophenotype, and morphology. Blood 1993;82:571–575.

82. Raghoebier S, Kibbelaar RE, Kleiverda K, et al. Mosaicism of trisomy 12 in chronic lymphocytic leukemia detected by non-radioactive in situ hybridisation. Leukemia 1992;6:1220–1226.

83. Bentz M, Huck K, du Manoir S, et al. Comparative genomic hybridization in chronic B-cell leukemias reveals a high incidence of chromosomal gains and losses. Blood 1995;85:3610–3618.

84. Merup M, Juliusson G, Wu X, et al. Amplification of multiple regions of chromosome 12, including 12q13-15, in chronic lymphocytic leukaemia. Eur J Haematol 1997;58:174–180.

85. Dierlamm J, Wlodarska I, Michaux L, et al. FISH identifies different types of duplications with 12q13-15 as the commonly involved segment in B-cell lymphoproliferative malignancies characterized by partial trisomy 12. Genes Chrom Cancer 1997;20:155–166.

86. Solinas-Toldo S, Lampel S, Stilgenbauer S, et al. Matrix-based comparative genomic hybridization: Biochips to screen for genomic imbalances. Genes Chrom Cancer 1997;20:399–407.

87. Pinkel D, Segraves R, Sudar D, et al. High resolution analysis of DNA copy number variation using comparative genomic hybridization to microarrays. Nat Genet 1998;20:207–211.

88. Wessendorf S, Schwaenen C, Barth Th, et al. Automated genomic profiling using microarray based hybridiza-tion (Matrix-CGH) - a powerful technique for the detection of DNA-amplification in aggressive lymphoma. Blood 2001;98(suppl 1):1940.

89. Schwaenen C, Nessling M, Wessendorf S, et al. Automated Genomic Profiling in Chronic Lymphocytic Leu-kemia using Array Based Comparative Genomic Hybridization (Matrix-CGH). 2003, submitted for publication.

90. Johansson B, Mertens F, Mitelman F. Cytogenetic deletion maps of hematologic neoplasms: circumstantial evidence for tumor suppressor loci. Genes Chrom Cancer 1993;8:205–218.

91. Offit K, Parsa NZ, Gaidano G, et al. 6q deletions define distinct clinico-pathologic subsets of non-Hodgkin's lymphoma. Blood 1993;82:2157–2162.

92. Offit K, Louie DC, Parsa NZ, et al. Clinical and morphologic features of B-cell small lymphocytic lymphoma with del(6)(q21q23). Blood 1994;83:2611–2618.

93. Merup M, Moreno TC, Heyman M, et al. 6q deletions in acute lymphoblastic leukemia and non-Hodgkin's lymphomas. Blood 1998;91:3397–4000.

94. Gaidano G, Newcomb EW, Gong JZ, et al. Analysis of alterations of oncogenes and tumor suppressor genes in chronic lymphocytic leukemia. Am J Pathol 1994;144:1312–1319.

95. Stilgenbauer S, Bullinger L, Benner A, et al. Indcidence and clinical significance of 6q deletions in B-cell chronic lymphocytic leukemia. Leukemia 1999;13:1331–1334.

96. Zhang Y, Matthiesen P, Harder S, et al. A 3-cM commonly deleted region in 6q21 in leukemias and lymphomas delineated by fluorescence in situ hybridization. Genes Chromosomes Cancer 2000;27:52–58.

97. Gaidano G, Ballerini P, Gong JZ, et al. p53 mutations in human lymphoid malignancies: association with Burkitt lymphoma and chronic lymphocytic leukemia. Proc Natl Acad Sci USA 1991;88:5413–5417.

98. El Rouby S, Thomas A, Costin D, et al. p53 gene mutation in B-cell chronic lymphocytic leukemia is associated with drug resistance and is independent of MDR1/MDR3 gene expression. Blood 1993;82:3452–3459.

99. Fenaux P, Preudhomme C, Laï JL, et al. Mutations of the p53 gene in B-cell chronic lymphocytic leukemia: a report on 39 cases with cytogenetic analysis. Leukemia 1992;6:246–250.

100. Döhner H, Fischer K, Bentz M, et al. p53 gene deletion predicts for poor survival and non-response to therapy with purine analogs in chronic B-cell leukemias. Blood 1995;85:1580–1589.

101. Geisler CH, Philip P, Egelund Christensen B, et al. In B-cell chronic lymphocytic leukaemia chromosome 17 abnormalities and not trisomy 12 are the single most important cytogenetic abnormalities for the prognosis: a cytogenetic and immunophenotypic study of 480 unselected newly diagnosed patients. Leuk Res 1997;21:1011–1023.

102. Kröber A, Scherer K, Leupolt E, Stilgenbauer S, Döhner H. p53 aberrations in B-CLL predict survival and are associated with in vivo resistance to therapy. Blood 2000;96(suppl 1):abstract 4463.

103. Bloomfield C, Arthur D, Frizzera G, Levine E, Peterson B, Gajl-Peczalska K. Nonrandom chromosome abnormalities in lymphoma. Cancer Res 1983;43:2975–2984.

104. Ueshima Y, Bird ML, Vardiman JW, Rowley JD. A 14;19 translocation in B-cell chronic lymphocytic leukemia: a new recurring chromosome aberration. Int J Cancer 1985;36:287–290.

105. Van den Berghe H, Parloir C, David G, Michaux JL, Sokal G. A new characteristic karyotypic anomaly in lymphoproliferative disorders. Cancer 1979;44:188–195.

106. Bosch F, Jares P, Campo E, et al. PRAD-1/Cyclin D1 gene overexpression in chronic lymphoproliferative disorders: a highly specific marker of mantle cell lymphoma. Blood 1994;84:2726–2732.

107. Rosenberg CL, Wong E, Petty EM, et al. PRAD1, a candidate BCL1 oncogene: Mapping and expression in centrocytic lymphoma. Proc Natl Acad Sci USA 1991;88:9638–9642.

108. Tsujimoto Y, Yunis J, Onorato-Showe L, Erikson J, Nowell PC, Croce CM. Molecular cloning of the chromosomal breakpoint of B-cell lymphomas and leukemias with the t(11;14) chromosome translocation. Science 1984;224:1403–1406.

109. Levy V, Ugo V, Delmer A, et al. Cyclin D1 overexpression allows identification of an aggressive subset of leukemic lymphoproliferative disorder. Leukemia 1999;13:1343–1351.

110. Withers DA, Harvey RC, Faust JB, Melnyk O, Carey K, Meeker TC. Characterization of a candidate bcl-1 gene. Mol Cell Biol 1991;11:4846–4853.

111. Raffeld M, Jaffe ES. bcl-1, t(11;14), and mantle cell-derived lymphomas. Blood 1991;78:259–263.

112. Medeiros J, van Krieken JH, Jaffe ES, Raffeld M. Association of bcl-1 rearrangements with lymphocytic lymphoma of intermediate differentiation. Blood 1990;76:2086-2090.

113. Newman RA, Peterson B, Davey FR, et al. Phenotypic markers and BCL1 rearrangements in B-cell chronic lymphocytic leukemia: a cancer and leukemia group B study. Blood 1993;82:1239–1246.

114. Raghoebier S, van Krieken JHJM, Kluin-Nelemans JC, et al. Oncogene rearrangements in chronic B-cell leukemia. Blood 1991;77:1560–1564.

115. Rechavi G, Katzir N, Brok-Simoni F, et al. A search for bcl1, bcl2, and c-myc oncogene rearrangements in chronic lymphocytic leukemia. Leukemia 1988;3:57-60.

116. Adachi M, Cossmna J, Longo D, Croce CM, Tsujimoto Y. Variant translocation of the bcl-2 gene to Ig in a chronic lymphocytic leukemia. Proc Natl Acad Sci USA 1989;86:2771–2774.

117. Crossen PE, Morrison MJ. Lack of 5'bcl2 rearrangements in B-cell leukemia. Cancer Genet Cytogenet 1993;69:72–73.
118. Dyer MJS, Zani VJ, Lu WZ, et al. BCL2 translocations in leukemias of mature B cells. Blood 1994;83:3682–3688.
119. Hanada M, Delia D, Aiello A, Stadtmauer E, Reed JC bcl-2 gene hypomethylation and high-level expression in B-cell chronic lymphocytic leukemia. Blood 1993;82:1820–1828.
120. McKeithan TW, Rowley JD, Shows T, Diaz M. Cloning of the chromosome translocation breakpoint junction of the t(14;19) in chronic lymphocytic leukemia. Proc Natl Acad Sci USA 1987;84:9257–9260.
121. McKeithan TW, Takimoto GS, Ohno H, et al. BCL3 rearrangements and t(14;19) in chronic lymphocytic leukemia and other B-cell malignancies: a molecular and cytogenetic study. Genes Chrom Cancer 1997;20:64–72.
122. Michaux L, Mecucci C, Stul M, et al. BCL3 rearrangements and t(14;19)(q32;q13) in lymphoproliferative disorders. Genes Chrom Cancer 1996;15:38–47.
123. Fais F, Ghiotto F, Hashimoto S, et al. Chronic lymphocytic leukemia B cells express restricted sets of mutated and unmutated antigen receptors. J Clin Invest 1998;102:1515–1525.
124. Küppers R, Klein U, Hansmann Ml, Rajewsky K. Cellular origin of human B-cell lymphomas. N Engl J Med 1999;341:1520–1529.
125. Schroeder HW, Dighiero G. The pathogenesis of chronic lymphocytic leukemia: analysis of the antibody repertoire. Immunol Today 1994;15:288–294.
126. Neilson JR, Auer R, White D, et al. Deletions at 11q identify a subset of patients with typical CLL who show consistent disease progression and reduced survival. Leukemia 1997;11:1929–1932.
127. Stilgenbauer S, Döhner H. Campath-1H induced complete remission of chronic lymphocytic leukemia despite p53 gene mutation and resistance to chemotherapy. N Engl J Med 2002;347:452–453 (lettter).
128. Damle JN, Wasil T, Allen SL, Schulman P, Rai KR, Chiorazzi N, Ferrarini M. Updated data on V gene mutation status and CD38 expression in CLL. Blood 2000;95:2456–2457 (letter).
129. Hamblin TJ, Orchard JA, Gardiner A, Oscier DG, Davis Z, Stevenson FK. Immunoglobulin V genes and CD38 expression in CLL. Blood 2000;95:2455–2456 (letter).
130. Hamblin TJ, Orchard JA, Ibbotson RE, et al. CD38 expression and immunoglobulin variable region mutations are independent prognostic variables in chronic lymphocytic leukemia, but CD38 expression may vary during the course of the disease. Blood 2002;99:1023–1029.
131. Thunberg U, Johnson A, Roos G, et al. CD38 expression is a poor predictor for VH gene mutational status and prognosis in chronic lymphocytic leukemia. Blood 2001;97:1892–1894.
132. Kröber A, Bühler A, Kienle D, Benner A, Döhner H, Stilgenbauer S. Analysis of VDJ rearrangement structure and VH mutation status in chronic lymphocytic leukemia. Blood 2001;98:abstract 1509.
133. Kipps TJ, Tomhave E, Pratt LF, Duffy S, Johnson T, Kobayashi R, Carson D. Developmentally restricted VH gene expressed at high frequency in chronic lymphocytic leukaemia. Proc Natl Acad Sci USA 1989;86:5913.
134. Küppers R, Gause A, Rajewsky K. B-cells of chronic lymphatic leukaemia express V genes in unmutated form. Leuk Res 1991;15:487–496.
135. Chang B, Casali P. The CDR1 sequences of a major proportion of human germline Ig VH genes are inherently susceptible to amino acid replacement. Immunol Today 1994;158:367–373.
136. Ibrahim S, Keating M, Do KA, et al. CD38 expression as an important prognostic factor in B-cell chronic lymphocytic leukemia. Blood 2001;98:181–186.
137. Matrai Z, Lin K, Dennis M, et al. CD38 expression and Ig VH gene mutation in B-cell chronic lymphocytic leukemia. Blood 2001;97:1902–1903.
138. Klein U, Tu Y, Stolovitzky GA, et al. Gene expression profiling of B cell chronic lymphocytic leukemia reveals a homogeneous phenotype related to memory B cells. J Exp Med 2001;194:1625–1638.
139. Rosenwald A, Alizadeh AA, Widhopf G, et al. Relation of gene expression phenotype to immunoglobulin mutation genotype in B cell chronic lymphocytic leukemia. J Exp Med 2001;194:1639–1647.
140. Oscier DG, Gardiner AC, Mould SJ, et al. Multivariate analysis of prognostic factors in CLL: clinical stage, IGVH gene mutational status, and loss or mutation of the p53 gene are independent prognostic factors. Blood 2002;100:1177–1184.
141. Lin K, Sherrington PD, Dennis M, Matrai Z, Cawley JC, Pettitt AR. Relationship between p53 dysfunction, CD38 expression, and IgV(H) mutation in chronic lymphocytic leukemia. Blood 2002;100:1404–1409.

3 Molecular Biology of Chronic Lymphocytic Leukemia

William G. Wierda, MD, PhD

1. INTRODUCTION

Discoveries in molecular biology are occurring rapidly, highlighted by new laboratory techniques, computers, and the sequencing of the human genome. These discoveries will shed new light on the etiology of diseases and the mechanisms that determine their clinical behavior. They will also help explain the diversity in disease progression and response to treatment and identify new therapeutic targets with the ultimate goal of cure.

Chronic lymphocytic leukemia is a monoclonal disease of mature-appearing lymphocytes that accumulate in blood, lymph nodes, spleen, liver, and bone marrow. Most cases (>95%) are characterized by monoclonal lymphocytes expressing normal B-cell surface proteins including immunoglobulin (Ig), CD19, and CD20 and aberrantly expressing CD5, a protein normally found on T-cells. A small minority (<5%) of cases are of T-cell origin, expressing T-cell surface markers such as CD3 and CD4 or CD8. These T-cell leukemias are not uncommon in individuals with ataxia telangiectasia. A thorough discussion of T-cell lymphocytic leukemia is beyond the scope of this text, since the molecular biology of this disease is distinct from that of B-cell CLL.

At the present time there is limited understanding of the molecular events that result in development and progression of B-cell CLL. One certainty is that irreversible changes occur in the B-cell genome in order for the cell to take on the malignant phenotype and biological behavior. Thus, a search is under way for *de novo* genome-based abnormalities uniformly associated with CLL that directly participate in the etiology and affect the clinical behavior of this disease. To date, no unifying chromosome abnormality has been identified.

Conventional cytogenetic analyses (Q-banding or G-banding) of blood- or bone marrow-derived cells arrested in metaphase have limited applicability and sensitivity in CLL since nearly all the leukemia cells are in G_0 phase of the cell cycle and therefore not amenable to metaphase arrest. Using this type of karyotype analysis, clonal chromosome abnormalities can be identified in 40–50% of CLL cases, the most common of which, in decreasing frequency, are trisomy 12 and deletions at 13q14 and 14q32 (1). Interphase cytogenetic analysis with fluorescence *in situ* hybridization (FISH) has increased the sensitivity for detecting specific chromosome abnormalities such as translocations, deletions, and even trisomy. Deletions of small portions of chromosomes not detected with standard karyotyping can readily be detected with FISH. This is clearly

From: *Contemporary Hematology*
Chronic Lymphocytic Leukemia: Molecular Genetics, Biology, Diagnosis, and Management
Edited by: G. B. Faguet © Humana Press Inc., Totowa, NJ

demonstrated for deletions of 13q, which are four times more prevalent when screened for by FISH vs metaphase karyotyping. By FISH analysis, Döhner and colleagues noted abnormalities in 268 of 325 (82%) cases of CLL *(2)*. Deletion at 13q (55%) is the most common abnormality in CLL, followed in order of frequency by deletion at 11q (18%), trisomy 12 (16%), deletion at 17p (7%), and deletion at 6q (6%) *(2)*. The association of loss of chromosomal material with malignancy suggests that the genetic lesion involves an inactivated tumor suppressor gene. To date, no tumor suppressor gene or relevant oncogene has been identified in CLL. Two important tumor suppressor genes, *P53* and *ATM,* have been noted to be abnormal in some cases of CLL and are discussed.

Although no ubiquitous chromosome abnormality has been identified to account for development of the disease, studies at the mRNA and protein levels have identified prevalent aberrations in the mediators of programmed cell death that may be fundamental to accumulation of the malignant B-cells. Although there must be a subpopulation of proliferating monoclonal B-cells, nearly all circulating leukemia cells are in G_0 phase of the cell cycle. Thus CLL is also characterized by a lack of normal programmed cell death or apoptosis typical for senescent cells. The majority (>85%) of CLL B-cells overexpress the anti-apoptotic protein bcl-2 and have abnormalities in levels of other members of the bcl-2 family of proteins. A genetic defect has not been shown to be directly responsible; however, this aberrant expression certainly influences the biological behavior of the disease. The relevance of these abnormalities to the natural history and response to therapy will be explored.

2. CHROMOSOME ABNORMALITIES

Although most of the chromosome abnormalities commonly observed in CLL have not been associated with specific genes, the clinical importance of such abnormalities is indicated by their influence on clinical course and survival (Table 1). Patients with structural or numerical chromosome abnormalities may have significantly shorter survival than comparably staged patients with a normal karyotype *(2)*. With the exception of the 13q deletion, chromosome abnormalities in CLL are associated with a poor prognosis compared with patients who have a normal karyotype. Multiple abnormalities, i.e. complex karyotypes, portend an even worse prognosis.

2.1. Chromosome 13

Deletion in the long arm of chromosome 13 at band 13q14 is the most frequently observed clonal abnormality, detected by interphase FISH in more than half (55%) of CLL cases *(2–5)*. Deletions at 13q have been associated with other lymphoid malignancies and with poor prognosis in these diseases, such as mantle cell lymphoma (50%) *(6,7)* and multiple myeloma (16–40%) *(8–10)*, as well as malignancies of other hematologic lineages *(11)*.

There is intense ongoing research to identify a putative tumor suppressor gene or genes involved in 13q deletion; several groups have identified the breakpoint at 13q14 *(3,12–15)*. The retinoblastoma *(RB-1)* gene (at 13q14) encodes a nuclear phosphoprotein involved in cell cycle control and transcription regulation *(16)* and was once considered a candidate tumor suppressor gene affected in CLL. However, *RB-1* is an unlikely candidate since homozygous mutations as well as loss of heterozygosity through mutation are very rare in CLL, and abnormal concentrations of *RB-1* protein are not reported in CLL *(14)*. Furthermore, analyses have indicated that the deleted region is approx 1.6 cM telomeric to the *RB-1* and centromeric to the D13S25 marker *(17–19)*.

Table 1
Influence of Chromosome Abnormalities in CLL

Chromosome abnormality	Frequency (%)	Significance
13q deletion	10–55	Most common
		Favorable prognosis
		Typical cell morphology
		Associated with mutated IgV$_H$ genes
Trisomy 12	20–30	Atypical morphology
		Acquired with clonal evolution
		Unfavorable prognosis
11q deletion	5–18	Associated with mutated *ATM* gene
		Atypical (prolymphocytic) morphology
		Unfavorable prognosis in age < 55 yr
17p deletion	10–15	Associated with mutated or deleted *P53* gene
		Atypical (prolymphocytic) morphology
		Associated with unmutated IgV$_H$ genes
		Resistant to chemotherapy
		Unfavorable prognosis
6q deletion	6–8	Atypical cell morphology
		May involve *TNF1* gene

The putative tumor suppressor gene located in this region (referred to as *DBM*, for *d*isrupted in *b*-cell *m*alignancies) remains to be confirmed. Several candidate genes have been suggested, including *LEU1*, *LEU2*, *LEU5*, *CLLD6*, *CLLD7*, *CLLD8*, *ALT1*, *BCMS*, and *FAM10A4* (Fig. 1) *(20–26)*. More recently, the supposed minimal deleted region, narrowed down to a 650–790 kb region between markers D13S319 and D13S25, has been completely sequenced *(27)*.

The candidate tumor suppressor genes that map to the 13q14 region, centromeric to D13S272, include *LEU1* and *LEU2 (20)*. The *LEU1* gene encodes a 1.1-kb mRNA transcript, and *LEU2* encodes two mRNA transcripts of 1.8 and 1.4 kb. CLL cells do not appear to have mutations in both alleles of these genes, making it unlikely that they are tumor suppressor genes in CLL *(28)*. *ALT1* and *BCMS* are splice variants encompassing the *LEU1* or *LEU2* gene and may prove to be important tumor suppressor genes *(24,25)*. Another candidate tumor suppressor gene is *LEU5 (22)*. This gene encodes a zinc-finger domain of the RING type and shares homology with genes involved in tumorigenesis, including the RET finger protein and BRCA1. The most recently reported gene, *FAM10A4*, maps to the minimally deleted region and may be an important tumor suppressor gene *(26)*. The search continues for one or more tumor suppressor genes at this location with functional confirmation.

Patients with 13q deletion have a similar survival as individuals with a diploid karyotype and significantly better than patients with 11q or 17p deletions *(1,2,29,30)*. Consistent with the favorable prognosis is the association of 13q deletion with other characteristics associated with favorable prognosis including low CD38 expression and somatic hypermutation of the Ig variable region (IgV$_H$) gene *(31–33)*.

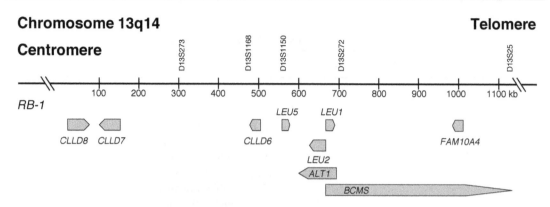

Fig. 1. Chromosome 13q14. Physical map of the critical region of chromosome 13q14 with relative size and position of proposed CLL-associated genes mapping to this region.

2.2. Chromosome 12

Trisomy 12 was the first recurring chromosome abnormality noted in CLL and was reported by Gahrton in 1980 *(34)*. Standard metaphase G-banding or Q-banding identified trisomy 12 as the most frequent chromosomal abnormality in CLL, present in the leukemia cells of 10–20% of patients *(35,36)*. However, when more sensitive techniques such as interphase FISH are applied (Fig.2), it is not the most frequent abnormality, but ranks second or third. Of note, a higher proportion (up to 35%) of CLL cases have trisomy 12 by FISH analysis than is noted by standard karyotyping methods, and it is commonly present in a subpopulation of leukemia cells *(37–42)*.

Duplication of one chromosome 12 and retention of the second is the usual mechanism for trisomy *(43,44)*. Localization studies indicate that 12q13-15 is the minimal duplication region needed for the expected clinical picture associated with trisomy 12 *(45)*. Partial trisomy 12 may occur by a mechanism of translocation or duplication of 12q13-22 *(45,46)*. A specific gene or genes associated with trisomy 12 has not been identified. One candidate gene that may be involved in leukemogenesis is the human homolog of the mouse double minute 2 (*MDM2*) gene, *HDM2*, located at 12q13-15 *(47,48)*. The *HDM2* gene is over-expressed in more than 30% of B-cell CLL cases *(49)*. MDM2 protein binds and inactivates p53 by promoting proteosome-mediated p53 degradation *(50,51)*.

Trisomy 12 was hypothesized to be a primary germline defect, occurring in CD34[+] hematopoietic progenitor cells *(52,53)*. However, subsequent studies failed to confirm this *(54)*. Furthermore, sequential karyotype studies suggest that trisomy 12 may be involved in disease progression or clonal evolution rather than primary leukemogenesis *(39,55,56)*. Trisomy 12 is most commonly noted in a subpopulation of leukemia cells, indicating that it may be a secondary event that occurs within an established leukemia clone *(39,56–59)*. Furthermore, the proportion of leukemia cells carrying trisomy 12 can vary by anatomic location, being highest in lymph nodes, followed by bone marrow and blood *(60,61)*. Trisomy 12 may occur singly or may be associated with complex karyotypic abnormalities *(36,42,55)*. One study employing FISH analysis found that nearly half of the cases with 13q14 deletions had trisomy 12 *(62)*. Multiple abnormalities combined with trisomy 12 carry a worse prognosis than trisomy 12 alone *(1,63)*.

Patients who have trisomy 12 have a worse prognosis than those with a diploid karyotype or 13q deletion *(1,35,36,63–65)*. In fact, univariable analysis indicates a shorter treatment-free interval and shorter overall survival in patients with trisomy 12 compared with the survival of

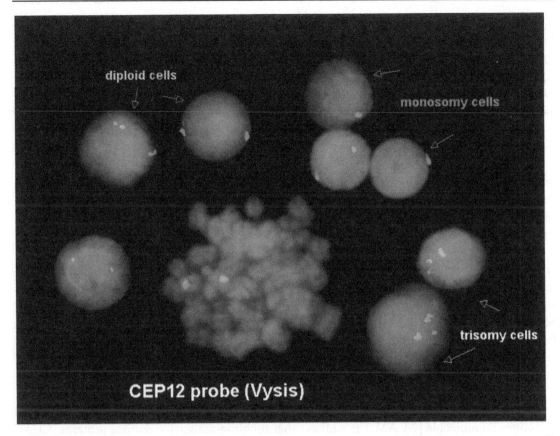

Fig. 2. Interphase FISH analysis for trisomy 12. FISH analysis was performed on blood mononuclear cells of a patient with B-cell CLL using a 12q probe (CEP12 probe [Vysis]). Cells displaying trisomy 12 (pink hybridization signals) are indicated in the figure. Cells with disomic and monosomic status are also noted for comparison. (Courtesy of Dr. Armand Glassman, Department of Hematopathology, U.T. M.D. Anderson Cancer Center, Houston, TX.)

patients with any other single chromosome abnormality *(1)*. Other studies do not confirm this report *(2,66,67)*. Trisomy 12 has been associated with several negative prognostic features such as atypical leukemia cell morphology (increased prolymphocytes), unmutated IgV_H gene, high CD38 expression, and advanced and progressive disease *(31,33,68–74)*. Trisomy 12 has also been associated with the presence of monoclonal paraprotein *(35,36,68)*.

2.3. Chromosome 11

Nearly a fifth (18%) of patients with CLL have leukemia cells with deletions in the long arm of chromosome 11, making this the next most common abnormality identified by interphase analysis *(2,29,75,76)*. Early reports identified 11q deletions at 11q13, the location of the *BCL-1* (cyclin D1 or CCND1) gene involved in the translocation t(11;14) associated with mantle cell lymphoma *(77–80)*. These reports may have included misclassified mantle cell cases; subsequent studies by the French-American-British system and by immunophenotyping have shown that 11q13 deletions are rare in CLL *(81)*. Regarding affected genes, one small study noted that in 3 of 14 CLL cases examined, there was deletion of *MEN1*, the tumor suppressor gene associated with multiple endocrine neoplasia syndrome type I, located in the 11q13 region *(82)*.

More commonly, 11q deletions involve a 2–3-Mb region at band 11q22.3-q23.1 *(83)*. The 11q14-24 region contains several important genes including *ATM* (ataxia telangiectasia mutated), *RDX* (radixin), and *FDX1* (ferredoxin 1), with *ATM* and *RDX* being potentially important tumor suppressor genes *(83)*. Ataxia telangiectasia is an autosomal recessive disease in which affected individuals have an increased incidence of T-cell lymphoproliferative disorders. Deletions and mutations that lead to disruption of both *ATM* alleles have been reported in T-cell prolymphocytic leukemia, indicating a tumor suppressor function for the *ATM* gene product which is lost in this leukemia *(84,85)*.

The *ATM* gene is located at 11q22-23 *(86)*. There is homology between unmutated ATM protein and proteins controlling cell cycle progression, telomere length, and response to DNA damage *(87)*. The ATM protein normally participates in phosphorylation of p53 protein in response to DNA damage and therefore may play a role in cell cycle regulation and repair of damaged DNA *(88)*.

Decreased ATM protein expression was initially described in association with loss of heterozygosity at the *ATM* gene *(89)*. Furthermore, a high proportion (34%) of CLL patients were reported to have decreased levels of ATM protein, even without loss of heterozygosity, and this was associated with shorter survival *(89)*. Analyses demonstrated mutations in the *ATM* gene, both in patients with 11q deletion and in patients without karyotypic abnormalities *(90–92)*. Furthermore, some of these individuals had germline *ATM* mutations, suggesting an inherited predisposition to develop CLL *(91,92)*. However, *ATM* mutations do not seem to account for familial clustering of the disease *(93,94)*.

The leukemia cells of CLL patients with deletions of chromosome 11q may express lower levels of surface adhesion molecules including CD11a/CD18, CD11c/CD18, and CD56 (neural cell adhesion molecule [NCAM]) as well as other function-associated surface proteins, CD31, CD48, and CD58, suggesting that such cells display distinct biological and clinical characteristics *(95,96)*. Deletion of the 11q 23.1 segment is also associated with prolymphocytic morphology *(97,98)*.

Patients with 11q deletions tend to be younger (<55 yr old) and have extensive lymphadenopathy, shorter time to treatment, and more aggressive disease than patients without 11q abnormalities *(29,75,89,99,100)*. In patients with 11q deletion, the median survival time is significantly shorter for patients younger than 55 yr. This is in contrast to patients over 55 yr of age, in whom there is no impact of 11q deletion on survival *(75)*. Multivariate survival analysis identified 11q deletion as an independent risk factor for poor prognosis *(2)*. *ATM* mutation or 11q deletion has been associated with other negative prognostic factors such as CD38 expression and unmutated IgV$_H$ genes *(32,33,101)*.

2.4. Chromosome 17

Structural abnormalities of the short arm of chromosome 17 may consist of either deletions or mutations and occur in 10–15% of B-cell CLL cases *(2,102)*. Deletions are seen in up to 10% of cases, and mutations are also seen in up to 10% of cases *(2,102–105)*. Abnormalities at 17p13.1 have been associated with deletion or mutation of *P53*, resulting in lack of or reduced p53 protein expression *(106)*.

The *P53* gene encodes a 53-kDa nuclear phosphoprotein that normally functions in surveying genomic integrity and eliminating DNA damage *(107,108)*. P53 protein targets genes involved in G$_1$/S arrest and genes that control apoptosis, and thus activated p53 may induce cell cycle arrest and/or apoptosis. Expression of proteins involved in cell cycle control including p21 is induced by p53. Expression of p21 normally leads to inhibition of cyclin-dependent kinase activity and results in cell cycle arrest *(109,110)*. In a complementary fashion, p53 can induce expression of pro-apoptotic proteins including CD95 and Bax *(110)*.

Mutations in *P53* reduce the sensitivity of leukemia cells to cell cycle control and apoptotic signals. p53 protein abnormalities have been reported in up to 10–15% of CLL cases *(103,104, 111)*. Mutations usually occur in exons 4–8 of the *P53* gene and are associated with loss of heterozygosity *(104,105,112–114)*. Point mutations in one allele combined with deletion of the second allele can be a mechanism of completely knocking out expression of a tumor suppressor gene such as *P53*.

Abnormalities in *P53* are associated with the evolution of CLL into prolymphocytic leukemia and Richter's transformation *(103,106)*. In fact, approximately half of patients with Richter's transformation or prolymphocytic leukemia have transformed cells with *P53* mutations *(103,113)*. Therefore, *P53* mutations acquired during disease progression may impart a growth advantage. Moreover, patients with CLL cells that have *P53* mutations generally have more advanced disease, a higher leukemia cell proliferative rate, resistance to first-line therapy with a purine analog, and shorter overall survival *(102,106,112,113,115–117)*.

2.5. Chromosome 6

Abnormalities involving the long arm of chromosome 6 (6q) are uncommon but recurrent in CLL, occurring in approx 6–8% of cases *(77,118–120)*. Deletions or translocations in the short arm of chromosome 6 (6p) have also been described in CLL but at a lower frequency *(118,119, 121)*. Abnormalities of the long arm of chromosome 6 involve breaks between 6q13 and 6q27, most frequently resulting in deletions at 6q21-23, 6q21-24, or 6q25-27 *(119,120,122–124)*. Not uncommonly, 6q deletions are associated with other recurrent chromosome abnormalities and may develop as a result of clonal evolution *(100,123)*. No specific gene or genes from this region has been implicated in the etiology of CLL. However, involvement of the gene encoding tumor necrosis factor-α (TNF-α), *TNF1*, located on chromosome 6q, has been described in CLL *(125)*. Patients with 6q deletion tend to have characteristics associated with poor prognosis including high white blood cell count, prolymphocyte morphology, advanced clinical stage, and diffuse pattern of bone marrow involvement and require treatment sooner *(118–120,122,126)*.

2.6. Chromosome 14

The gene encoding the Ig heavy chain is located on the long arm of chromosome 14 at 14q32. This region is frequently the site of translocations in B-cell malignancies. Breakpoints occur in the Ig heavy chain J segment or isotype switch region that then becomes juxtaposed to one of several genes that potentially participate in development of the malignant genotype *(127)*.

Mantle lymphoma cells, morphologically indistinguishable and phenotypically similar to CLL, expressing surface CD5 but not CD23, consistently have the t(11;14)(q13;q32) abnormality *(80,128)*. Mantle cell lymphoma tends to be refractory to treatment, and the clinical course of patients with mantle cell lymphoma tends to be more aggressive than that of CLL patients. The translocation t(11;14) juxtaposes the Ig heavy chain gene with the proto-oncogene *BCL-1* on chromosome 11 and results in constitutive overexpression of *BCL-1 (127,129)*. There have been several reports of t(11;14)(q13;q32) in CLL patients; however, many of these cases would probably be reclassified as mantle cell lymphoma based on immunophenotype *(77,78,128,130)*.

Recent studies of B-cell CLL show infrequent association with *BCL-1* overexpression or t(11;14) *(2)*. Rarely, cases of B-cell CLL have been reported with t(14;18), which juxtaposes the

Ig light chain gene with the *BCL-2* gene *(131,132)*. Overexpression of bcl-2 protein confers resistance to apoptosis. Translocation t(14;19)(q32;q13) is also a rare but recurrent finding in CLL and involves the Ig heavy chain isotype switch region on chromosome 14 and *BCL-3*, a member of the IκB family of transcription factors *(133–136)*. Nonetheless, patients with abnormalities affecting chromosome 14q have poorer prognosis and shorter survival than those with other cytogenetic abnormalities *(1,117,137)*.

The *TCL1* oncogene on human chromosome 14q32.1 is frequently involved in chromosome rearrangements in mature T-cell leukemias *(138,139)*. *TCL1* is also expressed in B-cell malignancies, and overexpression of Tcl1 protein has been demonstrated in CLL *(140,141)*. Aging transgenic mice that overexpress *TCL1* under control of the Ig gene promoter and enhancer develop CD5$^+$ B-cell lymphoproliferative disorders mimicking human CLL and implicating *TCL1* in the development or pathogenesis of CLL *(142)*. These transgenic mice may prove to be a valuable model in which to learn more about the biology of CLL and to test new therapeutic agents.

3. IMMUNOGLOBULIN GENES

Nearly all patients with CLL have leukemia cells that express low levels of surface monoclonal immunoglobulin, usually both IgM and IgD isotypes. Sixty percent of cases express κ, and 40% express λ light chain *(143)*. Rare cases of CLL (7%) lack allelic exclusion and therefore may express two different Ig heavy chain genes *(144)*. The immunoglobulins expressed by CLL cells usually have broad or overlapping antigen specificity, often with a propensity to bind self-antigens such as those on hematopoietic cells or the constant region of IgG *(145–148)*. One hypothesis to explain this association is that persistent low-level stimulation by ubiquitous antigen may participate in or predispose to B-cell malignant transformation. Consistent with this, certain IgV$_H$ genes are over-represented among CLL cases, indicating a selected or biased specificity *(149–152)*. Moreover, certain IgV$_H$ alleles (e.g., the 51p1 allele of V$_H$1-69) may be associated with a higher risk for developing CLL *(149)*.

CLL B-cells can be segregated into two groups that differ in the extent to which expressed IgV$_H$ gene has undergone somatic hypermutation. In about half of CLL cases, the leukemia cells express unmutated IgV$_H$ genes, whereas the rest express IgV$_H$ genes with base substitutions in more than 2% of the IgV$_H$ gene region compared with the germline counterpart and are considered mutated *(153–155)*. The IgV$_H$ genes expressed by CLL B-cells generally lack intraclonal sequence diversity, indicating lack of ongoing somatic hypermutation *(156–158)*. Some IgV$_H$ genes such as the 51p1 allele of IgV$_H$1-69 are expressed at high frequency and without mutation *(149)*.

Early studies indicated that patients with CLL B-cells that express unmutated IgV$_H$ genes might be clinically distinct for those with mutated IgV$_H$ genes. Oscier and colleagues *(73)* noted that cases with unmutated IgV$_H$ genes also had trisomy 12 and atypical morphology, whereas cases that expressed mutated IgV$_H$ genes tended to have abnormalities involving 13q14 and typical morphology. Two large studies have demonstrated the prognostic correlation of IgV$_H$ mutational status with survival *(74,159)*. Patients with unmutated IgV$_H$ genes have a more accelerated clinical course, with a median survival of 8 yr compared with 24 yr for patients with mutated IgV$_H$ genes *(74)*.

In addition to the immunoglobulin molecule, the B-cell receptor complex is composed of two accessory proteins, CD79a and CD79b, both required for intracellular assembly, surface expression, and signal transduction of the complex. Thompson and colleagues *(106,161)* reported that most cases of CLL cells had mutations in CD79b that could affect function. Also, recently a CD79b mRNA splice variant with a dominant negative affect on expression was shown to be overexpressed in CLL cases *(162)*. Defects in CD79 expression might explain the typical low-level expression of immunoglobulin on the surface of CLL B-cells.

4. DEFECTIVE APOPTOSIS

There are at least two corrupted processes in CLL resulting in accumulation of the malignant clone. First is unbridled proliferation of the clonal population of B-cells. This most likely occurs in proliferation centers of bone marrow, spleen, and/or lymph nodes, since nearly all leukemia cells in circulation are in the G_0 phase of the cell cycle. Circulating CLL B-cells express the cyclin-dependent kinase inhibitor $p27^{kip1}$, a protein that is ordinarily increased in cells arrested in the cell cycle. High p27 levels have been correlated with lymphocyte and total tumor mass doubling time and poor overall prognosis in CLL *(163)*.

Second is the failure of the expanded cells to undergo programmed cell death or apoptosis. The life span of CLL B-cells is five times that of normal B-cells *(164)*. The process of senescence leading to programmed cell death is tightly regulated in normal cells; governed by several pro- and anti-apoptotic proteins, particularly members of the bcl-2 family (reviewed in ref. *165*). The process is mediated by proteolytic enzymes called caspases that participate in a cascade of reactions culminating in irreversible DNA fragmentation and cell death.

The prototypic anti-apoptotic gene, *BCL-2*, located at 18q21, and the corresponding protein have been extensively studied in CLL. Leukemia B-cells overexpress the *BCL-2* gene, resulting in high levels of the anti-apoptotic protein in more than 80% of CLL cases *(166–170)*. The mechanism of *BCL-2* overexpression has not been delineated. Translocation t(14;18), juxtaposing the Ig heavy chain gene with the *BCL-2* gene, accounts for overexpression of *BCL-2* in follicular lymphoma but is rare in CLL *(171–173)*. Overexpression of *BCL-2* in CLL has rarely been associated with other translocations *(131,174,175)*. A recent study using pulsed-field gel electrophoresis found alterations in the large stretches of DNA on chromosome 18 containing the *BCL-2* gene *(176)*. This suggests that there may be previously undetected rearrangements in CLL involving chromosome 18 that are responsible for the high-level expression of the *BCL-2* gene. Other investigators have demonstrated hypomethylation of the *BCL-2* gene in CLL, which may play a role in overexpression *(167)*.

Bcl-2 protein forms a functional homodimer that has anti-apoptotic function and may also form heterodimers with other members of the bcl-2 family of proteins. Some of these family members promote anti-apoptotic activity, whereas others have pro-apoptotic activity when associated with bcl-2. As such, bcl-XL has anti-apoptotic activity with bcl-2 and is overexpressed in CLL *(177)*. Additionally, bag-1 and mcl-1, also anti-apoptotic proteins, are overexpressed in CLL *(178,179)*. Furthermore, high-level expression of mcl-1 protein has been associated with failure to achieve complete remission following single-agent chemotherapy *(178)*.

The *BAX* gene encodes a pro-apoptotic protein that can form a heterodimer with bcl-2 and thereby counter its anti-apoptotic activity. There is low level of expression of BAX in CLL, and resistance to apoptosis is associated with a high bcl-2/bax ratio *(169,170,177,178,180)*. Higher levels of bcl-2 and a high bcl-2/bax ratio have been noted in leukemia cells of patients with high leukemia cell blood counts *(177)*. Furthermore, a higher ratio of bcl-2 to bax protein has been correlated with resistance to chemotherapy and disease progression *(180,181)*.

CLL B-cells undergo apoptosis in vitro spontaneously and upon treatment with various drugs used to treat CLL such as chlorambucil and prednisone. This process involves activation of the proteolytic mediators of apoptosis including caspase-3, caspase-7, and caspase-8 *(182)*. However, CLL B-cells survive for long periods ex vivo when appropriately cultured with bone marrow stromal cells or blood-derived nurse-like cells *(183–186)*. The ability of stromal cells to inhibit ex vivo spontaneous apoptosis is not mediated by soluble factors, but apparently is dependent upon direct cell-cell contact involving β1 and β2 integrins. Programmed cell death may also be influenced in vitro and in vivo by cytokines such as TNF-α, interleukin-4 (IL-4), interferons, and basic fibroblast growth factor (bFGF) produced by the bone marrow, lymph node, or spleen microenvironment *(187–190)*. Ex vivo, TNF-α, IL-4, interferon-γ, and bFGF have been shown to sustain leukemia cell viability and elevated bcl-2 protein levels *(187–191)*. In vivo, chlorambucil and fludarabine, both used in the treatment of CLL, can downregulate expression of *BCL-2* mRNA and bcl-2 protein and can decrease the bcl-2/bax ratio, which may facilitate chemotherapy-induced apoptosis *(192–194)*. The sensitivity of leukemia cells to fludarabine-induced down-regulation of bcl-2 has been correlated with therapeutic response in vivo *(195)*. Other studies have not confirmed these findings *(196–198)*. Nevertheless, a high level of bcl-2 protein has been correlated with poor overall survival in patients with CLL *(199)*.

5. CONCLUSION

The fundamental molecular defects and events that result in transformation of a single normal B-cell into an expanded clonal population of long-lived B-cells are largely unknown. The development of this expanded population of malignant cells transforms a normal host into an individual with signs and symptoms of the disease of CLL. These defects and events must be rooted in the building blocks of a cell, the DNA sequence or genetic code. Many recurring chromosome abnormalities have been identified and are prevalent in CLL such as 13q deletion, trisomy 12, 11q deletion, 17p deletion, and 6q deletion; however, a unifying gene or genes has yet to be identified and confirmed. Genes such as *ATM* and *P53* are important in the biology of some cases of CLL, but these are also not unifying. Immunoglobulin genes also reflect the biology of the disease; however, the direct role in the etiology and clinical course remain unclear. Finally, resistance to senescence and normal programmed cell death can be explained in part by high expression of bcl-2 and expression of other members of this family of pro- and anti-apoptotic proteins, while the regulation of expression and mechanism of action of this family of proteins remains an area of active investigation. Intense research is under way to obtain a molecular understanding of the etiology of this disease, with biologic and clinical correlates, which will ultimately allow development of new therapies and cure.

REFERENCES

1. Juliusson G, Oscier DG, Fitchett M, et al. Prognostic subgroups in B-cell chronic lymphocytic leukemia defined by specific chromosomal abnormalities. N Engl J Med 1990;323:720–724.
2. Dohner H, Stilgenbauer S, Benner A, et al. Genomic aberrations and survival in chronic lymphocytic leukemia. N Engl J Med 2000;343:1910–1916.
3. Chapman RM, Corcoran MM, Gardiner A, Hawthorn LA, Cowell JK, Oscier DG. Frequent homozygous deletions of the D13S25 locus in chromosome region 13q14 defines the location of a gene critical in leukaemogenesis in chronic B-cell lymphocytic leukaemia. Oncogene 1994;9:1289–1293.
4. Jabbar SA, Ganeshaguru K, Wickremasinghe RG, Hoffbrand AV, Foroni L. Deletion of chromosome 13 (band q14) but not trisomy 12 is a clonal event in B-chronic lymphocytic leukaemia (CLL). Br J Haematol 1995;90:476–478.
5. Garcia-Marco JA, Price CM, Catovsky D. Interphase cytogenetics in chronic lymphocytic leukemia. Cancer Genet Cytogenet 1997;94:52–58.
6. Cuneo A, Bigoni R, Rigolin GM, et al. 13q14 deletion in non-Hodgkin's lymphoma: correlation with clinico-pathologic features. Haematologica 1999;84:589–593.

7. Cuneo A, Bigoni R, Rigolin GM, et al. Cytogenetic profile of lymphoma of follicle mantle lineage: correlation with clinicobiologic features. Blood 1999;93:1372–1380.

8. Sawyer JR, Waldron JA, Jagannath S, Barlogie B. Cytogenetic findings in 200 patients with multiple myeloma. Cancer Genet Cytogenet 1995;82:41–49.

9. Avet-Louseau H, Daviet A, Sauner S, Bataille R. Chromosome 13 abnormalities in multiple myeloma are mostly monosomy 13. Br J Haematol 2000;111:1116–1117.

10. Zojer N, Konigsberg R, Ackermann J, et al. Deletion of 13q14 remains an independent adverse prognostic variable in multiple myeloma despite its frequent detection by interphase fluorescence in situ hybridization. Blood 2000;95:1925–1930.

11. Knuutila S, Teerenhovi L, Larramendy ML, et al. Cell lineage involvement of recurrent chromosomal abnormalities in hematologic neoplasms. Genes Chromosomes Cancer 1994;10:95–102.

12. Brown AG, Ross FM, Dunne EM, Steel CM, Weir-Thompson EM. Evidence for a new tumour suppressor locus (DBM) in human B-cell neoplasia telomeric to the retinoblastoma gene. Nat Genet 1993;3:67–72.

13. Hawthorn LA, Chapman R, Oscier D, Cowell JK. The consistent 13q14 translocation breakpoint seen in chronic B-cell leukaemia (BCLL) involves deletion of the D13S25 locus which lies distal to the retinoblastoma predisposition gene. Oncogene 1993;8:1415–1419.

14. Liu Y, Szekely L, Grander D, et al. Chronic lymphocytic leukemia cells with allelic deletions at 13q14 commonly have one intact RB1 gene: evidence for a role of an adjacent locus. Proc Natl Acad Sci U S A 1993;90:8697–8701.

15. Hawthorn L, Roberts T, Verlind E, Kooy RF, Cowell JK. A yeast artificial chromosome contig that spans the RB1-D13S31 interval on human chromosome 13 and encompasses the frequently deleted region in B-cell chronic lymphocytic leukemia. Genomics 1995;30:425–430.

16. Weinberg RA. The retinoblastoma protein and cell cycle control. Cell 1995;81:323–330.

17. Bouyge-Moreau I, Rondeau G, Avet-Loiseau H, et al. Construction of a 780-kb PAC, BAC, and cosmid contig encompassing the minimal critical deletion involved in B cell chronic lymphocytic leukemia at 13q14.3. Genomics 1997;46:183–190.

18. Corcoran MM, Rasool O, Liu Y, et al. Detailed molecular delineation of 13q14.3 loss in B-cell chronic lymphocytic leukemia. Blood 1998;91:1382–1390.

19. Stilgenbauer S, Nickolenko J, Wilhelm J, et al. Expressed sequences as candidates for a novel tumor suppressor gene at band 13q14 in B-cell chronic lymphocytic leukemia and mantle cell lymphoma. Oncogene 1998;16:1891–1897.

20. Liu Y, Corcoran M, Rasool O, et al. Cloning of two candidate tumor suppressor genes within a 10 kb region on chromosome 13q14, frequently deleted in chronic lymphocytic leukemia. Oncogene 1997;15:2463–2473.

21. Bezieau S, Devilder MC, Rondeau G, Cadoret E, Moisan JP, Moreau I. Assignment of 48 ESTs to chromosome 13 band q14.3 and expression pattern for ESTs located in the core region deleted in B-CLL. Genomics 1998;52:369–373.

22. Kapanadze B, Kashuba V, Baranova A, et al. A cosmid and cDNA fine physical map of a human chromosome 13q14 region frequently lost in B-cell chronic lymphocytic leukemia and identification of a new putative tumor suppressor gene, Leu5. FEBS Lett 1998;426:266–270.

23. Mabuchi H, Fujii H, Calin G, et al. Cloning and characterization of CLLD6, CLLD7, and CLLD8, novel candidate genes for leukemogenesis at chromosome 13q14, a region commonly deleted in B-cell chronic lymphocytic leukemia. Cancer Res 2001;61:2870–2877.

24. Bullrich F, Fujii H, Calin G, et al. Characterization of the 13q14 tumor suppressor locus in CLL: identification of ALT1, an alternative splice variant of the LEU2 gene. Cancer Res 2001;61:6640–6648.

25. Wolf S, Mertens D, Schaffner C, et al. B-cell neoplasia associated gene with multiple splicing (BCMS): the candidate B-CLL gene on 13q14 comprises more than 560 kb covering all critical regions. Hum Mol Genet 2001;10:1275–1285.

26. Sossey-Alaoui K, Kitamura E, Head K, Cowell JK. Characterization of FAM10A4, a member of the ST13 tumor suppressor gene family that maps to the 13q14.3 region associated with B-cell leukemia, multiple myeloma, and prostate cancer. Genomics 2002;80:5–7.

27. Kitamura E, Su G, Sossey-Alaoui K, et al. A transcription map of the minimally deleted region from 13q14 in B-cell chronic lymphocytic leukemia as defined by large scale sequencing of the 650 kb critical region. Oncogene 2000;19:5772–5780.

28. Rondeau G, Moreau I, Bezieau S, Cadoret E, Moisan JP, Devilder MC. Exclusion of Leu1 and Leu2 genes as tumor suppressor genes in 13q14.3-deleted B-CLL. Leukemia 1999;13:1630–1632.

29. Neilson JR, Auer R, White D, et al. Deletions at 11q identify a subset of patients with typical CLL who show consistent disease progression and reduced survival. Leukemia 1997;11:1929–1932.

30. Hogan WJ, Tefferi A, Borell TJ, Jenkins R, Li CY, Witzig TE. Prognostic relevance of monosomy at the 13q14 locus detected by fluorescence in situ hybridization in B-cell chronic lymphocytic leukemia. Cancer Genet Cytogenet 1999;110:77–81.

31. D'Arena G, Musto P, Cascavilla N, et al. CD38 expression correlates with adverse biological features and predicts poor clinical outcome in B-cell chronic lymphocytic leukemia. Leuk Lymphoma 2001;42:109–114.

32. Krober A, Seiler T, Benner A, et al. V(H) mutation status, CD38 expression level, genomic aberrations, and survival in chronic lymphocytic leukemia. Blood 2002;100:1410–146.

33. Oscier DG, Gardiner AC, Mould SJ, et al. Multivariate analysis of prognostic factors in CLL: clinical stage, IGVH gene mutational status, and loss or mutation of the p53 gene are independent prognostic factors. Blood 2002;100:1177–1184.

34. Gahrton G, Robert KH, Friberg K, Zech L, Bird AG. Extra chromosome 12 in chronic lymphocytic leukaemia. Lancet 1980;1:146–147.

35. Sadamori N, Han T, Minowada J, Cohen E, Sandberg AA. Chromosome studies in stimulated lymphocytes of B-cell chronic lymphocytic leukemias. Hematol Oncol 1983;1:243–250.

36. Han T, Sadamori N, Ozer H, et al. Cytogenetic studies in 77 patients with chronic lymphocytic leukemia: correlations with clinical, immunologic, and phenotypic data. J Clin Oncol 1984;2:1121–1132.

37. Losada AP, Wessman M, Tiainen M, et al. Trisomy 12 in chronic lymphocytic leukemia: an interphase cytogenetic study. Blood 1991;78:775–779.

38. Anastasi J, Le Beau MM, Vardiman JW, Fernald AA, Larson RA, Rowley JD. Detection of trisomy 12 in chronic lymphocytic leukemia by fluorescence in situ hybridization to interphase cells: a simple and sensitive method. Blood 1992;79:1796–1801.

39. Raghoebier S, Kibbelaar RE, Kleiverda JK, et al. Mosaicism of trisomy 12 in chronic lymphocytic leukemia detected by non-radioactive in situ hybridization. Leukemia 1992;6:1220–1226.

40. Cuneo A, Wlodarska I, Sayed Aly M, et al. Non-radioactive in situ hybridization for the detection and monitoring of trisomy 12 in B-cell chronic lymphocytic leukaemia. Br J Haematol 1992;81:192–196.

41. Dohner H, Pohl S, Bulgay-Morschel M, Stilgenbauer S, Bentz M, Lichter P. Trisomy 12 in chronic lymphoid leukemias—a metaphase and interphase cytogenetic analysis. Leukemia 1993;7:516–20.

42. Escudier SM, Pereira-Leahy JM, Drach JW, et al. Fluorescent in situ hybridization and cytogenetic studies of trisomy 12 in chronic lymphocytic leukemia. Blood 1993;81:2702–2707.

43. Crossen PE, Horn HL. Origin of trisomy 12 in B-cell chronic lymphocytic leukemia. Cancer Genet Cytogenet 1987;28:185–186.

44. Einhorn S, Burvall K, Juliusson G, Gahrton G, Meeker T. Molecular analyses of chromosome 12 in chronic lymphocytic leukemia. Leukemia 1989;3:871–874.

45. Dierlamm J, Wlodarska I, Michaux L, et al. FISH identifies different types of duplications with 12q13-15 as the commonly involved segment in B-cell lymphoproliferative malignancies characterized by partial trisomy 12. Genes Chromosomes Cancer 1997;20:155–166.

46. Chena C, Sarmiento M, Palacios MF, Scolnik M, Slavutsky I. Dup(12)(q13-q22) and 13q14 deletion in a case of B-cell chronic lymphocytic leukemia. Acta Haematol 2000;104:197–201.

47. Huang YQ, Raphael B, Buchbinder A, Li JJ, Zhang WG, Friedman-Kien AE. Rearrangement and expression of MDM2 oncogene in chronic lymphocytic leukemia. Am J Hematol 1994;47:139–141.

48. Merup M, Juliusson G, Wu X, et al. Amplification of multiple regions of chromosome 12, including 12q13-15, in chronic lymphocytic leukaemia. Eur J Haematol 1997;58:174–180.

49. Watanabe T, Hotta T, Ichikawa A, et al. The MDM2 oncogene overexpression in chronic lymphocytic leukemia and low-grade lymphoma of B-cell origin. Blood 1994;84:3158–3165.

50. Haupt Y, Maya R, Kazaz A, Oren M. Mdm2 promotes the rapid degradation of p53. Nature 1997;387:296–299.

51. Kubbutat MH, Jones SN, Vousden KH. Regulation of p53 stability by Mdm2. Nature 1997;387:299–303.

52. Gahn B, Schafer C, Neef J, et al. Detection of trisomy 12 and Rb-deletion in CD34+ cells of patients with B-cell chronic lymphocytic leukemia. Blood 1997;89:4275–4281.

53. Gahn B, Schafer C, Neef J, et al. Detection of trisomy 12 in CD34+ progenitor cells in a patient with B-cell chronic lymphocytic leukemia by fluorescence in situ hybridization. Ann Oncol 1997;8(suppl 2):55–57.

54. Gahn B, Wendenburg B, Troff C, et al. Analysis of progenitor cell involvement in B-CLL by simultaneous immunophenotypic and genotypic analysis at the single cell level. Br J Haematol 1999;105:955–959.

55. Han T, Ohtaki K, Sadamori N, et al. Cytogenetic evidence for clonal evolution in B-cell chronic lymphocytic leukemia. Cancer Genet Cytogenet 1986;23:321–328.

56. Hjalmar V, Hast R, Kimby E. Sequential fluorescence in situ hybridization analyses for trisomy 12 in chronic leukemic B-cell disorders. Haematologica 2001;86:174–180.

57. Criel A, Wlodarska I, Meeus P, et al. Trisomy 12 is uncommon in typical chronic lymphocytic leukaemias. Br J Haematol 1994;87:523–528.

58. Cuneo A, Bigoni R, Balboni M, et al. Trisomy 12 in chronic lymphocytic leukemia and hairy cell leukemia: a cytogenetic and interphase cytogenetic study. Leuk Lymphoma 1994;15:167–172.

59. Garcia-Marco J, Matutes E, Morilla R, et al. Trisomy 12 in B-cell chronic lymphocytic leukaemia: assessment of lineage restriction by simultaneous analysis of immunophenotype and genotype in interphase cells by fluorescence in situ hybridization. Br J Haematol 1994;87:44–50.

60. Hjalmar V, Kimby E, Matutes E, et al. Trisomy 12 and lymphoplasmacytoid lymphocytes in chronic leukemic B-cell disorders. Haematologica 1998;83:602–609.

61. Liso V, Capalbo S, Lapietra A, Pavone V, Guarini A, Specchia G. Evaluation of trisomy 12 by fluorescence in situ hybridization in peripheral blood, bone marrow and lymph nodes of patients with B-cell chronic lymphocytic leukemia. Haematologica 1999;84:212–217.

62. Navarro B, Garcia-Marco JA, Jones D, Price CM, Catovsky D. Association and clonal distribution of trisomy 12 and 13q14 deletions in chronic lymphocytic leukaemia. Br J Haematol 1998;102:1330–1334.

63. Han T, Ozer H, Sadamori N, et al. Prognostic importance of cytogenetic abnormalities in patients with chronic lymphocytic leukemia. N Engl J Med 1984;310:288–292.

64. Sadamori N, Han T, Minowada J, Sandberg AA. Clinical significance of cytogenetic findings in untreated patients with B-cell chronic lymphocytic leukemia. Cancer Genet Cytogenet 1984;11:45–51.

65. Juliusson G, Gahrton G. Poor age-corrected survival of chronic lymphocytic leukaemia patients with trisomy 12. Eur J Haematol 1987;38:315–317.

66. Pittman S, Catovsky D. Prognostic significance of chromosome abnormalities in chronic lymphocytic leukaemia. Br J Haematol 1984;58:649–660.

67. Geisler CH, Philip P, Hansen MM. B-cell chronic lymphocytic leukaemia: clonal chromosome abnormalities and prognosis in 89 cases. Eur J Haematol 1989;43:397–403.

68. Han T, Sadamori N, Block AM, et al. Cytogenetic studies in chronic lymphocytic leukemia, prolymphocytic leukemia and hairy cell leukemia: a progress report. Nouv Rev Fr Hematol 1988;30:393–395.

69. Que TH, Marco JG, Ellis J, et al. Trisomy 12 in chronic lymphocytic leukemia detected by fluorescence in situ hybridization: analysis by stage, immunophenotype, and morphology. Blood 1993;82:571–575.

70. Knauf WU, Knuutila S, Zeigmeister B, Thiel E. Trisomy 12 in B-cell chronic lymphocytic leukemia: correlation with advanced disease, atypical morphology, high levels of sCD25, and with refractoriness to treatment. Leuk Lymphoma 1995;19:289–294.

71. Matutes E, Oscier D, Garcia-Marco J, et al. Trisomy 12 defines a group of CLL with atypical morphology: correlation between cytogenetic, clinical and laboratory features in 544 patients. Br J Haematol 1996;92:382–388.

72. Garcia-Marco JA, Price CM, Ellis J, et al. Correlation of trisomy 12 with proliferating cells by combined immunocytochemistry and fluorescence in situ hybridization in chronic lymphocytic leukemia. Leukemia 1996;10:1705–1711.

73. Oscier DG, Thompsett A, Zhu D, Stevenson FK. Differential rates of somatic hypermutation in V(H) genes among subsets of chronic lymphocytic leukemia defined by chromosomal abnormalities. Blood 1997;89:4153–4160.

74. Hamblin TJ, Davis Z, Gardiner A, Oscier DG, Stevenson FK. Unmutated Ig V(H) genes are associated with a more aggressive form of chronic lymphocytic leukemia. Blood 1999;94:1848–1854.

75. Dohner H, Stilgenbauer S, James MR, et al. 11q deletions identify a new subset of B-cell chronic lymphocytic leukemia characterized by extensive nodal involvement and inferior prognosis. Blood 1997;89:2516–2522.

76. Karhu R, Knuutila S, Kallioniemi OP, et al. Frequent loss of the 11q14-24 region in chronic lymphocytic leukemia: a study by comparative genomic hybridization. Tampere CLL Group. Genes Chromosomes Cancer 1997;19:286–290.

77. Nowell PC, Vonderheid EC, Besa E, Hoxie JA, Moreau L, Finan JB. The most common chromosome change in 86 chronic B cell or T cell tumors: a 14q32 translocation. Cancer Genet Cytogenet 1986;19:219–227.

78. Gahrton G, Juliusson G. Clinical implication of chromosomal aberrations in chronic B-lymphocytic leukaemia cells. Nouv Rev Fr Hematol 1988;30:389–392.

79. Koduru PR, Offit K, Filippa DA. Molecular analysis of breaks in BCL-1 proto-oncogene in B-cell lymphomas with abnormalities of 11q13. Oncogene 1989;4:929–934.

80. Raffeld M, Jaffe ES. bcl-1, t(11;14), and mantle cell-derived lymphomas. Blood 1991;78:259–263.

81. Brizard F, Dreyfus B, Guilhot F, Tanzer J, Brizard A. 11q13 rearrangement in B cell chronic lymphocytic leukemia. Leuk Lymphoma 1997;25:539–543.

82. Thieblemont C, Pack S, Sakai A, et al. Allelic loss of 11q13 as detected by MEN1-FISH is not associated with mutation of the MEN1 gene in lymphoid neoplasms. Leukemia 1999;13:85–91.

83. Stilgenbauer S, Liebisch P, James MR, et al. Molecular cytogenetic delineation of a novel critical genomic region in chromosome bands 11q22.3-923.1 in lymphoproliferative disorders. Proc Natl Acad Sci USA 1996; 93:11,837–11,841.

84. Stilgenbauer S, Schaffner C, Litterst A, et al. Biallelic mutations in the ATM gene in T-prolymphocytic leukemia. Nat Med 1997;3:1155–119.

85. Vorechovsky I, Luo L, Dyer MJ, et al. Clustering of missense mutations in the ataxia-telangiectasia gene in a sporadic T-cell leukaemia. Nat Genet 1997;17:96–99.

86. Savitsky K, Bar-Shira A, Gilad S, et al. A single ataxia telangiectasia gene with a product similar to PI-3 kinase. Science 1995;268:1749–1753.

87. Pandita TK. ATM function and telomere stability. Oncogene 2002;21:611–618.

88. Siliciano JD, Canman CE, Taya Y, Sakaguchi K, Appella E, Kastan MB. DNA damage induces phosphorylation of the amino terminus of p53. Genes Dev 1997;11:3471–3481.

89. Starostik P, Manshouri T, O'Brien S, et al. Deficiency of the ATM protein expression defines an aggressive subgroup of B-cell chronic lymphocytic leukemia. Cancer Res 1998;58:4552–4557.

90. Schaffner C, Stilgenbauer S, Rappold GA, Dohner H, Lichter P. Somatic ATM mutations indicate a pathogenic role of ATM in B-cell chronic lymphocytic leukemia. Blood 1999;94:748–753.

91. Stankovic T, Weber P, Stewart G, et al. Inactivation of ataxia telangiectasia mutated gene in B-cell chronic lymphocytic leukaemia. Lancet 1999;353:26–29.

92. Bullrich F, Rasio D, Kitada S, et al. ATM mutations in B-cell chronic lymphocytic leukemia. Cancer Res 1999;59:24–27.

93. Bevan S, Catovsky D, Marossy A, et al. Linkage analysis for ATM in familial B cell chronic lymphocytic leukaemia. Leukemia 1999;13:1497–1500.

94. Yuille MR, Condie A, Hudson CD, et al. ATM mutations are rare in familial chronic lymphocytic leukemia. Blood 2002;100:603–609.

95. Kobayashi H, Espinosa R, 3rd, Fernald AA, et al. Analysis of deletions of the long arm of chromosome 11 in hematologic malignancies with fluorescence in situ hybridization. Genes Chromosomes Cancer 1993;8:246–252.

96. Sembries S, Pahl H, Stilgenbauer S, Dohner H, Schriever F. Reduced expression of adhesion molecules and cell signaling receptors by chronic lymphocytic leukemia cells with 11q deletion. Blood 1999;93:624–631.

97. Lens D, Matutes E, Catovsky D, Coignet LJ. Frequent deletions at 11q23 and 13q14 in B cell prolymphocytic leukemia (B-PLL). Leukemia 2000;14:427–430.

98. Cuneo A, Bigoni R, Rigolin GM, et al. Late appearance of the 11q22.3-23.1 deletion involving the ATM locus in B-cell chronic lymphocytic leukemia and related disorders. Clinico-biological significance. Haematologica 2002;87:44–51.

99. Fegan C, Robinson H, Thompson P, Whittaker JA, White D. Karyotypic evolution in CLL: identification of a new sub-group of patients with deletions of 11q and advanced or progressive disease. Leukemia 1995;9:2003–2008.

100. Bigoni R, Cuneo A, Roberti MG, et al. Chromosome aberrations in atypical chronic lymphocytic leukemia: a cytogenetic and interphase cytogenetic study. Leukemia 1997;11:1933–1940.

101. Chevallier P, Penther D, Avet-Loiseau H, et al. CD38 expression and secondary 17p deletion are important prognostic factors in chronic lymphocytic leukaemia. Br J Haematol 2002;116:142–150.

102. Callet-Bauchu E, Salles G, Gazzo S, et al. Translocations involving the short arm of chromosome 17 in chronic B-lymphoid disorders: frequent occurrence of dicentric rearrangements and possible association with adverse outcome. Leukemia 1999;13:460–468.

103. Gaidano G, Ballerini P, Gong JZ, et al. p53 mutations in human lymphoid malignancies: association with Burkitt lymphoma and chronic lymphocytic leukemia. Proc Natl Acad Sci USA 1991;88:5413–5417.

104. Fenaux P, Preudhomme C, Lai JL, et al. Mutations of the p53 gene in B-cell chronic lymphocytic leukemia: a report on 39 cases with cytogenetic analysis. Leukemia 1992;6:246–250.

105. Gandini D, Aguiari GL, Cuneo A, Piva R, Castoldi GL, del Senno L. Novel small deletions of the p53 gene in late-stage B-cell chronic lymphocytic leukaemia. Br J Haematol 1994;88:881–885.

106. Lens D, De Schouwer PJ, Hamoudi RA, et al. p53 abnormalities in B-cell prolymphocytic leukemia. Blood 1997;89:2015–2023.

107. Hollstein M, Sidransky D, Vogelstein B, Harris CC. p53 mutations in human cancers. Science 1991;253:49–53.

108. Zambetti GP, Levine AJ. A comparison of the biological activities of wild-type and mutant p53. FASEB J 1993;7:855–865.

109. Harris CC. p53: at the crossroads of molecular carcinogenesis and risk assessment. Science 1993;262:1980–1981.
110. el-Deiry WS. Regulation of p53 downstream genes. Semin Cancer Biol 1998;8:345–357.
111. el Rouby S, Bayona W, Pisharody SM, Newcomb EW. p53 mutations in B-cell chronic lymphocytic leukemia. Curr Top Microbiol Immunol 1992;182:313–317.
112. Wattel E, Preudhomme C, Hecquet B, et al. p53 mutations are associated with resistance to chemotherapy and short survival in hematologic malignancies. Blood 1994;84:3148–3157.
113. Lens D, Dyer MJ, Garcia-Marco JM, et al. p53 abnormalities in CLL are associated with excess of prolymphocytes and poor prognosis. Br J Haematol 1997;99:848–857.
114. Barnabas N, Shurafa M, Van Dyke DL, Wolman SR, Clark D, Worsham MJ. Significance of p53 mutations in patients with chronic lymphocytic leukemia: a sequential study of 30 patients. Cancer 2001;91:285–293.
115. el Rouby S, Thomas A, Costin D, et al. p53 gene mutation in B-cell chronic lymphocytic leukemia is associated with drug resistance and is independent of MDR1/MDR3 gene expression. Blood 1993;82:3452–3459.
116. Dohner H, Fischer K, Bentz M, et al. p53 gene deletion predicts for poor survival and non-response to therapy with purine analogs in chronic B-cell leukemias. Blood 1995;85:1580–1589.
117. Geisler CH, Philip P, Christensen BE, et al. In B-cell chronic lymphocytic leukaemia chromosome 17 abnormalities and not trisomy 12 are the single most important cytogenetic abnormalities for the prognosis: a cytogenetic and immunophenotypic study of 480 unselected newly diagnosed patients. Leuk Res 1997;21:1011–1023.
118. Philip P, Geisler C, Hansen MM, et al. Aberrations of chromosome 6 in 193 newly diagnosed untreated cases of chronic lymphocytic leukemia. Cancer Genet Cytogenet 1991;53:35–43.
119. Glassman AB, Harper-Allen EA, Hayes KJ, Hopwood VL, Gutterman EE, Zagryn SP. Chromosome 6 abnormalities associated with prolymphocytic acceleration in chronic lymphocytic leukemia. Ann Clin Lab Sci 1998;28:24–29.
120. Stilgenbauer S, Bullinger L, Benner A, et al. Incidence and clinical significance of 6q deletions in B cell chronic lymphocytic leukemia. Leukemia 1999;13:1331–1334.
121. Cuneo A, Roberti MG, Bigoni R, et al. Four novel non-random chromosome rearrangements in B-cell chronic lymphocytic leukaemia: 6p24-25 and 12p12-13 translocations, 4q21 anomalies and monosomy 21. Br J Haematol 2000;108:559–564.
122. Offit K, Parsa NZ, Gaidano G, et al. 6q deletions define distinct clinico-pathologic subsets of non-Hodgkin's lymphoma. Blood 1993;82:2157–2162.
123. Finn WG, Kay NE, Kroft SH, Church S, Peterson LC. Secondary abnormalities of chromosome 6q in B-cell chronic lymphocytic leukemia: a sequential study of karyotypic instability in 51 patients. Am J Hematol 1998;59:223–229.
124. Amiel A, Mulchanov I, Elis A, et al. Deletion of 6q27 in chronic lymphocytic leukemia and multiple myeloma detected by fluorescence in situ hybridization. Cancer Genet Cytogenet 1999;112:53–56.
125. Demeter J, Porzsolt F, Ramisch S, Schmidt D, Schmid M, Messer G. Polymorphism of the tumour necrosis factor-alpha and lymphotoxin-alpha genes in chronic lymphocytic leukaemia. Br J Haematol 1997;97:107–112.
126. Oscier DG, Stevens J, Hamblin TJ, Pickering RM, Lambert R, Fitchett M. Correlation of chromosome abnormalities with laboratory features and clinical course in B-cell chronic lymphocytic leukaemia. Br J Haematol 1990;76:352–358.
127. Tsujimoto Y, Jaffe E, Cossman J, Gorham J, Nowell PC, Croce CM. Clustering of breakpoints on chromosome 11 in human B-cell neoplasms with the t(11;14) chromosome translocation. Nature 1985;315:340–343.
128. Hernandez JM, Mecucci C, Criel A, et al. Cytogenetic analysis of B cell chronic lymphoid leukemias classified according to morphologic and immunophenotypic (FAB) criteria. Leukemia 1995;9:2140–2146.
129. Hinds PW, Dowdy SF, Eaton EN, Arnold A, Weinberg RA. Function of a human cyclin gene as an oncogene. Proc Natl Acad Sci USA 1994;91:709–713.
130. Cuneo A, Bigoni R, Negrini M, et al. Cytogenetic and interphase cytogenetic characterization of atypical chronic lymphocytic leukemia carrying BCL1 translocation. Cancer Res 1997;57:1144–1150.
131. Adachi M, Cossman J, Longo D, Croce CM, Tsujimoto Y. Variant translocation of the bcl-2 gene to immunoglobulin lambda light chain gene in chronic lymphocytic leukemia. Proc Natl Acad Sci USA 1989;86:2771–2774.
132. Adachi M, Tefferi A, Greipp PR, Kipps TJ, Tsujimoto Y. Preferential linkage of bcl-2 to immunoglobulin light chain gene in chronic lymphocytic leukemia. J Exp Med 1990;171:559–564.
133. Ueshima Y, Bird ML, Vardiman JW, Rowley JD. A 14;19 translocation in B-cell chronic lymphocytic leukemia: a new recurring chromosome aberration. Int J Cancer 1985;36:287–290.

134. Kerr LD, Duckett CS, Wamsley P, et al. The proto-oncogene bcl-3 encodes an I kappa B protein. Genes Dev 1992;6:2352–2363.

135. Michaux L, Mecucci C, Stul M, et al. BCL3 rearrangement and t(14;19)(q32;q13) in lymphoproliferative disorders. Genes Chromosomes Cancer 1996;15:38–47.

136. McKeithan TW, Takimoto GS, Ohno H, et al. BCL3 rearrangements and t(14;19) in chronic lymphocytic leukemia and other B-cell malignancies: a molecular and cytogenetic study. Genes Chromosomes Cancer 1997; 20:64–72.

137. Juliusson G, Gahrton G. Chromosome aberrations in B-cell chronic lymphocytic leukemia. Pathogenetic and clinical implications. Cancer Genet Cytogenet 1990;45:143–160.

138. Virgilio L, Isobe M, Narducci MG, et al. Chromosome walking on the TCL1 locus involved in T-cell neoplasia. Proc Natl Acad Sci USA 1993;90:9275–9279.

139. Virgilio L, Narducci MG, Isobe M, et al. Identification of the TCL1 gene involved in T-cell malignancies. Proc Natl Acad Sci USA 1994;91:12,530–12,534.

140. Narducci MG, Pescarmona E, Lazzeri C, et al. Regulation of TCL1 expression in B- and T-cell lymphomas and reactive lymphoid tissues. Cancer Res 2000;60:2095–2100.

141. Yuille MR, Condie A, Stone EM, et al. TCL1 is activated by chromosomal rearrangement or by hypomethylation. Genes Chromosomes Cancer 2001;30:336–341.

142. Bichi R, Shinton SA, Martin ES, et al. Human chronic lymphocytic leukemia modeled in mouse by targeted TCL1 expression. Proc Natl Acad Sci U S A 2002;99:6955–6960.

143. Geisler CH, Larsen JK, Hansen NE, et al. Prognostic importance of flow cytometric immunophenotyping of 540 consecutive patients with B-cell chronic lymphocytic leukemia. Blood 1991;78:1795–1802.

144. Rassenti LZ, Kipps TJ. Lack of allelic exclusion in B cell chronic lymphocytic leukemia. J Exp Med 1997;185: 1435–1445.

145. Lewis CM, Pegrum GD. Autoimmune antibodies in chronic lymphatic leukaemia. Br J Haematol 1978;38:75–84.

146. Hamblin TJ, Oscier DG, Young BJ. Autoimmunity in chronic lymphocytic leukaemia. J Clin Pathol 1986; 39:713–716.

147. Broker BM, Klajman A, Youinou P, et al. Chronic lymphocytic leukemic (CLL) cells secrete multispecific autoantibodies. J Autoimmun 1988;1:469–481.

148. Caligaris-Cappio F. B-chronic lymphocytic leukemia: a malignancy of anti-self B cells. Blood 1996;87:2615–2620.

149. Kipps TJ, Tomhave E, Pratt LF, Duffy S, Chen PP, Carson DA. Developmentally restricted immunoglobulin heavy chain variable region gene expressed at high frequency in chronic lymphocytic leukemia. Proc Natl Acad Sci USA 1989;86:5913–5917.

150. Logtenberg T, Schutte ME, Inghirami G, et al. Immunoglobulin VH gene expression in human B cell lines and tumors: biased VH gene expression in chronic lymphocytic leukemia. Int Immunol 1989;1:362–366.

151. Mayer R, Logtenberg T, Strauchen J, et al. CD5 and immunoglobulin V gene expression in B-cell lymphomas and chronic lymphocytic leukemia. Blood 1990;75:1518–1524.

152. Deane M, Baker BW, Norton JD. Immunoglobulin VH4 gene usage in B lymphoid leukaemias. Br J Haematol 1993;84:242–249.

153. Ebeling SB, Schutte ME, Logtenberg T. Molecular analysis of VH and VL regions expressed in IgG-bearing chronic lymphocytic leukemia (CLL): further evidence that CLL is a heterogeneous group of tumors. Blood 1993;82:1626–1631.

154. Matolcsy A, Casali P, Nador RG, Liu YF, Knowles DM. Molecular characterization of IgA- and/or IgG-switched chronic lymphocytic leukemia B cells. Blood 1997;89:1732–1739.

155. Fais F, Ghiotto F, Hashimoto S, et al. Chronic lymphocytic leukemia B cells express restricted sets of mutated and unmutated antigen receptors. J Clin Invest 1998;102:1515–1525.

156. Korganow AS, Martin T, Weber JC, et al. Molecular analysis of rearranged VH genes during B cell chronic lymphocytic leukemia: intraclonal stability is frequent but not constant. Leuk Lymphoma 1994;14:55–69.

157. Aoki H, Takishita M, Kosaka M, Saito S. Frequent somatic mutations in D and/or JH segments of Ig gene in Waldenstrom's macroglobulinemia and chronic lymphocytic leukemia (CLL) with Richter's syndrome but not in common CLL. Blood 1995;85:1913–1919.

158. Schettino EW, Cerutti A, Chiorazzi N, Casali P. Lack of intraclonal diversification in Ig heavy and light chain V region genes expressed by CD5+IgM+ chronic lymphocytic leukemia B cells: a multiple time point analysis. J Immunol 1998;160:820–830.

159. Damle RN, Wasil T, Fais F, et al. Ig V gene mutation status and CD38 expression as novel prognostic indicators in chronic lymphocytic leukemia. Blood 1999;94:1840–1847.

160. Thompson AA, Talley JA, Do HN, et al. Aberrations of the B-cell receptor B29 (CD79b) gene in chronic lymphocytic leukemia. Blood 1997;90:1387–1394.
161. Thompson AA, Do HN, Saxon A, Wall R. Widespread B29 (CD79b) gene defects and loss of expression in chronic lymphocytic leukemia. Leuk Lymphoma 1999;32:561–569.
162. Cragg MS, Chan HT, Fox MD, et al. The alternative transcript of CD79b is overexpressed in B-CLL and inhibits signaling for apoptosis. Blood 2002;100:3068–3076.
163. Vrhovac R, Delmer A, Tang R, Marie JP, Zittoun R, Ajchenbaum-Cymbalista F. Prognostic significance of the cell cycle inhibitor p27Kip1 in chronic B-cell lymphocytic leukemia. Blood 1998;91:4694–4700.
164. Theml H, Love R, Begemann H. Factors in the pathomechanism of chronic lymphocytic leukemia. Annu Rev Med 1977;28:131-41.
165. Reed JC. Molecular biology of chronic lymphocytic leukemia: implications for therapy. Semin Hematol 1998;35:3–13.
166. Schena M, Larsson LG, Gottardi D, et al. Growth- and differentiation-associated expression of bcl-2 in B-chronic lymphocytic leukemia cells. Blood 1992;79:2981–2989.
167. Hanada M, Delia D, Aiello A, Stadtmauer E, Reed JC. bcl-2 gene hypomethylation and high-level expression in B-cell chronic lymphocytic leukemia. Blood 1993;82:1820–1828.
168. Robertson LE, Plunkett W, McConnell K, Keating MJ, McDonnell TJ. Bcl-2 expression in chronic lymphocytic leukemia and its correlation with the induction of apoptosis and clinical outcome. Leukemia 1996;10:456–459.
169. McConkey DJ, Chandra J, Wright S, et al. Apoptosis sensitivity in chronic lymphocytic leukemia is determined by endogenous endonuclease content and relative expression of BCL-2 and BAX. J Immunol 1996;156:2624–2630.
170. Aguilar-Santelises M, Rottenberg ME, Lewin N, Mellstedt H, Jondal M. Bcl-2, Bax and p53 expression in B-CLL in relation to in vitro survival and clinical progression. Int J Cancer 1996;69:114–119.
171. Rechavi G, Katzir N, Brok-Simoni F, et al. A search for bcl1, bcl2, and c-myc oncogene rearrangements in chronic lymphocytic leukemia. Leukemia 1989;3:57–60.
172. Medeiros LJ, Van Krieken JH, Jaffe ES, Raffeld M. Association of bcl-1 rearrangements with lymphocytic lymphoma of intermediate differentiation. Blood 1990;76:2086–2090.
173. Dyer MJ, Zani VJ, Lu WZ, et al. BCL2 translocations in leukemias of mature B cells. Blood 1994;83:3682–3688.
174. Adachi M, Tsujimoto Y. Juxtaposition of human bcl-2 and immunoglobulin lambda light chain gene in chronic lymphocytic leukemia is the result of a reciprocal chromosome translocation between chromosome 18 and 22. Oncogene 1989;4:1073–1075.
175. Tashiro S, Takechi M, Asou H, et al. Cytogenetic 2;18 and 18;22 translocation in chronic lymphocytic leukemia with juxtaposition of bcl-2 and immunoglobulin light chain genes. Oncogene 1992;7:573–577.
176. Laytragoon-Lewin N, Kashuba V, Mellstedt H, Klein G. bcl-2 rearrangement detected by pulsed-field gel electrophoresis (PFGF) in B-chronic lymphocytic leukemia (CLL) cells. Int J Cancer 1998;76:909–912.
177. Gottardi D, Alfarano A, De Leo AM, et al. In leukaemic CD5+ B cells the expression of BCL-2 gene family is shifted toward protection from apoptosis. Br J Haematol 1996;94:612–618.
178. Kitada S, Andersen J, Akar S, et al. Expression of apoptosis-regulating proteins in chronic lymphocytic leukemia: correlations with In vitro and In vivo chemoresponses. Blood 1998;91:3379–3389.
179. Kitada S, Zapata JM, Andreeff M, Reed JC. Protein kinase inhibitors flavopiridol and 7-hydroxy-staurosporine down-regulate antiapoptosis proteins in B-cell chronic lymphocytic leukemia. Blood 2000;96:393–397.
180. Pepper C, Bentley P, Hoy T. Regulation of clinical chemoresistance by bcl-2 and bax oncoproteins in B-cell chronic lymphocytic leukaemia. Br J Haematol 1996;95:513–517.
181. Molica S, Dattilo A, Giulino C, Levato D, Levato L. Increased bcl-2/bax ratio in B-cell chronic lymphocytic leukemia is associated with a progressive pattern of disease. Haematologica 1998;83:1122–1124.
182. King D, Pringle JH, Hutchinson M, Cohen GM. Processing/activation of caspases, -3 and -7 and -8 but not caspase-2, in the induction of apoptosis in B-chronic lymphocytic leukemia cells. Leukemia 1998;12:1553–1560.
183. Panayiotidis P, Jones D, Ganeshaguru K, Foroni L, Hoffbrand AV. Human bone marrow stromal cells prevent apoptosis and support the survival of chronic lymphocytic leukaemia cells in vitro. Br J Haematol 1996;92:97–103.
184. Lagneaux L, Delforge A, Bron D, De Bruyn C, Stryckmans P. Chronic lymphocytic leukemic B cells but not normal B cells are rescued from apoptosis by contact with normal bone marrow stromal cells. Blood 1998;91:2387–2396.
185. Burger JA, Tsukada N, Burger M, Zvaifler NJ, Dell'Aquila M, Kipps TJ. Blood-derived nurse-like cells protect chronic lymphocytic leukemia B cells from spontaneous apoptosis through stromal cell-derived factor-1. Blood 2000;96:2655–2663.

186. Pedersen IM, Kitada S, Leoni LM, et al. Protection of CLL B cells by a follicular dendritic cell line is dependent on induction of Mcl-1. Blood 2002;100:1795–1801.

187. Dancescu M, Rubio-Trujillo M, Biron G, Bron D, Delespesse G, Sarfati M. Interleukin 4 protects chronic lymphocytic leukemic B cells from death by apoptosis and upregulates Bcl-2 expression. J Exp Med 1992;176: 1319–1326.

188. Konig A, Menzel T, Lynen S, et al. Basic fibroblast growth factor (bFGF) upregulates the expression of bcl-2 in B cell chronic lymphocytic leukemia cell lines resulting in delaying apoptosis. Leukemia 1997;11:258–265.

189. Tangye SG, Raison RL. Human cytokines suppress apoptosis of leukaemic CD5+ B cells and preserve expression of bcl-2. Immunol Cell Biol 1997;75:127–135.

190. Bairey O, Zimra Y, Shaklai M, Rabizadeh E. Bcl-2 expression correlates positively with serum basic fibroblast growth factor (bFGF) and negatively with cellular vascular endothelial growth factor (VEGF) in patients with chronic lymphocytic leukaemia. Br J Haematol 2001;113:400–406.

191. Frankfurt OS, Byrnes JJ, Villa L. Protection from apoptotic cell death by interleukin-4 is increased in previously treated chronic lymphocytic leukemia patients. Leuk Res 1997;21:9–16.

192. Thomas A, El Rouby S, Reed JC, et al. Drug-induced apoptosis in B-cell chronic lymphocytic leukemia: relationship between p53 gene mutation and bcl-2/bax proteins in drug resistance. Oncogene 1996;12:1055–1062.

193. Pepper C, Hoy T, Bentley DP. Bcl-2/Bax ratios in chronic lymphocytic leukaemia and their correlation with in vitro apoptosis and clinical resistance. Br J Cancer 1997;76:935–938.

194. Pepper C, Thomas A, Hidalgo de Quintana J, Davies S, Hoy T, Bentley P. Pleiotropic drug resistance in B-cell chronic lymphocytic leukaemia—the role of Bcl-2 family dysregulation. Leuk Res 1999;23:1007–1014.

195. Gottardi D, De Leo AM, Alfarano A, et al. Fludarabine ability to down-regulate Bcl-2 gene product in CD5+ leukaemic B cells: in vitro/in vivo correlations. Br J Haematol 1997;99:147–157.

196. Bromidge TJ, Turner DL, Howe DJ, Johnson SA, Rule SA. In vitro chemosensitivity of chronic lymphocytic leukaemia to purine analogues—correlation with clinical course. Leukemia 1998;12:1230–1235.

197. Consoli U, El-Tounsi I, Sandoval A, et al. Differential induction of apoptosis by fludarabine monophosphate in leukemic B and normal T cells in chronic lymphocytic leukemia. Blood 1998;91:1742–1748.

198. Zaja F, Di Loreto C, Amoroso V, et al. BCL-2 immunohistochemical evaluation in B-cell chronic lymphocytic leukemia and hairy cell leukemia before treatment with fludarabine and 2-chloro-deoxy-adenosine. Leuk Lymphoma 1998;28:567–572.

199. Faderl S, Keating MJ, Do KA, et al. Expression profile of 11 proteins and their prognostic significance in patients with chronic lymphocytic leukemia (CLL). Leukemia 2002;16:1045–1052.

4

The Heterogeneous Origin of the B-CLL Cell

Terry Hamblin MB, DM

1. INTRODUCTION

It has long been recognized that chronic lymphocytic leukemia (CLL) may on the one hand adopt a benign aspect, scarcely troubling the patient over many years, or, on the other hand, may fiercely attack the patient, killing him (or, less commonly, her) within 2 years *(1)*. The two clinical staging systems introduced a generation ago *(2,3)* have been important prognostically. We know there is no advantage in the early treatment of Binet stage A or Rai stage 0 disease. Nevertheless, about half of such patients will eventually progress and require treatment. Despite the recognition of numerous prognostic factors, it has not, hitherto, been possible to predict reliably at diagnosis which patients will progress and which will not.

An attempt was made 25 years ago *(4)* to separate CLL into two different tumors, one arising from a cell early in maturation (and thus expressing surface IgD) and being more malignant, and one arising later in maturation (and thus lacking IgD) and being more benign. Unfortunately, this distinction fell foul of the poor reagents available at that time. The anti-IgD that was used was of low avidity and therefore only reacted with cells that had plentiful surface immunoglobulin. Such cells are seldom found in CLL, and in retrospect all that was being asserted was that the leukemic phase of mantle cell lymphoma is more malignant than is CLL.

Recently, a reliable method of distinguishing subtypes of CLL by sequencing the immunoglobulin variable region genes and searching for somatic mutations has revealed two forms of the disease with very different prognoses *(5,6)*. Again, the apparent difference between them is that one arises early in B-cell maturation and the other one later.

2. DISCERNABLE HETEROGENEITY IN CLL

2.1. Clinical Stage

Both the Binet *(3)* and Rai *(2)* staging systems are of immense value, and for a whole generation they have been the cornerstones of treatment decisions. It is disappointing that they make no distinction between genders over what constitutes anemia and do not insist that cytopenias should be caused by bone marrow suppression before assigning them a malign influence. Nevertheless, without these systems we would not be certain that early CLL does not benefit from early treatment with chlorambucil *(7)*.

From: *Contemporary Hematology*
Chronic Lymphocytic Leukemia: Molecular Genetics, Biology, Diagnosis, and Management
Edited by: G. B. Faguet © Humana Press Inc., Totowa, NJ

A more important problem with the staging system is that we must assume that every case of advanced CLL must pass through a phase of having early CLL. Up to half of all patients with early-stage disease eventually require treatment *(7)*. It would be useful to know in advance which half.

2.2. Complete Blood Count

Montserrat et al. *(8)* proposed a definition of "smoldering CLL" for a subset of stage A patients whose life expectancy was the same as for age-matched controls. An Hb of more than 13 g/dL, an absolute lymphocyte count of less than 30×10^9/L, a lymphocyte doubling time of more than 12 mo, and a nondiffuse pattern of bone marrow infiltration identified the subset. The requirement of knowing the lymphocyte doubling time means that a decision on nontreatment is necessarily delayed. The French Cooperative Group on CLL *(9)* defined a similar subset they deemed stage A'. The characteristics were Binet stage A, Hb 12 g/dL or more and a lymphocyte count less than 30×10^9/L.

2.3. Lymphocyte Morphology

CLL is characterized by a persistent lymphocytosis in blood and bone marrow. The leukemic lymphocytes are small, round, monomorphic cells. The nucleus contains heavily clumped basophilic chromatin, and sometimes an indistinct nucleolus can be discerned. The cytoplasm is scanty, agranular, pale blue, and apparently fragile, since "smudge" or "smear" cells are usually plentiful in blood films. There is some heterogeneity, however. A small percentage of the CLL cells are larger, with a prominent nucleolus (prolymphocytes). In some patients a small percentage of cells have a cleaved nucleus, and small numbers of lymphoplasmacytoid cells may also be seen. The French-American-British (FAB) group described three types of CLL: classical, mixed cell type with between 10 and 55% prolymphocytes, and a less well defined type with pleomorphic lymphocytes but fewer than 10% prolymphocytes *(10)*. This was further refined by Matutes et al. *(11)* into typical and atypical CLL. Patients whose cells have more 10% prolymphocytes or more than 15% cells with cleaved nuclei and lymphoplasmacytoid cells combined were defined as having atypical morphology. Atypical morphology correlates with progressive disease.

The bone marrow is inevitably infiltrated by small lymphocytes identical to those found in the blood. In bone marrow trephine biopsies, four histological patterns are described: interstitial, nodular, nodular and interstitial, and diffuse. Diffuse histology is associated with a poor prognosis *(12)*. In lymph nodes, normal nodal architecture is effaced by a diffuse infiltration of small lymphocytes identical to those seen in the bone marrow. Within both lymph nodes and bone marrow are foci of larger cells with prominent nucleoli that are referred to as proliferation centers.

2.4. Immunophenotype

Immunophenotyping has been critical in defining CLL as a clinical entity. In the past, clinical series have been contaminated by cases of spillover lymphoma, particularly mantle cell lymphoma (which shares the expression of CD5) and splenic marginal zone lymphoma (which does not always show the characteristic villi). The markers on CLL cells are distinct from those on normal B-cells and other B-cell tumors. In most cases the density of surface immunoglobulin is around 10% of that found on normal B-lymphocytes *(13)*, and the immunoglobulin-associated molecule, CD79b, is also only weakly expressed *(14)*. Again, there is some heterogeneity, with around 10% of cases expressing normal amounts of CD79b and 20–30% of cases expressing moderate amounts of surface immunoglobulin.

The other characteristic CLL markers are CD23, CD5, and rosettes with mouse red cells. There is no discernable heterogeneity with these markers; indeed, cells lacking CD23 and CD5 probably derive from a different type of tumor. Although CLL cells express cytoplasmic CD22, this molecule is absent from or only weakly expressed on the surface of the cells. Cases that express surface CD22 usually behave in a more aggressive manner. The antibody FMC7 has not been assigned a CD number, but it is still very useful in CLL. It reacts with only a very small percentage of CLL cells (usually <4%). Larger numbers indicate an adverse prognosis *(15)*. All CLLs express CD20, but it is generally less densely expressed than in other B-cell tumors. Bright CD20 expression is associated with atypical morphology and a worse prognosis *(16)*.

2.5. Serum Factors

Clinical staging is a surrogate for tumor mass. It says nothing about the virulence of the disease. A number of soluble factors have been proposed as markers of the aggressiveness of cell proliferation. Serum thymidine kinase is an enzyme reflecting cells entering division. Patients with early-stage CLL who had serum thymidine kinase levels greater than 7.0 U/L had a significantly shorter progression-free interval than those with a lower level *(17)*.

CD23 is rapidly cleaved from the cell membrane into a stable form in the serum. A faster doubling time of serum-soluble CD23 during follow-up correlates with a 3.2-fold increased risk of death *(18)*. Serum-soluble CD23 seems to reflect more than tumor mass, since its measurement can segregate Binet stage B disease into more or less aggressive forms *(19)*.

β_2-microglobulin, a protein noncovalently associated with the α-chain of MHC class I molecules, is normally present in the serum. Serum levels of β_2-microglobulin greater than 4.0 mg/L are adverse prognostic factors in a wide range of lymphoid malignancies *(20)* and probably relate to the rate of cell turnover. In this respect, CLL is no different *(21)*.

2.6. Cytogenetics

Although there is no archetypal chromosomal translocation in CLL, trisomy 12 occurs in 20–30% of cases *(22)* and deletions at 13q14 in up to 50% of cases *(22,23)*. Deletions at 11q23 occur in up to 15% of cases *(24)* and aberrations involving *p53* occur in around 10% *(25)*. There is a clear hierarchy of effect of these abnormalities. Patients with 13q14 deletions have a relatively benign disease, surviving longer than those with trisomy 12, who in turn have a better prognosis than those with 11q23 deletions, whereas those with *p53* aberrations do worst of all *(26)*.

Probably all these abnormalities are acquired during the course of the illness. For trisomy 12, the combined use of fluorescence *in situ* hybridization (FISH) and immunophenotyping with a surface light chain marker has shown that only 30–40% of the cells of the neoplastic clone have the extra chromosome *(27)*. In some cases, 13q14 deletions and trisomy 12 occur together. In such cases, subpopulations of the malignant clone may have both lesions together or either one separately, giving a confusing picture of which came first *(22)*. Abnormalities of *p53* are frequently late complications associated with a change in the pace of the disease *(28)*.

The inference is that, far from defining subtypes with different rates of progression, abnormal karyotypes are acquired during that progression and possibly acquired differentially because of different rates of progression.

2.7. Functional Heterogeneity

CLL is considered to result from the gradual accumulation of long-lived noncycling lymphocytes. There are a small number of "proliferating" cells denoted by positive Ki-67 staining *(29)*, but ethidium bromide staining shows these to be in G_1 and not in S phase *(29)*. Cordone et al. *(30)* showed a close correlation between the number of cells expressing Ki-67 and advanced clinical stage, and Del Giogli et al. *(31)* similarly correlated the expression of proliferating cell nuclear antigen (PCNA) with clinical stage and lymphocyte doubling time.

Interleukin-1 (IL-1) is a nonspecific mediator of inflammation. Cells from stable CLL spontaneously produce IL-1β, but this is reduced in cells from progressive CLL *(32)*. IL-6 is a multifunctional cytokine bearing many resemblances to IL-1. Cells from cases of advanced CLL lose their ability to produce high levels of IL-6 after stimulation by phorbol ester *(33)*. IL-8 is a chemokine with neutrophil chemoattractant properties. Patients with stage A CLL who have high levels of serum IL-8 are more likely to progress to advanced stages than those with low levels *(34)*. Interleukin-10 is an inhibitory cytokine. Although IL-10 mRNA expression correlates inversely with disease progression *(35)*, serum levels of IL-10 are higher in advanced stage than early stage disease *(36)*. Tumor necrosis factor-α (TNF-α) is a cytokine that shares many functions with IL-1. Serum levels of TNF-α and the TNF-α receptor increase with advancing stage *(37,38)*. Transforming growth factor-β (TGF-β) is a negative regulator of lymphocyte growth and development. About one-third of CLL cells are resistant to the inhibitory effects of TGF-β *(39)*.

CLL is the quintessential example of a tumor caused by a failure of apoptosis rather than uncontrolled proliferation. Examples of heterogeneity in the control of apoptosis can be demonstrated. Our knowledge of apoptosis derives from study of the nematode worm *Caenorhabditis elegans*. In this animal three essential genes have been identified, CED-3, CED-4, and CED-9.

CED-3 is the homolog of the mammalian caspase cascade (caspases-1–14). The downstream enzymes of this cascade eventually produce the biochemical and morphological features of apoptosis. At least one of these enzymes, caspase-3, which is involved in chemotherapeutic killing of CLL cells, is variably expressed in CLL *(40)*.

CED-4 activates CED-3. The human homolog of CED-4 is Apaf-1, although this gene is much more complex. Apaf-1 is activated by cytochrome C, which is released from mitochondria in response to a number of stimuli including cytotoxic drugs. Differential expression of Apaf-1 may equate with drug resistance in CLL *(41)*.

CED-9 binds to CED-4, preventing it from activating CED-3. The human homologs of CED-9 are the Bcl-2 family of apoptosis regulatory proteins. In the nematode, EGL-1 is an antagonist of CED-9; similarly, in the human there is a family of antagonists to Bcl-2 including Bcl-X_s and Bad. An additional class of pro-apoptotic Bcl-2 family proteins is not present in the nematode and is represented by Bax and Bid, which act directly on mitochondrial membranes, releasing cytochrome C. In CLL, high levels of Bcl-2 expression are seen, but higher levels or higher ratios of Bcl-2/Bax are seen in cases with progressive disease, chemorefractory disease, and short survival *(42)*. Another anti-apoptotic member of the Bcl-2 family, Mcl-1, is present in high levels in about half of CLL patients and is associated with a degree of chemorefractoriness *(43)*.

Apart from cytochrome C, the other main activators of caspases are the TNF family death receptors including Fas and Trail-1. CLL cells are resistant to Fas-induced apoptosis *(44)*. A caspase homolog, Flip, is an inhibitor of TNF family signaling and is dynamically regulated in CLL cells, being upregulated by CD40 signaling *(45)*.

CD40 is one of a number of molecules that is coexpressed with its ligand in a subset of CLL cells. CD40L is found in 15–30% of cases of CLL *(46)*. CD27 and its ligand CD70 are both expressed on CLL cells *(47)*. CLL cells express CD30 ligand, but CD30 is also present in a subset of CLL cells *(48)*. It is thought that the coexpression of receptor and ligand might lead to autocrine stimulation and stimulation of the transcription factor nerve factor-κB (NF-κB), levels of which are elevated in CLL *(49)*. NF-κB suppresses apoptosis by inducing the transcription of several anti-apoptotic genes including members of the Bcl-2 family *(50)*.

2.8. Immunoglobulin Genes

The raison d'être of B cells is the manufacture of immunoglobulin (Ig). Ig embedded in the surface membrane has the clear function of recognizing and responding to exogenous antigens. Recognition is via the variable (V) regions, which differ in sequence from one B-cell to another, and provide a complete catalog of potential antigen-combining sites. Cutting and pasting the component gene segments produces the extreme diversity of the B-cell receptor *(51,52)*. This recombinatorial process, which occurs in the bone marrow, is mediated by proteins encoded by the recombination-activating genes *RAG1* and *RAG2 (53)*.

For the heavy chain of Ig, selection takes place from the potentially functional genes of the unrearranged repertoire with 51 V_H genes divided into 7 families (V_H1–V_H7), 27 D genes, and 6 J_H genes. The junctions of V_H to D and D to J_H are imprecise, with the deletion by exonucleases of templated nucleotides or the insertion by terminal deoxytransferase (TdT) of nontemplated nucleotides in a random manner *(54)*. This introduces a further huge diversity into the shape of the Ig molecule, especially as the D segment can be read in any of the three frames *(55)*. The consequence is that the third complementarity-determining region (CDR3) of any given lymphocyte is virtually unique and provides a clonal signature for any tumor deriving from it.

The heavy chain genes also have a low degree of allelic polymorphism that has not been fully mapped *(56)*. The recombination of the constant regions (C_H and C_L) occurs following transcription; splicing of the transcribed RNA leads to a functional mRNA that can be translated into a μ heavy chain and κ or λ light chain proteins that combine to form whole IgM.

The usage of the 51 V_H genes is not random. Brezinschek et al. *(57)* analyzed the gene usage by individual normal B-cells in the blood of three individuals. Overusage of the V_H3 family was seen. The V_{3-23} gene was most commonly used, followed by $V_{3-30.3}$, V_{3-30}, and V_{3-07}. One possible reason for this predominance is the duplication of these segments in some haplotypes.

Rearrangement of the light chain variable region genes occurs in a similar manner, involving single-step recombinations of $V_κ/J_κ$ or $V_λ/J_λ$ gene segments but with no D segments. The B-cell receptor of pre-B-cells combines Ig heavy chains with the surrogate light chain encoded by the VpreB and λ5/14.1 genes *(58)*. Successful rearrangement of the light chain genes extinguishes expression of the pre-B-cell complex and suppresses further rearrangement. There are several checkpoints in B-cell maturation. Failure to produce a functional immunoglobulin induces apoptosis, as does an autoreactive specificity. Escape from apoptosis can occur by rearranging the other allele, most commonly of the light chain. This process is known as receptor editing. Occasionally B-cells express both κ and λ light chains, indicative of failure of allelic exclusion.

On completion of this maturation, the B-cell leaves the bone marrow for the periphery, where it may encounter antigen. It then undergoes affinity maturation, usually in the germinal centers of the peripheral lymphoid organs. Here, somatic mutation is induced under the influence of CD40+ T-cells, cytokines, and antigen-bearing follicular dendritic cells *(59)*. The rate of introduction of base pair changes is on the order of 10^{-4}–10^{-3} per generation. The mutations tend to cluster in the CDRs, possibly for structural reasons and possibly because of antigen selection.

A further genetic arrangement is necessary for Ig class switching from IgM plus IgD to IgG, IgA, or IgE. This process generally also occurs in the germinal center, although it may not be confined there *(59)*. The choice of isotype is cytokine determined *(60)*. The array of constant region genes at the heavy chain locus each has a 5' switch region that consists of tandem repeats.

Isotype switching conventionally occurs between two switch regions, looping out the intervening constant region genes, although RNA splicing, leading to the generation of multiple isotypes, may also occur (61).

Cells leaving the germinal center become either plasma cells or memory cells, the choice being directed by different cytokines. The plasma cells migrate mainly to bone marrow, but also to spleen, lymph nodes, and the mucosa-associated lymphoid tissue. Memory cells form part of the circulating pool but are also found in peripheral lymphoid organs and in the marginal zone of the spleen (62).

The peripheral blood B-cells of normal individuals comprise 60% naïve cells with unmutated IgV_H genes and 40% memory cells that carry somatically mutated IgV_H genes and express surface CD27 (63). Only a small proportion of naïve cells express CD5 (64), although this proportion is higher in early life. Most of circulating memory cells express surface IgM. (Some also express IgD.) Only a minority show evidence of class switching.

2.8.1. IMMUNOGLOBULIN V GENES IN CLL

Because CLL cells express CD5, many authorities had accepted that CLL cells derived from the minor population of CD5+ naïve B-cells. Early sequences of the IgV_H genes of tumor cells from patients with CLL found them to be in germline configuration (65–67), tending to confirm their origin from a naïve B-cell. However, reports began to appear in the literature detailing cases with evidence of somatic mutation, culminating in 1994 with a review of the literature by Schroeder and Dighiero (68), which found that 36/75 reported cases had IgV_H genes with less than 98% sequence homology to the appropriate germline gene. The figure of 98% was chosen because polymorphisms, which are quite common in V_H genes, can account for that degree of disparity (69). Schroeder and Dighiero (68) suspected that CLL might be a heterogeneous disorder but were unable to cull from the literature the comprehensive clinical details needed to establish this. They did report, however, that some of the cases with mutated V_H genes were CD5-negative and that there were a disproportionate number with class-switched IgV_H genes. These were not all cases of classical CLL.

More recently, a multicenter study of 64 patients with surface IgM+, CD5+ CLL also found two groups of roughly equal numbers with mutated and unmutated V_H genes (70). Although no clinical details were available otherwise to distinguish the two subsets, the authors were able to confirm the observation of Schroeder and Dighiero (68) that the presence or absence of somatic mutations was associated with the use of particular V_H genes.

In 1997 our group examined the V_H genes of 22 patients with classical B-cell CLL segregated according to karyotype. Tumors with trisomy 12 had unmutated V_H genes, but those with 13q14 abnormalities detected by conventional cytogenetics had evidence of somatic mutations (71). Since it has been previously shown that CLL patients with trisomy 12 have a poorer survival than those with abnormalities at 13q14 (26), this pointed to an association between clinical status and degree of somatic mutation.

The suspicion that the clinical heterogeneity of CLL might have a biological basis led us to extend this study. We examined the Ig V_H gene sequences in a series of 84 patients with classical B-cell CLL attending our hematology clinic and compared our results with various clinical characteristics of the patients and their survival. The striking finding to emerge was that the presence of IgV_H gene mutations placed the CLL patient in a disease group with a clearly better prognosis (4).

Patients with unmutated IgV_H genes had a median survival of 9.7 yr, whereas those with mutated IgV_H genes had a median survival of 24.4 yr. At the same time, Damle et al. (5), in a series

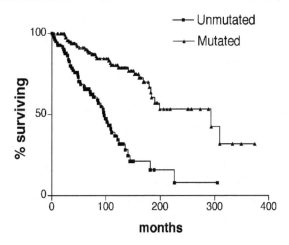

Fig. 1. Kaplan-Meier survival curve of 215 patients with chronic lymphocytic leukemia. Median survival for mutated cases was 293 mo; for unmutated cases, it was 93 mo ($p < 0.0001$).

of 64 patients published back to back with ours, found a median survival of 9 yr for the unmutated group and 17 yr for the mutated group. Others have since confirmed these findings in both CLL and small lymphocytic lymphoma *(72–74)*, and our own series, now extended to 215 patients, gives the same highly significant difference in survival (Fig. 1).

There are clear differences between the two subsets. Patients with unmutated V_H genes have characteristics associated with a more malignant type of disease than those with somatic mutations. They are significantly more likely to have advanced-stage disease, progressive disease, atypical morphology, and trisomy 12 as an isolated karyotypic abnormality, whereas those with somatic mutations were more likely to have stable stage A disease with typical morphology and chromosomal deletions or translocations at 13q14 *(4)*.

There is a significant tendency for V_H1 family genes and especially V1-69 to be used by the subset that lacks mutations *(4,70)*. A similar tendency toward the use of the D3-3 gene segment is also found in this subset. The biased use of the V1-69 gene, particularly the 51p1 allele, in CLL was first reported by Kipps et al. *(65)* and has since been confirmed by most workers in this field. In comparison with the normal IgV gene usage, V4-34 is also overused, especially in the mutated subset *(4,70)*.

The meaning of these biases is unclear. The control information derives from an examination of lymphocytes from three individuals, all under the age of 50 *(57)*, whereas most patients with CLL are much older. Inbred strains of mice show a biased usage of V_H gene usage with age *(75)*, and a similar bias has been suggested in elderly humans *(76)*. However, another possible explanation is that superantigen engages with framework regions of the B-cell receptor, stimulating the lymphocyte outside the germinal center *(4)*.

2.8.2. CD38

Damle et al. *(5)* suggested that expression of surface CD38 on CLL cells gave the same information as IgV gene mutations and might be a surrogate assay. However, in an analysis of 145 of our patients, although there was a highly significant association between CD38 expression and unmutated IgV_H genes, for individual patients there were important discordances *(77)*. Fifteen patients with unmutated IgV_H genes had less than 30% of cells expressing CD38, and 26 patients with mutated IgV_H genes had more than 30% of cells expressing CD38. The number of patients with discordant results for the two assays was 41/145 (28.3%). Discordant markers occurred as frequently in patients with stable disease as in those with progressive disease.

In a multivariate analysis of IgV_H status, CD38 positivity, Binet stage, typical or atypical morphology, progressive or stable disease (progressive disease included a lymphocyte doubling time of less than 12 mo as one of the criteria), and the two commonest karyotypic abnormalities, trisomy 12 and abnormalities at 13q14, only stage, IgV_H status, and CD38 positivity were independent prognostic factors (77).

Perhaps of more importance, CD38 expression did not remain constant throughout the course of the disease. Several patterns of CD38 positivity may be seen. Although in some cases all the cells are CD38-positive or CD38-negative, in many cases a mixture of CD38-positive and -negative cells is seen. The composition of this mixture changed in 24.4% of cases examined. In most cases, changes in CD38 expression were associated with treatment of the CLL, with a suggestion that chemotherapy selectively kills CD38-negative cells. In one patient the recovering cells after several rounds of chemotherapy were strongly CD38-positive, and the morphology of the cells had become atypical. In one case, stopping all therapy was associated with a recovery of CD38-negative cells. However, we also saw increases in the proportion of CD38-positive cells in patients with progressive disease without treatment (77).

In two of our patients, changes in the proportion of cells expressing CD38 were not associated with progression. One had stable disease but developed recurrent chest infections; the other developed concurrent chronic myelomonocytic leukemia. As the monocyte count rose, the expression of CD38 by the lymphocytes fell.

CD38 is a type II trans-membrane glycoprotein that acts as a complex ectoenzyme with ADP-ribosyl cyclase and cyclic ADP-ribose hydrolase activities (78). In the B-cell compartment, CD38 is not a lineage marker, but it is expressed at times during B-cell development when cell-to-cell interactions are crucial to development (79). Examples include an early bone marrow precursor cell, cells in the germinal center, and plasma cells (80). All the factors that signal its upregulation are as yet unknown, but they include both α- and γ-interferon (81). From the foregoing, it might be expected that expression of CD38 on b-cell CLL cells could vary, not only with disease progression, but also with the presence of intercurrent illness.

Because of the variability of CD38, it is risky to use it as a prognostic factor in early stage A disease. Nevertheless, patients who have both CD38-positive cells and unmutated IgV_H genes have a worse prognosis than those who are discordant for these markers (77). The independence of CD38 as an independent prognostic factor was lost when the series was extended to 215 patients, and loss or mutation of the p53 gene was included in the prognostic factors examined (82).

3. IS CLL ONE DISEASE OR TWO?

The separation of CLL into two subsets with widely differing prognoses and apparently arising from different stages of maturation suggests that they might be two different diseases with only superficial resemblances. The terms "naïve" and "memory" cells have been used to describe the cell of origin of the two types. This is probably a misrepresentation of the facts.

Evidence from gene expression profiles suggests that although the two subsets are different from each other and can be distinguished by the expression of around 30 genes, they bear more resemblances to each other than they do to other types of B-cell tumor or any normal B-cell (83,84). One of these studies suggests that they both bear some resemblance to memory B-cells

(84), and this is apparently confirmed by the fact that both subsets express CD27, a memory cell marker. However, CD27 was only designated as a marker of memory cells because it was found on cells that had undergone somatic mutation of the IgV$_H$ genes *(63)*.

How a cell without somatic mutations can be designated a memory cell is a semantic problem. What is it remembering? Chiorazzi and Ferrarini *(85)* have suggested that the unmutated subset might have encountered a T-independent antigen. Nagumo et al. *(86)* have recently demonstrated that CD27-negative "naïve" B cells may be induced to upregulate CD27 and to class switch their immunoglobulin expression, but not to generate somatic mutations, by CD40 signaling and B-cell receptor (BCR) engagement.

A further observation to be encompassed in the explanation is the finding of Tobin et al. *(87)* that patients whose CLL uses the gene V3-21 have a poor prognosis whether or not somatic mutations are present. These cases have a short, and sometimes identical, CDR3 and a preferential use of JH6. This suggests a unique binding of antigen or superantigen to the V3-21-encoded heavy chains.

4. A UNIFYING HYPOTHESIS

Gene expression profiling suggests that CLL is one disease. Sensitive probing for loss of the minimally deleted region at chromosome 13q14 shows loss of heterozygosity in over 80% of cases whether the IgV genes are mutated or not. The tumor cells are all anergic, partially activated, and anti-apoptotic *(88)*. Conventionally, the BCR should be stimulated by antigen on follicular dendritic cells in the presence of helper T-cells in the germinal center. A memory cell thus generated leaves the germinal center with somatic mutations and becomes part of the accumulation of long-lived, functionally incompetent lymphocytes described by Dameshek *(89)*. The cell never re-enters the germinal center, and therefore the chances of restimulation are remote.

Alternatively, the BCR complex may be stimulated outside the germinal center, either by a T-cell-independent antigen, or by a superantigen reacting with the BCR in framework regions outside the antibody-combining site. The conditions for somatic mutation are not met, so it does not occur. Nevertheless, the same process is set in train for partial activation with the expression of characteristic surface markers and the induction of anti-apoptotic pathways. Since the cell does not need to enter the germinal center for restimulation, restimulation will occur. The cell will therefore turn over more rapidly, albeit still very slowly, than its somatically mutated counterpart. Since it turns over more rapidly, it has a greater chance of accumulating further genetic errors and a greater chance of incapacitating the patient.

5. CONCLUSIONS

The discovery that the mutational status of the immunoglobulin genes separates CLL into two subsets with markedly different prognoses suggests that, although CLL may not be two different diseases, the pathway of differentiation that the malignant cell chooses determines in a major way the outcome of the disease. The two subsets are very similar to each other according to gene expression profiles, but the cells behave in markedly different ways. Those with unmutated IgV genes look more aggressive, infiltrate bone marrow more completely, progress more rapidly, double their white counts more quickly, express more surface CD38, and accumulate more and different karyotypic abnormalities.

Why some lymphocytes choose to enter germinal centers, the only place, we believe, where the IgV genes can undergo somatic mutation, is largely a matter of speculation. A major determining factor seems to be which particular V$_H$ gene is used by the cell, with V1-69 being mostly unmutated and V3-23 and V4-34 being mostly mutated. A possible explanation is that some gene products in their unmutated state might react either with T-independent antigens or via their framework regions with B-cell superantigens. Such cells seem predetermined to have a higher turnover rate than those that have passed through the germinal centers and thus to be at greater risk of accumulating further genetic errors.

The literature abounds with other characteristics in which CLL shows heterogeneity. The challenge of the future will be to see which, if any, of these correlate with IgV gene mutational status.

REFERENCES

1. Galton DAG. The pathogenesis of chronic lymphocytic leukaemia. Can Med Assoc J 1966;94:1005–1010.
2. Rai KR, Sawitsky, A, Cronkite ER, Chanana AD, Levy RN, Pasternack BS. Clinical staging of chronic lymphocytic leukemia. Blood 1975;46:219–234.
3. Binet J-L, Leporier M, Dighiero G, et al. A clinical staging system for chronic lymphocytic leukemia. Cancer 1977;40:855–864.
4. Hamblin TJ, Hough DW. Chronic lymphatic leukaemia: correlation of immunofluorescent characteristics and clinical features. Br J Haematol 1977;36:359–365.
5. Damle RN, Wasil T, Fais F, et al. Ig V gene mutation status and CD38 expression as novel prognostic indicators in chronic lymphocytic leukemia. Blood 1999;94:1840–1847.
6. Hamblin TJ, Davis Z, Gardiner A, Oscier DG, Stevenson FK. Unmutated Ig V(H) genes are associated with a more aggressive form of chronic lymphocytic leukemia. Blood 1999;94:1848–1854.
7. CLL Trialists' Collaborative Group. Chemotherapeutic options in chronic lymphocytic leukemia: a meta-analysis of the randomised trials. J Natl Cancer Inst 1999; 91:861–868.
8. Montserrat E, Vinolas N, Reverter JC, Rozman C. Natural history of chronic lymphocytic leukemia: on the progression and prognosis of early stages. Nouv Rev Fr Hematol 1988;30:359–361.
9. French Cooperative Group on Chronic Lymphocytic Leukemia. Natural history of stage A chronic lymphocytic leukemia untreated patients. Br J Hematol 1990;76:45–57.
10. Bennett JM, Catovsky D, Daniel MT, et al. French-American-British (FAB) Cooperative Group. Proposals for the classification of chronic (mature) B and T lymphoid leukaemias. J Clin Pathol 1989;42:567–584.
11. Matutes E, Oscier DG, Garcia-Marco J, et al. Trisomy 12 defines a group of CLL with atypical morphology: correlation between cytogenetic, clinical and laboratory features in 544 patients. Br J Haematol 1996;92:382–388.
12. Rozman C, Hernandez-Nieto L, Montserrat E, Brugues R. Prognostic significance of bone marrow patterns in chronic lymphocytic leukaemia. Br J Haematol 1981;47:529–537.
13. Ternynck T, Diaghiero G, Fallezou J, Binet JL. Comparison of normal and CLL lymphocyte surface Ig determinants using peroxidase-labelled antibodies. I. Detection and quantitation of light chain determinants. Blood 1974; 43:789–795.
14. Zomas AP, Matutes E, Morilla R, et al. Expression of immunoglobulin-associated protein B29 in B cell disorders with the monoclonal antibody SN8 (CD79b). Leukemia 1996;10:1966–1970.
15. Catovsky D, Cherchi M, Brooks J, Bradley J, Zola H. Heterogeneity of B cell leukemias demonstrated by the monoclonal antibody FMC7. Blood 1981;33:173–177.
16. Molica S, Levato D, Datillo A, Mannella A. Clinico-prognostic relevance of quantitative immunophenotyping in B-cell chronic lymphocytic leukemia with emphasis on the expression of CD20 antigen and surface immunoglobulins. Eur J Hematol 1998;60:47–52.
17. Hallek M, Langenmayer I, Nerl C, et al. Elevated serum thymidine kinase levels identify a subgroup at high risk of disease progression in early, non-smoldering chronic lymphocytic leukemia. Blood 1999;93:1732–1737.
18. Sarfati M, Chevet S, Chastang C, et al. Prognostic importance of serum levels of Cd23 in chronic lymphocytic leukemia. Blood 1996;88:4259–4264.
19. Molica S, Levato D, Dell'Olio M, et al. Cellular expression and serum circulating levels of CD23 in B-cell chronic lymphocytic leukemia. Implications for prognosis. Haematologica 1996;81:428–433.
20. Kantarjian HM, Smith T, Estey E, et al. Prognostic significance of elevated serum beta-2-microglobulin levels in adult acute lymphocytic leukemia. Am J Med 1994;93:599–604.
21. Ibrahim S, Keating M, Do KA, et al. CD38 expression as an important prognostic factor in B-cell chronic lymphocytic leukemia. Blood 2001;98:181–186.
22. Oscier D. Cytogenetic and molecular abnormalities in chronic lymphocytic leukaemia. Blood Rev 1994;8:88–97.

23. Hogan WJ, Tefferi A, Borell TJ, Jenkins R, Li CY, Witzig TE. Prognostic relevance of monosomy at the 13q14 locus detected by fluorescence in situ hybridization in B-cell chronic lymphocytic leukemia. Cancer Genet Cytogenet 1999;110:77–81.

24. Dohner H, Stilgenbauer S, James MR, et al. 11q deletions identify a new subset of B-cell chronic lymphocytic leukemia characterized by extensive nodal involvement and inferior prognosis. Blood 1997;89:2516–2522.

25. Gaidano G, Newcombe EW, Gong JZ, et al. Analysis of alterations of oncogenes and tumor suppressor genes in chronic lymphocytic leukemia. Am J Pathol 1994;144:1312–1319.

26. Juliusson G, Oscier DG, Fitchett M, et al. Prognostic subgroups in B-cell chronic lymphocytic leukemia defined by specific chromosomal abnormalities. N Engl J Med 1990;323:720–724.

27. Garcia-Marco J, Matutes E, Morilla R, et al. Trisomy 12 in B-cell chronic lymphocytic leukaemia: assessment of lineage restriction by simultaneous analysis of immunophenotype and genotype in interphase cells by fluorescence in situ hybridization. Br J Haematol 1994;83:44–50.

28. Leupolt E, Stilgenbauer S, Krober A, et al. Clonal evolution in B-CLL: acquisition of deletions involving 6q21, 11q22 and 17p13 (TP53) associated with disease progression. Blood 2001;98(suppl 1):471a, abstract 1968.

29. Orchard JA, Oscier DG. Prognostic value of Ki 67 and cell cycle analysis in chronic lymphocytic leukaemia. Br J Haematol 1996;93(suppl 2):116.

30. Cordone I, Matutes E, Catovsky. Monoclonal antibody Ki-67 identifies B and T cells in cycle in chronic lymphocytic leukaemia. Leukemia 1992;6:902–906.

31. Del Giglio A, O'Brien S, Ford RJ Jr, et al. Proliferating cell nuclear antigen (PCNA) expression in chronic lymphocytic leukaemia (CLL) Leuk Lymphoma 1993;10:265–271.

32. Anguilar-Santelises M, Amador JF, Mellstedt H, Jondal M. Low IL-1 beta production in leukemia cells from progressive B-cell chronic leukemia (B-CLL). Leuk Res 1989;13:937–942.

33. Hulkkonen J, Vilpo J, Vilpo L, Hurme M. Diminished production of IL-6 in chronic lymphocytic leukaemia (B-CLL) cells from patients with advanced stages of disease. Br J Haematol 1998;100:478–483.

34. Molica S, Vitelli G, Levato D, Datillo A, Gandolfo GM. Clinico-biological implications of increased serum levels of Interleukin-8 in B-cell chronic lymphocytic leukemia. Haematologica 1999;84:208–211.

35. Sjoberg J, Anguilar-Santelises M, Sjogren AM, et al. Interleukin-10 mRNA expression in B-cell chronic lymphocytic leukaemia inversely correlates with progression of disease. Br J Haematol 1996;92:393–400.

36. Egle A, Marschitz I Posch B, Herold M, Griel R. IL-10 serum levels in B-cell chronic lymphocytic leukaemia. Br J Haematol 1996;94:211–212.

37. Anguilar-Santelises M, Giglliotti D, Osorio LM, et al. Cytokine expression in B-CLL in relation to disease progression and in vitro activation. Med Oncol 1999;16:289–295.

38. Waage A, Especik T. TNF receptors in chronic lymphocytic leukemia. Leuk Lymphoma 1994;3:41–46.

39. Israels LG, Israels SJ, Begleiter A, et al. Role of transforming growth factor-beta in chronic lymphocytic leukemia. Leuk Res 1993;17:81–87.

40. Bellosillo B, Dalmau M, Colomer D, Gil J. Involvement of CED-3/ICE proteases in the apoptosis of B-chronic lymphocytic leukemia cells. Blood 1997;89:3378–3384.

41. Leoni L Chao Q, Cottam H, et al. Induction of an apoptotic program in cell-free extracts by 2-chloro-2'-deoxyadenosine 5'-triphosphate and cytochrome c. Proc Natl Acad Sci USA 1998;95:9567–9571.

42. Reed J. Chronic lymphocytic leukemia: a disease of disregulated programmed cell death. Clin Immunol Newslett 1998;17:125–140.

43. Kitada S, Andersen J, Akar S, et al. Evidence of apoptosis regulating proteins in chronic lymphocytic leukemia; correlations with in vitro and in vivo chemoresponses. Blood 1998;91:3379–3389.

44. Panayiotidis P, Ganeshaguru K, Foroni L, Hoffbrand AV. Expression and function of the FAS antigen in B chronic lymphocytic leukemia and hairy cell leukemia. Leukemia 1995;9:1227–1232.

45. Kitada S, Zapata J, Andreef M, Reed J. Bryostatin and CD40-ligand enhance apoptosis resistance and induce expression of cell survival genes in B-cell chronic lymphocytic leukaemia. Br J Haematol 1999;106:995–1004.

46. Schattner E, Mascarenhas J Reyfman I, et al. CLL B cells can express CD40 ligand and demonstrate T cell type costimulatory activity. Blood 1998;91:2689–2697.

47. Ranhein EA, Cantwell MJ, Kipps TJ. Expression of CD27 and its ligand, CD70, on chronic lymphocytic leukemia B cells. Blood 1995;85:3556–3565.

48. Trentin L, Zambello R, Sancetta R, et al. B lymphocytes from patients with chronic lymphoproliferative disorders are equipped with different co-stimulatory molecules. Cancer Res 1997;57:4940–4947.

49. Furman RR, Asgary Z, Mascarenhas J, Liou H-C, Schattner E. Modulation of NFκB activity and apoptosis in chronic lymphocytic leukemia B cells. J Immunol 2000;164:2200–2206.

50. Gheng G, Lee H, Dadgostar H, Cheng Q, Shu J. NFκB-mediated up-regulation of bcl-x and bfl-1/al is required for CD40 survival signaling in B lymphocytes. Proc Natl Acad Sci USA 1999;96:9136–9141.

51. Tonegawa S. Somatic generation of antibody diversity. Nature 1983;302:575–581.

52. Alt FW, Oltz EM, Young F, Gorman J, Taccioli G, Chen J. VDJ recombination. Immunol Today 1992;13:306–314.

53. Lewis S, Gellert M.The mechanism of antigen receptor gene assembly. Cell 1989;59:585–588.

54. Desiderio SV, Yancopoulos GD, Paskind M, et al. Insertion of N regions into heavy chain genes is correlated with the expression of terminal deoxytransferase in B cells. Nature 1984;311:752–755.

55. Corbett SJ, Tomlinson IM, Sonnhammer EL, Buck D, Winter G. Sequence of the human immunoglobulin diversity (D) segment locus: a systematic analysis provides no evidence for the use of DIR segments, inverted D segments, "minor" D segments or D-D recombination. J Mol Biol 1997;270:587–597.

56. Cook GP, Tomlinson IM. The human immunoglobulin VH repertoire. Immunol Today 1995;16:237–242.

57. Brezinschek HP, Brezinschek RI, Lipsky PE. Analysis of the heavy chain repertoire of human peripheral B cells using single-cell polymerase chain reaction. J Immunol 1995;155:190–202.

58. Wang YH, Nomura J, Faye-Petersen OM, Cooper MD. Surrogate light chain production during B cell differentiation: differential intracellular versus cell surface expression. J Immunol 1998;161:1132–1139.

59. MacLennan IC. Germinal centers. Annu Rev Immunol 1994;12:117–139

60. Stavnezer J, Sirlin S, Abbott J. Induction of immunoglobulin isotype switching in cultured I.29 B lymphoma cells. Characterization of the accompanying rearrangements of heavy chain genes. J Exp Med 1985;161: 577–601.

61. Matsuoka M, Yoshida K, Maeda T, Usuda S, Sakano H. Switch circular DNA formed in cytokine-treated mouse splenocytes: evidence for intramolecular DNA deletion in immunoglobulin class switching. Cell 1990;62: 135–142.

62. Liu YJ, Zhang J, Lane PJ, Can EY, MacLennan IC. Sites of specific B cell activation in primary and secondary responses to T-cell dependent and T-cell independent antigens. Eur J Immunol 1991;21:2951–2962.

63. Klein U, Rajewsky K, Kuppers R. Human immunoglobulin (Ig)M+IgD+ peripheral blood B cells expressing the CD27 cell surface antigen carry somatically mutated variable region genes: CD27 as a general marker for somatically mutated (memory) B cells. J Exp Med 1998;188:1679–1689.

64. Brezinschek HP, Foster SJ, Brezinschek RI, Dorner T, Domiati-Saad R, Lipsky PE. Analysis of the human VH gene repertoire. Differential effects of selection and somatic hypermutation on human peripheral CD5(+)/IgM+ and CD5(-)/IgM+ B cells. J Clin Invest 1997;99:2488–2501.

65. Kipps TJ, Tomhave E, Pratt LF, Duffey S, Chen PP, Carson DA. Developmentally restricted immunoglobulin heavy chain variable region gene expressed at high frequency in chronic lymphocytic leukemia. Proc Natl Acad Sci USA 1989;86:5913–5917.

66. Deane M, Norton JD. Preferential rearrangement of developmentally regulated immunoglobulin V_H1 genes in human B-lineage leukaemias. Leukemia 1991;5:646.

67. Ebeling SB, Schutte MEM, Akkermans-Koolhaas KE, Bloem AC, Gmelig-Meyling FHJ, Logtenberg T. Expression of members of the immunoglobulin V_H3 gene families is not restricted at the level of individual genes in human chronic lymphocytic leukemia. Int Immunol 1992;4:313.

68. Schroeder HWJr, Dighiero G. The pathogenesis of chronic lymphocytic leukemia: analysis of the antibody repertoire. Immunol Today 1994;15:288.

69. Matsuda F, Shin EK, Nagaoka H, et al. Structural and physical map of the 64 variable segments in the 3' 0.8 megabase region of the human immunoglobulin heavy chain locus. Nat Genet 1993;3:88.

70. Fais F, Ghiotto F, Hashimoto S, et al. Chronic lymphocytic leukemia B cells express restricted sets of mutated and unmutated antigen receptors. J Clin Invest 1998;102:1515.

71. Oscier DG, Thompsett A, Zhu D, Stevenson FK. Differential rates of somatic hypermutation in V_H genes among subsets of chronic lymphocytic leukemia defined by chromosomal abnormalities. Blood 1997;89:4153.

72. Maloum K, Davi F, Merle-Beral H, et al. expression of unmutated V_H genes is a detrimental prognostic factor in chronic lymphocytic leukemia. Blood 2000;96:377–378.

73. Bahler DW, Aguilera NS, Chen CC, Abbondanzo SL, Swerdlow SH. Histological and immunoglobulin VH gene analysis of interfollicular small lymphocytic lymphoma provides evidence for two types. Am J Pathol 2000;157: 1063–1070.

74. Kroeber A, Seiler T, Leupolt E, Dohner H, Stilgenbauer S, IgV_H mutated and unmutated B-CLL tumors show distinct genetic aberration patterns. Blood 2000;96:3609a, abstract.

75. Viale AC, Chies JA, Huetz F, et al. VH-gene family dominance in ageing mice. Scand J Immunol 1994;39:184–188.

76. Wang X, Stollar BD. Immunoglobulin VH gene expression in human aging. Clin Immunol 1999;93:132–142.

77. Hamblin TJ, Orchard JA, Ibbotson RE, et al. CD38 expression and immunoglobulin variable region mutations are independent prognostic variables in chronic lymphocytic leukemia, but CD38 expression may vary during the course of the disease. Blood 2002;99:1023–1029.

78. Howard M, Grimaldi JC, Bazan JF, et al. Formation and hydrolysis of cyclic ADP-ribose catalyzed by lymphocyte antigen CD38. Science 1993;262:1056–1059.

79. Malavasi F, Funaro A, Roggero S, Horenstein A, Calosso L, Mehta K. Human CD38: a glycoprotein in search of a function. Immunol Today 1994;15:95–97.

80. Deaglio S, Mehta K, Malavasi F. Human CD38: a (r)evolutionary story of enzymes and receptors. Leuk Res 2001; 25:1–12.

81. Bauvois B, Durant L, Laboureau J, et al. Upregulation of CD38 gene expression in leukemic B cells by interferon types I and II. J Interferon Cytokine Res 1999;19:1059–1066.

82. Oscier DG, Gardiner AC, Mould SJ, et al. Multivariate analysis of prognostic factors in CLL: clinical stage, V_H gene mutational status, and loss or mutation of the p53 gene are independent prognostic factors. Blood 2002,100: 1177–1184.

83. Rosenwald A, Alizadeh AA, Widhopf G, et al. Relation of gene expression phenotype to immunoglobulin mutation genotype in B cell chronic lymphocytic leukemia. J Exp Med 2001;194:1639–1647.

84. Klein U, Tu Y, Stolovitzky GA, et al. Gene expression profiling of B cell chronic lymphocytic leukemia reveals a homogeneous phenotype related to memory B cells. J Exp Med 2001;194:1625–1638.

85. Chiorazzi N, Ferrarini M. Immunoglobulin variable region gene characteristics and surface membrane phenotype define B-CLL subgroups with distinct clinical courses. In: Cheson BD, ed. Chronic Lymphoid Leukemias, 2nd ed. Marcel Dekker, New York, 2001, pp. 81–109.

86. Nagumo H, Agematsu K, Kobayashi N, et al. The different process of class switching and somatic mutation; a novel analysis by CD27-naïve B cells. Blood 2002;99:567–575.

87. Tobin G, Thunberg U, Johnson A, et al. Somatically mutated Ig VH3-21 genes characterize a new subset of chronic lymphocytic leukemia. Blood 2002;99:2262–2264.

88. Caligaris-Cappio F, Hamblin TJ. B-cell chronic lymphocytic leukemia: a bird of a different feather. J Clin Oncol 1999;17:399–408.

89. Dameshek W. Chronic lymphocytic leukemia: an accumulative disease of immunologically incompetent lymphocytes. Blood 1967:29:566–584.

5

Pathogenesis of Impaired Cellular Immune Function in CLL

Patrick B. Johnston, MD *and Neil E. Kay,* MD

1. INTRODUCTION

B-cell chronic lymphocytic leukemia (B-CLL) is defined as a monoclonal B-cell malignancy with a characteristic cell surface phenotype including expression of both CD19 and CD5 antigens (*see* Chapter 7). The clinical events characterizing the patients who eventually progress are most often linked to an accumulation of clonal CD5+ leukemic cells, particularly in the bone marrow, lymph nodes, and spleen. Although the hallmark of the leukemic CLL B-cell is its resistance to apoptosis, there is no significant insight into the exact biological reasons for that seminal biological event. It is probably true that critical genetic events are primary and lead to the B-cell resistance to apoptosis. However, we would hypothesize that the role of the microenvironment, including tissue-specific stroma, cytokine levels, vascular supply, and the host immune system, contribute to the augmentation and/or stabilize CLL B-cell apoptotic resistance. Thus, we have been interested in the study of both the qualitative and quantitative nature of the immune system in B-CLL.

An additional rationale for understanding the immune system in B-CLL patients is the frequent occurrence of clinical complications that may be related to the presence of an expanding leukemic B-cell clone and/or to a dysfunctional immune system.

B-CLL patients exhibit a range of infections resulting from a number of infectious agents (i.e., bacterial, viral), suggesting defects in humoral and cellular immunity. B-CLL patients with advanced but sometimes with early-stage disease may have hypogammaglobulinemia. In addition, this can be accompanied by recurrent, severe infections in diverse organ sites. Most of the infections are bacterial, and the various strains include *Streptococcus pneumoniae, Staphylococcus aureus,* and *Escherichia coli.* Although the bacterial infections could be linked to a simple deficiency in humoral immunity, B-CLL patients also have increasing problems with viral and fungal infections, particularly as the disease progresses. In addition, early reports have suggested that there are significant increases in certain malignancies (i.e., skin, colon) *(1).* A more recent publication *(2)* has found that second cancer risks for patients who received chemotherapy up front were similar to risks for CLL patients who received no initial therapy. Interestingly the most common second cancers in that series included Kaposi's sarcoma, malignant melanoma, and cancers of the lung and larynx. In addition, there are frequent autoimmune complications (i.e., immune hemolysis, idiopathic throbocytopenia [ITP]) in B-CLL patients. These latter clinical complications could at least in part be related to extensive deficiencies in the humoral and/or

From: *Contemporary Hematology*
Chronic Lymphocytic Leukemia: Molecular Genetics, Biology, Diagnosis, and Management
Edited by: G. B. Faguet © Humana Press Inc., Totowa, NJ

cellular components of the B-CLL immune system. Finally, with increasing use of potent chemo-therapeutic agents such as the purine nucleoside analogs, there will be additional cellular immune defects for the B-CLL patient.

In summary, the underlying biology of the disease and its clinical correlates have prompted a wide array of in vitro studies of the immune system in B-CLL patients. These latter studies have shown that there are significant recurring abnormalities in the nonmalignant immune cells of these patients. The increasingly refined information regarding the specific abnormalities of these immune cells is reviewed here with emphasis on the potential relationship of these findings to clinical complications often associated with B-CLL. The lessons learned from studying these relationships may lead to future unique therapeutic applications in the management of B-CLL patients.

2. OVERVIEW OF THE IMMUNE DEFICITS IN B-CLL

To set the stage for a description of the immune deficits in B-CLL, we provide a brief, relevant review of the normal immune system. An intact immune system will include both humoral and cellular components. The humoral component is comprised of circulating antibodies (i.e., IgA, IgG, IgM) that have reactivity to specific antigens and are important in the host defense against infectious microbes. A polyclonal population of B-lymphocytes residing primarily in the lymph nodes, spleen, and gastrointestinal tract produces these antibodies. These antibodies react with antigens, including those on the surface of the infectious microbe (particularly with encapsulated bacteria), allowing the innate cellular immune system to recognize and destroy the infectious agent. Antibodies can also trigger the cellular release (i.e., by mast cells, monocytes) of inflam-matory mediators (i.e., cytokines, chemokines) that are important in recruiting additional immune cells to participate and compete for the host response.

The cellular components of the immune system involve numerous cell types, including T-lymphocytes, natural killer (NK) cells, and dendritic cells (DCs). Those of potential clinical importance in B-CLL are briefly discussed here. T-lymphocytes have memory and specificity to particular infectious agents (viral and bacterial), whereas NK cells are capable of spontaneous and nonspecific killing of viral infected cells and tumor cells. NK function is often referred to as innate immunity. T-lymphocytes can be divided into two functionally distinct groups, CD4+ (Th) helper and CD8+ cytolytic/suppressor cells (Ts). Both subsets can be divided on the basis of cytokine secretion profiles. Thus, T1 T-cells (Th1, Ts1) secrete predominantly interleukin-2 (IL-2) and/or interferon-γ vs IL-4, IL-5, and IL-10 for the T2 cells (Th2, Ts2 type cells). It is important for host defense to have a complete T-cell repertoire of both CD4+ and CD8+ subsets. An important aspect of activated CD4+ helper T-cells includes the release of an array of cytokines (i.e., IL-2, interferon-γ) with many disparate functions, including activation of B- and T-lymphocytes. This stimulation is critical in initiating and amplifying the proliferation and differentiation of these cells. An important role for activated CD8+ cytolytic T-lymphocytes is to react with the target cell and induce cell lysis. This latter activity is particularly important in the destruction of intracellular infectious agents, including viruses and intracellular bacteria. In addition, these cells can release cytokines such as interferon and tumor necrosis factor.

In the normal immune response, T-cell activation is mediated by interactions between antigen-presenting cells (APCs) like B-cells and dendritic cells (DC). These interactions involve a pathway of highly regulated events critical for specific activation and control of both B- and T-cells (Fig. 1). T-cells that encounter antigen in conjunction with APCs have cell-cell contact via at least the leukocyte function associated antigen-1 (LFA-1; CD11a) and intercellular adhesion

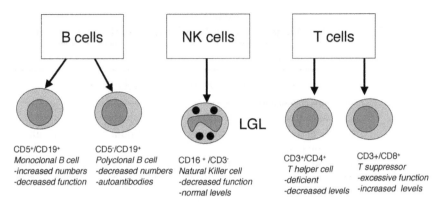

Fig. 1. Immune cell compartments known to be abnormal in B-CLL. Only the most well-characterized defects are listed here. Thus, both the polyclonal and malignant B-cells are deficient and at least contribute to the hypogammaglobulinemia often seen in this disease. The natural killer (NK) cells are consistently abnormal and may represent a significant defect in innate immunity for these patients. Finally, T-cells in this disease have many complex defects that in total give many B-CLL patients considerable difficulty both in resisting infections and in generating an effective antitumor impact. LGL, large granular lymphocyte.

molecule-1 (ICAM-1; CD54) interaction. At that time cell binding is still nonspecific and of low affinity. The LFA-1/ICAM-1 interaction is a major contributor to adhesion between T-cells and other lymphoid cells. The binding of LFA-1 (CD11a)/ICAM-1 (CD54) allows the cells to be brought into close proximity for antigen recognition to take place via the T-cell receptor (TCR)/ CD3 complex. T-cell response (T-cell activation) is enhanced via interactions between HLA antigens and the TCR, a process that is upregulated by the CD3 complex and strengthened by CD4 (MHC class II) or CD8 (MHC class I) binding. TCR/CD3 complex signals lead to the initiation of key T-cell immune responses, including cytokine production and surface marker upregulation. The T-cell surface marker CD28 interacts with the CD80/CD86 receptors on the B-cells, and increased expression of CD154 on the T-cell leads to binding with its B-cell surface ligand, CD40. Production of IL-2 occurs, and receptors for this cytokine (CD25/IL-2R) are expressed some 2 d post activation, facilitating recruitment of other T-cells with continued activation and clonal expansion. It is believed that expression of CTLA-4 (CD152) sends a negative "off" signal to the T-cell, which serves to control the immune response via cessation of T-cell proliferation or by inducing apoptosis.

B-CLL is notable in that a significant proportion of patients develop infectious complications, which are associated with impaired immune responses. Because of the frequent bacterial infections seen early on in the disease course of B-CLL and the viral/fungal infections seen later on or with therapy in B-CLL, investigations into the underlying causes have been undertaken. Early studies identified defects in both the humoral and cellular immune responses. Hypogammaglobulinemia detected by serum protein electrophoresis has been noted to occur in up to 70% of these patients *(3)*, and significant declines in certain antibody classes have been demonstrated to correlate with disease severity *(4)*. It is likely that up to 50% of patients with B-CLL sustain infectious complications during the course of their disease. Patients with hypogammaglobulinemia have more frequent infections with encapsulated bacteria, including *Streptococcus pneumoniae* and *Hemophilus influenza (5,6)*. Not only is the overall level of circulating antibodies reduced in B-CLL, but antibody responses to individual vaccination appears to decline with

Table 1
B-CLL Immune Cell Dysfunction and Associated Clinical Complications

Affected cell type	Associated defect
B-cell	Hypogammaglobulinemia—increased bacterial infections
	Decreased vaccination response
T-cell	Increased viral and intracellular bacterial infections
Natural killer cell	Possible association with increased autoimmune phenomena and/or second malignancies
Dendritic cell	? Unknown, possible dysfunction

progressive disease (7). Recent in vitro data suggest that the B-CLL cells inhibit spontaneous immunoglobulin production by bone marrow cells, suggesting an etiology for the hypogamma-globulinemia (8). In addition, the monoclonal B-CLL B-cells often produce antibodies, which are reactive with self antigens (9). These antibodies may contribute to immune abnormalities seen with this disorder (10).

Components of the cellular immune system are also known to be impaired/altered in patients with B-CLL. Figure 1 summarizes the different immune cell subsets known to be abnormal in patients with B-CLL. Most prominently, blood T-cell dysfunction has been well documented with B-CLL patients. The blood CD4/CD8 ratio, with a relative decrease in helper phenotype, has been reported in patients with B-CLL (11,12). A clinical manifestation of this defect in T-lymphocyte function may include the decreased responsiveness or anergy noted on skin recall antigen tests to common antigens. NK cells in B-CLL have a significant deficit in their ability to be activated and to lyse appropriate cellular targets (13). Less information is available for DCs/APCs, although some recent information suggests that these cells are also defective in B-CLL (reviewed below in Subheading 3.5.). These in vitro immune defects and their potential relationship to clinical and/or immune defects seen in vivo in B-CLL are listed in Table 1.

3. IMMUNE CELL PROFILES IN B-CLL

3.1. Malignant B-Cells (CD5+/CD19+)

The malignant B-CLL B-cell has been well characterized by surface immunophenotype. This latter feature gives us a potential clue as to its origin and functional capacity. In addition to the common B-cell antigens CD19, CD20, and CD21, these malignant cells have been demonstrated to express CD5 and variable amounts of surface-bound immunoglobulin (sIg). In normal hosts, CD5+ B-cells occur at the edge of germinal centers in the mantle zone of lymphoid follicles (14) and are found in cord blood. This latter marker on the malignant B-CLL clone may provide insight into the level of arrest in development of the monoclonal CLL B-cell. The faint expression of sIgs on the B-CLL B-cells is also common to normal B-cells at the edge of germinal centers. The sIgs in B-CLL are usually IgM and/or IgD, and rarely IgG or IgA (15). The sIgs often have reactivity for multiple self-antigens (polyreactive autoantibodies) with low avidity and frequently behave like rheumatoid factor (9). Up to 25% of patients with B-CLL have associated autoimmune phenomena, including autoimmune hemolytic anemia and autoimmune thrombocytopenia (10). Interestingly, the offending autoantibodies are of the IgG type and do not appear to be a direct product of the B-CLL B-cells. Thus, there is a discrepancy between the B-CLL-associated cell-bound, low-affinity IgM antibodies and the circulating, cytopenia-inducing IgG autoantibodies. To date it is not clear whether the CLL B-cell sIg plays a role in the induction of the IgG autoantibodies.

Investigations into the nature of modulation of B-cell surface receptors and other molecules on the monoclonal B-cell have provided insight into the etiology of some aspects of the cellular immune dysfunction seen with B-CLL. Recent studies have identified the presence of CD95 ligand (CD95L) on the cell surface of B-CLL cells. CD95 (Fas) is a known death receptor protein expressed on the surface of cells, and its interaction with CD95L results in apoptosis of the CD95-expressing cell. Panayiotidis et al. *(16)* demonstrated decreased levels of CD95 on the leukemic B-cells in CLL patients. However, subsequent work demonstrated increased Fas ligand (CD95L) on the surface of the monoclonal CLL B-cell *(17)*. The exact nature of CD95–CD95L interaction on CLL B-cells needs to be more fully delineated, since this is an important death pathway. Recent work by Sampalo et al. *(8)*. detected the spontaneous inhibition of autologous bone marrow cell production of Ig by normal B-cells via a mechanism involving B-CLL B-cells. Cocultivation of CD5+-depleted bone marrow cells with autologous B-CLL B-cells resulted in decreased Ig production by the bone marrow cells, and this effect increased when the leukemic B-cells were stimulated with phorbol myristate acetate (PMA). The bone marrow plasma cells were demonstrated to express CD95, whereas the monoclonal CLL B-cells were found to express CD95L. Most importantly, increased apoptosis was detected when the bone marrow plasma cells were incubated with the monoclonal CLL B-cells. This CD95-CD95L interaction could result in increased apoptosis of the normal Ig-producing B-cells and suggests a unique cellular mechanism for the hypogammaglobulinemia noted in B-CLL patients. Additional work has also demonstrated the increased expression of CD95 on both CD4+ and CD8+ T-cells in B-CLL *(17)*. The implications of this work with regard to its effect on the cellular immune system in B-CLL will be discussed in more detail below.

CD23 is a protein expressed on the surface of most of B-CLL B-cells. The protein is a low-affinity receptor for IgE and is an adhesion molecule expressed on activated mature B-cells. CD23 expression appears to be upregulated when immature B-cells are exposed to IL-4 *(18)*. Proteolysis of CD23 results in increased concentrations of soluble CD23. Indeed, most patients with B-CLL have been noted to have increased levels of soluble CD23. Furthermore, the plasma level of CD23 correlates with disease activity *(19,20)*. Interestingly, soluble CD23 can induce cell growth and differentiation of B- and T-cells as well as myeloid cell lines *(21,22)*. CD21 is the natural ligand for CD23 *(23)*, and their interaction is involved in cell adhesion, B-cell activation, and proliferation. Since these two molecules are coexpressed on B-CLL B-cell membranes, their interaction may promote growth or cellular viability of the leukemic cells.

The monoclonal CLL B-cell appears to be an ineffective APC. Normal activated B-cells are effective APCs, which interact with T-cells to elicit an immune response. The inability of CLL B-cells to act as effective APCs can be explained in part by their diminished expression of membrane CD80 (B7-1) and CD86 (B7-2), costimulatory molecules required for T-cell activation *(24)*. Activation of the T-cell requires at least two receptor-receptor ligand interactions. First, the antigen/major histocompatibility complex must bind to the T-cell receptor (TCR). In addition, the CD80/CD86 complex must bind to CD28 on the T-cell surface to elicit activation of the T-cell *(25)*. Stimulation of the TCR without CD28 interaction with CD80/CD86 results in T-cell anergy *(26)*.

CLL B-cells, as well as normal B-lymphocytes, express CD40 on their cell surface. CD40, a member of the tumor necrosis factor (TNF) receptor superfamily, interacts with CD40 ligand (CD154), which is transiently expressed on activated T-cells, leading to B-cell activation with

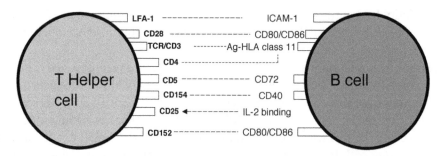

Fig. 2. Membrane profile of the B-cell and the T-helper cell with respect to expression of the critical activation or receptor/receptor ligand interactions that are probably involved in the efficient and complete activation of the the the T-cell. Since the CLL B-cell is often deficient in several of these important receptors (reviewed in text and briefly in Fig. 3) the T-cell may not be properly activated in patients with B-CLL. ICAM, intercellular adhesion molecule; LFA-1, leukocyte function-associated antigen-1.

upregulation of various molecules, including CD80 *(27)*. Incubation of CLL B-cells with activated T-cells similarly resulted in upregulation of CD80 in the leukemic cells *(28,29)* Kato et al. *(30)* noted that the CD4+ T-cells of patients with CLL failed to express surface CD154 after CD3 ligation despite adequate levels of mRNA for CD154. These investigators determined that CLL B-cells could also block the induction of CD154 in normal T-cells by a CD40-directed mechanism.

Thus, a negative complex feedback mechanism appears to exist in B-CLL, in which the decreased APC ability of the leukemic B-cell pool results in T-cell anergy, whereas the absence of activated T-cells results in deficient B-cell activation. Figure 2 illustrates the spectrum of membrane antigens on B-cells known to be crucial to efficient and vigorous T-cell helper activation. A novel strategy to break this "immunodeficiency" cycle has involved the introduction of transgenic CD154 expression in CLL B-cells. This generates CD154 on the membrane of CLL B-cells, resulting in a more efficient leukemic APC and subsequent induction of cytolytic T-cell activity *(30)*. This approach for the transformation of leukemic CLL B-cells into effective APCs is currently undergoing clinical trials.

An additional set of T-cell costimulatory molecules, CD27 and CD70, appear to be regulated in a matter similar to CD40/CD154 *(31)*. CD27 expressed on the surface of B-cells appears to interact with CD70 on the surface of T-cells. This interaction, in concert with TCR activation, results in T-cell proliferation. Ranheim et al. *(31)* demonstrated the coexpression of CD70 and CD27 on the surface of leukemic B-cells, and soluble CD27 was also detectable. A CD40-dependent downmodulation of CD27 with reciprocal upregulation of CD70 was noted in the B-CLL B-cells. The latter work has suggested that the CD27-CD70 interactions on CLL B-cells may be an important and distinct costimulatory signal for T-cell proliferation. The possible role of soluble CD27 in disturbing this costimulation exists in B-CLL since there are increased levels of soluble CD27 in B-CLL. Finally, there are complex and contrary changes for CD70 on CLL B-cells in relation to the cytokine(s) present in the microenvironment. Thus, the complex interplay between various surface molecules necessary for efficient T-cell activation may not occur because of membrane abnormalities present on CLL B-cells. Some of the contributing factors that probably impact on T-cell function in B-CLL are illustrated in Fig. 3. This defective B/T-cell interaction probably has implications for the cellular immune arm of the B-CLL patient. Table 2 summarizes the aberrant expression of surface molecules on B-CLL cells and their role in immune dysfunction.

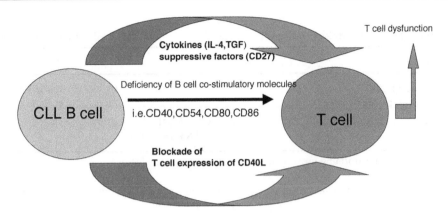

Fig. 3. Multiple causes of T-cell immunodeficiency in B-CLL. Both B-cell secreted cytokines and defective membrane receptor profiles of B-cells can lead to significant T-cell dysfunction including decreased CD40 ligand and ultimately T-cell functional defects that include poor proliferative response to mitogens and defective helper and cytotoxic function. IL, interleukin; TGF, transforming growth factor.

Table 2
Aberrant Expression of Surface Molecules on B-CLL Cells and Their Role in Immune Dysfunction

Surface molecule	Effect on immune cells
Increased CD95 ligand	Apoptosis of CD95-expressing cells: possible role in development of hypogammaglobulinemia owing to interaction with CD95+ B-cells, resultant decrease in CD95+ T-cells
Increased CD5	Unknown function
Increased CD23 (cell-bound and soluble)	Induction of B-cell proliferation
Increased CD21	Receptor for CD23, coexpression may promote leukemic cell growth
Decreased CD80	Coexpression with CD86 and interaction with T-cell required for T-cell activation
Decreased CD86	*See* CD80 above
Increased soluble CD27	May have role in interrupting normal CD27/CD70 interaction necessary for T-cell activation
Increased interleukin-4 receptor	Decreased apoptosis

3.2. Nonmalignant B-Cells

The nonmalignant B-cell population (i.e., polyclonal cells) in B-CLL is not well characterized. The proportion and overall number of nonmalignant B-cells in patients with B-CLL is often significantly reduced. It has been postulated that this may, however, represent a dilutional effect. Regardless, B-cell function in many patients with B-CLL is abnormal, as exemplified by the frequent hypogammaglobulinemia and decreased antibody response to immunization seen in B-CLL patients. Multiple factors may contribute to the abnormal polyclonal B-cell function in B-CLL. As discussed above, CD95-CD95L interactions may contribute to the decreased number of antibody-producing cells in these patients *(8)*. Also, CD5+ B-CLL cells can produce elevated levels of transforming growth factor-β, which may contribute to hyporesponsiveness of the normal B-cells *(32)*. Since the autoantibodies responsible for the autoimmune disease are prob-

Table 3
Cytokine Production and Cytokine Receptor Changes in T- and B-CLL Cells of Patients With B-CLL

Cytokine alterations	CLL B-cells	T-cells
Elevated cytokine levels[a]	IL-4, TGF-β	IL-4, TNF-α, IL-2
Decreased cytokine levels[a]		IL-10
Elevated cytokine receptor levels	CD25, CD119, CD124, IL-4 receptor, IL-6 receptor, TNF receptor	

IL, interleukin; TGF, transforming growth factor; TNF, tumor necrosis factor.
Modified from ref. 33.
[a]Cytokine alteraltions have been described as altered in the cell's culture medium or in the cytoplasm or in both.

ably produced by the residual pool of normal B-cells in B-CLL, further work needs to be done to examine the functional capacity of these B-cells. This work should provide additional clues regarding the etiology of these autoimmune disorders.

3.3. T-Cells

In addition to the polyclonal B-cell defects noted in patients with B-CLL, numerical and functional abnormalities exist in the T (CD3+) cell population in these patients. Because of the increased number of malignant B-cells, the percentage of T-lymphocytes is reduced; however, the absolute number of blood T-lymphocytes is often increased. Interestingly, a relative decrease in CD4+ T-cells is noted, with a relative increase in CD8+ T-cells in these patients (33; Table 3). A possible factor in the development of this CD4+ T-cell deficit may relate to the membrane expression of CD95 discussed above. Work by Tinhofer et al. (17) identified increased levels of CD95 (Fas) on the surface of CD4+ T-cells and CD8+ T-cells derived from patients with B-CLL (17). Stimulation of CD95 with monoclonal antibodies to Fas resulted in apoptosis of the CD4+ T-cells, but not the CD8+ T-cells.

Early studies identified oligoclonal T-cell populations in the blood of most B-CLL patients, utilizing molecular cloning techniques that detail the T-cell receptor repertoire (34,35). Further investigation with polymerase chain reaction (PCR) identified oligoclonal expansion in both the CD4+ and CD8+ T-cell subsets (36,37). Although initial studies by Rezany et al. (36) suggested that the T-cell clonality occurred primarily within the CD4+ T-cell subset, more recent studies have suggested that these perturbations are primarily restricted to the CD8+ T-cell population (38). In this study, Goolsby et al. (38) used multicolor flow cytometric techniques to assess the presence of oligoclonal T-cell populations directly in the blood of B-CLL patients. Nine of 19 patients were found to have clonal/oligoclonal expansion of a T-cell subset, based on flow cytometry. Molecular analysis of the T-cell receptor gene utilizing PCR was used to complement these findings. Of the 16 patients who underwent molecular testing, 12 were found to have clonal/oligoclonal patterns. In addition, based on the flow cytometric analysis, it was demonstrated that this occurred primarily within the CD8+ T-cell subset. It is perhaps relevant that certain T-cell subsets with oligoclonal expansion in the CD8+ T-cell population may be associated with an increased risk of disease progression in early-stage B-CLL (R.L. Bjork, Jr., personal communication).

Expansion of CD8+ T-cells detected by other methods have been described in B-CLL. Two separate investigations (39,40) demonstrated the presence of CD8+ B-CLL T-cells with a polarized cytokine profile for IL-4. In addition these T-cells were able to release IL-4 spontaneously. Since the latter cytokine is able to enhance CLL B-cell resistance to apoptosis, it is possible this

45. Huang R, Tsuda H, Takatsuki K. Interleukin-2 prevents programmed cell death in chronic lymphocytic leukemia cells. Int J Hematol 1993;58:83–92.

46. Buschle M, Campana D, Carding S, Richard C, Hoffbrand A, Brenner M. Interferon gamma inhibits apoptotic cell death in B cell chronic lymphocytic leukemia. J Exp Med 1993;177:213–218.

47. Mainou-Fowler T, Craig V, Copplestone J, Hamon M, Prentice A. Interleukin-5 (IL-5) increases spontaneous apoptosis of B-cell chronic lymphocytic leukemia cells in vitro independently of bcl-2 expression and is inhibited by IL-4. Blood 1994;84:2297–2304.

48. Fluckiger A, Durand I, Banchereau J. Interleukin 10 induces apoptotic cell death lymphocytic leukemia cells. J Exp Med 1994;179:91–99.

49. Foa R, Massaia M, Cardona S, et al. Production of tumor necrosis factor-alpha by B-cell chronic lymphocytic leukemia cells: a possible regulatory role of TNF in the progression of the disease. Blood 1990;76:393–400.

50. Mainou-Fowler T, Miller S, Proctor SJ, Dickinson AM. The levels of TNF-α, IL-4 and IL-10 production by T-cells in B-cell chronic lymphocytic leukemia (B-CLL). Leuk Res 2001;25:157–163.

51. Scrivener S, Kaminski ER, Demaine A, Prentice AG. Analysis of the expression of critical activation/interaction markers on peripheral blood T-cells in B-cell chronic lymphocytic leukaemia: evidence of immune dysregulation. Br J Hematol 2001;112:959–964.

52. Kaleem Z, White G, Zutter MM. Aberrant expression of T-cell associated antigens on B-cell non-Hodgkin lymphomas. Am J Clin Pathol 2001;115:396–403.

53. Dieckmann D, Plottner H, Berchtold S, Berger T, Schuler G. Ex vivo isolation and characterization of CD4+CD25+ T-cells with regulatory properties from human blood. J Exp Med 2001;193:1303–1310.

54. Vuillier F, Tortevoye P, Binet JL, Dighiero G. CD4, CD8 and NK subsets in B-CLL. Nouv Rev Fr Hematol 1988; 30:331–334.

55. Apostolopoulos A, Symeonidis A, Zoumbos N. Prognostic significance of immune function parameters in patients with chronic lymphocytic leukaemia. Eur J Haematol 1990;44:39–44.

56. Frolova E, Richards S, Jones R, et al. Immunophenotypic and DNA genotypic analysis of T-cell and NK-cell subpopulations in patients with B-cell chronic lymphocytic leukaemia (B-CLL). Leuk Lymph 1995;16:307–318.

57. Ziegler H, Kay NE, Zarling J. Deficiency of natural killer cell activity in patients with chronic lymphocytic leukemia. Int J Cancer 1981;27:321–327.

58. Alvarez de Mon M, Casas J, Laguna R, Toribio M, deLandazuri M, Durantez A. Lymphokine induction of NK-like cytotoxicity in T-cells from B-CLL. Blood 1986;67:228–232.

59. Katrinakis G, Kyriakou D, Papadaki H, Kalokyri I, Markidou F, Eliopoulos G. Defective natural killer cell activity in B-cell chronic lymphocytic leukaemia is associated with impaired release of natural killer cytotoxic factor(s) but not of tumour necrosis factor-alpha. Acta Haematol 1996;96:16–23.

60. Gunzer M, Janich S, Varga G, Grabbe S. Dendritic cells and tumor immunity. Semin Immunol 2001;13:291–302.

61. Bleijs DA, Geijtenbeek TB, Figdor CG, van Kooyk Y. DC-SIGN and LFA-1: a battle for ligand. Trends Immunol 2001;22:457–463.

62. Vuillier F, Maloum K, Thomas E, Jouanne C, Dighiero G, Scott-Algara D. Monocyte-derived dendritic cells from CLL patients display normal phenotypic and functional properties but spontaneously secrete IL-10. Blood 2001;98:287b.

63. Chilosi M, Pizzolo G, Caligaris-Cappio F, et al. Immunohistochemical demonstration of follicular dendritic cells in bone marrow involvement of B-cell chronic lymphocytic leukemia. Cancer 1985;56:328–332.

64. Stadelmeyer E, Grube R, Chraust S, Linkesch W, Strunk D. Alteration of dendritic cell function in B-CLL. Blood 2001;98:287b.

65. Orsini E, Chiaretti S, Mauro F, Guarini A, Foa R. Defective dendritic cell compartment in chronic lymphocytic leukemia patients. Blood 2001;98:731a.

20. Sarfati M. Prognostic importance of serum soluble CD23 level in chronic lymphocytic leukemia. Blood 1996; 88:4259–4264.
21. Liu Y, Cairns J, Holder M, et al. Recombinant 25-kDa CD23 and interleukin 1 alpha promote the survival of germinal center B-cells: evidence for bifurcation in the development of centrocytes rescued from apoptosis. Eur J Immunol 1991;21:1107–1114.
22. Mossalayi M, Arock M, Bertho J, et al. Proliferation of early human myeloid precursors induced by interleukin-1 and recombinant soluble CD23. Blood 1990;75:1924–1927.
23. Aubry JP, Pochon S, Graber P, Jansen KU, Bonnefoy JY. CD21 is a ligand for CD23 and regulates IgE production. Nature 1992;358:505–507.
24. Dorfman DM, Schultze JL, Shahsafaei A, et al. In vivo expression of B7-1 and B7-2 by follicular lymphoma cells can prevent induction of T-cell anergy but is insufficient to induce significant T-cell proliferation. Blood 1997;90:4297–4306.
25. Linsley P, Brady W, Grosmaire L, Aruffo A, Damle N, Ledbetter J. Binding of the B cell activation antigen B7 to CD28 costimulates T cell proliferation and interleukin 2 mRNA accumulation. J Exp Med 1991;173:721–730.
26. Schwartz R. Costimulation of lymphocyites: the role of CD28, CTLA-4, and B7/BB1 in interleukin-2 production and immunotherapy. Cell 1992;71:1065–1068.
27. Eris J, Basten A, Brink R, Doherty K, Kehry M, Hodgkin P. Anergic self-reactive B-cells present self antigen and respond normally to CD40-dependent T-cell signals but are defective in antigen-receptor-mediated functions. Proc Natl Acad Sci USA 1994;91:4392–4396.
28. Ranheim E, Kipps T. Activated T-cells induce expression of B7/BB1 on normal or leukemic B-cells through a CD40-dependent signal. J Exp Med 1993;177:925–935.
29. Yellin M, Sinning J, Covey L, et al. T lymphocyte T cell-B cell-activating molecule/CD40-L molecules induce normal B-cells or chronic lymphocytic leukemia B-cells to express CD80 (B7/BB-1) and enhance their costimulatory activity. J Immunol 1994;153:666–674.
30. Kato K, Cantwell MJ, Sharma S, Kipps TJ. Gene transfer of CD40-ligand induces autologous immune recognition of chronic lymphocytic leukemia B-cells. J Clin Invest 1998;101:1133–1141.
31. Ranheim E, Cantwell MJ, Kipps TJ. Expression of CD27 and its ligand, CD70, on chronic lymphocytic leukemia B-cells. Blood 1995;85:3556–3565.
32. Lotz M, Ranheim E, Kipps T. Transforming growth factor beta as endogenous growth inhibitor of chronic lymphocytic leukemia B-cells. J Exp Med 1994;179:999–1004.
33. Zaknoen S, Kay N. Immunoregulatory cell dysfunction in chronic B-cell leukemias. Blood Review 1990;4:165–174.
34. Farace F, Orlanducci F, Dietrich P, et al. T cell repertoire in patients with B chronic lymphocytic leukemia: evidence for multiple in vivo T cell clonal expansions. J Immunol 1994;153:4281–4290.
35. Wen T, Mellstedt H, Jondal M. Presence of clonal T cell populations in chronic B lymphocytic leukemia and smoldering myeloma. J Exp Med 1990;171:659–666.
36. Rezvany M-R, Jeddi-Tehrani M, Osterborg A, Kimby E, Wigzell H, Mellstedt H. Oligoclonal TCRBV gene usage in B-cell chronic lymphocytic leukemia: major perturbations are preferentially seen within the CD4 T-cell subset. Blood 1999;94:1063–1069.
37. Serrano D, Monteiro J, Allen S, et al. Clonal expansion within the CD4+ CD57+ and CD8+ CD57+ T cell subsets in chronic lymphocytic leukemia. J Immunol 1997;158:1482–1489.
38. Goolsby CL, Kuchnio M, Finn WG, Peterson L. Expansions of clonal and oligoclonal T-cells in B-cell chronic lymphocytic leukemia are primarily restricted to the CD3+CD8+ T-cell population. Cytometry 2000;42:188–195.
39. Mu X, Kay NE, Gosland MP, Jennings CD. Analysis of blood T-cell cytokine expression in B-chronic lymphocytic leukaemia: evidence for increased levels of cytoplasmic IL-4 in resting and activated CD8 T-cells. Br J Haematol 1997;96:733–735.
40. de Totero D, Reato G, Mauro F, et al. IL4 production and increased CD30 expression by a unique CD8+ T-cell subset in B-cell chronic lymphocytic leukemia. Br J Haematol 1999;104:589–599.
41. Kay NE, Han L, Bone ND, Williams G. Interleukin 4 content in chronic lymphocytic leukaemia (CLL) B-cells and blood CD8+ T-cells from B-CLL patients: impact on clonal B-cell apoptosis. Br J Hematol 2001;112:760–767.
42. Dancescu M, Rubio-Trujillo M, Biron G, Bron D, Delespesse G, Sarfati M. Interleukin 4 protects chronic lymphocytic leukemic B-cells from death by apoptosis and upregulates Bcl-2 expression. J Exp Med 1992;176:1319–1326.
43. Mainou-Fowler T, Craig V, Copplestone J, Hamon M, Prentice A. Effect of anti-APO1 on spontaneous apoptosis of B-cells in chronic lymphocytic leukaemia: the role of bcl-2 and interleukin 4. Leuk Lymph 1995;19:301–308.
44. Mainou-Fowler T, Copplestone J, Prentice A. Effect of interleukins on the proliferation and survival of B cell chronic lymphocytic leukaemia cells. J Clin Pathol 1995;48:482–487.

tioning in B-CLL has provided further targets for therapeutic intervention. For example, the identification of the defective CD40/CD154 interaction leading to poor APC ability has resulted in the design and introduction of gene therapy intended to make the leukemic cells "visible" to the innate immune system. Other opportunities include the judicious exploration and testing of cytokines such as IL-2 to improve NK function or interruption of cytokine pathways like IL-4 that impact on CLL B-cell apoptosis. Newer technologies, including gene array profiling, may lgive us insight into the nature of the complex interplay between cells in the immune system. Innovative strategies designed to treat B-CLL appearing on the near horizon include peptide and cellular vaccines and the use of cytokines or donor lymphocyte infusions. Given that these vaccines require a competent immune system to yield optimum clinical results, we need to develop strategies specifically designed to activate, enhance, and replete the host immune system. This latter activity probably represents the most significant challenge in our long-term management and care of B-CLL patients.

REFERENCES

1. Manusow D, Weinerman BH, Hisada M, et al. Subsequent neoplasia in chronic lymphocytic leukemia. JAMA 1975;232:267–269.
2. Hisada M, Biggar RJ, Greene MH, Fraumeni JF, Jr., Travis LB. Solid tumors after chronic lymphocytic leukemia. Blood 2001;98:1979–1981.
3. Rozman C, Montserrat E, Vinolas N. Serum immunoglobulins in B-CLL: natural history and prognostic significance. Cancer 1988;61:279–283.
4. Rozman C, Montserrat E. Chronic lymphocytic leukemia. N Engl J Med 1995;333:1052–1057.
5. Shaw R, Szwed C, Boggs D. Infection and immunity in chronic lymphocytic leukemia. Arch Intern Med 1960; 106:467–477.
6. Twomey J. Infections complicating multiple myeloma and chronic lymphocytic leukemia. Arch Intern Med 1973; 132:562–565.
7. Hartkamp A, Mulder A, Rijkers G. Antibody responses to pneumococcal and hemophilus vaccinations in patients with B-cell chronic lymphocytic leukemia. Vaccine 2001;19:1671–1677.
8. Sampalo A, Navas G, Medina F, Segundo C, Camara C, Brieva JA. Chronic lymphocytic leukemia B-cells inhibit spontaneous Ig production by autologous bone marrow cells: role of CD95-CD95L interaction. Blood 2000; 96:3168–3174.
9. Kipps T, Carson D. Autoantibodies in chronic lymphocytic leukemia and related systemic autoimmune diseases. Blood 1993;81:2475–2487.
10. Hamblin T, Oscier D, Young B. Autoimmunity in chronic lymphocytic leukemia. J Clin Pathol 1986;39:713–716.
11. Kay N. Abnormal T-cell subpopulation function in CLL: excessive suppressor (T gamma) and deficient helper (T mu) activity with respect to B-cell proliferation. Blood 1981;57:418–420.
12. Kay NE, Perri RT. Immunobiology of malignant B-cells and immunoregulatory cells in B-chronic lymphocytic leukemia. Clin Lab Med 1988;8:163–177.
13. Kay N, Zarling J. Impaired natural killer activity in patients with chronic lymphocytic leukemia is associated with a deficiency of azurophilic cytoplasmic granules in putative NK cells. Blood 1984;63:305–309.
14. Caligaris-Cappio F, Gobbi M, Bofill M. Infrequent normal B-lymphocytes express features of B-chronic lymphocytic leukemia. J Exp Med 1982;155:623–628.
15. Hashimoto S, Dono M, Watai M. Somatic diversification and selection of immunoglobulin heavy and light chain variable region genes in IgG+, CD5+ chronic lymphocytic leukemia B-cells. J Exp Med 1995;181:1507–1517.
16. Panayiotidis P, Ganeshaguru K, Dforoni L, Hoffbrand A. Expression and function of the FAS antigen in B chronic lymphocytic leukemia and hairy cell leukemia. Leukemia 1995;9:1227.
17. Tinhofer I, Marschitz I, Kos M, et al. Differential sensitivity of CD4+ and CD8+ T-lymphocytes to the killing efficacy of Fas (Apo-1/CD95) ligand+ tumor cells in B chronic lymphocytic leukemia. Blood 1998;91:4273–4281.
18. Conrad D, Waldschmidt T, Lee W, et al. Effect of B cell stimulatory factor-1 (interleukin 4) on Fc epsilon and Fc gamma receptor expression on murine B-lymphocytes and B cell lines. J Immunol 1987;139:2290–2296.
19. Knauf WU, Langenmayer I, Ehlers B, et al. Serum levels of soluble CD23, but not soluble CD25, predict disease progression in early stage B-cell chronic lymphocytic leukemia. Leuk Lymph 1997;27:523–532.

6 Cytokines and Soluble Molecules in CLL

Enrica Orsini, MD *and Robin Foa,* MD, PhD

1. INTRODUCTION

The pathogenesis of B-cell chronic lymphocytic leukemia (CLL) and the mechanisms regulating the growth, survival, and expansion of the leukemic clone are still largely unknown, but there is growing evidence of the important role played by cytokine networks and soluble mediators in the leukemic process. Leukemic CLL cells represent the most prominent population in CLL, but not the only one. Accessory non-neoplastic hematopoietic cells circulate in the peripheral blood and bone marrow of CLL patients, and cells of stromal origin are in strict contact with the tumor clone. The crosstalk between all these cell populations is mediated by soluble factors that may influence the pattern of survival and expansion of the disease, as well as the function of the normal compartment. The peculiar and in many ways unique clinical picture of CLL is likely to arise from the complex interactions of different networks, in which the action of one cytokine may strongly influence the production of, and response to, another. In the present chapter we discuss the role that different cytokines and soluble molecules may play, alone or through complex interactions, both on the leukemic clone and on the clinical course of the disease. For the sake of clarity, we discuss separately cytokines that induce cell survival, inhibitory cytokines, and soluble molecules.

2. SURVIVAL CYTOKINES

CLL is an accumulative disorder, characterized by low proliferative activity and by the progressive accumulation of clonal B-lymphocytes blocked in the early phases (G_0/G_1) of the cell cycle (1). In the pathogenesis of the disease an important role is thus played by the dysregulation of cellular mechanisms that control the progression through the cell cycle and the activation of programmed cell death (2). Abnormal cytokine loops may favor the survival and expansion of the leukemic clone through induction of cell proliferation or protection from apoptosis. In fact, defective apoptosis is considered to play a major role in the pathogenesis of the disease, and most cytokines capable of sustaining the leukemic cell growth act by inhibiting programmed cell death. Also, the cellular mechanisms that mediate these effects are shared by different cytokine networks that in many cases are thought to involve the regulation of the anti-apoptotic gene *bcl-2*, as will be discussed below in Subheadings 2.3., 2.5., and 2.8. Furthermore, many of these cytokines are members of the cytokine receptor family, which utilizes a common family of signal transduction molecules; the Janus kinase (JAK) kinases and signal transducer and activation of transcripton (STAT) signal transduction molecules (3). In CLL patients, several cytokines are secreted by the non-neoplastic accessory cell compartment, and the in vivo survival advantage is induced by

From: *Contemporary Hematology*
Chronic Lymphocytic Leukemia: Molecular Genetics, Biology, Diagnosis, and Management
Edited by: G. B. Faguet © Humana Press Inc., Totowa, NJ

Table 1
Cytokines in CLL

Cytokine	Activities
Survival cytokines	
IL-1β	Inhibits apoptosis
IL-2	Costimulates proliferation
IL-4	Inhibits or increases proliferation
	Protects from apoptosis
IL-6	Protects from apoptosis
IL-8	Inhibits apoptosis
IL-10	Contrasting data: may induce or prevent apoptosis
TNF-α	Contrasting data: may increase or inhibit proliferation
	May suppress apoptosis
IFN-α/γ	Inhibits apoptosis
G-CSF/GM-CSF	Decrease apoptosis
Inhibitory cytokines	
IL-5	Induces apoptosis
TGF-β	Inhibits proliferation

GM-CSF, granulocyte/macrophage colony-stimulating factor; IFN, interferon; IL, interleukin; TNF, tumor necrosis factor; TGF, transforming growth factor.

increased serum levels or by the peculiar response of the leukemic cells; there is, however, growing evidence that CLL cells themselves are capable of producing many autocrine factors that enhance their life span.

Finally, as in many hematological malignancies, a relevant role in disease control could be played by the antitumor immunological response. A permissive role may then be played by dysregulated cytokine pathways that could influence the function of the residual non-neoplastic immune system.

Below, we will individually discuss some of the cytokines and soluble molecules that have gained more attention, and their possible involvement in CLL. A short summary of potential activities of different cytokines in B-CLL is reported in Table 1.

2.1. Interleukin-1

Interleukin-1 (IL-1) was initially described as lymphocyte-activating factor (LAF) and endogenous pyrogen (EP) for its proinflammatory, immunostimulant, and chemotactic properties (4,5). The genes of the IL-1 complex code for three proteins: IL-1α, IL-1β, and the IL-1 receptor antagonist (IL-1Ra). The net plasma IL-1 activity is influenced by the balance between the levels of IL-1β, the major extracellular agonist, and that of IL-1 Ra (6).

Leukemic CLL cells spontaneously produce IL-1β (7–9) and also express the IL-1β receptor (10). Although this cytokine does not induce proliferation of CLL cells, it is capable of protecting CLL lymphocytes from apoptosis, both spontaneous and induced by hydrocortisone, supporting its potential role as an autocrine survival factor in CLL (11).

However, the production of IL-1 by CLL lymphocytes correlates inversely with the stage of the disease. In fact, whereas cells from patients with stable disease have been shown to secrete near normal levels of IL-1β, B-cells from patients with progressive CLL produce lower amounts of the cytokine (12,13). Given the immunomodulatory activities of IL-1, this reduced production in progressive CLL patients might have a role in the reduced immunological control of the disease, although this aspect of the role of IL-1 in CLL has been less investigated.

2.2. Interleukin-2

IL-2, a glycoprotein secreted mainly by activated T-cells, plays a critical role in the development of immune responses. In addition to inducing the proliferation and activation of T-lymphocytes and cytotoxic cells, it may promote the production of other cytokines such as granulocyte/ macrophage colony-stimulating factor (GM-CSF), interferon-γ (IFNγ), and tumor necrosis factor-α (TNFα) *(14,15)*.

The direct effect of IL-2 on CLL leukemic cells is exerted through the IL-2 receptors, whose presence has been demonstrated on the surface of CLL B-lymphocytes *(16)*. IL-2 has a costimulatory effect on CLL cells, following a primary signal: CLL B-cells preactivated with anti-IgM and anti-CD40 have been shown to increase the incorporation of thymidine, a marker of proliferative activity *(17,18)*. Proliferation was also observed in CLL cells upon culture with IL-2 alone *(19)*.

The IL-2 pathway may also be involved in the survival of the leukemic clone through an indirect effect on the non-neoplastic T-cell compartment. Not only do CLL B-lymphocytes express IL-2 receptor on their surface, but they may also absorb exogenous IL-2 *(20)*. In addition, CLL patients show increased levels of the soluble IL-2 receptor *(21,22)*. Given the overwhelming number of CLL B-cells in the peripheral blood of CLL patients, both these circumstances may decrease the availability of IL-2 for the accessory T- and cytotoxic lymphocytes, thus impairing the efficacy of physiological immune responses *(23)*. This may contribute to the numerous functional defects recorded within the T- and cytotoxic compartments of patients with CLL *(24)*.

2.3. Interleukin-4

IL-4 is a T-cell-derived lymphokine capable of promoting the proliferation and differentiation of normal B-cells following activation by other mechanisms, such as anti-IgM and anti-CD40 antibodies *(25–27)*.

The ability of IL-4 to induce proliferation of CLL leukemic B-cells has been controversial. In fact, IL-4 has been reported to both inhibit and induce a proliferative effect on neoplastic cells from CLL patients in vitro *(18,28,29)*. These contrasting data can possibly be explained by the influence of the different signaling pathways used by various authors for the in vitro activation studies.

It has, instead, been convincingly shown that IL-4 is capable of protecting CLL cells from apoptotic death, both spontaneous and induced by steroids, IL-5, and Fas signaling *(30–32)*. The inhibition of apoptosis mediated by IL-4 was found to correlate with increased levels of bcl-2 *(30,32)*, an association not confirmed by all authors *(31)*. The stage of the disease has no effect on the level of apoptosis inhibition by IL-4, but doses of IL-4 capable of protecting cells from previously treated CLL patients from spontaneous apoptosis were reported to have very little effect on cells from untreated patients. It was thus suggested that increased sensitivity to the anti-apoptotic effect of IL-4 might be one of the mechanisms of acquired drug resistance in CLL *(33)*. This anti-apoptotic effect might have a particular relevance in vivo since non-neoplastic CLL T-cells have been reported to produce increased levels of IL-4, potentially supporting the expansion and accumulation of the neoplastic clone *(34–37)*. Moreover, an autocrine pathway can also be hypothesized: CLL B-cells have in fact been recently found capable of secreting detectable amounts of IL-4 *(37)*.

Despite these preclinical studies, in a recently published phase I/II study, IL-4 was administered to CLL patients. In most of them, IL-4 promoted an increase in the number of circulating CLL lymphocytes (38). In accordance with most of the in vitro data, the in vivo administration of IL-4 may thus induce a stimulatory or anti-apoptotic effect on the leukemic CLL clone.

2.4. Interleukin-6

IL-6, a pleiotropic cytokine produced by a variety of cell types, is a well-characterized B-cell growth and differentiation factor, known to be essential for normal B-cell development and megakaryocyte maturation, and involved in the pathogenesis of several B-cell malignancies (39–41).

In contrast with what is observed in other B-cell neoplasms, IL-6 does not induce CLL cell proliferation in vitro (42–44), and, when administered in vivo in an attempt to increase sensitivity to chemotherapy, no growth-stimulatory effects have been observed (45). Nevertheless, this cytokine may have a role in sustaining the survival of the leukemic clone, as suggested by its effects on apoptosis of CLL cells and by the relationship between IL-6 serum levels and disease progression. With regard to the anti-apoptotic activity of IL-6 on CLL leukemic cells, the results are controversial: some researchers have found no effect, whereas others have described the inhibition of apoptosis by IL-6 (11,19,30,43). The mechanism proposed for this effect would be a delay in downregulation of bcl-2 in vitro (32). Recently, the anti-apoptotic activity of IL-6 has been ascribed to the dimeric, but not monomeric, form of this cytokine (46). In the report by Moreno et al. (46), although both the monomeric and dimeric forms of IL-6 bound IL-6R with comparable affinity, only the latter was capable of prolonging the survival of CLL lymphocytes in vitro. Moreover, in the same paper, the authors identify dimeric IL-6 as the soluble factor responsible for the anti-apoptotic effect exerted by endothelial cells on CLL B-lymphocytes in vitro. This cytokine, then, would be one of the soluble agents that mediate the interactions between stromal cells and CLL lymphocytes, a network that growing evidence indicates as pivotal in supporting the survival of the leukemic clone in vivo (47,48).

Serum levels of IL-6 have been found to be elevated in CLL patients compared with normal controls (13,22,43). Although CLL leukemic cells are known to produce a biologically active IL-6 protein, the non-neoplastic compartment could also be a source of IL-6 in CLL (49). A correlation between serum IL-6 levels and clinical features and survival has been recently described (50). Elevated IL-6 levels correlated with unfavorable features, such as advanced Rai stage, older age, and previous treatment, and patients with elevated serum IL-6 levels had a worse survival. Other groups have reported similar results, but it should be recalled that a reduced ability to produce IL-6 in CLL cells from patients with advanced disease has also been described (13,51).

As is the case with several cytokines in CLL, the mechanisms and modalities that influence the effects of IL-6 in vivo need to be further elucidated to obtain a more precise picture of the role of this cytokine in the pathogenesis of the disease.

2.5. Interleukin-8

IL-8/NAP-1 is a member of the proinflammatory supergene family with potent and specific neutrophil activation and chemoattractant properties (52–54). IL-8 is constitutively expressed by CLL leukemic cells and released in the serum, contributing through an autocrine pathway to the process of cell accumulation characteristic of this disease (55,56). In fact, the addition of IL-8 at doses comparable to the levels released constitutively by CLL cells can prolong their survival, whereas endogenous IL-8 neutralization by anti-IL-8 antibodies is capable of inducing the in vitro death of CLL cells. Moreover, IL-8 has the ability to upmodulate IL-8 mRNA in CLL B-lymphocytes (57).

The survival activity of IL-8 on CLL cells is not based on its ability to stimulate proliferation, but rather on its ability to inhibit apoptosis in CLL leukemic cells. In fact, IL-8 belongs to the number of cytokines that exert their anti-apoptotic role through a bcl-2-dependent pathway. Circulating levels of IL-8 have been found to parallel the mRNA expression of bcl-2 by CLL cells *(58)*, and this cytokine is experimentally capable of increasing bcl-2 expression in CLL lymphocytes *(57)*.

Beside its ability to sustain the survival of the leukemic clone, IL-8 may also have a role in the pathogenesis of the disease as a potential mediator of CLL cell motility, as discussed below in the chemokine section (Subheading 4.2.). Taken together, these findings may justify the prognostic role proposed for this cytokine in CLL. Clinically, stage A patients with levels of IL-8 above the median value were shown to be more likely to progress to a more advanced clinical stage than those with levels below the median value *(58)*. With a different and more sophisticated approach, the IL-8 coding gene was identified as one of the genes whose expression levels significantly correlated with patient survival or clinical stage in a recent microarray gene expression analysis of peripheral blood samples from 54 CLL patients *(59)*.

2.6. Interleukin-10

IL-10 is a cytokine produced by type 2 helper T-cells, as well as by monocytes and B-lymphocytes, with strong immunosuppressive effects via inhibition of Th1-type cytokines, including IFN-γ and IL-2 *(60–62)*. It has a potent stimulating effect on B-cells and is capable of inducing proliferation and differentiation *(63)*.

The role of IL-10 in the pathogenesis and clinical course of CLL is one of the more controversial within the cytokines potentially connected with this disease (Fig. 1). Leukemic CLL lymphocytes express both the IL-10 mRNA and its receptor *(64,65)*; thus, an autocrine role in sustaining the leukemic clone survival has been proposed for this cytokine. As a matter of fact, IL-10 has been reported to inhibit proliferation and to both inhibit and induce apoptosis of CLL lymphocytes *(66–68)*. In the study by Fluckiger et al. *(67)*, IL-10 was found to be capable of inducing CLL cells to die from apoptosis with a concomitant decrease in bcl-2 protein levels. In contrast, other authors reported a spontaneous release of IL-10 by CLL cells and a survival effect through inhibition of apoptotic cell death *(69)*. Consistent with the latter data, Jurlander and collegues *(70)* also found that IL-10 could prolong survival of CLL cells, with a pattern of STAT protein phosphorylation similar to that induced through the receptors for IFN-α and IFN-γ, proteins known to inhibit apoptosis in CLL cells. More suggestions come from a murine model of CLL, the B-1 malignant clones in NZB mice. In this spontaneously arising malignancy, IL-10 acts as an autocrine growth factor, and its gene expression levels increase with disease progression *(71)*. The role of IL-10 in B-1 cells, investigated by means of antisense IL-10 oligonucleotides, would lie in its ability to inhibit apoptosis induction through the maintenance of sustainable cell cycle progression *(72)*.

Just as equivocal are literature data on the in vivo production of IL-10: the ability to express IL-10 mRNA by CLL leukemic cells has been found to be associated with stable disease and to be lost in patients with progressive CLL *(65)*, whereas serum levels seem to follow an inverse pattern. CLL patients in more advanced stages of their disease show higher levels of IL-10 compared with normal controls and with patients in Rai stages 0–II *(73,74)*. Moreover, in the recent report by Fayad et al. *(50)*, elevated levels of IL-10 were an independent prognostic factor for survival, directly correlated with unfavorable features such as advanced Rai stage, older age, and previous treatment. Based on these data, the source of IL-10 in CLL might be the polyclonal normal cells rather than the leukemic clone.

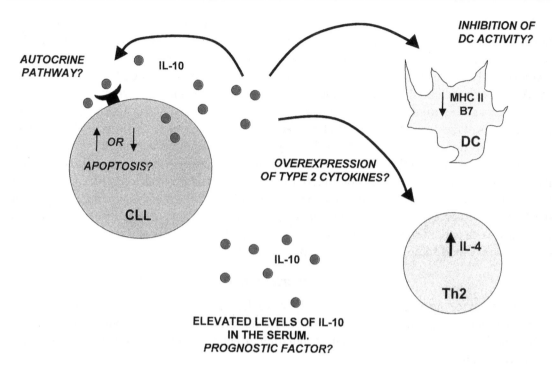

Fig. 1. Controversial role of interleukin-10 (IL-10) in CLL. The ability of IL-10 to either inhibit or induce apoptosis of CLL lymphocytes needs to be further investigated, as well as the suggested prognostic role of IL-10 serum levels in CLL patients, since contrasting data have been reported in the literature. In addition, IL-10 may exert a direct inhibitory effect on the antigen-presenting cell compartment and induce predominantly Th-2 type T-cell responses. DC, dendritic cell.

Finally, the elevated levels of IL-10 in CLL may also influence the growth and survival of the leukemic clone through its effects on the residual accessory compartment. Indeed, IL-10 production could represent a factor that affects the shift toward a Th-2-type response and the overexpression of type 2 cytokines reported in CLL patients (34,36). In addition, IL-10 exerts a direct inhibitory effect on the antigen-presenting cell compartment and is capable of inducing a downmodulation of MHC class II and B7 expression of peripheral blood dendritic cells. Further investigations will clarify whether these mechanisms are effective in CLL patients.

2.7. Tumor Necrosis Factor-α

TNF-α is a proinflammatory cytokine with heterogeneous activities, including immune modulation and regulation of tumor cell growth. In addition, it is also a growth factor for different normal cell populations, such as T- and B-lymphocytes (75,76).

TNF-α belongs to the group of multiple cytokines produced and released by CLL cells (77,78), which also express TNF-α receptors (79,80). Moreover, elevated serum levels of TNF-α are detectable in patients with CLL compared with normal controls, with a progressive increase in relation to the stage of disease (81,82). However, CLL patients also have elevated serum levels of soluble TNF-α receptor, and the latter appears to be more pronounced in advanced disease. In this situation, owing to the competitive effects of the soluble receptor form, the net effect of TNF-α on the surface of the neoplastic cells could be less relevant (80).

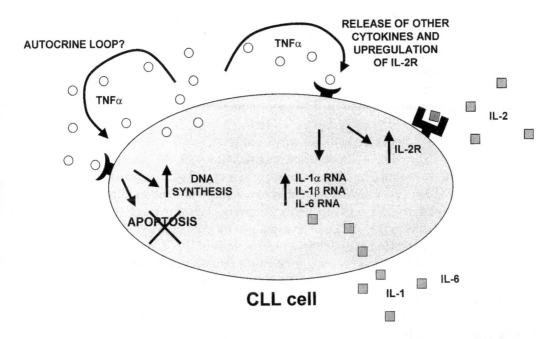

Fig. 2. TNF-α in CLL cell survival and cytokine loops. CLL cells spontaneously release TNF-α in vitro and respond to this cytokine, increasing their proliferative rate and suppressing apoptosis. The elevated serum levels of TNF-α in CLL patients may also induce the release of other cytokines and regulate the expression of IL-2 receptors (IL-2R).

The potential role of TNF-α as an autocrine growth factor in CLL is supported by observations reporting the ability of this cytokine to increase CLL B-lymphocyte proliferation *(77,83)* and to suppress apoptosis through a delay in downregulation of bcl-2 *(32)* (Fig. 2). It has to be noted, however, that other studies have not confirmed, or confirmed only partially, these data *(11,78,79,84)*, so that the real role of TNF-α in influencing the proliferation and survival of CLL cells has still to be conclusively established. However, the elevated serum levels of TNF-α in CLL patients may play a pivotal role in regulating different cytokine pathways: the synthesis of IL-1α, IL-1β, and IL-6, as well as the expression of the p55 IL-2 receptor *(79)*, is induced in CLL cells treated in vitro with TNF-α *(85)*. Recently, TNF-α has also been shown to be capable of increasing CD20 expression significantly on CLL leukemic cells, a finding potentially exploitable in the treatment of CLL patients with the anti-CD20 monoclonal antibody *(86,87)*.

2.8. Interferon α and β

IFN type I (α and β) and type II (γ) were initially described as proteins capable of conferring resistance to viral infections in uninfected cells, but they have a broad variety of cellular effects, including regulation of cell proliferation and differentiation, as well as modulation of immune functions *(88–90)*. The demonstration of its antineoplastic effects has led to the use of IFN-α as a therapeutic agent for different malignant diseases, including CLL *(91,92)*.

The potential role of IFN-γ as a clinically relevant anti-apoptotic cytokine in the pathogenesis of CLL has been suggested on the basis of experimental evidence. IFN-γ inhibits programmed cell death and promotes survival of CLL cells in culture *(93–95)*, an effect associated with a delay in downregulation of bcl-2 *(32)*. Sera from CLL patients have increased levels of IFN-γ compared with sera from healthy donors *(93,96)*. In addition, leukemic CLL cells are capable of synthesizing this cytokine *(93,96)*, suggesting an autocrine source of IFN-γ beyond the amounts produced by the T-cell populations in CLL. In the report by Rojas et al. *(94)*, the inhibitory effect of IFN-γ on CLL cell apoptosis correlated directly with the stage of the disease, and this was explained by a marked upregulation of IFN-γ receptors in cells from patients in the high-risk group.

IFN-α can likewise protect CLL cells not only from spontaneous apoptotic death in vitro, but also from apoptosis induced by hydrocortisone or irradiation *(97,98)*. This protection has been alternatively reported to be bcl-2-independent *(99)* or associated with increased bcl-2 expression in CLL cells *(97,98)*. However, IFN-α is an effective therapy in a subset of patients with CLL, capable of inducing partial remissions in patients with early-stage disease *(100)*. Thus, the clinical responses of CLL patients to IFN-α cannot be explained by a direct cytotoxic effect of IFN-α on circulating CLL cells and different direct or indirect actions of IFN-α might mediate this antitumor effect in vivo *(101,102)*. It has been suggested, for example, that IFN-α may act by interrupting autocrine growth loops in CLL, particularly by interfering with an autocrine production of TNF-α *(85)*. In addition, IFN-α may induce the differentiation of the malignant cell to a more mature phenotype *(103,104)* and may also modulate the expression of adhesion molecules on the cell surface, altering the homing pattern of CLL cells in the body *(105,106)*. Both these actions might affect numerically the malignant clone and the clinical course of the disease and may have a relevant immunomodulatory effect on T-cell and NK cell functions. The therapeutic effectiveness, although partial, of a cytokine capable of supporting the survival of the leukemic clone in vitro underlines the importance of the complex interactions of different intercellular networks in determining the net effect in vivo of each single cytokine.

2.9. Granulocyte Colony-Stimulating Factor and Granulocyte/Macrophage Colony-Stimulating Factor

Although the best-known functions of G-CSF and of GM-CSF are their stimulatory effects on myelopoiesis and on mature myeloid cell function, these agents have pleiotropic effects on multiple cell types *(107–109)*. In particular, they can exert a number of different effects on both immature and mature B-cells *(110,111)*. Therefore, the role of these cytokines in lymphoproliferative disorders has been actively investigated.

In earlier studies, GM-CSF production by CLL cells remained a matter of controversy. One group showed constitutive GM-CSF production in some cases but not in others *(112)*, whereas in a different report no GM-CSF mRNA was detectable by reverse transcriptase-polymerase chain reaction (RT-PCR) in 10 cases of CLL *(56)*. More recently, the constitutive production of a biologically active GM-CSF by leukemic CLL lymphocytes has been reported *(113)*. CLL B-cells were shown to express both the α and β chains of the GM-CSF receptor, and a role for this cytokine in sustaining cell survival was suggested. If these observations are confirmed, GM-CSF might be added to the number of cytokines capable of regulating the survival of CLL B-cells in an autocrine fashion.

Similar results have been reported for G-CSF, although CLL B-cells have to be stimulated with *Staphylococcus aureus* Cowan I (SAC) or the anti-CD40 antibody in combination with IL-2 or IL-4 to produce G-CSF in vitro *(114)*. Moreover, leukemic CLL cells bear receptors for G-CSF that are upregulated in vitro by IL-2 and that have been reported to mediate an anti-apoptotic effect in some CLL cell samples *(115,116)*.

3. INHIBITORY CYTOKINES

Cytokines capable of reducing the growth of the leukemic clone, (through induction of apoptosis or inhibition of proliferation), have also been identified, although in small numbers. By definition, they are not capable of blocking the neoplastic process, but their role in the control of the disease and in influencing the expansion of tumor cells cannot be ruled out. Moreover, their potential therapeutic use could be investigated further.

3.1. Interleukin-5

IL-5 is recognized as a growth factor involved in hematopoiesis that specifically stimulates growth and differentiation of human eosinophils and is produced by helper T-cells (117,118). Although IL-5 has some specific effects on normal peripheral blood B-cells, such as the increase in IgM production, a lack of responsiveness of CLL leukemic cells to the differentiation activity of IL-5 has been reported (119). Also controversial is the proliferative response of CLL B-lymphocytes to IL-5: a lack of response (as well as proliferation in the presence of IL-2 or inhibition of CLL cell responses to IL-2) has been described by different authors (19,120,121).

IL-5 is the only cytokine to have unanimously been described to induce apoptosis in leukemic CLL cells. IL-5 is capable of increasing the spontaneous apoptosis of CLL cells in vitro in a dose-dependent manner, an effect specific to the CLL clone and not observed in normal peripheral blood B-cells (19,122). This pro-apoptotic activity of IL-5 appears to be independent of bcl-2 levels and is significantly reduced in the presence of IL-4.

3.2. Transforming Growth Factor-β

TGF-β has been described as a potent inhibitor of various cell types, capable of depressing B-cell proliferation and IgG and IgM synthesis. A role as a negative autocrine regulator of normal lymphocyte growth and differentiation has been proposed for this cytokine (123,124).

TGF-β is produced by CLL cells and is present in the serum of patients (125–127). Since CLL lymphocytes are sensible to TGF-β-induced inhibition of DNA synthesis, although in a variable way and in general to a lesser extent than normal B-cells (128), some investigators have proposed that TGF-β may serve as an endogenous growth inhibitor for CLL cells, contributing to the slow progression of the leukemia in vivo (127). However, CLL lymphocytes may escape from TGF-β growth inhibition through a downregulation of the surface-specific type I receptor (129,130), and about one-third of CLL cases in the different studies are reported to be insensitive to the antiproliferative effect of TGF-β (127,128). The clinical significance of CLL cell sensitivity to TGF-β has to be assessed, since no correlation between loss of TGF-β receptor expression and stage of the disease has been reported (129,130).

At variance from other cytokines, TGF-β has no effect on programmed cell death in CLL leukemic cells. Although this cytokine may promote apoptosis in various cell types, including normal and leukemic B-cells, CLL lymphocytes have consistently shown resistance to the pro-apoptotic effects of TGF-β (131,132).

4. SOLUBLE MOLECULES

4.1. Vascular Endothelial Growth Factor and Angiogenesis

In the last few years, a considerable amount of work has been dedicated to elucidating the relationship between angiogenesis and tumor growth. It has been established that the expansion and dissemination of primary solid tumors is supported by the ability of tumor cells to generate vascularization intimately connected to the tumor (133,134). The release of pro-angiogenic vascular factors is essential in this process. Although the role of angiogenesis in hematopoietic malignancies is less clear, several recent observations have suggested that the release of angiogenic growth factors and abnormal angiogenesis may be intimately related to the leukemic process (135–137).

In CLL, there is growing experimental evidence that various angiogenic molecules and receptors may be linked to the pathogenesis of the disease. The expression of vascular factors and their receptors by leukemic CLL B-cells could be essential to induce the tumor vasculature required for disease progression in the bone marrow and in secondary lymphoid tissues. Even more intriguing is the question of whether it could also result in the generation of autocrine or paracrine loops that directly modulate the biology of the leukemic clone, through modifications of CLL cell survival or acquisition of drug resistance.

An abnormal angiogenesis, with increased microvessel density compared with normal controls, has been described in the bone marrow of CLL patients (138). A recent study also demonstrated a high blood vessel density in lymph nodes infiltrated by CLL cells, and this abnormal vasculature was reported to be intimately connected to the leukemic CLL infiltration (139). In the same report, CLL B-cells were reported to be capable of inducing the proliferation of endothelial cells and of enhancing angiogenesis in vitro. Thus, in CLL, the leukemic clone appears to be able to induce the genesis of the blood vessels required to supply oxygen and nutrients to the tumor tissue, through the secretion of vascular growth factors.

Among the several molecules with angiogenic or endothelial cell-activating properties, vascular endothelial growth factor (VEGF) is considered one of the most relevant, and many studies on the role of angiogenesis in CLL have chosen to focus on this molecule (Fig. 3). VEGF is a multifunctional protein that, upon binding to its receptors on endothelial cells, affects vascular permeability and cell proliferation, migration, and survival, all of which are required for angiogenesis (140,141). Serum levels of VEGF have been reported to be abnormally elevated in CLL, with higher values more frequently detected in advanced clinical stage patients and capable of predicting the risk of disease progression in early CLL (142). VEGF is produced by the leukemic B-cells (139,143), which also express the VEGF-specific receptors Flt1 and Tie1 (144). Recently, peripheral blood CLL cells were also found to express higher than normal levels of another VEGF receptor, VEGFR-2, also termed KDR (145). These findings are interesting in that they raise the question of a possible autocrine VEGF pathway, with several biological implications for CLL cell survival and proliferation. In fact, higher levels of Tie1 and KDR were both found to be associated with a significantly shorter survival in CLL patients, suggesting a possible role in the proliferation of leukemic CLL cells (144,145).

Endothelial cells are capable of secreting several CSFs in response to cytokines such as IL-1 (146). In the study of Bellamy et al. (147), human endothelial cells exposed to VEGF were found to be capable of increasing the message for a number of hematopoietic growth factors, including G-CSF, M-CSF, IL-6, and stem cell factor (SCF). The role of some of these cytokines in the pathogenesis and clinical course of CLL has already been discussed. Thus, it is possible that endothelial cells may, in response to angiogenic factors, release cytokines capable of influencing the growth and survival of the leukemic CLL clone. The possible autocrine and paracrine pathways associated with the release of vascular growth factors in CLL need to be elucidated by future studies, as does the possibility that modulation of vascular growth factor synthesis could be helpful in the management of these patients.

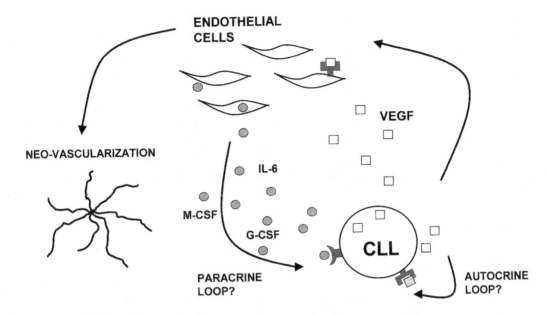

Fig. 3. Vascular endothelium-derived growth factor (VEGF): role in CLL-induced neo-angiogenesis and CLL cell survival. VEGF released by CLL neoplastic cells can induce the proliferation of endothelial cells and enhance angiogenesis in vivo. In addition, it might be involved in autocrine and paracrine loops: CLL cells express surface receptors for VEGF itself and for several VEGF-induced cytokines released by endothelial cells. G-CSF, granulocyte colony-stimulating factor; IL-6, interleukin-6; M-CSF, macrophage colony-stimulating factor.

4.2. Stromal Cell-Derived Factor 1 and Chemokines

The importance of the mechanisms regulating lymphocyte trafficking and adhesion in the pathogenesis of CLL is underlined by well-known clinical observations (in patients with CLL, the marrow is invariably infiltrated with leukemia cells, and the extent of marrow infiltration correlates with clinical stage and prognosis) *(148,149)*, as well as by more recent experimental data. The results of a study in which cDNA microarrays were employed to compare gene expression profiles with clinical features in CLL have been recently published. The authors were able to identify genes whose expression levels correlated significantly with patient survival and/or with clinical staging. Surprisingly, most of these genes coded either for cell adhesion molecules or for factors inducing cell adhesion molecules, suggesting that prognosis of this disease may be related to a defect in lymphocyte trafficking *(59)*.

The superfamily of chemokines consists of an array of chemoattractant proteins capable of regulating the trafficking of immune cells during hematopoiesis and inflammatory responses. In addition, they also stimulate leukocyte degranulation, have a pivotal role in the signaling of integrin activation, and promote angiogenesis or angiostasis *(150,151)*. Evidence is increasing that through binding to their specific membrane receptors, chemokines may regulate many aspects of immune responses, in part because cell migration is intimately related to lymphocyte function *(152,153)*. Like to their normal counterparts, it is conceivable that the functional behavior of CLL B-cells may be influenced by chemokine and chemokine receptor expression.

Most of the recent studies investigating the relationship between chemokines and CLL have focused on the mechanisms of extravasation of leukemic cells and of bone marrow infiltration.

Although the effects of many chemokines are largely redundant, and several chemokines can usually bind the same receptor, stromal-derived factor-1 (SDF-1) is a chemokine with the unique features of nonredundant functions (mutant mice die perinatally) and capable of binding to a single receptor, CXCR4 (154,155). SDF-1, initially designated as pre-B-cell growth-stimulating factor (PBSF), plays an important role in B-cell development, retaining B-cell precursors in close contact with bone marrow stromal cells, and it may also function as a B-cell growth factor (156,157). SDF-1 is constitutively produced by bone marrow stromal cells and acts as a chemoattractant, supporting the homing of hematopoietic cells, on which the chemokine receptor CXCR4 is broadly distributed (158,159). On circulating CLL cells, CXCR4 was found to be consistently expressed at a fluorescence intensity fourfold greater than that of normal B-cells and threefold greater than that of normal bone marrow CD19+/CD5+ cells. Migration of CLL cells was also more efficiently stimulated by recombinant SDF-1 compared with migration of normal B-cells (160). Burger et al. (161) have confirmed these findings in a study that investigated the function of CXCR4 expression on CLL cells. The critical role of the chemokine receptor CXCR4 for heterotypic adherence to marrow stromal cells was demonstrated by experiments in which CLL B-cells were cocultured with a murine cell line that secretes SDF-1: CLL B-cells spontaneously migrated beneath such stromal cells, and this migration could be inhibited by anti-CXCR4 monoclonal antibodies. In addition to this role in CLL B-cell migration, the same authors proposed in a recent paper a new role for SDF-1 in sustaining CLL leukemic cell survival. In fact, they identified a new population of stromal cells in the peripheral blood of CLL patients, named blood-derived nurse-like cells, capable of adhering to CLL B-cells in vitro and protecting them from undergoing spontaneous apoptosis. The process was SDF-1-dependent, since neutralizing antibodies to SDF-1 inhibited this protecting effect, and it could be partially mimicked, in the absence of the nurse cells, by exogenous SDF-1 (162) (Fig. 4).

At variance from the ubiquitous expression of CXCR4, the recently cloned chemokine receptor CXCR3 has been reported to be expressed on activated T-cells, but it is usually lacking in resting T-lymphocytes and most CD5+ and CD5- B-cells (163,164). This receptor is also expressed on the surface of leukemic CLL cells and is fully functional (165). In fact, malignant B-cells from patients with CLL show a definite in vitro migration in response to IFN-inducible protein 10 (IP-10) and IFN-γ-induced monokine (Mig), two chemokines that bind the CXCR3 receptor. CXCR3 expression appears to be a specific marker of CLL leukemic cells, since cells from patients with other B-cell malignancies, such as mantle cell lymphoma, follicular lymphoma, and hairy cell leukemia, were found to be generally negative (165,166). The same authors report that the CXCR3 ligand, Mig, is coexpressed on the leukemic cells in many cases of CLL. Coexpression of CXCR3 and its ligand, Mig, may play an important functional role in CLL, which needs to be further investigated.

The chemokine and chemokine receptor family is growing. According to NH_2-terminal cysteine motifs, chemokines are divided into the C, CC, CXC, and CX_3C subfamilies, and new members are being constantly added (167). Well-known molecules with chemotactic properties have been included in this classification and renamed following these criteria. This is the case for IL-8, now called CXCL8, whose role in sustaining CLL leukemic cell survival has already been discussed. In addition, IL-8 is capable of inducing motility of CLL cells on hyaluronan and thus is likely to be important for CLL cell migration through lymphoid tissues (168). In this context, future studies are likely to define additional factors that may have a role in mediating CLL leukemic cell trafficking and adhesion mechanisms. Assessing the relevance of these

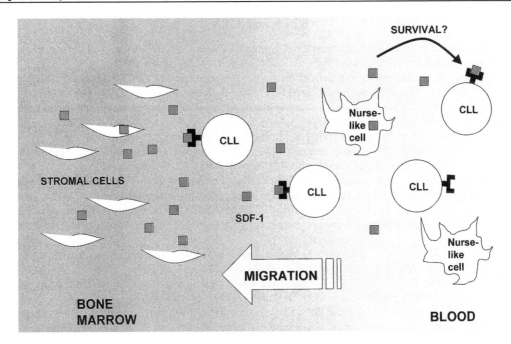

Fig. 4. Stromal-derived factor-1 (SDF-1) and bone marrow infiltration by CLL cells. CLL lymphocytes express high levels of SDF-1 receptor CXCR4 and may be attracted in the bone marrow by stromal cell-derived SDF-1. In the peripheral blood, SDF-1 released by "nurse-like" cells might also function as a CLL cell survival factor.

processes on CLL cell survival and disease spreading might lead to new therapeutic avenues for patients with CLL.

5. CONCLUSIONS

Based on accumulated data, it is now evident that several cytokines and soluble molecules play an important role in both the leukemic population and the host immune compartment of CLL patients. This opens new conceptual and applied scenarios. First, we have a better understanding of the biological mechanisms regulating the accumulation process that takes place in B-CLL, a unique feature of this disease that appears to be largely caused by decreased apoptotic machinery of the leukemic B-cell populations. From a clinical point of view, we are beginning to appreciate that the marked heterogeneity in the clinical course of patients with apparently similar features may be partly caused by a differential action exerted by cytokines and soluble molecules. It is foreseeable that in the near future we could use this knowledge to identify new prognostic indices and to differentiate early in the disease process CLL patients with a stable or progressive clinical picture. Finally, new therapeutic prospects based on strategies aimed at correcting an identified defect or interrupting a given cytokine loop could be designed, as well as more targeted therapeutic protocols according to objective biological parameters.

ACKNOWLEDGMENTS

This work was supported by the Associazione Italiana per la Ricerca sul Cancro (AIRC), Milan, the Istituto Superiore di Sanità, Rome, and the Ministero dell'Istruzione, dell'Università e della Ricerca, Rome, Italia.

REFERENCES

1. Andreeff M, Darzynkiewicz Z, Sharpless TK, Clarkson BD, Melamed MR. Discrimination of human leukemia subtypes by flow cytometric analysis of cellular DNA and RNA. Blood 1980;55:282–293.
2. Jurlander J. The cellular biology of B-cell chronic lymphocytic leukemia. Crit Rev Oncol Hematol 1998;27:29–52.
3. Ihle JN, Kerr IM. Jaks and Stats in signaling by the cytokine receptor superfamily. Trends Genet 1995;11:69–74.
4. Auron PE, Webb AC, Rosenwasser LJ, et al. Nucleotide sequence of human monocyte interleukin 1 precursor cDNA. Proc Natl Acad Sci USA 1984;81:7907–7911.
5. Dinarello CA. Biologic basis for interleukin-1 in disease. Blood 1996;87:2095–2147.
6. Hurme M, Santtila S. IL-1 receptor antagonist (IL-1Ra) plasma levels are co-ordinately regulated by both IL-1Ra and IL-1beta genes. Eur J Immunol 1998;28:2598–2602.
7. Pistoia V, Cozzolino F, Rubartelli A, Torcia M, Roncella S, Ferrarini M. In vitro production of interleukin 1 by normal and malignant human B-lymphocytes. J Immunol 1986;136:1688–1692.
8. Morabito F, Prasthofer EF, Dunlap NE, Grossi CE, Tilden AB. Expression of myelomonocytic antigens on chronic lymphocytic leukemia B-cells correlates with their ability to produce interleukin 1. Blood 1987;70:1750–1757.
9. Uggla C, Aguilar-Santelises M, Rosen A, Mellstedt H, Jondal M. Spontaneous production of interleukin 1 activity by chronic lymphocytic leukemic cells. Blood 1987;70:1851–1857.
10. Plate JM, Knospe WH, Harris JE, Gregory SA. Normal and aberrant expression of cytokines in neoplastic cells from chronic lymphocytic leukemias. Hum Immunol 1993;36:249–258.
11. Jewell AP, Lydyard PM, Worman CP, Giles FJ, Goldstone AH. Growth factors can protect B-chronic lymphocytic leukaemia cells against programmed cell death without stimulating proliferation. Leuk Lymphoma 1995;18:159–162.
12. Aguilar-Santelises M, Amador JF, Mellstedt H, Jondal M. Low IL-1 beta production in leukemic cells from progressive B cell chronic leukemia (B-CLL). Leuk Res 1989;13:937–942.
13. Hulkkonen J, Vilpo J, Vilpo L, Koski T, Hurme M. Interleukin-1 beta, interleukin-1 receptor antagonist and interleukin-6 plasma levels and cytokine gene polymorphisms in chronic lymphocytic leukemia: correlation with prognostic parameters. Haematologica 2000;85:600–606.
14. Smith KA. Interleukin-2: inception, impact, and implications. Science 1988;240:1169–1176.
15. Theze J, Alzari PM, Bertoglio J. Interleukin 2 and its receptors: recent advances and new immunological functions. Immunol Today 1996;17:481–486.
16. de Totero D, Francia di Celle P, Cignetti A, Foa R. The IL-2 receptor complex: expression and function on normal and leukemic B-cells. Leukemia 1995;9:1425–1431.
17. Lantz O, Grillot-Courvalin C, Schmitt C, Fermand JP, Brouet JC. Interleukin 2-induced proliferation of leukemic human B-cells. J Exp Med 1985;161:1225–1230.
18. Fluckiger AC, Rossi JF, Bussel A, Bryon P, Banchereau J, Defrance T. Responsiveness of chronic lymphocytic leukemia B-cells activated via surface Igs or CD40 to B-cell tropic factors. Blood 1992;80:3173–3181.
19. Mainou-Fowler T, Copplestone JA, Prentice AG. Effect of interleukins on the proliferation and survival of B cell chronic lymphocytic leukaemia cells. J Clin Pathol 1995;48:482–487.
20. Foa R, Giovarelli M, Jemma C, et al. Interleukin 2 (IL 2) and interferon-gamma production by T-lymphocytes from patients with B-chronic lymphocytic leukemia: evidence that normally released IL 2 is absorbed by the neoplastic B cell population. Blood 1985;66:614–619.
21. Semenzato G, Foa R, Agostini C, et al. High serum levels of soluble interleukin 2 receptor in patients with B chronic lymphocytic leukemia. Blood 1987;70:396–400.
22. Callea V, Morabito F, Luise F, et al. Clinical significance of sIL2R, sCD23, sICAM-1, IL6 and sCD14 serum levels in B-cell chronic lymphocytic leukemia. Haematologica 1996;81:310–315.
23. Foa R, Fierro MT, Giovarelli M, et al. Immunoregulatory T-cell defects in B-cell chronic lymphocytic leukemia: cause or consequence of the disease? The contributory role of decreased availability of interleukin 2 (IL-2). Blood Cells 1987;12:399–412.
24. Bartik MM, Welker D, Kay NE. Impairments in immune cell function in B cell chronic lymphocytic leukemia. Semin Oncol 1998;25:27–33.
25. Howard M, Farrar J, Hilfiker M, et al. Identification of a T cell-derived B cell growth factor distinct from interleukin 2. J Exp Med 1982;155:914–923.
26. Banchereau J, Bidaud C, Fluckiger AC, et al. Effects of interleukin 4 on human B-cell growth and differentiation. Res Immunol 1993;144:601–605.

27. Llorente L, Mitjavila F, Crevon MC, Galanaud P. Dual effects of interleukin 4 on antigen-activated human B-cells: induction of proliferation and inhibition of interleukin 2-dependent differentiation. Eur J Immunol 1990; 20:1887–1892.
28. Karray S, DeFrance T, Merle-Beral H, Banchereau J, Debre P, Galanaud P. Interleukin 4 counteracts the interleukin 2-induced proliferation of monoclonal B-cells. J Exp Med 1988;168:85–94.
29. van Kooten C, Rensink I, Aarden L, van Oers R. Interleukin-4 inhibits both paracrine and autocrine tumor necrosis factor-alpha-induced proliferation of B chronic lymphocytic leukemia cells. Blood 1992;80:1299–1306.
30. Dancescu M, Rubio-Trujillo M, Biron G, Bron D, Delespesse G, Sarfati M. Interleukin 4 protects chronic lymphocytic leukemic B-cells from death by apoptosis and upregulates Bcl-2 expression. J Exp Med 1992;176:1319–1326.
31. Mainou-Fowler T, Craig VA, Copplestone AJ, Hamon MD, Prentice AG. Effect of anti-APO1 on spontaneous apoptosis of B-cells in chronic lymphocytic leukaemia: the role of bcl-2 and interleukin 4. Leuk Lymphoma 1995;19:301–308.
32. Tangye SG, Raison RL. Human cytokines suppress apoptosis of leukaemic CD5+ B-cells and preserve expression of bcl-2. Immunol Cell Biol 1997;75:127–135.
33. Frankfurt OS, Byrnes JJ, Villa L. Protection from apoptotic cell death by interleukin-4 is increased in previously treated chronic lymphocytic leukemia patients. Leuk Res 1997;21:9–16.
34. de Totero D, Reato G, Mauro F, et al. IL4 production and increased CD30 expression by a unique CD8+ T-cell subset in B-cell chronic lymphocytic leukaemia. Br J Haematol 1999;104:589–599.
35. Reyes E, Prieto A, Carrion F, et al. Altered pattern of cytokine production by peripheral blood CD2+ cells from B chronic lymphocytic leukemia patients. Am J Hematol 1998;57:93–100.
36. Mainou-Fowler T, Miller S, Proctor SJ, Dickinson AM. The levels of TNF alpha, IL4 and IL10 production by T-cells in B-cell chronic lymphocytic leukaemia (B-CLL). Leuk Res 2001;25:157–163.
37. Kay NE, Han L, Bone N, Williams G. Interleukin 4 content in chronic lymphocytic leukaemia (CLL) B-cells and blood CD8+ T-cells from B-CLL patients: impact on clonal B-cell apoptosis. Br J Haematol 2001;112:760–767.
38. Lundin J, Kimby E, Bergmann L, Karakas T, Mellstedt H, Osterborg A. Interleukin 4 therapy for patients with chronic lymphocytic leukaemia: a phase I/II study. Br J Haematol 2001;112:155–160.
39. Kishimoto T. The biology of interleukin-6. Blood 1989;74:1–10.
40. Hsu SM, Xie SS, Waldron JA Jr. Functional heterogeneity and pathogenic significance of interleukin-6 in B-cell lymphomas. Am J Pathol 1992;141:915–923.
41. Seymour JF, Talpaz M, Cabanillas F, Wetzler M, Kurzrock R. Serum interleukin-6 levels correlate with prognosis in diffuse large-cell lymphoma. J Clin Oncol 1995;13:575–582.
42. Aderka D, Maor Y, Novick D, et al. Interleukin-6 inhibits the proliferation of B-chronic lymphocytic leukemia cells that is induced by tumor necrosis factor-alpha or -beta. Blood 1993;81:2076–2084.
43. Reittie JE, Yong KL, Panayiotidis P, Hoffbrand AV. Interleukin-6 inhibits apoptosis and tumour necrosis factor induced proliferation of B-chronic lymphocytic leukaemia. Leuk Lymphoma 1996;22:83–90.
44. Bussing A, Stein GM, Stumpf C, Schietzel M. Release of interleukin-6 in cultured B-chronic lymphocytic leukaemia cells is associated with both activation and cell death via apoptosis. Anticancer Res 1999;19:3953–3959.
45. Brown PD, Diamant M, Jensen PO, Geisler CH, Mortensen BT, Nissen NI. S-phase induction by interleukin-6 followed by chemotherapy in patients with chronic lymphocytic leukemia and non-Hodgkin's lymphoma. Leuk Lymphoma 1999;34:325–333.
46. Moreno A, Villar ML, Camara C, et al. Interleukin-6 dimers produced by endothelial cells inhibit apoptosis of B-chronic lymphocytic leukemia cells. Blood 2001;97:242–249.
47. Panayiotidis P, Jones D, Ganeshaguru K, Foroni L, Hoffbrand AV. Human bone marrow stromal cells prevent apoptosis and support the survival of chronic lymphocytic leukaemia cells in vitro. Br J Haematol 1996;92:97–103.
48. Lagneaux L, Delforge A, Bron D, DeBruyn C, Stryckmans P. Chronic lymphocytic leukemic B-cells but not normal B-cells are rescued from apoptosis by contact with normal bone marrow stromal cells. Blood 1998;91: 2387–2396.
49. Biondi A, Rossi V, Bassan R, et al. Constitutive expression of the interleukin-6 gene in chronic lymphocytic leukemia. Blood 1989;73:1279–1284.
50. Fayad L, Keating MJ, Reuben JM, et al. Interleukin-6 and interleukin-10 levels in chronic lymphocytic leukemia: correlation with phenotypic characteristics and outcome. Blood 2001;97:256–263.
51. Hulkkonen J, Vilpo J, Vilpo L, Hurme M. Diminished production of interleukin-6 in chronic lymphocytic leukaemia (B-CLL) cells from patients at advanced stages of disease. Tampere CLL Group. Br J Haematol 1998; 100:478–483.

52. Baggiolini M, Walz A, Kunkel SL. Neutrophil-activating peptide-1/interleukin 8, a novel cytokine that activates neutrophils. J Clin Invest 1989;84:1045–1049.

53. Mukaida N. Interleukin-8: an expanding universe beyond neutrophil chemotaxis and activation. Int J Hematol 2000;72:391–398.

54. Hermouet S, Corre I, Lippert E. Interleukin-8 and other agonists of Gi2 proteins: autocrine paracrine growth factors for human hematopoietic progenitors acting in synergy with colony stimulating factors. Leuk Lymphoma 2000;38:39–48.

55. Srivastava MD, Srivastava R, Srivastava BI. Constitutive production of interleukin-8 (IL-8) by normal and malignant human B-cells and other cell types. Leuk Res 1993;17:1063–1069.

56. Francia di Celle P, Carbone A, Marchis D, et al. Cytokine gene expression in B-cell chronic lymphocytic leukemia: evidence of constitutive interleukin-8 (IL-8) mRNA expression and secretion of biologically active IL-8 protein. Blood 1994;84:220–228.

57. Francia di Celle P, Mariani S, Riera L, Stacchini A, Reato G, Foa R. Interleukin-8 induces the accumulation of B-cell chronic lymphocytic leukemia cells by prolonging survival in an autocrine fashion. Blood 1996;87:4382–4389.

58. Molica S, Vitelli G, Levato D, Levato L, Dattilo A, Gandolfo GM. Clinico-biological implications of increased serum levels of interleukin-8 in B-cell chronic lymphocytic leukemia. Haematologica 1999;84:208–211.

59. Stratowa C, Loffler G, Lichter P, et al. cDNA microarray gene expression analysis of B-cell chronic lymphocytic leukemia proposes potential new prognostic markers involved in lymphocyte trafficking. Int J Cancer 2001;91: 474–480.

60. Fiorentino DF, Zlotnik A, Mosmann TR, Howard M, O'Garra A. IL-10 inhibits cytokine production by activated macrophages. J Immunol 1991;147:3815–3822.

61. Del Prete G, De Carli M, Almerigogna F, Giudizi MG, Biagiotti R, Romagnani S. Human IL-10 is produced by both type 1 helper (Th1) and type 2 helper (Th2) T cell clones and inhibits their antigen-specific proliferation and cytokine production. J Immunol 1993;150:353–360.

62. Mosmann TR, Moore KW. The role of IL-10 in crossregulation of TH1 and TH2 responses. Immunol Today 1991;12:A49–53.

63. Levy Y, Brouet JC. Interleukin-10 prevents spontaneous death of germinal center B-cells by induction of the bcl-2 protein. J Clin Invest 1994;93:424–428.

64. Finke J, Ternes P, Lange W, Mertelsmann R, Dolken G. Expression of interleukin 10 in B-lymphocytes of different origin. Leukemia 1993;7:1852–1857.

65. Sjoberg J, Aguilar-Santelises M, Sjogren AM, et al. Interleukin-10 mRNA expression in B-cell chronic lympho-cytic leukaemia inversely correlates with progression of disease. Br J Haematol 1996;92:393–400.

66. Tangye SG, Weston KM, Raison RL. Interleukin-10 inhibits the in vitro proliferation of human activated leukemic CD5+ B-cells. Leuk Lymphoma 1998;31:121–130.

67. Fluckiger AC, Durand I, Banchereau J. Interleukin 10 induces apoptotic cell death of B-chronic lymphocytic leukemia cells. J Exp Med 1994;179:91–99.

68. Castejon R, Vargas JA, Romero Y, Briz M, Munoz RM, Durantez A. Modulation of apoptosis by cytokines in B-cell chronic lymphocytic leukemia. Cytometry 1999;38:224–230.

69. Kitabayashi A, Hirokawa M, Miura AB. The role of interleukin-10 (IL-10) in chronic B-lymphocytic leukemia: IL-10 prevents leukemic cells from apoptotic cell death. Int J Hematol 1995;62:99–106.

70. Jurlander J, Lai CF, Tan J, et al. Characterization of interleukin-10 receptor expression on B-cell chronic lymphocytic leukemia cells. Blood 1997;89:4146–4152.

71. Peng B, Zhang M, Sun R, et al. The correlation of telomerase and IL-10 with leukemia transformation in a mouse model of chronic lymphocytic leukemia (CLL). Leuk Res 1998;22:509–516.

72. Yen Chong S, Lin YC, et al. Cell cycle effects of IL-10 on malignant B-1 cells. Genes Immun 2001;2:239–247.

73. Egle A, Marschitz I, Posch B, Herold M, Greil R. IL-10 serum levels in B-cell chronic lymphocytic leukaemia. Br J Haematol 1996;94:211–212.

74. Kamper EF, Papaphilis AD, Angelopoulou MK, et al. Serum levels of tetranectin, intercellular adhesion mol-ecule-1 and interleukin-10 in B-chronic lymphocytic leukemia. Clin Biochem 1999;32:639–645.

75. Brenner MK. Tumour necrosis factor. Br J Haematol 1988;69:149–152.

76. Gehr G, Gentz R, Brockhaus M, Loetscher H, Lesslauer W. Both tumor necrosis factor receptor types mediate proliferative signals in human mononuclear cell activation. J Immunol 1992;149:911–917.

77. Cordingley FT, Bianchi A, Hoffbrand AV, et al. Tumour necrosis factor as an autocrine tumour growth factor for chronic B-cell malignancies. Lancet 1988;1:969–971.

78. Foa R, Massaia M, Cardona S, et al. Production of tumor necrosis factor-alpha by B-cell chronic lymphocytic leukemia cells: a possible regulatory role of TNF in the progression of the disease. Blood 1990;76:393–400.
79. Trentin L, Zambello R, Agostini C, et al. Expression and regulation of tumor necrosis factor, interleukin-2, and hematopoietic growth factor receptors in B-cell chronic lymphocytic leukemia. Blood 1994;84:4249–4256.
80. Waage A, Espevik T. TNF receptors in chronic lymphocytic leukemia. Leuk Lymphoma 1994;13:41–46.
81. Adami F, Guarini A, Pini M, et al. Serum levels of tumour necrosis factor-alpha in patients with B-cell chronic lymphocytic leukaemia. Eur J Cancer 1994;30A:1259–1263.
82. Aguilar-Santelises M, Gigliotti D, Osorio LM, Santiago AD, Mellstedt H, Jondal M. Cytokine expression in B-CLL in relation to disease progression and in vitro activation. Med Oncol 1999;16:289–295.
83. Digel W, Stefanic M, Schoniger W, et al. Tumor necrosis factor induces proliferation of neoplastic B-cells from chronic lymphocytic leukemia. Blood 1989;73:1242–1246.
84. Burke F, Griffin D, Elwood N, et al. The effect of cytokines on cultured mononuclear cells from patients with B cell chronic lymphocytic leukemia. Hematol Oncol 1993;11:23–33.
85. Heslop HE, Bianchi AC, Cordingley FT, et al. Effects of interferon alpha on autocrine growth factor loops in B lymphoproliferative disorders. J Exp Med 1990;172:1729–1734.
86. Sivaraman S, Deshpande CG, Ranganathan R, et al. Tumor necrosis factor modulates CD20 expression on cells from chronic lymphocytic leukemia: a new role for TNF alpha? Microsc Res Tech 2000;50:251–257.
87. Venugopal P, Sivaraman S, Huang XK, Nayini J, Gregory SA, Preisler HD. Effects of cytokines on CD20 antigen expression on tumor cells from patients with chronic lymphocytic leukemia. Leuk Res 2000;24:411–415.
88. Rubin BY, Gupta SL. Differential efficacies of human type I and type II interferons as antiviral and antiproliferative agents. Proc Natl Acad Sci USA 1980;77:5928–5932.
89. Nakamura M, Manser T, Pearson GD, Daley MJ, Gefter ML. Effect of IFN-gamma on the immune response in vivo and on gene expression in vitro. Nature 1984;307:381–382.
90. Sen GC, Lengyel P. The interferon system. A bird's eye view of its biochemistry. J Biol Chem 1992;267:5017–5020.
91. Goldstein D, Laszlo J. Interferon therapy in cancer: from imaginon to interferon. Cancer Res 1986;46:4315–4329.
92. The Italian Cooperative Study Group on Chronic Myeloid Leukemia. Interferon alfa-2a as compared with conventional chemotherapy for the treatment of chronic myeloid leukemia. N Engl J Med 1994;330:820–825.
93. Buschle M, Campana D, Carding SR, Richard C, Hoffbrand AV, Brenner MK. Interferon gamma inhibits apoptotic cell death in B cell chronic lymphocytic leukemia. J Exp Med 1993;177:213–218.
94. Rojas R, Roman J, Torres A, et al. Inhibition of apoptotic cell death in B-CLL by interferon gamma correlates with clinical stage. Leukemia 1996;10:1782–1788.
95. Zaki M, Douglas R, Patten N, Bachinsky M, Lamb R, Nowell P, Moore J. Disruption of the IFN-gamma cytokine network in chronic lymphocytic leukemia contributes to resistance of leukemic B-cells to apoptosis. Leuk Res 2000;24:611–621.
96. Mainou-Fowler T, Prentice AG. Modulation of apoptosis with cytokines in B-cell chronic lymphocytic leukaemia. Leuk Lymphoma 1996;21:369–377.
97. Panayiotidis P, Ganeshaguru K, Jabbar SA, Hoffbrand AV. Alpha-interferon (alpha-IFN) protects B-chronic lymphocytic leukaemia cells from apoptotic cell death in vitro. Br J Haematol 1994;86:169–173.
98. Jewell AP, Worman CP, Lydyard PM, Yong KL, Giles FJ, Goldstone AH. Interferon-alpha up-regulates bcl-2 expression and protects B-CLL cells from apoptosis in vitro and in vivo. Br J Haematol 1994;88:268–274.
99. Chaouchi N, Wallon C, Taieb J, et al. Interferon-alpha-mediated prevention of in vitro apoptosis of chronic lymphocytic leukemia B-cells: role of bcl-2 and c-myc. Clin Immunol Immunopathol 1994;73:197–204.
100. McSweeney EN, Giles FJ, Worman CP, et al. Recombinant interferon alfa 2a in the treatment of patients with early stage B chronic lymphocytic leukaemia. Br J Haematol 1993;85:77–83.
101. Heslop HE, Brenner MK, Ganeshaguru K, Hoffbrand AV. Possible mechanism of action of interferon alpha in chronic B-cell malignancies. Br J Haematol 1991;79(suppl 1):14–16.
102. Jewell AP. Interferon-alpha, Bcl-2 expression and apoptosis in B-cell chronic lymphocytic leukemia. Leuk Lymphoma 1996;21:43–47.
103. Ostlund L, Einhorn S, Robert KH, Juliusson G, Biberfeld P. Chronic B-lymphocytic leukemia cells proliferate and differentiate following exposure to interferon in vitro. Blood 1986;67:152–159.
104. Totterman TH, Carlsson M, Nilsson K. Induction of IgM secretion by chronic B-lymphocytic leukaemia cells in serum-free medium: effects of interferon-alpha, -gamma and phorbol ester. Clin Exp Immunol 1988;71:187–192.

105. Jewell AP, Yong KL, Worman CP, Giles FJ, Goldstone AH, Lydyard PM. Cytokine induction of leucocyte adhesion molecule-1 (LAM-1) expression on chronic lymphocytic leukaemia cells. Leukemia 1992;6:400–404.
106. Csanaky G, Vass JA, Losonczy H, Schmelczer M. Expression of an adhesion molecule and homing in B-cell chronic lymphocytic leukaemia: II. L-selectin expression mediated cell adhesion revealed by immobilized analogue carbohydrates in B-cell chronic lymphocytic leukaemia and monoclonal lymphocytosis of undetermined significance. Med Oncol Tumor Pharmacother 1993;10:173–180.
107. Lieschke GJ, Burgess AW. Granulocyte colony-stimulating factor and granulocyte-macrophage colony-stimulating factor (1). N Engl J Med 1992;327:28–35.
108. Khwaja A, Linch DC. Effects of granulocyte colony-stimulating factor and granulocyte-macrophage colony-stimulating factor on neutrophil formation and function. Curr Opin Hematol 1994;1:216–220.
109. Nishijima I, Nakahata T, Hirabayashi Y, et al. A human GM-CSF receptor expressed in transgenic mice stimulates proliferation and differentiation of hemopoietic progenitors to all lineages in response to human GM-CSF. Mol Biol Cell 1995;6:497–508.
110. Ni K, O'Neill HC. Proliferation of the BCL1 B cell lymphoma induced by IL-4 and IL-5 is dependent on IL-6 and GM-CSF. Immunol Cell Biol 1992;70:315–322.
111. Till KJ, Burthem J, Lopez A, Cawley JC. Granulocyte-macrophage colony-stimulating factor receptor: stage-specific expression and function on late B-cells. Blood 1996;88:479–486.
112. Zupo S, Perussia B, Baldi L, et al. Production of granulocyte-macrophage colony-stimulating factor but not IL-3 by normal and neoplastic human B-lymphocytes. J Immunol 1992;148:1423–1430.
113. Harris RJ, Pettitt AR, Schmutz C, et al. Granuloctye-macrophage colony-stimulating factor as an autocrine survival factor for mature normal and malignant B-lymphocytes. J Immunol 2000;164:3887–3893.
114. Corcione A, Corrias MV, Daniele S, Zupo S, Spriano M, Pistoia V. Expression of granulocyte colony-stimulating factor and granulocyte colony-stimulating factor receptor genes in partially overlapping monoclonal B-cell populations from chronic lymphocytic leukemia patients. Blood 1996;87:2861–2869.
115. Corcione A, Pistoia V. B-cell-derived granulocyte-colony stimulating factor (G-CSF). Methods 1997;11:143–147.
116. Handa A, Kashimura T, Takeuchi S, et al. Expression of functional granulocyte colony-stimulating factor receptors on human B-lymphocytic leukemia cells. Ann Hematol 2000;79:127–131.
117. Lopez AF, Sanderson CJ, Gamble JR, Campbell HD, Young IG, Vadas MA. Recombinant human interleukin 5 is a selective activator of human eosinophil function. J Exp Med 1988;167:219–224.
118. Sanderson CJ. Interleukin-5, eosinophils, and disease. Blood 1992;79:3101–3109.
119. Hayes TG, Tan XL, Moseley AB, Huston MM, Huston DP. Abnormal response to IL-5 in B-cell chronic lymphocytic leukemia. Leuk Res 1993;17:777–783.
120. Carlsson M, Totterman TH, Rosen A, Nilsson K. Interleukin-2 and a T cell hybridoma (MP6) derived B cell-stimulatory factor act synergistically to induce proliferation and differentiation of human B-chronic lymphocytic leukemia cells. Leukemia 1989;3:593–601.
121. Tavernier J, Devos R, Van der Heyden J, et al. Expression of human and murine interleukin-5 in eukaryotic systems. DNA 1989;8:491–501.
122. Mainou-Fowler T, Craig VA, Copplestone JA, Hamon MD, Prentice AG. Interleukin-5 (IL-5) increases spontaneous apoptosis of B-cell chronic lymphocytic leukemia cells in vitro independently of bcl-2 expression and is inhibited by IL-4. Blood 1994;84:2297–2304.
123. Massague J. The transforming growth factor-beta family. Annu Rev Cell Biol 1990;6:597–641.
124. Wallick SC, Figari IS, Morris RE, Levinson AD, Palladino MA. Immunoregulatory role of transforming growth factor beta (TGF-beta) in development of killer cells: comparison of active and latent TGF-beta 1. J Exp Med 1990;172:1777–1784.
125. Kremer JP, Reisbach G, Nerl C, Dormer P. B-cell chronic lymphocytic leukaemia cells express and release transforming growth factor-beta. Br J Haematol 1992;80:480–487.
126. Schena M, Gaidano G, Gottardi D, et al. Molecular investigation of the cytokines produced by normal and malignant B-lymphocytes. Leukemia 1992;6:120–125.
127. Lotz M, Ranheim E, Kipps TJ. Transforming growth factor beta as endogenous growth inhibitor of chronic lymphocytic leukemia B-cells. J Exp Med 1994;179:999–1004.
128. Israels LG, Israels SJ, Begleiter A, et al. Role of transforming growth factor-beta in chronic lymphocytic leukemia. Leuk Res 1993;17:81–87.
129. DeCoteau JF, Knaus PI, Yankelev H, et al. Loss of functional cell surface transforming growth factor beta (TGF-beta) type 1 receptor correlates with insensitivity to TGF-beta in chronic lymphocytic leukemia. Proc Natl Acad Sci USA 1997;94:5877–5881.

130. Lagneaux L, Delforge A, Bron D, Massy M, Bernier M, Stryckmans P. Heterogenous response of B-lympho-cytes to transforming growth factor-beta in B-cell chronic lymphocytic leukaemia: correlation with the expression of TGF-beta receptors. Br J Haematol 1997;97:612–620.

131. Douglas RS, Capocasale RJ, Lamb RJ, Nowell PC, Moore JS. Chronic lymphocytic leukemia B-cells are resistant to the apoptotic effects of transforming growth factor-beta. Blood 1997;89:941–947.

132. Lagneaux L, Delforge A, Bernier M, Stryckmans P, Bron D. TGF-beta activity and expression of its receptors in B-cell chronic lymphocytic leukemia. Leuk Lymphoma 1998;31:99–106.

133. Folkman J. Angiogenesis in cancer, vascular, rheumatoid and other disease. Nat Med 1995;1:27–31.

134. Ellis LM, Fidler IJ. Angiogenesis and metastasis. Eur J Cancer 1996;32A:2451–2460.

135. Perez-Atayde AR, Sallan SE, Tedrow U, Connors S, Allred E, Folkman J. Spectrum of tumor angiogenesis in the bone marrow of children with acute lymphoblastic leukemia. Am J Pathol 1997;150:815–821.

136. Hussong JW, Rodgers GM, Shami PJ. Evidence of increased angiogenesis in patients with acute myeloid leukemia. Blood 2000;95:309–313.

137. Fiedler W, Graeven U, Ergun S, et al. Vascular endothelial growth factor, a possible paracrine growth factor in human acute myeloid leukemia. Blood 1997;89:1870–1875.

138. Kini AR, Kay NE, Peterson LC. Increased bone marrow angiogenesis in B cell chronic lymphocytic leukemia. Leukemia 2000;14:1414–1418.

139. Chen H, Treweeke AT, West DC, et al. In vitro and in vivo production of vascular endothelial growth factor by chronic lymphocytic leukemia cells. Blood 2000;96:3181–3187.

140. Leung DW, Cachianes G, Kuang WJ, Goeddel DV, Ferrara N. Vascular endothelial growth factor is a secreted angiogenic mitogen. Science 1989;246:1306–1309.

141. Thomas KA. Vascular endothelial growth factor, a potent and selective angiogenic agent. J Biol Chem 1996; 271:603–606.

142. Molica S, Vitelli G, Levato D, Gandolfo GM, Liso V. Increased serum levels of vascular endothelial growth factor predict risk of progression in early B-cell chronic lymphocytic leukaemia. Br J Haematol 1999;107: 605–610.

143. Aguayo A, O'Brien S, Keating M, et al. Clinical relevance of intracellular vascular endothelial growth factor levels in B-cell chronic lymphocytic leukemia. Blood 2000;96:768–770.

144. Aguayo A, Manshouri T, O'Brien S, et al. Clinical relevance of Flt1 and Tie1 angiogenesis receptors expression in B-cell chronic lymphocytic leukemia (CLL). Leuk Res 2001;25:279–285.

145. Ferrajoli A, Manshouri T, Estrov Z, et al. High levels of vascular endothelial growth factor receptor-2 correlate with shortened survival in chronic lymphocytic leukemia. Clin Cancer Res 2001;7:795–799.

146. Griffin JD, Rambaldi A, Vellenga E, Young DC, Ostapovicz D, Cannistra SA. Secretion of interleukin-1 by acute myeloblastic leukemia cells in vitro induces endothelial cells to secrete colony stimulating factors. Blood 1987;70:1218–1221.

147. Bellamy WT, Richter L, Frutiger Y, Grogan TM. Expression of vascular endothelial growth factor and its receptors in hematopoietic malignancies. Cancer Res 1999;59:728–733.

148. Han T, Barcos M, Emrich L, et al. Bone marrow infiltration patterns and their prognostic significance in chronic lymphocytic leukemia: correlations with clinical, immunologic, phenotypic, and cytogenetic data. J Clin Oncol 1984;2:562–570.

149. Pangalis GA, Roussou PA, Kittas C, et al. Patterns of bone marrow involvement in chronic lymphocytic leukemia and small lymphocytic (well differentiated) non-Hodgkin's lymphoma. Its clinical significance in relation to their differential diagnosis and prognosis. Cancer 1984;54:702–708.

150. Rollins BJ. Chemokines. Blood 1997;90:909–928.

151. Mackay CR. Chemokines: immunology's high impact factors. Nat Immunol 2001;2:95–101.

152. Baggiolini M. Chemokines and leukocyte traffic. Nature 1998;392:565–568.

153. Moser B, Loetscher P. Lymphocyte traffic control by chemokines. Nat Immunol 2001;2:123–128.

154. Nagasawa T, Hirota S, Tachibana K, et al. Defects of B-cell lymphopoiesis and bone-marrow myelopoiesis in mice lacking the CXC chemokine PBSF/SDF-1. Nature 1996;382:635–638.

155. Zou YR, Kottmann AH, Kuroda M, Taniuchi I, Littman DR. Function of the chemokine receptor CXCR4 in haematopoiesis and in cerebellar development. Nature 1998;393:595–599.

156. Kawabata K, Ujikawa M, Egawa T, et al. A cell-autonomous requirement for CXCR4 in long-term lymphoid and myeloid reconstitution. Proc Natl Acad Sci USA 1999;96:5663–5667.

157. Nishii K, Katayama N, Miwa H, et al. Survival of human leukaemic B-cell precursors is supported by stromal cells and cytokines: association with the expression of bcl-2 protein. Br J Haematol 1999;105:701–710.

158. Bleul CC, Fuhlbrigge RC, Casasnovas JM, Aiuti A, Springer TA. A highly efficacious lymphocyte chemoattractant, stromal cell-derived factor 1 (SDF-1). J Exp Med 1996;184:1101–1109.
159. Ma Q, Jones D, Springer TA. The chemokine receptor CXCR4 is required for the retention of B lineage and granulocytic precursors within the bone marrow microenvironment. Immunity 1999;10:463–471.
160. Mohle R, Failenschmid C, Bautz F, Kanz L. Overexpression of the chemokine receptor CXCR4 in B cell chronic lymphocytic leukemia is associated with increased functional response to stromal cell-derived factor-1 (SDF-1). Leukemia 1999;13:1954–1959.
161. Burger JA, Burger M, Kipps TJ. Chronic lymphocytic leukemia B-cells express functional CXCR4 chemokine receptors that mediate spontaneous migration beneath bone marrow stromal cells. Blood 1999;94:3658–3667.
162. Burger JA, Tsukada N, Burger M, Zvaifler NJ, Dell'Aquila M, Kipps TJ. Blood-derived nurse-like cells protect chronic lymphocytic leukemia B-cells from spontaneous apoptosis through stromal cell-derived factor-1. Blood 2000;96:2655–2663.
163. Loetscher M, Gerber B, Loetscher P, et al. Chemokine receptor specific for IP10 and mig: structure, function, and expression in activated T-lymphocytes. J Exp Med 1996;184:963–969.
164. Piali L, Weber C, LaRosa G, et al. The chemokine receptor CXCR3 mediates rapid and shear-resistant adhesion-induction of effector T-lymphocytes by the chemokines IP10 and Mig. Eur J Immunol 1998;28:961–972.
165. Trentin L, Agostini C, Facco M, et al. The chemokine receptor CXCR3 is expressed on malignant B-cells and mediates chemotaxis. J Clin Invest 1999;104:115–121.
166. Jones D, Benjamin RJ, Shahsafaei A, Dorfman DM. The chemokine receptor CXCR3 is expressed in a subset of B-cell lymphomas and is a marker of B-cell chronic lymphocytic leukemia. Blood 2000;95:627–632.
167. Zlotnik A, Yoshie O. Chemokines: a new classification system and their role in immunity. Immunity 2000;12: 121–127.
168. Till KJ, Zuzel M, Cawley JC. The role of hyaluronan and interleukin 8 in the migration of chronic lymphocytic leukemia cells within lymphoreticular tissues. Cancer Res 1999;59:4419–4426.

III CLINICAL ASPECTS: *DIAGNOSIS*

7

Immunophenotypic Differential Diagnosis and Cell Cycle Analysis

Vonda K. Douglas, MD and Raul C. Braylan, MD

1. IMMUNOPHENOTYPIC DIFFERENTIAL DIAGNOSIS OF CLL

1.1. Introduction

Chronic lymphocytic leukemia (CLL), including its tissue expression designated as small lymphocytic lymphoma (SLL), is a disease that, although first clinically described over 175 years ago, continues to evolve as an entity. As a result, the list of differential diagnoses for CLL also continues to evolve. Before the advent of immunophenotyping, the diagnosis of CLL included an assortment of diseases from circulating follicular lymphoma to large granular lymphocytic leukemia. The emergence of immunophenotyping as a diagnostic tool heralded a vast improvement in the definition and reproducibility of the diagnosis of CLL. Immunophenotypic characterization of this disease first began in the early 1970s, and by the late 1970s a fairly well-defined immunophenotypic profile for CLL was established that, although refined, probably still included many non-CLL entities. The expansion of cytogenetic and molecular information provided further tools in refining CLL as a distinct entity. For example, in 1989, the entity of mantle cell lymphoma (MCL) was separated from CLL/SLL as a distinct disease *(1)*. Thus, more than 30 years after its first phenotypic description, the definition of CLL is still a matter of debate. Although CLL has been significantly narrowed as a disease category, it is likely that CLL as it is currently defined still represents more than one disease. Consequently, the diagnosis of CLL and the differentiation from related entities can still present a diagnostic dilemma, and numerous points of controversy are raised.

Depending on the cell of origin, CLL is classified into T- and B-cell types. T-CLL is not a well-defined entity and includes a diverse group of indolent and rare post-thymic T-cell lymphoproliferative disorders that are currently given a number of different names, including T-prolymphocytic leukemia, large granular lymphocytosis, and circulating cutaneous T-cell lymphomas *(2)*. If these disorders are excluded, the frequency of a well-defined entity that could be named T-CLL is extremely low, and its existence is questionable. As a matter of fact, the recently published World Health Organization (WHO) classification of hematopoietic and lymphoid tumors does not include T-CLL as a distinct entity *(3)*. Therefore, the discussions in this chapter will refer exclusively to CLL of the B-cell type.

From: *Contemporary Hematology*
Chronic Lymphocytic Leukemia: Molecular Genetics, Biology, Diagnosis, and Management
Edited by: G. B. Faguet © Humana Press Inc., Totowa, NJ

1.2. Immunophenotypic Differential Diagnosis of CLL

1.2.1. Background

As mentioned above, immunophenotyping has emerged as an essential tool in the diagnosis of CLL *(4–6)*. A classic phenotype of typical CLL has been defined (*see* Subheading 1.2.2.). When demonstrated, this characteristic phenotype does not present diagnostic difficulties. The caveat lies in the fact that, absent this characteristic pattern, the overlap with other lymphoid proliferations may be quite substantial. Diagnostic dilemmas most often arise when the diagnostician is faced with a case of presumed CLL that does not fully demonstrate the requisite characteristic pattern, or in the setting of nontypical CLL lymphoid proliferations that express CD5. Although only two entities are defined by CD5 positivity (CLL and MCL), a number of mature B-cell neoplasms that may also demonstrate CD5 positivity. It should be noted, however, that a differential diagnosis of CLL based exclusively on immunophenotype is substantially broader than that of one that incorporates other parameters including clinical presentation, microscopy, cytogenetics, and molecular genetics. For example, entities that warrant consideration based solely on immunophenotypic profile can easily be eliminated with even cursory morphologic examination of the cells in question.

1.2.2. Immunophenotype of Classical Chronic Lymphocytic Leukemia

CLL, when it does demonstrate the classic pattern, is quite distinctive *(2,7)*. Useful markers in the evaluation for CLL include CD5, CD10, CD11c, CD19, CD20, CD22, CD23, CD79b, FMC7, and surface immunoglobulin (sIg) expression. Diagnosis can be rendered based on the presence or absence of the expression of these markers in combination with the intensity of their expression. CLL demonstrates bright CD45 intensity, as do the most mature B-lymphocytic neoplasms. However, downregulation of CD45 with a spectrum of positivity, although still bright, is not an uncommon finding in CLL. CD19 expression is greater than CD20 expression in typical CLL. CD19 is bright and CD20 is classically dim or downregulated compared with CD19 and also compared with normal B-cells in the sample that may serve as internal controls. CD20 also shows more variability, i.e., broader distribution, compared with CD19 and normal internal B-cell controls. Typically CLL demonstrates dim sIg expression. CD23 is expressed in classical CLL and is perhaps the most useful single marker in distinguishing CLL from MCL *(4)*. CLL is usually negative for CD79b *(8,9)* or, when present, expression is dim *(10)*. FMC7 is also usually negative in CLL or dimly expressed *(11,12)*. Lack of expression of these two latter markers is also very helpful in distinguishing CLL from MCL. Three markers are of paramount importance in making the diagnosis of typical CLL–CD5, CD10, and CD23. The sensitivity and specificity of a CD5+, CD10–, CD23+ chronic B-cell lymphoproliferative process for the diagnosis of CLL is extremely high. The combination of bright CD19, dim CD20, CD5, and CD23, and dim immunoglobulin expression in a monomorphopus small lymphocyte population is virtually pathognomonic for CLL.

1.3. Atypical CLL

1.3.1. Immunophenotype

Atypical CLL (aCLL) is an ill-defined term applied to cases that mimic CLL but do not have the classical morphological or immunophenotypic features. Uniformly accepted criteria for aCLL do not exist. Historically the term aCLL has been used primarily for lymphocytosis with morphologically atypical cells (lymphoplasmacytoid features, irregular/clefted nuclei) *(13)*. Numerous studies have attempted to correlate the morphological definition of aCLL with immunophenotype *(7,14,15)*, but these studies have failed to identify an immunophenotypic pattern that is pathognomonic for aCLL. Some authors have defined aCLL by the presence of any deviation from the typical phenotype or morphology of CLL in a setting that is otherwise consistent with CLL *(16)*. Others include CD5 negativity in the definition in a morphological and phenotypic picture that is otherwise characteristic of CLL *(17)*, whereas other authors prefer to separate CD5– lymphoproliferative disorders from aCLL, using the term CD5–CLL *(18)*. Some have argued that the entity of aCLL by definition should be CD5+, CD19+, CD23+, monotypic sIg+ and make the distinction solely based on the morphological criteria outlined by the French-American-British (FAB) Group *(19)*. No clear link with CD38 expression has been demonstrated *(19)*.

More recent reports have stressed the importance of specifically evaluating the density of various surface antigens by quantitative flow cytometry, vs. just the percentage of positive cells, in distinguishing between classical (cCLL) and aCLL *(4)*. Accordingly, an increased intensity, or increased numbers of molecules, of CD20 and CD22 compared with cCLL, as well as increased percentages of CD79b and FMC7, with compared with cCLL cells, are used to define aCLL immunophenotypically. D'Arena et al. *(20)* found no differences in CD23, CD79b, CD11c, and CD5 in terms of number of molecules/per cell between cCLL and aCLL. It is obvious that further studies are necessary to establish a clear definition of aCLL and to determine whether it is a unique clinical and/or pathological entity.

1.3.2. MOLECULAR GENETICS/CYTOGENETICS

The distinction between cCLL and aCLL can be aided by molecular/cytogenetic evaluation. aCLL, largely classified on the basis of morphological definition, is associated with an increased incidence of trisomy 12 and poorer survival than typical CLL *(21,22)*. As such, the presence of trisomy 12 is a useful adjunct in separating aCLL from cCLL. Molecular and cytogenetic data are also important in the differential diagnosis between aCLL and MCL *(23,24)*.

1.4. CD5– CLL

1.4.1. DEFINITION

Cases of CD5– CLL are quite rare *(25)*. Some authors have historically included CD5– CLL as part of the CLL group, but this inclusion is somewhat controversial. The current recommendation is that CD5– CLL be viewed as distinct from both cCLL and aCLL, owing to its more aggressive clinical picture, with more severe cytopenias, higher stage at presentation, and increased incidence of cytogenetic abnormalities *(13,18)*.

1.4.2. CRITERIA FOR CD5– CLL

Although CD5– CLL does not represent a well-defined entity, and cases are rare, criteria for rendering this diagnosis have been proposed. These include: (1) SLL or CLL/prolymphocytic leukemia morphology; (2) absence of immunophenotypic, cytogenetic or molecular markers for MCL or follicular lymphoma (e.g., negative for CD10, cyclin D1, t(11;14), t(14;18); and (3) absence of significant serum proteinemia (e.g., <10 g/L). The presence of CD23 strengthens the case for CD5– CLL but is not sufficient for diagnosis since other entities are also CD5–/CD23+ *(26,27)*.

1.5. Mantle Cell Lymphoma

1.5.1. IMMUNOPHENOTYPE

MCL is perhaps most common in the differential diagnosis of CLL. MCL, like CLL, is a CD5+ B-cell clonal process of small lymphocytes. Although MCL is mainly a lymph node-based neoplasm, it may invade bone marrow and circulate, creating a diagnostic dilemma in distinguishing it from CLL. Like CLL, MCLs are positive for CD19 and CD20, but, unlike CLL, CD20 is usually expressed more intensely than CD19 in MCL. Also, unlike CLL, MCL is CD23–, CD79b+, and FMC7+. The lack of CD23 is the most useful immunological criterion in distinguishing CLL from MCL *(4)*. The utility of CD23 expression lies in the context of CD5+ B-cell neoplasms, since other mature B-cell lymphoproliferative processes that are CD5–, such as follicular center lymphoma (FCL) and marginal zone lymphoma (MZL), may express CD23. FMC7 and CD11c are useful to a lesser extent. More than 95% of MCLs are FMC7+/CD11c–. Thus, the absence of FMC7 or the presence of CD11c, particularly in combination with other markers, also provides a useful discriminator for ruling out MCL *(12,28,29)*.

1.5.2. MOLECULAR GENETICS AND CYTOGENETICS

Although CD23 is a highly useful immunophenotypic marker to discriminate CLL from MCL, Cyclin D1 protein expression or demonstration of the t(11;14) are the most useful discriminators between CLL and MCL and are especially useful in differentiating between MCL and aCLL.

1.5.3. OTHER FEATURES THAT AID IN DISTINGUISHING MCL FROM CLL

Morphologically, the cells in MCL are more pleomorphic than those seen in cCLL, both in size and in nuclear irregularities. Clinically, patients with MCL often have more extensive adenopathy and severity of disease at presentation, consistent with a more aggressive course.

1.6. Chronic Lymphocytic Leukemia/Prolymphocytic Leukemia and B-Prolymphocytic Leukemia

1.6.1. DEFINITION

CLL/prolymphocytic leukemia (CLL/PLL) and B-prolymphocytic leukemia (PLL) are disorders that are distinguished from CLL and from each other based on morphological determination of the percentage of prolymphocytes (large lymphoid cells with ample cytoplasm and nuclei with prominent central nucleoli). PLL is usually a *de novo* process without a prodromic chronic phase. CLL/PLL is arbitrarily defined as CLL demonstrating between 10 and 55% prolymphocytes, and PLL is defined as more than 55% prolymphocytes. Consequently, PLL exhibits a more morphologically monomorphous population of cells than those of CLL/PLL, which are uniformly larger than the lymphocytes seen in CLL.

1.6.2. IMMUNOPHENOTYPE

The prolymphocytic component in CLL/PLL or PLL has a highly variable phenotype, reflecting the vague definition of CLL/PLL or PLL. PLL is described as CD5–, CD10–, CD23–, CD19+, and intense expression of CD20, CD22 and sIg compared with CLL *(30)*. However, prolymphocytes may demonstrate expression of CD5, which adds difficulty in clearly delineating PLL from CLL.

1.7. Lymphoplasmacytic Lymphoma

1.7.1. IMMUNOPHENOTYPE

Lymphoplasmacytic lymphoma (LPL) is a morphologically defined small lymphocytic process that, unlike most of the other entities discussed in the differential diagnosis of CLL, presents a more compelling diagnostic dilemma morphologically than immunophenotypically. As with many small lymphocytic processes, there is a lack of a clear definition and thus a resultant lack of reproducibility in the diagnosis of this so-called entity. Typically, LPLs are CD5–, CD10–, CD23–, CD11c– and may show variable CD20 and sIg depending on the degree of plasma cell differentiation. LPLs may occasionally demonstrate CD5+, raising the possibility of CLL and (when expressing bright sIg and no CD23) creating diagnostic difficulties with other processes such as MCL.

1.7.2. OTHER FEATURES THAT AID IN DISTINGUISHING LPL FROM CLL

Morphologically, the cells in LPL have a lymphoplasmacytoid morphology, and a plasma cell component is usually present, although this component may be absent or less apparent in the peripheral blood. Clinically, patients usually demonstrate a high serum monoclonal IgM (>10 g), often accompanied by hyperviscosity syndrome.

1.7.3. μ HEAVY CHAIN DISEASE

μ heavy chain disease is a variant of LPL in which the patient may demonstrate small lymphocytes that are similar in morphology to CLL. The plasma cells in these cases are often vacuolated. Immunophenotypically, however, the lymphocytes are quite distinctive from CLL in that they are CD5– and sIg light chain– but μ positive *(31)*.

1.8. Splenic Lymphoma With Villous Lymphocytes/ Splenic Marginal Zone Lymphoma

1.8.1. IMMUNOPHENOTYPE

The clonal B-lymphocytes in splentic lymphoma with villous lymphocytes (SLVL) are classically CD5– and CD10–; however, some authors report that approximately 20% of SLVLs are CD5+ *(32)*, although this is not a universal experience. Matutes et al. also reported that these neoplastic B-cells are usually FMC7(+) and strong CD22(+) *(32,33)*.

1.8.2. OTHER FEATURES THAT AID IN DISTINGUISHING SLVL FROM CLL

Morphologically, the lymphocytes in SLVL are distinctive from those of CLL. SLVL demonstrates lymphocytes with abundant pale cytoplasm, often with irregular cytoplasmic borders and with polar villous projections. The nuclear chromatin is condensed, and often visible nucleoli are present. Thus these cells morphologically bear a closer resemblance to PLL than CLL. Clinically, the distinction between SLVL and PLL may be a difficult one, as both may present with splenomegaly.

1.9. CD5+ Diffuse Large Cell Lymphoma

Diffuse large B-cell lymphomas (DLBCL) rarely, if ever, present a diagnostic dilemma in the morphological evaluation of CLL, since the large size and nuclear characteristics of DLBCL readily distinguish this entity from CLL. From an immunophenotypic standpoint, however, CD5 positivity can be see in up to 10% of cases of DLBCL *(34,35)*. CD5+ DLBCL can be divided into two broad categories: (1) primary or *de novo* DLBCL; and (2) DLBCL secondary to transformation of CLL/SLL. Most *de novo* DLBCL demonstrate bright expression of the pan-B-cell markers CD19, CD20, CD22, and CD79b, as well as FMC7, and expression of CD23, minimizing confusion with CLL. Rare cases of CD5+ Burkitt's lymphomas have also been described *(36)*. Cyclin D1 negativity distinguishes these lymphomas from the blastic variant of MCL, which demonstrates similar morphology and a virtually identical phenotype. Differentiation of *de novo* CD5+ DLBCL from that arising from CLL is also difficult in the absence of a known history of CLL. Useful tools in determining the presence of antecedent CLL include partial involvement by CLL or a disease phenotype that more resembles CLL than DLBCL (CD23+, dim to no expression of FMC7, dim sIg, dim CD20) *(37)*. An important exception to this latter phenotype is that of the DLBCL with plasmacytoid/immunoblast features. Due to the plasmacytic features, this entity may demonstrate dim to absent sIg and dim CD20; however, this variant of DLBCL does not express CD5.

1.10. Hairy Cell Leukemia

Hairy cell leukemia (HCL) is an entity that is not immunophenotypically difficult to distinguish from CLL, but it is included in the differential diagnosis of CLL in this chapter because of its historic inclusion in the differential diagnosis of chronic lymphoproliferative disorders. Immunophenotypically, HCL demonstrates very little overlap with CLL. HCL exhibits bright expression of the pan-B-cell markers CD19, CD20, and CD22, whereas CD5 and CD23 are negative. Classical features of HCL also include positivity for CD11c, CD25, and CD103. The pattern of CD11c/CD20 positively is highly characteristic of this disease *(38)*.

1.11. CD5+ Follicular Lymphoma

Although not frequent, CD5 expression has been reported in FCLs. CD5 positivity has been reported to correlate histologically with the floral variant of FCL *(39)*. CD5+ FCLs are typically also CD10+, CD23– and demonstrate IgG heavy chain, distinguishing them from most CLLs.

1.12. Summary

Classification and the proposed differential diagnosis of CLL yield the conundrum of trying to classify disorders that often do not lend themselves to strict subclassification. Despite the many categories of lymphoproliferative disorders discussed in this chapter, the fact remains that many of their definitions are still somewhat imprecise.

Thus, in tackling the differential diagnosis of CLL and other B-cell lymphoproliferative disorders, it is important to take a global approach. Often what appears to be a diagnostic dilemma based solely on morphological or immunophenotypic data can be easily resolved when all the information (clinical and genetic data as well as microscopy and immunophenotyping) is taken into consideration comprehensively. Conversely, the most critical and unnecessary diagnostic errors occur when only one modality or source of information is utilized for diagnosis. Finally, in resolving the differential diagnosis in CLL, the clinical course of the disease provides perhaps the most relevant information, since this is the information that is more important with regard to treatment than a specific name for a disease.

2. CELL CYCLE KINETICS OF CLL

2.1. Techniques to Determine Cell Growth Kinetics

Cell growth kinetics is an important parameter in assessing the potential aggressiveness of tumors and in the prediction of clinical outcome of patients with neoplastic diseases. Slowly proliferating tumors generally have a longer course and a better prognosis than rapidly growing ones, which may require a more aggressive therapy for their control. Different methods have been used over the years to measure the proliferation characteristics of neoplastic cells with the purpose of providing a quantitative means of determining tumor growth potential and prognosis. Using histological preparations, pathologists estimate tumor "aggressiveness" by simply observing the frequency of mitosis that could be quantitated as a mitotic index. This approach, however, is subjective and limited to the mitotic phase only.

2.1.1. Thymidine Incorporation

More objective assessment of dividing cells was made possible by the use of radiolabeled thymidine analogs, which are incorporated into S-phase cells in proliferating populations and can easily be revealed by measuring radioactivity or by autoradiography. The latter procedure allows the percentage of cells that incorporate the analog to be counted. This fraction is called the labeling index (LI), and it has been used extensively in classical cell cycle kinetic studies. Furthermore, the length of the S phase could be estimated by determining the time it takes for the radioactivity to decrease to one-half of the initial level.

2.1.2. Bromodeoxyuridine Incorporation

Bromodeoxyuridine (BrdU) incorporation is currently more widely used than thymidine for the study of cell proliferation. With BrdU, cells that have synthesized DNA are identified by fluorochrome-conjugated antibodies against BrdU, which are readily available commercially. The results are based on either fluorescent microscopic counts or flow cytometry. Anti-BrdU antibodies can be used in combination with other antibodies to select specific cell populations and thus provide information on the proliferation of subgroups of cells.

Most studies using thymidine or BrdU incorporation in humans have been performed in vitro. This approach assumes that cells in short-term culture would behave like those within their natural environment. Some studies using radiolabeled thymidine or BrdU have also been conducted in vivo *(40)*. Although less artificial, the in vivo human studies are complicated by the potential toxicity of the chemicals used and also by factors such as cell traffic, organ distribution and compartmentalization, and sampling impediments.

2.1.3. Cell Cycle Analysis by Flow Cytometry

Cell cycle phase fractions can be rapidly computed by flow cytometry based on measurements of fluorescence from DNA-binding fluorochromes. As cells traverse the S phase, the DNA content of each cell increases from G_1 to G_2, doubling before mitosis. Thus, the quantitation of fluorescence from each cell allows the enumeration of cells in G_{0-1}, S, and G_2-M phases. Because of its relative simplicity, this approach has been used extensively in a variety of solid tumors as well as hematological malignancies. Provided that the neoplastic cells are well represented in the sample analyzed, or that they can be identified by an independent parameter such as size, ploidy level, or specific antigen, the measurement of cell cycle fractions by this technique should reflect the true in vivo condition of the neoplastic cells.

2.1.4. Antibody Detection of Cycle-Dependant Proteins

Although thymidine or BrdU incorporation and cell cycle fraction calculations by DNA-binding fluorochromes provide a reasonable estimation of S-phase cells, the neoplastic growth fraction, defined as the total number of cells in the G_1, S, and G_2-M phases, is more difficult to measure. This is because these methods cannot easily distinguish nonproliferating cells in G_0 phase from proliferating cells. Such a distinction can be made by newer approaches based on the use of antibodies to markers expressed exclusively in cycling cells. The most commonly used markers are the proliferating cell nuclear antigen (PCNA) *(41)* and Ki-67 *(42)*. Both of these molecules have been used as proliferating cell markers. PCNA is a nuclear DNA-binding protein, with multiple functions in nucleic acid replication and repair; its concentration is indicative of the proliferative state of the cell. PCNA levels correlate with Ki-67 and BrdU incorporation *(43)*. Ki-67 is a nuclear antigen that is present only in cycling cells passing through G_1, S, G_2, and M phases; it is absent in G_0. Its function, however, is not well defined.

2.1.5. Other Methods

Other approaches have been used to assess cell proliferation in neoplasia. For example, the quantitation of argyrophilic protein sites of the nucleolar organizer region (AgNORs) has been used as a reliable indicator of the rapidity of cell duplication (44) and has been shown to correlate with Ki-67 labeling and the fraction of S-phase cells as measured by flow cytometry. Even serum markers such as serum deoxythymidine kinase may be used to assess the proliferative activity of leukemic cells and discriminate between progressive and indolent CLL (45).

2.1.6. Cell Cycle Analysis in Combination With Antigen Detection

Procedures for the measurement of DNA content and/or DNA synthesis simultaneously with cell surface antigens are available (46). Also, combined analysis of surface antigens and cell cycle-dependent proteins is possible (47). These multiparametric techniques provide valuable data regarding the specific cell cycle kinetics of leukemic cells in heterogeneous samples that contain irrelevant cells.

Each of the above approaches to determine the kinetics of tumor growth has advantages and disadvantages, but in general they are complementary. CLL cells, which are easily obtainable from the blood, are ideal for kinetic studies, and, since they are naturally suspended as single cells, are particularly suitable for flow cytometry-based analysis.

2.2. Growth Kinetics of CLL in the Blood

2.2.1. Cell Proliferation

CLL is a clonal expansion of leukemic cells that results from the slow and progressive accumulation of ineffectual long-lived lymphocytes arrested in G_0. The notion that CLL is an accumulative disorder dates back many decades ago (48,49). In the absence of significant cell death (see below), the slow pace of the disease indicates a relatively low proliferative capacity. This slow proliferation has been repeatedly documented using a variety of methods to determine cell cycle kinetics, both in vivo and in vitro. In early studies, the classical approach to the analysis of cell proliferation was based on the determination of thymidine incorporation into dividing cells. Theml et al. (50), using continuous infusion of 3H-thymidine and autoradiography in two patients with CLL, demonstrated that cell production was low and that the vast majority of the lymphocytes in the blood were long lived, with a turnover time longer than 1 year. Although lymphocyte proliferation was virtually absent in the blood and very low in the marrow, it was relatively high in the enlarged nodes. The exchange of lymphocytes seems partially intact between lymph nodes and blood but impaired between marrow and blood. Also, there is a reduced capability of CLL lymphocytes to recirculate from blood to blood via the lymph node and the thoracic duct (51). The disturbance of exchange of cells between the intra- and extravascular pools in CLL could explain some of their clinical manifestations (52,53). In vitro ^{3}H-thymidine LI of marrow leukemic cells determined at diagnosis in CLL also demonstrated little labeling of leukemic lymphocytes, with a median LI as low as 0.05% (54). This initial LI was unrelated to age, sex, absolute number of circulating lymphocytes, degree of marrow lymphocytosis, or clinical staging.

The low proliferative capacity of CLL has also been demonstrated by other techniques. Using acridine orange as a fluorescent dye, Andreeff et al. (55) showed that CLL cells have diploid DNA, very low proliferation, and a low RNA content, similar to that found in normal B-cells. Likewise, de Melo et al. (56) demonstrated a very low percentage of proliferating cells by Ki-67 staining (1.4%).

Applying double-color immunofluorescence methods to determine BrdU incorporation and the expression of the nuclear proliferation-associated antigen, Ki-67, together with the phenotypic profile of the cells, Stephenson et al. *(57)* also showed that unstimulated B-CLL cells are primarily in G_0, like to peripheral blood lymphocytes. Lin et al. *(58)* measured PCNA and BrdU incorporation as surrogate markers for proliferation and found a very low level of proliferation in CLL. Even PLL, a process characterized by the presence of numerous circulating large cells with immunophenotypic features reminiscent of CLL, demonstrated only slightly higher proliferative potential, either by S-phase *(59)* or Ki-67 analysis *(56)*.

The reasons for the low proliferative capacity of CLL cells, even after stimulation by a variety of polyclonal B-cell activators, are not completely understood, although it is likely that alteration in the expression of genes that participate in cell cycle control and progression may be in part responsible *(60)*. Of interest was the observation that cases with trisomy 12 were associated with a higher percentage of Ki-67-positive cells and that most Ki-67-positive cells were trisomic for chromosome 12, as determined by fluorescence *in situ* hybridization (FISH) analysis *(61)*. Also, thymidine uptake following mitogenic stimulation was significantly greater in CLL cells with an extra chromosome 12 than in those with normal karyotypes *(62)*. These findings suggest that growth control mechanisms in CLL may reside at this chromosome location, at least in some cases.

2.2.2. Clinical Correlation

Although the circulating cells in most patients with CLL demonstrate little capacity to grow, some evidence of more active proliferation may be observed in some cases. This variability in growth capacity has been correlated with clinical variables to determine whether it has potential prognostic value. In one study, the initial in vitro ^{3}H-thymidine labeling in marrow leukemic cells did not show prognostic significance *(54)*. Likewise, in another study, relative thymidine uptake (radioactivity per 10^3 lymphocytes) did not prove to be a useful prognostic parameter *(63)*. However, the latter authors showed that an absolute higher in vitro uptake of thymidine (by leukocytes in a standard volume of peripheral blood) was associated with a higher lymphocyte count, a more advanced stage, greater frequency of functional impairment, and shorter survival, suggesting that thymidine uptake by circulating leukocytes in CLL provides useful prognostic information. Similarly, Simonsson et al. *(64)* demonstrated a strong correlation between proliferation index (^{3}H-thymidine uptake-based LI × WBC) and clinical disease progression.

Using flow cytometry, high numbers of circulating lymphocytes in S phase had a shorter therapy-free and total survival compared with those with fewer S-phase cells *(65)*. Also, Orfao et al. *(66)* showed that a high absolute count of circulating S-phase leukocytes was associated with a higher incidence of hepatosplenomegaly, anemia, and thrombocytopenia, a higher number of lymphocytes in blood and bone marrow, advanced clinical stages, lower serum IgG and IgM, and poorer survival. Moreover, the fraction of circulating Ki-67-labeled cells in CLL correlated with the proportion of prolymphocytes and was higher in resistant CLL than in indolent cases *(67)*. Even high proliferative in vitro responses to B-cell mitogens were significantly associated with poor survival, whereas unstimulated thymidine uptake did not predict outcome *(62)*. Studies of lymphocyte doubling time (LDT) confirmed the above data. LDT is defined as the period needed for the peripheral lymphocyte count to double the original count and has been associated with prognosis. A low LDT (< 12 mo) is associated with a poor survival and predicts rapid disease progression *(68)*.

Other proliferative markers such as PCNA concentration were significantly lower in earlier stage CLL, and the level of this marker, which correlates with proliferative phase and LDT, also correlated with known prognostic factors such as disease stage in CLL patients (69). Similarly, both the percentage and absolute number of Ki-67-expressing cells were found to increase with disease stage (70).

High expression of the cyclin-dependent kinase inhibitor p27, which contributes to cell cycle arrest, may also be a valuable kinetic marker in B-CLL, since stable CLL patients usually express low levels of p27, whereas progressive CLL patients show a significant overexpression of this cyclin-dependent kinase inhibitor (71).

2.3. The Proliferative Sites

The studies mentioned above prove unequivocally that the circulatory cell component in most CLL patients has little capacity to proliferate. Where then are the CLL cells produced? Although lymphocyte proliferation is virtually absent in the blood and very low in the marrow, morphological and kinetic data indicate that lymph nodes contain growth sites (72) consisting of relative circumscribed areas with clusters of large cells (growth centers). These areas are generally small and represent a relatively small proliferating pool. Using Ki-67 labeling by immunohistochemistry, numerous studies of lymph nodes infiltrated by CLL—a process also designated a small lymphocytic lymphoma (SLL)—have shown that these tumors are the least proliferative lymphomas (73–75). The same finding was observed by BrdU (LI) (76) and PCNA immunohistochemistry (77). An increased proportion of Ki-67-positive cells in SLL is associated with a higher number of large cells, higher stage of disease, and treatment resistance (67,70). Similarly, a greater number of S-phase cells correlated with a significantly shorter survival in these patients (78).

The mechanisms underlying the CLL proliferative events in the lymph node are not understood. Of interest, Survivin, a member of the family of inhibitor of apoptosis proteins expressed in proliferating elements that coexpress Bcl-2, is confined within the lymph node pseudofollicles (growth centers). This suggests that growth and expansion of dividing CLL cells in the lymph node within the small proliferating pseudofollicles is governed by the expression of Survivin. These cells are bound to accumulate because they also express Bcl-2 (79).

2.4. Large Cell Transformation

As disease progresses, the number of proliferative large cells in the relatively indolent SLL may increase and even convert in some cases into a more rapidly growing large cell lymphoma, a transformation that has been designated Richter's syndrome. Richter's syndrome occurs in a small fraction of patients with CLL during the course of the disease and is associated with systemic symptoms, progressive lymphadenopathy, increased lactate dehydrogenase levels, and multiple chromosomal abnormalities (80). As expected, the large lymphoma cells in this syndrome are Ki-67-positive (70) and contain larger AgNORs, a pattern consistent with proliferation (81). The molecular events leading to the development of B-cell diffuse large cell lymphoma in CLL are not well known, although it is likely that multiple cell cycle regulator gene disruptions may facilitate this transformation (82).

2.5. Role of Apoptosis in CLL

As mentioned above, the proliferative capacity of classical CLL is low, and the leukemic cells expand mainly because of a prolonged life span caused by a dysregulation of apoptosis. Both intrinsic and extrinsic cellular factors have been held responsible for this abnormality.

2.5.1. INTRINSIC FACTORS

The progressive expansion of CLL in the face of its poor proliferative capacity has led to the notion that the neoplastic cells in this disease enjoy increased longevity owing to defective apoptosis rather than to alterations in cell cycle regulation. Apoptosis, or programmed cell death, consists of a cascade of biochemical events leading to cell destruction that plays a critical role both in normal tissue development and in malignancy *(83)*. The apoptotic failure of CLL has been studied extensively, and numerous mechanisms have been proposed to explain this deficiency. Of course, most investigations have been centered on the *Bcl-2* gene family and their proteins *(84–86)*. The importance of the anti-apoptosis *Bcl-2* oncogene in B-cell malignancies was established more than 20 years ago in follicular lymphomas with the t(14;18). However, in contrast to follicular lymphomas, translocations of the *Bcl-2* gene are relatively infrequent in CLL *(87)*. Indeed, unlike other B-cell lymphoproliferative disorders, CLL is not associated with specific molecular defects, although many show deletions of the long arm of chromosome 13 or trisomy 12, possibly deregulating genes encoding for proteins involved in apoptosis *(88)*. Despite the infrequent *Bcl-2* gene rearrangements, high expression of *Bcl-2* mRNA and protein are quite common in CLL *(89,90)*. Apparently, the mechanism of *bcl-2* overexpression in CLL is not owing to gene rearrangement, but rather to hypomethylation of *Bcl-2* promoter region DNA *(90)*. Bcl-2 is only one member of a large family of apoptosis-regulating proteins. Some of these proteins function like *Bcl-2* as inhibitors of apoptosis, whereas others are cell death promoters. The level of expression of apoptosis-related genes other than *Bcl-2* was also investigated in CLL. Elevated *BCL-2* and Bax expression was associated with apoptosis resistance *(91)*. Gottardi et al. *(85)* detected high message and protein Bax expression in most B-CLL cases. They also showed high levels of Bcl-xL in many but not all cases, whereas Bcl-xS was detectable only in very low amounts in some patients, a pattern that is skewed toward prevention of apoptosis. Similarly, Krajewski et al. *(92)*, using specific antibodies, showed that *Bcl-2*, Mcl-1, Bax, Bak, BAG-1, and Caspase-3 were commonly expressed in circulating B-CLLs, whereas the Bcl-X and BAD proteins were not present at detectable levels.

Some studies suggest that Bax is the critical protein in determining the fate of CLL cells following apoptotic signals and that *Bcl-2* and Bax interaction, rather than the absolute level of *Bcl-2* expression, is a more important determinant of B-CLL cell apoptosis *(93)*. In this regard it was shown that levels of *Bcl-2* correlate with those of the pro-apoptotic protein Bax *(86)*.

2.5.2. EXTRINSIC FACTORS

The fact that despite their prolonged survival in vivo, a substantial proportion of CLL cells only survive a few days when cultured in vitro has intrigued investigators *(94)*. This observation has prompted the notion that the genetic abnormalities of the CLL cell do not entirely account for all aspects of cell accumulation, which may also be influenced by external stimuli. Numerous studies have shown that host elements extrinsic to the neoplastic cells may provide survival signals to the neoplastic cells in vivo. When these elements are absent, i.e., in culture, CLL cells have the propensity to undergo spontaneous apoptosis. These survival factors in CLL would include cytokines and soluble molecules, such as interferon-α and -γ, interleukin-2, -4, -6, -8, and -13 *(95–100)*, the ligand for β2 integrins *(101)*, tumor necrosis factor-α *(102)*, immune complexes in the context of accessory leukocytes *(103)*, inflammatory elements such as CD40 ligand (CD154) *(104)*. and antigen for which the malignant clone has affinity *(105)*.

At the cellular level, receptor abnormalities may contribute to the long-lived status of B-CLL cells. For example, B-CLL cells show a defective CD40-mediated signal transduction and a downregulated expression of the apoptosis-inducer CD95 (Fas). As a consequence, no apoptosis could be induced in B-CLL cells by a soluble anti-CD95 monoclonal antibody (106). Also, perturbed T-cell/B-cell interactions have been described in this disease (107).

A large body of experimental data emphasizes the protective role of the stromal microenvironment that exerts a strong influence in vivo on the promotion of progressive accumulation of the CLL cell (108). Cell-to-cell and matrix interactions mediated by adhesion molecules prevent the death of B-CLL cells (94). Also, B-CLL cell-to-matrix binding results in an increased Bcl-2/Bax ratio and prevents apoptosis (109). Binding of stromal cells from bone marrow to B-CLL cells was shown to prevent B-CLL apoptotic cell death in vitro (110,111). Blood-derived "nurse-like" cells also show similar effects (112). These studies suggest that direct cell-to-cell contact and/or cell-to-matrix- or membrane-bound cytokines rather than soluble factors may be important for the in vivo survival of CLL cells.

2.5.3. CLINICAL CORRELATION

The role of apoptosis and cell kinetics in CLL progression were investigated by Ricciardi et al. (113), who observed that CLL cells from patients with progressive disease were more quiescent and exhibited much lower susceptibility to apoptosis than those from patients with stable disease, even in the presence of autologous serum. These investigators speculated that higher quiescence may be responsible for the decreased susceptibility of cells from patients with progressive disease to enter apoptosis. The clinical impact of apoptotic-related gene expression has also been investigated. High Bcl-2 levels have been associated with the presence of adverse prognostic factors (114). Kitada et al. (115) studied a large number of Bcl-2 family proteins including Bcl-2, Bcl-X$_L$, Mcl-1, Bax, Bak, Baf, the Bcl-2 binding protein Bag-1, and the protease caspase-3 with regard to therapy response. These authors found that overexpression of the Mcl-1 protein was strongly associated with lower patient response rate.

Another gene implicated in the regulation of cell cycle arrest and apoptosis is p53, a tumor suppressor gene that is commonly mutated in a variety of human cancers (116). A large study demonstrated that p53 mutations in CLL correlate with a much higher frequency of disease progression, inferior survival, and poor response to therapy (117).

2.6. Conclusions

The typical CLL cell represents an accumulation of clonal, mostly small, mature lymphocytes that exhibit a distinctive immunophenotype, circulate, and home in on lymphoid organs and bone marrow. Circulating cells have little capacity to proliferate, whereas small islands of dividing cells are usually present in lymph nodes, accounting for the slow cell production that is characteristic of this neoplasia. Putative genetic as well as soluble and other cellular factors may contribute to the remarkable resistance of these neoplastic cells to apoptosis. Although generally phenotypically uniform, kinetically quiescent, and resilient, CLL cells sometimes manifest biological variability, a feature that may be useful in predicting disease progression and therapy response.

REFERENCES

1. De Oliveira MS, Jaffe ES, Catovsky D. Leukaemic phase of mantle zone (intermediate) lymphoma: its characterisation in 11 cases. J Clin Pathol 1989;42:962–972.
2. Bartlett NL, Longo DL. T-small lymphocyte disorders. Semin Hematol 1999;36:164–170.
3. Jaffe ES, Ralfkiaer E. Mature T-cell and NK-cell neoplasms. In: Jaffe ES, Harris NL, Stein H, Vardiman JW, eds. World Health Organization Classification of Tumours (WHO): Pathology and Genetics; Tumours of Haematopoietic and Lymphoid Tissues. IARC Press, Lyon, 2001, p. 190.

4. D'Arena G, Musto P, Cascavilla N, et al. Quantitative flow cytometry for the differential diagnosis of leukemic B-cell chronic lymphoproliferative disorders. Am J Hematol 2000;64:275–281.
5. DiGiuseppe JA, Borowitz MJ. Clinical utility of flow cytometry in the chronic lymphoid leukemias. Semin Oncol 1998;25:6–10.
6. Rothe G, Schmitz G. Consensus protocol for the flow cytometric immunophenotyping of hematopoietic malignancies. Working Group on Flow Cytometry and Image Analysis. Leukemia 1996;10,:877–895.
7. Matutes E, Polliack A. Morphological and immunophenotypic features of chronic lymphocytic leukemia. Rev Clin Exp Hematol 2000;4:22–47.
8. Cabezudo E, Carrara P, Morilla R, Matutes E. Quantitative analysis of CD79b, CD5 and CD19 in mature B-cell lymphoproliferative disorders. Haematologica 1999;84:413–418.
9. Zomas AP, Matutes E, Morilla R, et al. Expression of the immunoglobulin-associated protein B29 in B cell disorders with the monoclonal antibody SN8 (CD79b) Leukemia 1996;10:1966–1970.
10. Alfarano A, Indraccolo S, Circosta P, et al. An alternatively spliced form of CD79b gene may account for altered B- cell receptor expression in B-chronic lymphocytic leukemia. Blood 1999;93:2327–2335.
11. Catovsky D, Cherchi M, Brookss D, Bradely J, Zola H. Heterogeneity of B-cell leukemias demonstrated by the monoclonal antibody FMC7. Blood 1981;58:406–408.
12. Huh YO, Pugh WC, Kantarjian HM, et al. Detection of subgroups of chronic B-cell leukemias by FMC7 monoclonal antibody. Am J Clin Pathol 1994;101:283–289.
13. Bennett JM, Catovsky D, Daniel MT, et al. Proposals for the classification of chronic (mature) B and T lymphoid leukaemias. French-American-British (FAB) Cooperative Group. J Clin Pathol 1989;42:567–584.
14. Criel A, Verhoef G, Vlietinck R, et al. Further characterization of morphologically defined typical and atypical CLL: a clinical, immunophenotypic, cytogenetic and prognostic study on 390 cases. Br J Haematol 1997;97:383–391.
15. Finn WG, Thangavelu M, Yelavarthi KK, et al. Karyotype correlates with peripheral blood morphology and immunophenotype in chronic lymphocytic leukemia. Am J Clin Pathol 1996;105:458–467.
16. Criel A, Michaux L, Wolf-Peeters C. The concept of typical and atypical chronic lymphocytic leukaemia. Leuk Lymph 1999;33:33–45.
17. Cartron G, Linassier C, Bremond JL, et al. CD5 negative B-cell chronic lymphocytic leukemia: clinical and biological features of 42 cases. Leuk Lymph 1998;31:209–216.
18. Shapiro JL, Miller ML, Pohlman B, Mascha E, Fishleder AJ. CD5- B-cell lymphoproliferative disorders presenting in blood and bone marrow. A clinicopathologic study of 40 patients. Am J Clin Pathol 1999;111: 477–487.
19. Frater JL, McCarron KF, Hammel JP, et al. Typical and atypical chronic lymphocytic leukemia differ clinically and immunophenotypically. Am J Clin Pathol 2001;116:655–664.
20. D'Arena G, Dell'Olio M, Musto P, et al. Morphologically typical and atypical B-cell chronic lymphocytic leukemias display a different pattern of surface antigenic density. Leuk Lymph 2001;42:649–654.
21. Matutes E, Oscier D, Garcia-Marco J, et al. Trisomy 12 defines a group of CLL with atypical morphology: correlation between cytogenetic, clinical and laboratory features in 544 patients. Br J Haematol 1996;92:382–388.
22. Oscier DG, Matutes E, Copplestone A, et al. Atypical lymphocyte morphology: an adverse prognostic factor for disease progression in stage A CLL independent of trisomy 12. Br J Haematol 1997;98:934–939.
23. Matutes E, Carrara P, Coignet L, et al. FISH analysis for BCL-1 rearrangements and trisomy 12 helps the diagnosis of atypical B cell leukaemias. Leukemia 1999;13:1721–1726.
24. Cuneo A, Bigoni R, Negrini M, et al. Cytogenetic and interphase cytogenetic characterization of atypical chronic lymphocytic leukemia carrying BCL1 translocation. Cancer Res 1997;57:1144–1150.
25. Huang JC, Finn WG, Goolsby CL, Variakojis D, Peterson LC. CD5- small B-cell leukemias are rarely classifiable as chronic lymphocytic leukemia. Am J Clin Pathol 1999;111:123–130.
26. Carey JL. Immunophenotyping in diagnosis and prognosis of mature lymphoid leukemias and lymphomas. In: Keren D, McCoy JP, Carey JL, eds. Flow Cytometry in Clinical Diagnosis. ASCP Press, Chicago, 2001, pp. 227–378.
27. Bennett JM, Catovsky D, Daniel MT, et al. Proposals for the classification of chronic (mature) B and T lymphoid leukaemias. French-American-British (FAB) Cooperative Group. J Clin Pathol 1989;42:567–584.
28. Kilo MN, Dorfman DM. The utility of flow cytometric immunophenotypic analysis in the distinction of small lymphocytic lymphoma/chronic lymphocytic leukemia from mantle cell lymphoma. Am J Clin Pathol 1996;105:451–457.
29. Wormsley SB, Baird SM, Gadol N, Rai KR, Sobol RE. Characteristics of CD11c+CD5+ chronic B-cell leukemias and the identification of novel peripheral blood B-cell subsets with chronic lymphoid leukemia immunophenotypes. Blood 1990;76:123–130.

30. Matutes E, Owusu-Ankomah K, Morilla R, et al. The immunological profile of B-cell disorders and proposal of a scoring system for the diagnosis of CLL. Leukemia 1994;8:1640–1645.

31. Fermand JP, Brouet JC. Heavy-chain diseases. Hematol Oncol Clin N Am 1999;13:1281–1294.

32. Matutes E, Morilla R, Owusu-Ankomah K, Houlihan A, Catovsky D. The immunophenotype of splenic lymphoma with villous lymphocytes and its relevance to the differential diagnosis with other B-cell disorders. Blood 1994;83:1558–1562.

33. Ferry JA, Yang WI, Zukerberg LR, et al. CD5+ extranodal marginal zone B-cell (MALT) lymphoma. A low grade neoplasm with a propensity for bone marrow involvement and relapse. Am J Clin Pathol 1996;105:31–37.

34. Yamaguchi M, Seto M, Okamoto M, et al. De novo CD5+ diffuse large B-cell lymphoma: a clinicopathologic study of 109 patients. Blood 2002;99:815–821.

35. Harada S, Suzuki R, Uehira K, et al. Molecular and immunological dissection of diffuse large B cell lymphoma: CD5+, and CD5- with CD10+ groups may constitute clinically relevant subtypes. Leukemia 1999;13:1441–1447.

36. Lin CW, O'Brien S, Faber J, et al. De novo CD5+ Burkitt lymphoma/leukemia. Am J Clin Pathol 1999;112:828–835.

37. Kroft SH, Dawson DB, Mckenna RW. Large cell lymphoma transformation of chronic lymphocytic leukemia/ small lymphocytic lymphoma. A flow cytometric analysis of seven cases. Am J Clin Pathol 2001;115:385–395.

38. Cornfield DB, Mitchell Nelson DM, Rimsza LM, Moller-Patti D, Braylan RC. The diagnosis of hairy cell leukemia can be established by flow cytometric analysis of peripheral blood, even in patients with low levels of circulating malignant cells. Am J Hematol 2001;67:223–226.

39. Tiesinga JJ, Wu CD, Inghirami G. CD5+ follicle center lymphoma. Immunophenotyping detects a unique subset of "floral" follicular lymphoma. Am J Clin Pathol 2000;114:912–921.

40. Raza A, Alvi S, Broady-Robinson L, et al. Cell cycle kinetic studies in 68 patients with myelodysplastic syndromes following intravenous. Exp Hematol 1997;25:530–535.

41. Kelman Z. PCNA: structure, functions and interactions. Oncogene 1997;14:629–640.

42. Gerdes J, Lemke H, Baisch H, Wacker HH, Schwab U, Stein H. Cell cycle analysis of a cell proliferation-associated human nuclear antigen defined by the monoclonal antibody Ki-67. J Immunol 1984;133:1710–1715.

43. van Dierendonck JH, Wijsman JH, Keijzer R, van de Velde CJ, Cornelisse CJ. Cell-cycle-related staining patterns of anti-proliferating cell nuclear antigen monoclonal antibodies. Comparison with BrdUrd labeling and Ki-67 staining. Am J Pathol 1991;138:1165–1172.

44. Trere D. Quantitative analysis of AgNOR proteins: a reliable marker of the rapidity of cell duplication and a significant prognostic parameter in tumour pathology. Adv Clin Path 1998;2:261–270.

45. Kallander CF, Simonsson B, Gronowitz JS, Nilsson K. Serum deoxythymidine kinase correlates with peripheral lymphocyte thymidine uptake in chronic lymphocytic leukemia. Eur J Haematol 1987;38:331–337.

46. Holm M, Thomsen M, Hoyer M, Hokland P. Optimization of a flow cytometric method for the simultaneous measurement of cell surface antigen, DNA content, and in vitro BrdUrd incorporation into normal and malignant hematopoietic cells. Cytometry 1998;32:28–36.

47. Glasova M, Konikova E, Kusenda J, Babusikova O. Evaluation of different fixation-permeabilization methods for simultaneous detection of surface, cytoplasmic markers and DNA analysis by flow cytometry in some human hematopoietic cell lines. Neoplasma 1995;42:337–346.

48. Bierman HR. The leukemias—proliferative or accumulative? Blood 1967;30:238–250.

49. Dameshek W. Chronic lymphocytic leukemia—an accumulative disease of immunolgically incompetent lymphocytes. Blood 1967;29(suppl):566–584.

50. Themi H, Trepel F, Schick P, Kaboth W, Begemann H. Kinetics of lymphocytes in chronic lymphocytic leukemia: studies using continuous 3H-thymidine infusion in two patients. Blood 1973;42:623–636.

51. Stryckmans PA, Debusscher L, Collard E. Cell kinetics in chronic lymphocytic leukaemia (CLL). Clin Haematol 1977;6:159–167.

52. Theml H, Love R, Begemann H. Factors in the pathomechanism of chronic lymphocytic leukemia. Annu Rev Med 1977;28:131–141.

53. Matsuda S, Uchida T, Kariyone S. Kinetic studies on lymphocytes labelled with indium 111-oxine in patients with chronic lymphocytic leukaemia. Scand J Haematol 1985;35:210–218.

54. Petti MC, Testa MG, Deb G, Amadori S. Cytokinetic studies in chronic lymphocytic leukemia. Relationship to other variables at diagnosis and survival. Biomedicine 1980;33:188–190.

55. Andreeff M, Darzynkiewicz Z, Sharpless TK, Clarkson BD, Melamed MR. Discrimination of human leukemia subtypes by flow cytometric analysis of cellular DNA and RNA. Blood 1980;55:282–293.

56. de Melo N, Matutes E, Cordone I, Morilla R, Catovksy D. Expression of Ki-67 nuclear antigen in B and T cell lymphoproliferative disorders. J Clin Pathol 1992;45:660–663.

57. Stephenson CF, Desai ZR, Bridges JM. The proliferative activity of B-chronic lymphocytic leukaemia lymphocytes prior to and after stimulation with TPA and PHA. Leuk Res 1991;15:1005–1012.

58. Lin CW, Manshouri T, Jilani I, et al. Proliferation and apoptosis in acute and chronic leukemias and myelodysplastic syndrome. Leuk Res 2002;26:551–559.

59. Diamond LW, Bearman RM, Berry PK, et al. Prolymphocytic leukemia: flow microfluorometric, immunologic, and cytogenetic observations. Am J Hematol 1980;9:319–330.

60. Decker T, Schneller F, Hipp S, et al. Cell cycle progression of chronic lymphocytic leukemia cells is controlled by cyclin D2, cyclin D3, cyclin-dependent kinase (cdk) 4 and the cdk inhibitor p27. Leukemia 2002;16:327–334.

61. Garcia-Marco JA, Price CM, Ellis J, et al. Correlation of trisomy 12 with proliferating cells by combined immunocytochemistry and fluorescence in situ hybridization in chronic lymphocytic leukemia. Leukemia 1996; 10:1705–1711.

62. Juliusson G, Gahrton G. Clinical implications of CLL cell proliferation in vitro. Nouv Rev Fr Hematol 1988; 30:399–401.

63. Moayeri H, Sokal JE. In vitro leukocyte thymidine uptake and prognosis in chronic lymphocytic leukemia. Am J Med 1979;66:773–778.

64. Simonsson B, Nilsson K. 3H-thymidine uptake in chronic lymphocytic leukaemia cells. Scand J Haematol 1980; 24:169–173.

65. Kimby E, Mellstedt H, Nilsson B, et al. Blood lymphocyte characteristics as predictors of prognosis in chronic lymphocytic leukemia of B-cell type. Hematol Oncol 1988;6:47–55.

66. Orfao A, Ciudad J, Gonzalez M, et al. Prognostic value of S-phase white blood cell count in B-cell chronic lymphocytic leukemia. Leukemia 1992;6:47–51.

67. Astsaturov IA, Samoilova RS, Iakhnina EI, Pivnik AV, Vorobiov AI. The relevance of cytological studies and Ki-67 reactivity to the clinical course of chronic lymphocytic leukemia. Leuk Lymph 1997;26:337–342.

68. Vinolas N, Reverter JC, Urbano-Ispizua A, Montserrat E, Rozman C. Lymphocyte doubling time in chronic lymphocytic leukemia: an update of its prognostic significance. Blood Cells 1987;12:457–470.

69. del Giglio A, O'Brien S, Ford R, et al. Prognostic value of proliferating cell nuclear antigen expression in chronic lymphoid leukemia. Blood 1992;79:2717–2720.

70. Cordone I, Matutes E, Catovsky D. Monoclonal antibody Ki-67 identifies B and T cells in cycle in chronic lymphocytic leukemia: correlation with disease activity. Leukemia 1992;6:902–906.

71. Vrhovac R, Delmer A, Tang R, Marie JP, Zittoun R, Ajchenbaum-Cymbalista F. Prognostic significance of the cell cycle inhibitor p27Kip1 in chronic B-cell lymphocytic leukemia. Blood 1998;91:4694–4700.

72. Dormer P, Theml H, Lau B. Chronic lymphocytic leukemia: a proliferative or accumulative disorder? Leuk Res 1983;7:1–10.

73. Schwartz BR, Pinkus G, Bacus S, Toder M, Weinberg DS. Cell proliferation in non-Hodgkin's lymphomas. Digital image analysis of Ki-67 antibody staining. Am J Pathol 1989;134:327–336.

74. Gerdes J, Dallenbach F, Lennert K, Lemke H, Stein H. Growth fractions in malignant non-Hodgkin's lymphomas (NHL) as determined in situ with the monoclonal antibody Ki-67. Hematol Oncol 1984;2:365–371.

75. Weiss LM, Strickler JG, Medeiros LJ, Gerdes J, Stein H, Warnke RA. Proliferative rates of non-Hodgkin's lymphomas as assessed by Ki-67 antibody. Hum Pathol 1987;18:1155–1159.

76. Witzig TE, Gonchoroff NJ, Greipp PR, et al. Rapid S-phase determination of non-Hodgkin's lymphomas with the use of an immunofluorescence bromodeoxyuridine labeling index procedure. Am J Clin Pathol 1989;91:298–301.

77. Sebo TJ, Roche PC, Witzig TE, Kurtin PJ. Proliferative activity in non-Hodgkin's lymphomas. A comparison of the bromodeoxyuridine labeling index with PCNA immunostaining and quantitative image analysis. Am J Clin Pathol 1993;99:668–672.

78. Lindh J, Jonsson H, Lenner P, Roos G. 'Aggressive' low grade lymphocytic lymphomas can be identified by flow cytometric S-phase determinations. Hematol Oncol 1992;10:171–179.

79. Granziero L, Ghia P, Circosta P, et al. Survivin is expressed on CD40 stimulation and interfaces proliferation and apoptosis in B-cell chronic lymphocytic leukemia. Blood 2001;97:2777–2783.

80. Robertson LE, Pugh W, O'Brien S, et al. Richter's syndrome: a report on 39 patients. J Clin Oncol 1993;11:1985–1989.

81. Nikicicz EP, Norback DH. Spectrum of argyrophilic nucleolar organizer region (AgNOR) staining patterns in chronic and transformed B-cell leukemias. Arch Pathol Lab Med 1992;116:265–268.

82. Cobo F, Martinez A, Pinyol M, et al. Multiple cell cycle regulator alterations in Richter's transformation of chronic lymphocytic leukemia. Leukemia 2002;16:1028–1034.

83. Wickremasinghe RG, Hoffbrand AV. Biochemical and genetic control of apoptosis: relevance to normal hematopoiesis and hematological malignancies. Blood 1999;93:3587–3600.

84. Reed JC. Double identity for proteins of the Bcl-2 family. Nature 1997;387:773–776.
85. Gottardi D, Alfarano A, De Leo AM, et al. In leukaemic CD5+ B cells the expression of BCL-2 gene family is shifted toward protection from apoptosis. Br J Haematol 1996;94:612–618.
86. Klein A, Miera O, Bauer O, Golfier S, Schriever F. Chemosensitivity of B cell chronic lymphocytic leukemia and correlated expression of proteins regulating apoptosis, cell cycle and DNA repair. Leukemia 2000;14:40–46.
87. Raghoebier S, van Krieken JH, Kluin-Nelemans JC, et al. Oncogene rearrangements in chronic B-cell leukemia. Blood 1991;77:1560–1564.
88. Reed JC. Molecular biology of chronic lymphocytic leukemia. Semin Oncol 1998;25:11–18.
89. Schena M, Larsson LG, Gottardi D, et al. Growth- and differentiation-associated expression of bcl-2 in B-chronic lymphobytic leukemia cells. Blood 1992;79:2981–2989.
90. Hanada M, Delia D, Aiello A, Stadtmauer E, Reed JC. bcl-2 gene hypomethylation and high-level expression in B-cell chronic lymphocytic leukemia. Blood 1993;82:1820–1828.
91. McConkey DJ, Chandra J, Wright S, et al. Apoptosis sensitivity in chronic lymphocytic leukemia is determined by endogenous endonuclease content and relative expression of BCL-2 and BAX. J Immunol 1996;156:2624–2630.
92. Krajewski S, Gascoyne RD, Zapata JM, et al. Immunolocalization of the ICE/Ced-3-family protease, CPP32 (Caspase-3), in non-Hodgkin's lymphomas, chronic lymphocytic leukemias, and reactive lymph nodes. Blood 1997;89:3817–3825.
93. Pepper C, Hoy T, Bentley P. Elevated Bcl-2/Bax are a consistent feature of apoptosis resistance in B-cell chronic lymphocytic leukaemia and are correlated with in vivo chemoresistance. Leuk Lymph 1998;28:355–361.
94. Collins RJ, Verschuer LA, Harmon BV, Prentice RL, Pope JH, Kerr JF. Spontaneous programmed death (apoptosis) of B-chronic lymphocytic leukaemia cells following their culture in vitro. Br J Haematol 1989;71:343–350.
95. Mainou-Fowler T, Prentice AG. Modulation of apoptosis with cytokines in B-cell chronic lymphocytic leukaemia. Leuk Lymph 1996;21:369–377.
96. Aguilar-Santelises M, Magnusson KP, Wiman KG, Mellstedt H, Jondal M. Progressive B-cell chronic lymphocytic leukaemia frequently exhibits aberrant p53 expression. Int J Cancer 1994;58:474–479.
97. Tangye SG, Raison RL. Human cytokines suppress apoptosis of leukaemic CD5+ B cells and preserve expression of bcl-2. Immunol. Cell Biol 1997;75:127–135.
98. Buschle M, Campana D, Carding SR, Richard C, Hoffbrand AV, Brenner MK. Interferon gamma inhibits apoptotic cell death in B cell chronic lymphocytic leukemia. J Exp Med 1993;177:213–218.
99. Dancescu M, Rubio-Trujillo M, Biron G, Bron D, Delespesse G, Sarfati M. Interleukin 4 protects chronic lymphocytic leukemic B cells from death by apoptosis and upregulates Bcl-2 expression. J Exp Med 1992;176:1319–1326.
100. Molica S, Vitelli G, Levato D, Levato L, Dattilo A, Gandolfo GM. Clinico-biological implications of increased serum levels of interleukin-8 in B-cell chronic lymphocytic leukemia. Haematologica 1999;84:208–211.
101. Plate JM, Long BW, Kelkar SB. Role of beta2 integrins in the prevention of apoptosis induction in chronic lymphocytic leukemia B cells. Leukemia 2000;14:34–39.
102. Cordingley FT, Bianchi A, Hoffbrand AV, et al. Tumour necrosis factor as an autocrine tumour growth factor for chronic B-cell malignancies. Lancet 1988;1:969–971.
103. Gamberale R, Geffner JR, Trevani A, et al. Immune complexes inhibit apoptosis of chronic lymphocytic leukaemia B cells. Br J Haematol 1999;107:870–876.
104. Schattner EJ. Cd40 ligand in cll pathogenesis and therapy. Leuk Lymph 2000;37:461–472.
105. Bernal A, Pastore RD, Asgary Z, et al. Survival of leukemic B cells promoted by engagement of the antigen receptor. Blood 2001;98:3050–3057.
106. Laytragoon-Lewin N, Duhony E, Bai XF, Mellstedt H. Downregulation of the CD95 receptor and defect CD40-mediated signal transduction in B-chronic lymphocytic leukemia cells. Eur J Haematol 1998;61:266–271.
107. Kneitz C, Goller M, Wilhelm M, et al. Inhibition of T cell/B cell interaction by B-CLL cells. Leukemia 1999;13:98–104.
108. Ghia P, Caligaris-Cappio F. The indispensable role of microenvironment in the natural history of low-grade B-cell neoplasms. Adv Cancer Res 2000;79:157–173.
109. de la Fuente MT, Casanova B, Garcia-Gila M, Silva A, Garcia-Pardo A. Fibronectin interaction with alpha4beta1 integrin prevents apoptosis in B cell chronic lymphocytic leukemia: correlation with Bcl-2 and Bax. Leukemia 1999;13:266–274.

110. Panayiotidis P, Jones D, Ganeshaguru K, Foroni L, Hoffbrand AV. Human bone marrow stromal cells prevent apoptosis and support the survival of chronic lymphocytic leukaemia cells in vitro. Br J Haematol 1996;92:97–103.
111. Lagneaux L, Delforge A, Bron D, De Bruyn C, Stryckmans P. Chronic lymphocytic leukemic B cells but not normal B cells are rescued from apoptosis by contact with normal bone marrow stromal cells. Blood 1998;91: 2387–2396.
112. Burger JA, Tsukada N, Burger M, Zvaifler NJ, Dell'Aquila M, Kipps TJ. Blood-derived nurse-like cells protect chronic lymphocytic leukemia B cells from spontaneous apoptosis through stromal cell-derived factor-1. Blood 2000;96:2655–2663.
113. Ricciardi MR, Petrucci MT, Gregorj C, et al. Reduced susceptibility to apoptosis correlates with kinetic quiescence in disease progression of chronic lymphocytic leukaemia. Br J Haematol 2001;113:391–399.
114. Robertson LE, Plunkett W, McConnell K, Keating MJ, McDonnell TJ. Bcl-2 expression in chronic lymphocytic leukemia and its correlation with the induction of apoptosis and clinical outcome. Leukemia 1996;10:456–459.
115. Kitada S, Andersen J, Akar S, et al. Expression of apoptosis-regulating proteins in chronic lymphocytic leukemia: correlations with In vitro and In vivo chemoresponses. Blood 1998;91:3379–3389.
116. Hollstein M, Sidransky D, Vogelstein B, Harris CC. p53 mutations in human cancers. Science 1991;253:49–53.
117. Cordone I, Masi S, Mauro FR, et al. p53 expression in B-cell chronic lymphocytic leukemia: a marker of disease progression and poor prognosis. Blood 1998;91:4342–4349.

8   Common Cytogenetic Abnormalities

Gunnar Juliusson, MD

1. INTRODUCTION

Since the description by Nowell and Hungerford *(1)*, in 1960 of the Philadelphia (Ph) chromosome in chronic myelogeneous leukemia, exploration of recurrent chromosomal abnormalities has been the most successful method for the identification of new genes that are important in cancer development (such as the *bcr/abl* hybrid gene) and also in the biology of normal cells (such as the gene *BCL2*). Chromosome abnormalities in tumor cells were first described by Boveri in 1914 *(2)*, but the major prerequisites for the identification of specific abnormalities were the chromosome banding techniques developed by Caspersson in 1971 *(3)*. Previously, chromosomes could be classified only from their size and the proportions between the short (p for *petit*) and long (q) arms. A large number of genes of great physiological importance, such as *bcl-2*, have been identified through analysis of the breakpoints in recurrent chromosome translocations in tumor cells. Currently, chromosome abnormalities are mandatory in the diagnostic evaluation of patients with acute leukemia, partly for the documentation of specific subtypes for individualized therapy, such as the t(15;17) translocation in acute promyelocytic leukemia, but not less importantly for the prediction of prognosis, such as the Ph chromosome in acute lymphocytic leukemia.

Good-quality metaphases are required for chromosome analysis, which is a problem in chronic lymphocytic leuukemia (CLL), owing to the extremely low spontaneous mitotic index. No valid cytogenetic data were available before Robèrt et al. in 1978 *(4)* successfully activated CLL B-cells through culture with polyclonal B-cell mitogens, such as lipopolysaccharides from *E. coli*. During the 1990s, molecular techniques including fluorescence *in situ* hybridization (FISH) were developed that confirmed the cytogenetic data and gave additional information about abnormalities on the gene level. Unfortunately, we are still awaiting a breakthrough in regard to specific genes involved in the pathogenesis of CLL. The hard work and technical difficulties involved in cytogenetic analyses in CLL have largely resulted in the replacement of cytogenetics with molecular techniques, which is regrettable since chromosome analysis remains the major technique for screening of the entire tumor cell genome.

2. CHROMOSOME ABNORMALITIES IN CLL

With proper mitogen stimulation in vitro in dedicated laboratories, most CLL samples present mitotic cells, and clonal chromosome abnormalities are found in about one-half of the cases studied *(5,6)*. In more than one-half of cases with clonal abnormalities, there is only one single chromosome aberration, and in one-fourth of those with clonal abnormalities there are complex

From: *Contemporary Hematology*
Chronic Lymphocytic Leukemia: Molecular Genetics, Biology, Diagnosis, and Management
Edited by: G. B. Faguet © Humana Press Inc., Totowa, NJ

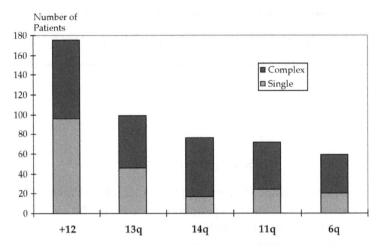

Fig. 1. Chromosomes involved in the most common clonal abnormalities in CLL, divided into single abnormalities and complex (here, two or more) abnormalities. Data are from the International Working Party on Chromosomes in CLL, for 662 CLL patients *(6)*.

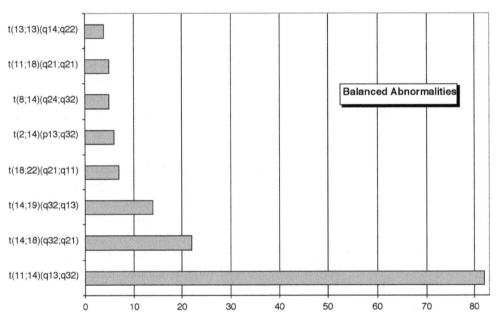

Fig. 2. Balanced clonal chromosomal abnormalities in CLL. All translocations reported in at least four CLL-patients in the Mitelman Database of Chromosome Abnormalities in Cancer 2001 *(26)*.

karyotypes with three or more clonal cytogenetic events. Subclones, i.e., cells with some but not all the clonal abnormalities of a certain population, are commonly found.

The pattern of chromosomal abnormalities in CLL is quite different from that of most other leukemias and lymphoproliferative disorders. In CLL, specific balanced translocations are distinctly rare, whereas trisomies (mainly +12) and deletions (mainly involving 13q, 11q, and 6q) are common (Fig. 1). The most common translocation is the t(11;14) (Fig. 2), which is the characteristic finding of mantle cell lymphoma.

2.1. Trisomy 12

The first nonrandom chromosome abnormality discovered in CLL was trisomy 12 (+12) *(7)*, which is found in about one-third of those who show clonal abnormalities, i.e., about 17% of all patients (Fig. 1). Using FISH analysis, a somewhat higher percentage is achieved *(8)*; about 24% of over 600 CLL patients studied showed evidence of trisomy 12 (for review, *see* ref. *9*), whereas 16% had +12 in the German FISH study *(10)*. Half of all patients with trisomy 12 have no additional abnormality, and although +12 may occasionally be seen in other tumors, it is most common in CLL, indicating a significant role in the pathophysiology of this disease. Interestingly, it is rare that trisomy 12 is found in all leukemia cells of an individual patient *(11)*. The median percentage of CLL cells with trisomy 12 in a patient with such an abnormality is 50%, whether the analysis is performed by cytogenetics or by FISH, and some have +12 in only a few percent of their CLL cells.

The finding of a proportion of CLL cell samples with a normal karyotype is likely to represent a failure to activate leukemia cells and a subsequent analysis of normal cells. In others, small deletions and other submicroscopic changes are beyond detection by cytogenetics. A finding of cells with normal chromosomes coexisting with cells with clonal changes may indicate a clonal evolution, i.e., a secondary event occurring during the subsequent clonal development of the disease. However, if so, trisomy 12 should commonly appear in follow-up samples taken during the course of the disease, and in fact, this has not been the case in several cytogenetic studies in which repeated samples have been collected during progression of CLL *(12)*. CLL cell clones are usually cytogenetically stable during progressive disease, which was recently confirmed using FISH techniques *(13)*. This contrasts to chronic myelogeneous leukemia in blastic phase and follicular lymphoma in transformation, in which additional abnormalities are frequent. Additional abnormalities in CLL usually lead to an increased complexity of the karyotype in cells that already had multiple abnormalities at first analysis. These data indicate that chromosome abnormalities are not exclusively formed at a single transforming event but represent disturbed mitotic procedures during clonal evolution.

Trisomy 12 occurs more frequently together with some additional abnormalities, i.e., +18, +19, or +3, whereas it is rare to find +12 together with del(13q) *(11)*. This observation is likely to have biological significance, although the subcellular mechanisms remains totally unclear.

It is also of major interest that, although rare, structural abnormalities involving chromosome 12 in CLL almost always lead to an increased gene dosage through partial trisomies, i.e., duplications of parts of the chromosome, a finding that is distinctly uncommon with structural abnormalities involving other chromosome sites. One of our patients had CLL cells with five copies of the segment 12q13-15 when presenting with a very aggressive relapse *(14)* following autologous bone marrow transplantation. This and other cases suggest that genes of pathophysiological importance in CLL may be localized to this region. Trisomies are likely to occur through nondisjunction during mitosis. However, it is distinctly difficult to assess which mechanisms (and which genes) are involved in the survival and/or proliferation advantage of trisomic cells, and there are so far no valid data on the role of any trisomy in human tumors.

Trisomy 12 may be slightly more common in patients with the common pregerminal type of CLL with unmutated V_H genes and poorer survival *(15)*. It has also been associated with CLL having atypical morphology *(16,17)*; we had already shown in 1985 that +12 was common in CLL with lymphoplasmacytoid cells *(16)*, termed immunocytoma according to the Kiel classification.

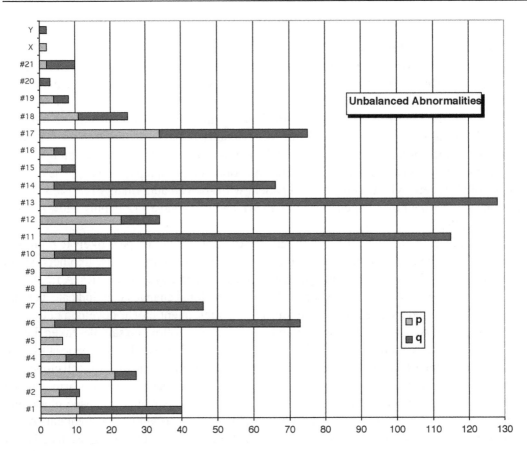

Fig. 3. Unbalanced clonal chromosomal abnormalities in CLL according to chromosome arm. All breakpoints reported in CLL-patients in the Mitelman Database of Chromosome Abnormalities in Cancer 2001 *(26)*. There is an uneven distribution, considering that the chromosomes are ordered according to size (#1 is the largest and #22 the smallest; X is large and Y is small).

2.2. Deletions of Chromosome 13

The most common structural abnormalities in CLL are deletions of the long arm of chromosome 13 *(5)* (Fig. 3). These deletions may be terminal and involve most of the long arm but may also be interstitial with variable breakpoints (Figs. 4 and 5). Small interstitial deletions are difficult or impossible to identify by cytogenetic techniques, and their frequency was underestimated in many early studies, mainly before the FISH techniques were utilized. The most commonly deleted region is 13q14, which is the site for the retinoblastoma (*Rb*) tumor suppressor gene, which, however, does not seem to be involved in CLL. Major efforts from several groups *(18,19)* have made sequencing of the entire region possible, but still there are no indisputable candidates for a CLL gene.

Deletions of 13q have been associated with CLL of the less common postgerminal type with mutated V_H genes and better prognosis *(13)*.

2.3. Deletions of Chromosome 11

The long arm of chromosome 11 is also frequently deleted in CLL (Fig. 3), sometimes as terminal deletions with variable breakpoints (Fig. 4), but also as interstitial deletions *(6)*, without

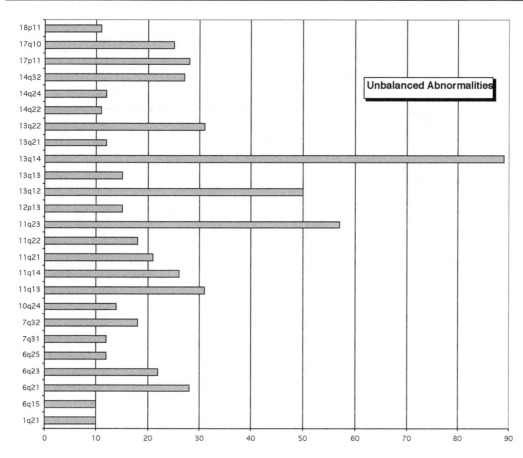

Fig. 4. Unbalanced clonal chromosomal abnormalities in CLL according to specific band. All breakpoints reported in at least 10 CLL patients in the Mitelman Database of Chromosome Abnormalities in Cancer 2001 *(26)*.

a clear-cut minimally deleted region. The only commonly recurring translocation in CLL involves the *cyclin D1/BCL-1* gene on 11q13, which by translocation is juxtaposed to the immunoglobulin heavy chain genes on chromosome 14 band q32. This abnormality is more typically found in mantle cell lymphoma than in CLL, but there are phenotypically well-defined CLLs reported to have this translocation, indicating a relationship between these two CD5+ chronic B-cell malignancies. Chromosome 11 abnormalities rarely occur as single abnormalities (Fig. 1), and, thus, in the so-called hierarchical model of chromosomal abnormalities in CLL proposed by Döhner et al. *(10)*, the designation 11q deletion is likely to be a surrogate marker for a complex karyotype.

Deletions of 11q have been found in younger patients with more aggressive disease and more lymphadenopathy *(20)*, whereas the prognostic impact was not seen among the older population that constitutes most CLL patients.

2.4. 14q+ Chromosomes

B-cells must rearrange their immunoglobulin heavy chain genes at chromosome 14 at band q32 to create their idiotype specificity. This predisposition of normal B-cells may be the cause of the common finding in all B-cell malignancies that chromosome translocations involving 14q32 are common. Since 14q32 is at the telomeric end of the long arm, most balanced trans-

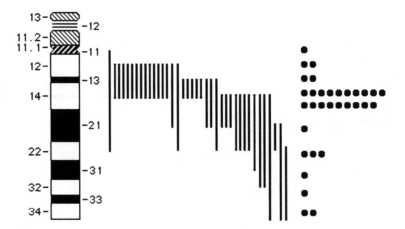

Fig. 5. Chromosome 13. Left, schematic view. Middle, deletions: each line indicates the part of chromosome 13 that has been deleted in one patient. Right, structural abnormalities: each dot indicates a clonal breakpoint in one patient. Note that there are two rows of dots for 13q14. Data from the International Working Party on Chromosomes in CLL *(6)*.

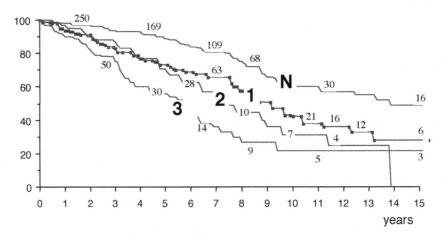

Fig. 6. Impact of the complexity of the karyotype on overall survival for CLL patients. Normal karyotype (*n* = 293), 1, one abnormality (*n* = 176), 2, two clonal abnormalities (*n* = 64), 3, complex karyotypes with three or more abnormalities (*n* = 71). Data from the International Working Party on Chromosomes in CLL *(6)*.

locations give rise to an elongation of the chromosome, called 14q+ chromosomes. However, the translocation partner may be very different in various diseases: the *BCL-2* gene at 18q21 in follicular lymphoma, the *BCL-1/cyclin D1* gene on 11q13 in mantle cell lymphoma, and the *MYC* gene on 8q24 in Burkitt's lymphoma, as well as many other less common translocation partners are seen. In CLL, these translocations are rarely found as the only abnormality (Fig. 1) and might be regarded as an additional finding with no specific role in the pathogenesis. However, the presence of additional abnormalities has an adverse prognostic impact in CLL (Fig. 6).

In follicular lymphoma, *BCL-2* is almost always translocated to the immunoglobulin heavy chain gene on 14q32. However, when *BCL-2* translocations occur in CLL, it more commonly translocates to the light chain genes on 2p13 and 22q11 instead (Fig. 2) *(21)*. The biological significance of this finding is unclear.

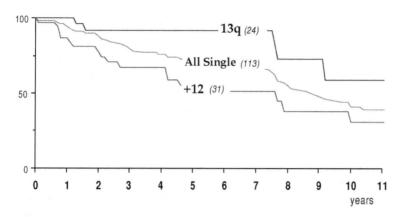

Fig. 7. Impact of specific karyotypic abnormality on overall survival of CLL patients; only single aberrations. Data from the International Working Party on Chromosomes in CLL *(6)*.

3. CHROMOSOME ABNORMALITIES AND PROGNOSIS

Patients with clonal cytogenetic abnormalities have a poorer overall survival than those with normal karyotypes *(5,6)*, and the survival becomes increasingly poorer with more clonal abnormalities (Fig. 6). This prognostic variable is independent of clinical stage and of CLL cell kinetics in vitro *(22)*. In studies from the early 1980s, we found that patients with trisomy 12 had CLL with a higher progression rate, requiring early therapy *(16)*. If only patients with single chromosomal abnormalities were studied, we found that those with trisomy 12 did worse than those with other single abnormalities (Fig. 7), whereas patients with structural abnormalities of chromosome 13 did as well as those with a normal karyotype *(5,6)*. However, patients with a complex karyotype did poorly whether or not the karyotype included trisomy 12. The association of certain karyotypes with mutational status of the immunoglobulin V_H genes, as well as the CLL cell morphology *(17)*, could in part explain the prognostic impact.

p53, localized to 17p13, is a tumor suppressor gene frequently deleted in human cancer and associated with poor prognosis. *p53* deletions are rare in CLL, but they identify drug-resistant leukemia and patients with a poor prognosis *(23–25)*.

A German study evaluated CLL cells from 325 patients in a single center (Ulm) with FISH and a set of fluorescent probes detecting 3q26, 6q21, 8q24, 11q22-q23, 12q13, 13q14, 14q32, and 17p13 *(10)* and identified abnormal karyotypes in 82%. The higher incidence of abnormal karyotypes compared with cytogenetic studies is almost exclusively because of a high rate of 13q14 deletions (55%), since the FISH technique can pick up small deletions, using two probes detecting RB1 and D13S25 *(10)*. FISH analysis only identifies abnormalities that are precisely detected by the probes used, in contrast to cytogenetic analysis. This would be sufficient if all relevant genes were known and evaluated. However, unfortunately, there are no known specific genes influencing the development, course, or prognosis of CLL. In the current situation, it is likely that FISH analysis underestimate complex karyotypes, although it has a greater sensitivity than cytogenetics for small deletions in established regions.

The greatest prognostic impact of the Ulm study was the poor survival of the 7% of the patients who had *p53* deletions (identified through multiple cosmids detecting 17p13). In addition, the authors constructed a hierarchical model of chromosomal abnormalities, confirming the good overall survival of patients with 13q14 deletions as the sole abnormality (among the evaluated gene sites). However, this study seems to indicate an adverse prognostic impact of 11q22-q23 deletions, although this is an abnormality that is uncommon as a single marker, and thus 11q deletions in the German study are likely to be associated with complex karyotypes. In the International Working Party on Chromosomes in CLL study, we compared the overall survival for those few who had 11q abnormalities as a single abnormality with those of other single abnormalities. The results showed an intermediate prognosis for 11q deletions, in contrast to those who had 13q deletions, who did better, and those with +12, who did worse (*see* Fig. 10:1 in ref. 9).

The difference in categorization between the German hierarchical model and those previously reported from cytogenetic studies may well influence interpretation of the prognostic impact of trisomy 12. Thus, it is hazardous to interpret prognostic information established in one diagnostic system for use in another. It would be extremely valuable if more investigators would evaluate cytogenetics and a broad set of FISH markers simultaneously in prospective studies of CLL. In addition, the search for pathophysiologically relevant genetic events and not only surrogate genetic events must proceed. Hopefully, we will learn in the future how to do narrower, simpler, and more specific analyses to identify the genetic status with the greatest clinical importance.

It is commonly claimed that genetic data as well as other prognostic markers are important to assess in clinical practice for the benefit of our patients. This is certainly true for several types of acute leukemias and lymphomas. However, in CLL, such information is still solely of theoretical interest, since no data indicate that overall therapeutic results will improve by knowing the likelihood of clinical progression before it has actually showed up, or that any specific mode of therapy will benefit patients with certain risk factors or clinical characteristics.

4. CONCLUSIONS

With proper CLL cell culture and cytogenetic technique, clonal chromosome abnormalities are found in one-half of patients with CLL, and they indicate poor prognosis. In contrast to most hematological tumors, in which chromosomal abnormalities are mainly balanced structural abnormalities (translocations), the most common aberrations in CLL are unbalanced deletions with variable breakpoints involving chromosomes 13q, 11q, and 6q, as well as trisomy of chromosome 12. Of these, only +12 and del(13q) frequently occur as single abnormalities. The deletions may be small and require FISH analysis for detection. However, cytogenetic techniques are required for evaluating the entire genome and to assess complex karyotypes properly. No defined genetic event behind these aberrations has been identified. Cytogenetics as well as FISH analyses thus indicate surrogate genetic abnormalities than a true underlying genetic event of biological importance. Cytogenetic data indicate that complex karyotypes are associated with poor prognosis. *p53* deletions, although rare, also indicate poor prognosis. The hierarchical model of genetic events detected by FISH proposes a poor prognosis for patients with deletions 11q22-q23, although these are mostly found in younger patients and are probably associated with complex karyotypes. 13q deletions are more common in the postgerminal type of CLL with mutated IgV_H genes and are associated with a good overall survival.

REFERENCES

1. Nowell PC, Hungerford DA. A minute chromosome in human chronic granulocytic leukemia (letter). Science 1960;132:1497.
2. Boveri T. Zur Frage der Entstehung Maligner Tumoren. Fischer, Jena, 1914.
3. Caspersson T, Lomakka G, Zech L. The 24 fluorescence patterns of the human metaphase chromosomes - distinguishing charcaters and variability. Hereditas 1971;67:89–102.

4. Robèrt K-H, Möller E, Gahrton G, Eriksson H, Nilsson B. B-cell activation of peripheral blood lymphocytes from patients with chronic lymphatic leukemia. Clin Exp Immunol 1978;33:302.

5. Juliusson G, Oscier DG, Fitchett M, et al. Prognostic subgroups in B-cell chronic lymphocytic leukemia defined by specific chromosomal abnormalities. N Engl J Med 1990;323:720–724.

6. Juliusson G, Oscier D, Gahrton G for the International Working Party on Chromosomes in Chronic Lymphocytic Leukemia (IWCCLL). Cytogenetic findings and survival in B-cell chronic lymphocytic leukemia. Second international compilation of data on 662 patients. Leuk Lymphoma 1991;5(suppl):21–25.

7. Gahrton G, Robèrt K-H, Friberg K, Zech L, Bird AG. Nonrandom chromosomal aberrations in chronic lymphocytic leukemia revealed by polyclonal B-cell-mitogen stimulation. Blood 1980;56:640.

8. Anastasi J, Le Beau MM, Vardiman JW, et al. Detection of trisomy 12 in chronic lymphocytic leukemia by fluorescence in situ hybridisation to interphase cells: a simple and sensitive method. Blood 1992;79:1796–1801.

9. Juliusson G. Chronic lymphoid leukemias. In: Kurzrock R, Talpaz M, eds. Molecular Biology in Cancer Medicine, 2nd ed. Martin Dunitz, London, 1999, pp. 191–209.

10. Döhner H, Stilgenbauer S, Brenner A, et al. Genomic aberrations and survival in chronic lymphocytic leukemia. N Engl J Med 2000;343:1910–1916.

11. Juliusson G, Merup M. Cytogenetics in chronic lymphocytic leukemia. Semin Oncol 1998;25:19–26.

12. Juliusson G, Friberg K, Gahrton G. Consistency of chromosomal aberrations in chronic B-lymphocytic leukemia. A longitudinal cytogenetic study of 41 patients. Cancer 1988;62:500–506.

13. Döhner H. Prognostic implications of findings from cytogenetic and molecular genetics. In: Chronic Lymphocytic Leukemia: Case-Based Session. American Society of Hematology Education Program Book, 2001, pp. 141–145.

14. Merup M, Juliusson G, Wu X, Stenman G, Gahrton G, Einhorn S. Amplification of multiple regions of chromosome 12, including 12q13-15, in chronic lymphocytic leukemia. Eur J Haematol 1997;58:174–180.

15. Hamblin TJ, Davis Z, Gardiner A, Oscier DG, Stevenson FK. Unmutated Ig VH genes are associated with a more aggressive form of chronic lymphocytic leukemia. Blood 1999;94:1848–1854.

16. Juliusson G, Robèrt K-H, Öst Å, et al. Prognostic information from cytogenetic analysis in chronic B-lymphocytic leukemia and leukemic immunocytoma. Blood 1985;65:134–141.

17. Matutes E, Oscier D, Garcia-Marco J, et al. Trisomy 12 defines a group of CLL with atypical morphology: correlation between cytogenetic, clinical and laboratory features in 544 patients. Br J Haematol 1996;92:382–388.

18. Liu Y, Corcoran M, Rasool O, et al. Cloning of two candidate tumor suppressor genes within a 10 kb region on chromosome 13q14, frequently deleted in chronic lymphocytic leukemia. Oncogene 1997;15:2463–2473.

19. Bullrich F, Veronese ML, Kitada S, et al. Minimal region of loss at 13q14 in B-cell chronic lymphocytic leukemia. Blood 1996;88:3109–3115.

20. Neilson JR, Auer R, White D, et al. Deletions at 11q identify a subset of patients with typical CLL who show consistent disease progression and reduced survival. Leukemia 1997;11:1929–1932.

21. Adachi M, Tefferi A, Greipp PR, Kipps TJ, Tsujimoto Y. Preferential linkage of bcl-2 to immunoglobulin light chain gene in chronic lymphocytic leukemia. J Exp Med 1990;171:559.

22. Juliusson G. Immunological and cytogenetic studies improve prognosis prediction in chronic B-lymphocytic leukemia: a multivariate analysis of 24 parameters. Cancer 1986;58:688–692.

23. el Rouby S, Thomas A, Costin D, et al. p53 gene mutation in B-cell chronic lymphocytic leukemia is associated with drug resistance and is independent of MDR1/MDR3 gene expression. Blood 1993;82:3452–3459.

24. Lens D, Dyer MJS, Garcia-Marco JM, et al. P53 abnormalities in CLL are associated with excess of prolymphocytes and poor prognosis. Br J Haematol 1997;99:848–857.

25. Geisler CH, Philip P, Egelund Christiansen B, et al. In B-cell chronic lymphocytic leukaemia chromosome 17 abnormalities and not trisomy 12 are the single most important cytogenetic abnormalities for the prognosis: a cytogenetic and immunphenotypic study of 480 unselected newly diagnosed patients. Leuk Res 1997;21:1011–1023.

26. Mitelman F, Johansson B, Mertens F, eds. Mitelman Database of Chromosome Aberrations in Cancer 2001. http://cgap.nci.nih.gov/Chromosomes/Mitelman

9

Immunophenotypic Diagnosis of Leukemic B-Cell Chronic Lymphoproliferative Disorders Other Than Chronic Lymphocytic Leukemia

Alberto Orfao, MD, PhD, Julia Almeida, MD, PhD, Maria Luz Sanchez, PhD, and Jesus F. San Miguel, MD, PhD

1. INTRODUCTION

Leukemic B-cell chronic lymphoproliferative disorders (B-CLPD) are a relatively heterogeneous group of diseases, all of which exhibit a clonal expansion of mature-appearing B-lymphoid cells in the peripheral blood (PB). Both primary leukemias and the leukemic phase of primary lymphomas are included in this category *(1)*. Among the primary B-cell leukemias, chronic lymphocytic leukemia (CLL), prolymphocytic leukemia (PLL), and hairy cell leukemia (HCL) are usually considered; within the primary lymphomas, follicular lymphoma (FL), mantle cell lymphoma (MCL), marginal zone splenic lymphoma (MZSL), lymphoplasmacytic lymphoma (LPL), and the large B-cell lymphomas (LCLs) exhibit PB involvement more frequently *(1)*.

At present, analysis of the immunophenotypic features of the clonal B-cells and study of their cytomorphological and histopathological characteristics are the most valuable tools for the diagnosis of this group of diseases *(1,2)*. More recently, the information provided by conventional cytogenetic, molecular, and fluorescence *in situ* hybridization (FISH) studies has further contributed to a detailed characterization of these entities, providing the tools for an integrated classification of B-cell CLPD *(1,2)*.

Immunophenotypic studies have now been applied for more than two decades to the study of B-cell CLPD. From the diagnostic point of view, immunophenotyping has long been used for the screening of B-cell clonality and for the phenotypic characterization and subclassification of B-cell CLPD *(3–6)*. More recently, it has also been employed for additional clinical purposes including staging of the disease *(7)*, prognostic evaluation *(8)*, monitoring of residual leukemic cells *(9)*, and prediction of response to specific therapies such as those that use anti-CD20 monoclonal antibodies *(10–12)*.

Initially, most of the studies dedicated to the analysis of antigen expression in CLPD used microscopy-based techniques *(13)*. However, in the last decade, multiparameter flow cytometry has progressively replaced the microscope, and it is now the preferred method for the immunophenotypic identification, enumeration, and characterization of neoplastic B-cells in PB,

From: *Contemporary Hematology*
Chronic Lymphocytic Leukemia: Molecular Genetics, Biology, Diagnosis, and Management
Edited by: G. B. Faguet © Humana Press Inc., Totowa, NJ

bone marrow (BM), and other body fluids *(3,4,14,15)*. In addition, flow cytometry-based immunophenotypic techniques are also increasingly used for the study of biopsy samples, fine-needle aspirates, and single-cell suspensions obtained from lymph nodes, spleen, and other lymphoid tissue specimens employed in the diagnosis of CLPD. Such extended use of flow cytometry for the evaluation of immunostainings relates to the unique analytical features of this technology *(16)*. Among other advantages, flow cytometry is rather simple and rapid, allowing multiparameter analysis of high numbers of cells in relatively short periods, information being specifically recorded for each individual cell analyzed; in addition, assessment of antigen expression by flow cytometry is performed in both a qualitative and quantitative objective fashion.

In this chapter we review the diagnostic utility of immunophenotyping of leukemic B-cell CLPD other than CLL, which is discussed in detail in Chapter 7.

2. IMMUNOPHENOTYPIC IDENTIFICATION OF LEUKEMIC B-CELLS FOR DIAGNOSTIC PURPOSES

Classically, the first step used for immunophenotypic identification of leukemic B-cells in a given sample is based on analysis of the restricted expression of surface (sIg) and/or cytoplasmic immunoglobulin (cIg) κ or λ light chains on B-cells *(3,17–19)*. For many years, this approach has been used for the diagnostic screening of B-cell clonality in several different types of samples, whenever the presence of mature-appearing clonal leukemic B-cells was suspected or had to be ruled out. This is particularly relevant when cytomorphological and histopathological studies could not distinguish between leukemic and normal/reactive B-cells or when they could not establish the lineage and clonal nature of an expanded population of lymphoid cells.

The use of Ig light chain restriction as a marker for B-cell clonality relies on the fact that in different human samples containing normal/reactive polyclonal B-cells, both κ+ and λ+ B-cells are found at rather stable frequencies of around 1.5 κ+ for each λ+ cell *(3,4,18,19)* (Fig. 1A); infiltration by a population of clonal B-cells induces an imbalanced ratio between the number of κ+ and λ+ cells owing to the restricted use of either κ or λ Ig light chains by the population of clonal B-cells (Fig. 1B). The greater the proportion of clonal vs normal polyclonal B-cells is in the sample, the higher the probability of detecting an imbalanced κ+/λ+ ratio. Accordingly, κ+/λ+ ratios either lower than 0.5 or higher than 3 indicate the presence of a population of clonal B-cells in the sample *(17,19)*. Usually this strategy does not allow for a specific identification of neoplastic cells on the basis of uniquely aberrant phenotypic features. Even so in practice, such an approach, based on an imbalanced excess of either κ+ or λ+ B-cells, has proved to be highly valuable for the diagnostic screening of B-CLPD in PB, BM, lymph node, spleen, and other types of samples containing increased numbers of mature lymphocytes *(3,4,18,19)*. In contrast, determination of the ratio between κ+ and λ+ B-cells has proved to be of limited value for the identification of low numbers of clonal B-cells among a major population of normal B-lymphocytes (indicating minimal disease levels) because of the relatively low sensitivity of this approach: between 10^{-1} and 10^{-2} in lymphoid tissue specimens and between 10^{-2} and 10^{-3} in PB and BM samples *(18,19)*. Moreover, recent studies *(20,21)* show that in around 5% of leukemic B-cell CLPD, two or even more clones of neoplastic B-cells showing different and unique IgH gene rearrangements coexist in the same individual *(20,21)*; in these patients, one clone is frequently κ+ and the other λ+, which may translate into a normal κ+/λ+ B-cell ratio, even in the presence of substantial tumor burden (Fig. 1C). All together, these observations pointed to the need for more specific immunophenotypic criteria for the identification of leukemic vs normal/reactive

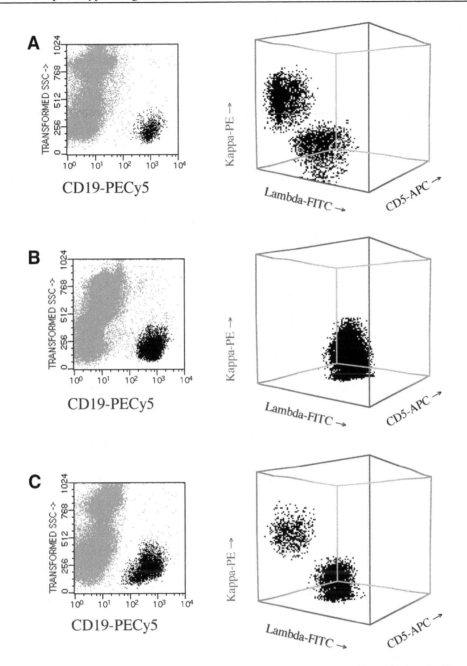

Fig. 1. Representative dot plots of sIg κ, sIg λ, and CD5 expression on normal (**A**) and leukemic (**B** and **C**) PB B-cells. (**B**) A case with a monoclonal expansion of CD5+/sIg λ+ B-cells. (**C**) A B-CLPD other than CLL carrying two different B-cell clones. One clone is CD5+/sIg λ+ and the other of CD5–/sIg κ+. APC, allophycocyanin; FITC, fluorescein isothiocyanate; PE, phycoerythrin.

B-cells than an imbalanced κ+/λ+ ratio alone, particularly for cases with low tumor infiltration or two different clones of B-cells.

Following previous observations in acute leukemias *(22–24)*, in recent years several different groups have clearly shown that not only in CLL patients *(9,25–27)*, but also in most CLPD other than CLL, neoplastic B-cells frequently display aberrant phenotypes *(25–28)*. For each disease entity, slight differences have been reported in the incidence of aberrant phenotypes, ranging from 80% in PLL up to virtually all (99%) cases in MCL, HCL, LPL, and SMZL *(25)*. Interestingly, in most of these patients (90%), two or more aberrant phenotypes are detected *(25)*. The combined analysis of aberrant phenotypes and restricted Ig light chain expression significantly increases the specificity and sensitivity of the second parameter, since light chain restriction would be specifically evaluated within the tumor cell compartment (those B-cells that display aberrant phenotypes) (Fig. 1). The sensitivity of this approach is between 10^{-4} and 10^{-5} (detection of at least one leukemic cell among 10^4 to 10^5) *(25)*. Table 1 summarizes the most frequently observed phenotypic aberrations in the different diagnostic groups of leukemic B-CLPD other than CLL.

3. IMMUNOPHENOTYPIC SUBCLASSIFICATION OF B-CLPD OTHER THAN CLL

Phenotypic features of leukemic cells are considered to reflect the maturation stage at which the neoplastic cell accumulates; at the same time aberrant patterns of protein expression presumably relate to the genetic abnormalities carried by the tumor cells *(17)*. Accordingly, leukemic cells from patients suffering from B-CLPD would display, at least to a certain extent, phenotypic features similar to those of mature B-cells, which would allow subclassification of CLPD according to the degree of maturation of neoplastic B-cells; in turn, the aberrant phenotypes of these leukemic B-cells, would provide a unique screening tool for the identification of underlying genetic abnormalities. Although the former concept appears to be true *(29,30)*, the latter still remains to be confirmed in leukemic B-CLPD.

These data highlight the need to know in advance the exact immunophenotypic features of normal mature PB and/or BM B-cells, including the phenotype of naive, memory, and antibody-secreting B-cells; in line with this, knowledge of the phenotypic features of normal B-cells present in lymph nodes, spleen, and other lymphoid tissues is also essential for an accurate subclassification of primary lymphomas with PB involvement.

3.1. Immunophenotypic Characteristics of Normal Mature B-Cells

Many studies have been reported, in which the phenotypic features of normal, mature PB *(25,28,31)*, and/or BM B-cells *(32–36)* have been analyzed. These studies systematically show that virtually all PB and a substantial part of BM B-cells are mature sIg+ lymphocytes. Most of these correspond to naive sIgM+/sIgD+ (80–90%) and, to a lesser extent (10–15%), immature sIgM+ B-lymphocytes *(37–43)*. In contrast, sIgM+, sIgG+, or sIgA+ memory B-cells only represent a minor fraction of the total sIg+ lymphocytes (<10%) *(28)*. These different B-cell populations have in common expression of cytoplasmic CD79a and surface CD19, CD79b, CD21, CD22, FMC7/CD20, CD37, CD40, CD44, CD21, CD18, CD53, and CD81, and they are strongly positive for surface CD45 and cytoplasmic bcl2 *(8,25,28,44–48)*; in contrast, they are negative for CD10 and CD103 *(25,44–48)*. Other antigens like CD5, CD23, CD24, CD27, CD38, CD11c, CD25, CD43, CD62L, CD80, and CD148 show variable expression within the sIg+ mature PB and/or BM B-cells *(32–36)*. Based on these latter markers, several different subsets of normal mature PB and/or BM B-cells can be identified. As an example, expression of both CD27 and CD148 have been shown to identify the population of memory B-cells generated by germinal center reaction *(39–41)*; among these memory B-cells both Ig class-switched sIgG+ or sIg A+ B-cells and either sIgM+ or sIgM+/sIgD+ memory B-lymphocytes are included *(39–41)*.

Table 1
Incidence and Type of the Most Common Aberrant Phenotypes Detected in Leukemic B-Cell Chronic Lymphoproliferative Disorders Other Than CLL

	PLL	HCL	LPL	MCL	FL	SMZL
Incidence of aberrant phenotypes (%)	80	100	100	100	97	100
Type and frequency of the most common aberrant phenotypes (% in parentheses)[a]						
Antigen overexpression	sIg (60)	CD103 (92) CD19 (69) CD11c (69)			CD10 (80) bcl2 (80)	FMC7 (57)
Asynchronous antigen expression			CD22−/+(weak)/CD10− (67)	CD22−/+(weak)/CD5+ (100) CD22−/+(weak)/CD10− (100) CD22−/+(weak)/sIg+ (68) CD22−/+(weak)/FMC7+ (64)	CD22−/+(weak)/sIg+ (59)	
Aberrant FSC/SSC		↑ FSC/SSC (85)				↑FSC/SSC (57)

PLL, prolymphocytic leukemia; HCL, hairy cell leukemia; LPL, lymphoplasmacytic lymphoma; MCL, mantle-cell lymphoma; FL, follicular lymphoma; SMZL, splenic marginal zone B-cell lymphoma; FSC, forward light scatter; SSC, sideward light scatter (flow cytometry).
[a]Present in more than 50% of cases within each group.

177

Table 2
Phenotypic Subsets of Mature Peripheral Blood (PB) and Bone Marrow (BM)
B-Cells From Normal Healthy Adults

	PB[a]	BM[a]
sIg–/CD22+(weak)/CD23– CD10+	ND	4.9–46
CD11c– CD19+ FSC/SSC(int) (precursor B-cells)		
sIg+ CD19+ FSC/SSC(int) (mature naive/memory B-cells)	97–100	53.9–95.1
SIg M+/D–	1.3–4.3	5–60
SIg M+/D+	71-90	NR
SIg G+ or A+	0.8–36.9	NR
CD5+	2.5–43	6.3–49.2
CD11c+	4.6–39.5	0.8–11.7
CD19+/CD20+ or ++/CD22+	97–100	53.9–95.1
CD23+	11.7–83.9	4–63.1
CD24+ or ++	92–97	98–100
CD25+	5.4–44	0.8–12
CD27+	31.9–89.4	NR
CD38+ or ++	74–88	84.5–99.5
CD43+	8–21	NR
CD62L+	24–52	NR
CD80+	10–22	NR
CD103+	0–6	0
FMC7+	64.2–98	51–88.2
CD10–/CD11c++/FMC7++/CD22++	0.3–6.8	0.3–9.2
CD103–/CD25–/CD5–/CD23–/CD19++/FSC/SSC(hi)		
(mature memory B-cells)		

[a]Results expressed as the range (minimum–maximum) of the percentage of the total B-cells.
ND, not detected (constantly < 0.001%); NR, not reported; int, intermediate lymphoid FSC/
SSC values; hi, high lymphoid FSC/SSC values; –, negative; +(weak), weakly positive; +, positive;
++, strongly positive.

Although for those markers showing a variable expression on mature sIg+ B-cells, the percentage of positive cells depends on the sensitivity of the method used for their evaluation; an estimation of their relative representation on PB mature B-cells is shown in Table 2.

Until now, information on the exact phenotypic features of mature B-cells from lymphoid tissues, as assessed by flow cytometry-based methods for the quantitative evaluation of antigen expression, has been scanty. Even so, recent studies based on the analysis of reactive lymph nodes show that germinal center and mantle zone-derived normal B-cells display clearly different phenotypes (4) (Table 3). Accordingly, germinal center B-cells are usually negative for CD5, CD23, and cytoplasmic bcl2, they express sIg of the IgG subtype and they are strongly positive for CD20, CD10, CD38, and the Ki67 proliferation-associated nuclear antigen. In addition, these cells are CD27+, which supports the notion that they would correspond to memory B-cells (37). In contrast, normal B-cells derived from the mantle zone of the lymphoid follicles are typically sIg M/D+, bcl2+, and CD23+, and display lower reactivity for CD38 and CD20 and variable CD5 expression, in the absence of positivity for CD10 and CD27 (49). This phenotype suggests that mantle zone B-cells would correspond to naive B-cells. In addition, these latter B-cells usually

Table 3
Phenotypic Differences Between Germinal Center and Mantle Zone Normal B-Cells Derived From Reactive Lymph Nodes

	CD5	CD10	CD20	CD23	CD27	CD38	cy-bcl2	Ki67	sIgG	sIgM/D
Germinal center-derived normal B-cells	–	++	++	–	+	++	–	++	+(weak)	–
Mantle zone-derived normal B-cells	–/+	–	+(weak)/+	+	–	+(weak)/+	+	–/+(weak)	–	+

–, negative; +(weak), weakly positive; +, positive; ++, strongly positive; Cy, cytoplasmic.

show negativity or low reactivity for Ki67, supporting the notion that they would correspond to resting B-lymphocytes.

3.2. Immunophenotypic Characteristics of Leukemic B-Cells in CLPD Other Than CLL

Among the B-CLPD, CLL is the most common disease, its differential diagnosis from other leukemic B-cell CLPD being a constant challenge. Typically, CLL exhibits a highly characteristic phenotype, different from that found in other B-CLPD (44–48), including weak expression of CD22, CD20/FMC7, CD79b and sIg, together with a relatively high reactivity for the CD5 and CD23 antigens (for more details, see Chapter 7). In the last decade, scoring systems based on the above mentioned markers (46,48) have been proposed for the diagnosis of CLL; these have proved to be extraordinarily helpful in distinguishing typical CLL cases from other leukemic B-CLPD. Accordingly, whereas CLL patients usually (>90% of cases) display either 5/6 or 6/6 of these markers, only a few other B-CLPD (<5%) exhibit them in such high numbers (44,46, 50,51).

Information provided by these and other additional phenotypic markers is also essential for the diagnostic subclassification of B-CLPD other than CLL. Of all antigens tested in the past, a general consensus exists that CD5, CD19, sIg light chains, CD20, CD23, bcl2, and CD10 are essential for the evaluation of B-CLPD (52). Additional markers such as CD22, FMC7, CD11c, CD103, CD38, CD25, CD79b, and sIg heavy chains would be needed for the full characterization of these disease entities (52). In tissue lymphoma, CD30, terminal deoxynucleotidyl transferase (Tdt), CD71, and CD34 might be useful as well, in specific cases (52).

In the following sections the phenotype of each individual diagnostic subgroup of leukemic B-CLPD is described (Table 4).

3.2.1. PROLYMPHOCYTIC LEUKEMIA

PLL was initially described in 1974 by Galton et al. (53) as a disorder characterized by the presence of massive splenomegaly (in the absence of extensive lymph node involvement) and high white blood cell counts, PB leukocytes corresponding to large lymphocytes with a prominent nucleoli. Despite their apparent morphological immaturity, B-prolymphocytes typically display phenotypic patterns consistent with a more advanced maturation stage than that of the typically small lymphocytes from CLL (8,54) (Table 4). Accordingly, PLL B-prolymphocytes show strong sIg, CD79b, CD22, and CD20/FMC7 expression, they are CD23–, CD24+, and they display a lower reactivity for CD5 than CLL B-cells (8,47,53–55). In addition, prolymphocytes from PLL patients are typically negative for CD103, HC2, and CD10, although they may frequently show weak CD11c expression (8,47,53–56).

It should be noted that intermediate variant forms between CLL and PLL have been described, either presenting at the diagnostic onset of the disease, or as progression from a CLL (1,54,57). In any case, morphologically, these patients have a mixed population of small mature-appearing B-cells and B-prolymphocytes and display intermediate phenotypic features between typical CLL and PLL cases, the relationship to PLL remaining unclear (57,58).

3.2.2. Hairy Cell Leukemia

HCL was initially described in 1958 under the term "leukemic reticulosis" (59). Because of the unique morphologic features of the leukemic B-cells, with their highly characteristic "hairy" cytoplasmic projections, the term hairy cell leukemia was finally accepted in 1966 (60). HCL

Table 4
Immunophenotypic Patterns of the Most Common Leukemic B-Cell Chronic Lymphoproliferative Disorders Other Than CLL

	CD19	CD22	CD20/FMC7	CD5	CD10	CD23	CD79b	sIg	CD103	CD11c	CD43	CD24	HC2	CD25	CD38
Primary leukemias															
PLL	+	+	+	-/+	-	-	+	++	-	-/+(weak)	-	+	-	-	-
HCL	++	++	++	-	-	-	+	+	+	++	-	-	+	+	-/+(weak)
HCLv	++	++	++	-	-	-	+	+	+	+/++	-	-	-	-	-/+(weak)
Primary lymphomas															
LPL	+	+	+	-/+(weak)	-/+(weak)	-	-/+	-/+	-	-/+(weak)	-/+	+	-	-	+
MCL	+	+	+	+	-/+	-	+	+	-	-	-/+	+	-	-	-/+
FL	+	+	+	-	++	-/+	+	+	-	-	-	+	-	-	+
SMZL	+	+	+	-	-	-	+	+	-/+(weak)	+/-	-/+(weak)	+	-	-/+(weak)	-
LCL	+	+	+	-/+	-/+	-/+	-/+	-/+	-	-	+	+	-	-/+(weak)	+

PLL, prolymphocytic leukemia; HCL, hairy cell leukemia; HCLv, HCL variant; LPL, lymphoplasmacytic lymphoma; MCL, mantle cell lymphoma; FL, follicular lymphoma; SMZL, splenic marginal zone B-cell lymphoma, LCL, large B-cell lymphoma; –, negative; +(weak), weakly positive; +, positive; ++, strongly positive.

presentation is different from that of other chronic B-cell leukemias: patients have cytopenias and splenomegaly, villous large lymphocytes in a PB smear and a dry BM aspirate *(61–64)*.

To the best of our knowledge, the potential normal counterpart of hairy cells has not been identified so far, in either PB or BM or in lymphoid tissues such as the spleen. From the phenotypic point of view, typical hairy cells show unique features, which include coexpression of CD103, CD25, and HC2 and strong reactivity for CD11c *(8,45,47,53,61–65)* (Table 4). In addition, overexpression of several pan-B antigens such as CD19 and CD22 together with CD20/FMC7 is also a frequent finding *(3,46,65,66)*. Most cases are CD5–, CD23–, and CD24– and show sIg expression of the IgG and/or the IgA isotypes, with strong reativity for CD79b *(17,44,48)*. Based on their flow cytometry light scatter properties—forward (FSC) and sideward light scatter (SSC)—hairy cells are larger than normal B-cells from both PB and BM *(3,4,25,26)*.

A variant form of HCL has been reported *(61–64)*. Like classical HCL, variant cases frequently display splenomegaly, anemia, and thrombocytopenia but in association with leukocytosis and in the absence of monocytopenia *(61–64)*. In these patients, leukocytosis is at the expense of atypical hairy cells that, together with the characteristic "hairy" cytoplasmic projections, may show a prominent nucleoli *(61–64)*. Phenotypically, these B-cells are similar to typical hairy cells, except that they are usually CD25– and HC2– *(46,47)*.

3.2.3. FOLLICULAR LYMPHOMA

Of all the primary lymphomas displaying PB involvement, FL is the most frequently observed. Although the overall incidence of PB involvement in FL has been estimated to be around 10–40% of all cases *(68)*, the use of sensitive techniques [such as multiparameter antigen stainings analyzed by flow cytometry and the polymerase chain reaction (PCR)], shows that neoplastic B-cells are already detectable in PB at diagnosis, or they will appear later in the evolution of the disease, in a substantially higher proportion of FL cases *(68,69)*. From the morphological point of view, these patients, in contrast to CLL cases, frequently show the presence of small lymphocytes with a cleaved nuclei or a certain degree of polymorphism with both small and large lymphocytes in the absence of smudged cells *(68)*. Phenotypic analysis of clonal B-cells (Table 4) shows strong sIg, CD22, and CD20/FMC7 expression, together with reactivity for CD38; CD79b is usually expressed at levels intermediate between CLL and HCL *(4,8,45,47,53)*. In addition, these cells are typically CD10+ *(52)* and negative for CD11c, CD23, CD5, CD43, CD103, and HC2 *(4,8,25,45,47,53)*. It should be noted that different patterns of reactivity for the CD10 antigen have been reported, not only in FL *(1,25,70)* but also in multiple myeloma *(71,72)*, such variability probably being associated with the use of different monoclonal antibody clones and fluorochrome conjugates *(72)*. In this sense, for assessment of CD10 expression in FL either the J5 or the 5-1B4 monoclonal antibody clones conjugated to the most sensitive fluorochromes—phycoerythrin (PE) or PE/cyanin 5—should be used as the reference reagents *(72,73)*.

From the genetic point of view, a high proportion (60–80%) of patients with FL have the t(14;18) translocation *(68)*, in which the *bcl2* gene from chromosome 18 is translocated into chromosome 14, close to the region where the Ig heavy chain gene is located *(68,74)*; this translates into a very high cytoplasmic expression of the bcl2 protein *(75)*.

Overall, the existence of neoplastic B-cells in the PB of patients with FL does not seem to influence disease outcome, except if it is associated with high white blood cell counts (> 50 × 10^9/L) *(68)*. Even so, clearance of PB B-cells after treatment has been associated with a better clinical outcome in FL *(76)*.

3.2.4. MANTLE CELL LYMPHOMA

Around one-third of all MCLs show PB and/or BM infiltration the latter usually consisting of either a paratrabecular or a diffuse pattern (77). In these cases, differential diagnosis with B-CLL represents a major challenge. MCL is usually morphologically associated with small lymphocytes, but, in contrast to typical CLL cases, these cells show an irregular nuclei contour, with even some cleaved nuclei and nucleoli, in the absence of Gumprecht's shadows (77). Even though in both entities clonal B-cells are CD5+, CD24+, CD22+(weak), and CD11c-/+(weak) (1,8,50,45–48), different patterns of expression are found in MCL compared with CLL for other phenotypic markers. Accordingly, MCL B-cells are characteristically CD23– and show high expression of sIgM+ (with or without sIgD+), CD79b, and FMC7/CD20 together with variable reactivity for CD38 and CD43 (1,2,25,50,52) (Table 4). In addition, CD54 and CD18 expression has been suggested to be particularly useful in the differential diagnosis between MCL and atypical CLL, the reactivity for both markers being higher in MCL (50). In the blastic variant of MCL (1,77), B-cells show FSC and SSC values higher than those of normal B-cells, and they are usually associated with a greater proliferative rate (77). Typically, in both the classical and variant forms of MCL, B-cells carry the t(11;14) (q13;q32) translocation, which involves the bcl1 and IgH genes (77) and translates into overexpression of the PRAD1/cyclin D1 protein (77,78). Although overexpression of cyclin D1 represents a characteristic phenotypic feature of MCL, until now, no reliable technique has been reported that would allow its assessment by conventional flow cytometry (79).

In MCL, the presence of neoplastic B-cells in the PB has been suggested to be associated with a worse clinical outcome (77).

3.2.5. MARGINAL ZONE SPLENIC LYMPHOMA

MZSL has been extensively studied from both the clinical and the phenotypic point of view (80,81). MZSL frequently affects adult patients around the fifth decade of life who show a large splenomegaly in the absence of lymph node involvement (81,82); in PB, lymphocytes larger than those found in CLL patients with round nuclei, sometimes with nucleoli, basophilic cytoplasm, and characteristic "hairy" cytoplasmic projections shorter than those observed in HCL, are frequently found (81). Leukocytosis is usually moderate (between 10 and 30 × 10⁹/L), and mild anemia and thrombocytopenia are detected in up to 20–30% of all cases, owing to hypersplenism (81). Up to 50% of SZML cases have been reported to have a serum monoclonal component typically of the IgM isotype, which is sometimes associated with the presence of Ig light chains in the urine (81).

From the phenotypic point of view, MZSL probably represents one of the most heterogeneous B-CLPD (2,80). Typically these cells show strong sIg and CD79b expression, together with reactivity for pan-B cell markers such as CD19 and CD22; in contrast to HCL, SMZL is usually CD24+ (8,45–48,53,83,84). In addition, clonal SMZL B-cells are FMC7+/CD20+ but negative or weakly positive (<25% of the cases) for CD38, CD43, and CD25 (52,80–82). Surface antigens characteristic of other B-CLPD such as CD5, CD10, CD23, CD103, and HC2 are frequently absent in MZSL (<20% positive cases) (2,80–82). In contrast, CD54 is expressed at similar levels as in MCL and FL (50).

3.2.6. LYMPHOPLASMACYTIC LYMPHOMA

LPL frequently shows BM involvement, with the presence of clonal B-cells in PB being less common (8,45–48,53). In PB, low to moderate numbers of clonal small B-lymphocytes frequently coexist with typical lymphoplasmacytes or even with plasma cells *(8,45–48,53)*. A serum monoclonal component is detected in most cases, although the use of sensitive methods such as immunofixation is frequently required for its detection *(1,2,85)*. From the phenotypic point of view, the most characteristic features of clonal PB B-cells from patients with LPL include the absence or weak expression of CD5 and CD10 together with reactivity for pan-B-markers—CD79a+, CD19+, CD22+, and FMC7/CD20+—and CD38, associated with the presence of cytoplasmic IgM and high CD54 expression *(2,8,50,45–48)* (Table 4). Around half of all LPL patients have been reported to carry the t(9;14)(p13;q32) translocation *(86)*, which involves the *PAX5* gene *(86)* and might be of help for the differential diagnosis between this and other variants of non-Hodgkin's lymphomas (NHL).

3.2.7. LARGE CELL LYMPHOMA

Only a small proportion of all B-large cell lymphomas (<5%) show PB involvement at diagnosis *(68)*. Typically, large immunoblasts and/or centroblasts in the PB are present that display high light scatter characteristics (FSC and SSC) and show strong reactivity for pan-B-markers such as CD19—overexpressed in immunoblastic lymphomas *(87)*, FMC7/CD20, CD22, CD79b, and sIg *(2,45–47,53)*; in up to 50% of the cases, neoplastic B-cells are CD10+ *(52)*. Although most patients have a CD5–, CD23– phenotype, cases have been reported in which clonal B-cells show variable expression for these antigens *(1,2)* (Table 4). Some LCL cases display DNA aneuploidy by flow cytometry *(88)*, and they typically show intermediate to high proliferative rates *(88,89)*, which helps in the differential diagnosis with other leukemic B-CLPD. Because of the morphological appearance of the large leukemic B-cells, in some cases the myeloid (monocytic/dendritic cell) origin of the neoplastic cells has to be ruled out.

3.3. Immunophenotypic Investigation of Minimal Disease Levels in B-CLPD Other Than CLL

Assessment of minimal disease in already diagnosed B-CLPD is of utility not only for the evaluation of response to treatment but also, in primary lymphomas, to identify small numbers of neoplastic B-cells in PB, BM, and other body fluids for either diagnostic or staging purposes *(25–27,90–92)*. Until recently, assessment of the quality of remission in B-CLPD using immunophenotyping has been almost restricted to CLL patients and mainly based on monitoring either the κ+/λ+ B-cell ratio or the number of cells showing CD5 overexpression *(91,92)*. As discussed above in Subheading 2., the balance between κ+ and λ+ B-lymphocytes is not a specific marker for leukemic B-cells, and its sensitivity is relatively low (10^{-2}–10^{-3}), being limited by the presence of normal B-cells in the sample *(3,94)*. In turn, CD5 overexpression, although a useful marker for the detection of minimal disease levels in CLL *(91)*, can only be applied to a minor subset of other leukemic B-CLPDs (<15%) *(25)*; the same applies for CD79b *(93)*.

Information currently available on the incidence and type of aberrant phenotypes displayed by neoplastic B-cells in CLPD other than CLL is limited to a few reports. In a recent study *(25)* based on the analysis of 85 B-CLPD other than CLL, we have clearly shown that PB and/or BM B-cells from most patients (99%) display aberrant phenotypes. Serial dilutional experiments demonstrated that, based on these aberrant phenotypes, unequivocal identification of neoplastic B-cells can be achieved even once they are present at frequencies as low as one neoplastic B-cell among 10^4 to 10^5 normal PB or BM cells (10^{-4}–10^{-5}) *(25)* (Fig. 2). Interestingly, distinct patterns of phenotypic aberrations were found in the different diagnostic subgroups. Accordingly, antigen overexpression was the most common aberration in PLL (80%), HCL (100%), and SMZL (79%),

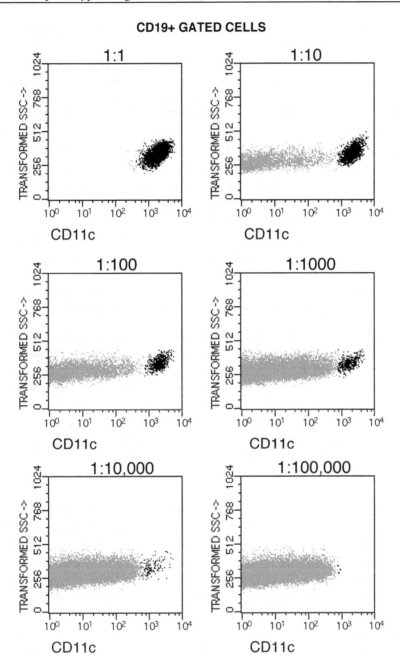

CD19+ GATED CELLS

Fig. 2. Representative dilutional experiment of neoplastic B-cells in normal peripheral blood cells. This case corresponds to a hairy cell leukemia in which neoplastic B-cells overexpress CD11c. Aberrant B-cells could be detected at a level of 10^{-4} (one aberrant B-cell among 10,000 normal PB cells).

whereas in LPL, FL, and MCL the most frequent abnormality consisted of the presence of asynchronous antigen expression: 83, 95, and 100% of the cases, respectively *(25)*. The most frequently overexpressed markers *(25)* included sIg (60%) and FMC7 (40%) in the context of abnormally high FSC/SSC values (85%) in HCL and FMC7 (57%) in SMZL *(25)*. In turn, the most frequent patterns of asynchronous antigen expression involved CD22–(weak)/CD10–/ CD19+ B-cells found in 67 and 100%, respectively, of the LPL and MCL analyzed; in addition, in MCL, neoplastic B-cells frequently showed coexpression of CD5 on B-cells showing abnormally low levels of CD22 *(25)*. Additional aberrations that have been reported as rather frequent in FL (>80% of cases) include CD10 and bcl2 overexpression on CD20 strongly positive B-cells *(4,50,52)* and abnormally low CD44 expression on CD38+ clonal B-cells *(50)*.

Despite the apparently high applicability of immunophenotyping for the detection of minimal disease in leukemic B-CLPD other than CLL, few studies have explored its potential clinical utility. Wells et al. *(26)* have clearly shown that occult B-cell malignancies can be successfully detected by multiparameter flow cytometry in patients with cytopenias, mainly including the diagnosis of HCL and, to a lesser extent, other primary B-cell lymphomas. In a similar way, Subira et al. *(90)* have demonstrated that multiparameter flow cytometry immunophenotyping is a rather sensitive and specific approach for the detection of central nervous system involvement by B-cell neoplasias. Further studies are still necessary to confirm and potentially extend these observations.

3.4. Other Clinical Applications of the Immunophenotypic Characterization of B-CLPD Other Than CLL

Flow cytometric analysis of the immunophenotype of leukemic B-cells has proved to be of additional value in the study of CLPD, especially as regards prognostic assessment. In this area, expression of several cell surface and intracellular immunophenotypic markers has been correlated with prognosis in B-CLPD. As an example, proliferation-associated markers—evaluated either as the proportion of CD71+ and Ki67+/MIB1+ cells or the percentage of S-phase cells— have proved to be of prognostic relevance in B-CLPD other than CLL *(4,88,89)*: high numbers of proliferating cells correlate with a higher tumor grade in NHL and worse clinical outcome *(4,88)*. Similarly, recent studies suggest that quantitative evaluation of β-integrin levels expression on neoplastic B-cells correlates with the metastatic potential of the disease in patients with B-cell NHL *(95)*.

The use of new treatment strategies based on protein targets present on the surface of neoplastic B-cells will potentially expand the prognostic utility of immunophenotyping in CLPD as regards prediction of response to therapy. As an example, large multicenter studies *(10)* have recently shown higher response rates to anti-CD20 therapy in patients with FL, MCL, and LPL, compared with CLL/SLL cases. These findings suggest the existence of an association between the levels of CD20 expression on neoplastic B-cells and response to anti-CD20 therapy, as the number of CD20 molecules per cell is typically lower in CLL/SLL than in the other groups of B-CLPD patients *(11,12,52)*. Also, further studies are necessary in this field both to confirm such preliminary observations and to determine whether this also applies to other treatment protocols that directly target markers expressed on the surface membrane of the neoplastic B-cells such as CD52 *(9,96)*.

4. CONCLUSIONS

At present, general consensus exists on the utility of immunophenotyping of leukemic B-cell CLPD, multiparameter flow cytometry being the preferred method for analysis of body fluids and single-cell suspensions presumably containing the neoplastic cells. Immunophenotyping is essential for both the diagnosis of B-cell clonality and the phenotypic subclassification of leukemic B-CLPD. To detect B-cell clonality, the analysis of Ig light chain restricted expression on phenotypically aberrant B-cells results in an especially powerful tool. In turn, for the phenotypic subclassification of leukemic B-CLPD, an extended panel of monoclonal antibodies is necessary, some of which are particularly useful (CD19, FMC7/CD20, CD5, CD23, sIg light chains, CD10, bcl2, CD103, CD11c, CD79b, CD22, CD25) for identification of unique phenotypic patterns characteristic of a specific disease entity. Accumulating evidence shows that flow cytometry based on immunophenotyping is quite a sensitive and specific technique for the detection of minimal numbers of leukemic cells in B-CLPD other than CLL; the clinical utility of its application, for either monitoring residual disease after treatment or evaluating disease extension, largely remains to be explored. Finally, increasing evidence supports the need to develop standardized flow cytometry methods for quantitative evaluation of the expression on leukemic cells of antigens that will be targeted by specific monoclonal antibody based therapies.

REFERENCES

1. Harris N, Jaffe E, Diebold J, et al. World Health Organization Classification of Neoplastic Diseases of the Hematopoietic and Lymphoid Tissues: Report of the Clinical Advisory Committee Meeting—Airlie House, Virginia, November 1997. J Clin Oncol 1999;17:3835–3849.
2. Harris NL, Jaffe ES, Stein H, et al. A revised european-american classification of lymphoid neoplasms: a proposal from the international lymphoma study group. Blood 1994;84:1361–1392.
3. Di Giuseppe JA, Borowitz MJ. Clinical utility of flow cytometry in the chronic lymphoid leukemias. Semin Oncol 1998;25:6–10.
4. Stetler-Stevenson M, Braylan RC. Flow cytometric analysis of lymphomas and lymphoproliferative disorders. Semin Hematol 2001;38:2111–2123.
5. Jennings CD, Foon KA. Recent advances in flow cytometry: application to the diagnosis of hematologic malignancy. Blood 1997;90:2863–2892.
6. Matutes E, Polliack A. Morphological and immunophenotypic features of chronic lymphocytic leukemia. Rev Clin Exp Hematol 2000;4:22–47.
7. Matutes E. Contribution of immunophenotype in the diagnosis and classification of haemapoietic malignancies. J Clin Pathol 1995;48:194–197.
8. Montserrat E. Chronic lymphoproliferative disorders. Curr Opin Oncol 1997;9:34–41.
9. Rawstron AC, Kennedy B, Evans PA, et al. Quantification of minimal residual disease levels in chronic lymphocytic leukemia using a sensitive flow cytometric assay improves the prediction of outcome and can be used to optimize therapy. Blood 2001;98:29–35.
10. Foran JM, Rohatiner AZ, Cunningham D, et al. European phase II study of rituximab (chimeric anti-CD20 monoclonal antibody) for patients with newly diagnosed mantle cell lymphoma and previously treated mantle-cell lymphoma, immunocytoma and small B-cell lymphocytic lymphoma. J Clin Oncol 2000;18:317–324.
11. Davis TA, Czerwinski DK, Levy R. Therapy of B-cell lymphoma with anti-CD20 antibodies can result in loss of CD20 antigen expression. Clin Cancer Res 1999;5:611–615.
12. Foran JM, Norton AJ, Micallef IN, et al. Loss of CD20 expression following treatment with rituximab (chimaeric monoclonal anti-CD20): a retrospective cohort analysis. Br J Haematol 2001;114:881–883.
13. Samoilava RS. Possibilities of differential diagnosis of B-cell chronic lymphoproliferative diseases using monoclonal antibodies. Gematol Transfuzion 1990;35:24–27.
14. Rothe G, Schmitz G. Consensus protocol for the flow cytometric immunophenotyping of hematopoietic malignancies. Working Group on Flow Cytometry and Image Analysis. Leukemia 1996;10:877–895.
15. Davis BH, Foucar K, Szczarkowski W, et al. U.S.-Canadian Consensus recommendations on the immunophenotypic analysis of hematologic neoplasia by flow cytometry: medical indications. Cytometry 1997;30:249–263.
16. Whiteside TL. Basic techniques for the detection of human T and B lymphocytes in tissues. Clin Immunol News 1980;1:1–15.
17. Orfao A, Schmitz G, Brando B, et al. Clinically useful information provided by the flow cytometric immunophenotyping of haematological malignancies: current status and future directions. Clin Chem 1999;45:1708–1717.
18. Geary W, Frierson HF, Innes DJ, et al. Quantitative criteria for clonality in the diagnosis of B-cell non-Hodgkin's lymphoma by flow cytometry. Mod Pathol 1993;6:155–161.

19. Peters R, Janossy G, Ivory K, et al. Leukemia-associated changes identified by quantitative flow cytometry. III. B-cell gating in CD37 κ/λ clonality test. Leukemia 1994;8:1864–1870.

20. Fend F, Quintanilla-Martinez L, Kumar S, et al. Composite low grade B-cell lymphomas with two immuno-phenotypically distinct cell populations are true biclonal lymphomas. A molecular analysis using laser capture microdissection. Am J Pathol 1999;154:1857–1866.

21. Sanchez ML, Almeida J, Gonzalez D, et al. Incidence and clinico-biologic characteristics of biclonality in leuke-mic B-cell Chronic lymphoproliferative disorders (B-CLPD). In: Proceedings of the 7th Congress of the European Hematology Association (abstract).

22. Ciudad J, San Miguel JF, Lopez-Berges MC, et al. Prognostic value of immunophenotypic detection of minimal residual disease in acute lymphoblastic leukemia. J Clin Oncol 1998;16:3774–3781.

23. San Miguel JF, Martinez A, Macedo A, et al. Immunophenotyping investigation of minimal residual disease is a useful approach for predicting relapse in acute myeloid leukemia patients. Blood 1997;90:2465–2470.

24. Coustan-Smith E, Behm FG, Sanchez J, et al. Immunological detection of minimal residual disease in children with acute lymphoblastic leukaemia. Lancet 1998;351:550–554.

25. Sanchez ML, Almeida J, Vidriales B, et al. Incidence of phenotypic aberrations in a series of 467 patients with B-chronic lymphoproliferative disorders: basis for the design of specific 4-color stainings to be used for minimal residual disease investigation. Leukemia 2002;16:1460–1469.

26. Wells DA, Hall MC, Shulman HM, Loken MR. Occult B cell malignancies can be detected by three-color flow cytometry in patients with cytopenias. Leukemia 1998;12:2015–2023.

27. Chan LC, Lam CK, Yeung TC, et al. The spectrum of chronic lymphoproliferative disorders in Hong Kong. A prospective study. Leukemia 1997;11:1964–1972.

28. Deneys V, Mazzon AM, Marques JL, Benoit H, De Bruyere M. Reference values for peripheral blood B-lympho-cyte subpopulations: a basis for multiparametric immunophenotyping of abnormal lymphocytes. J Immunol Methods 2001;253:23–36.

29. Haase D, Feuring-Buske M, Schafer C, et al. Cytogenetic analysis of CD34+ subpopulations in AML and MDS characterized by the expression of CD38 and CD117. Leukemia 1997;11:674–679.

30. Wuchter C, Harbott J, Schoch C, et al. Detection of acute leukemia cells with mixed lineage leukemia (MLL) gene rearrangements by flow cytometry using monoclonal antibody 7.1. Leukemia 2000;14:1232–1238.

31. Groeneveld K, te Marvelde JG, van den Beemd MW, Hooijkaas H, van Dongen JJ. Flow cytometric detection of intracellular antigens for immunophenotyping of normal and malignant leukocytes. Leukemia 1996;10:1383–1389.

32. Lucio P, Parreira A, van den Beemd MWM, et al. Flow cytometric analysis of normal B cell differentiation: a frame of reference for the detection of minimal residual disease in precursor-B ALL. Leukemia 1999;13:419–427.

33. Dworzak MN, Fritsch G, Froschl G, Printz D, Gadner H. Four-color flow cytometric investigation of terminal deoxynucleotidyl transferase-positive lymphoid precursors in pediatric bone marrow: CD79a expression pre-cedes CD19 in early B-cell ontogeny. Blood 1998;92:3203–3209.

34. Ciudad J, Orfao A, Vidriales B, et al. Immunophenotypic analysis of CD19+ precursors in normal human adult bone marrow: implications for minimal residual disease detection. Haematologica 1998;83:1069–1075.

35. De Waele M, Renmans W, Jochmans K, et al. Different expression of adhesion molecules on CD34+ cells in AML and B-lineage ALL and their normal bone marrow counterparts. Eur J Haematol 1999;63:192–201.

36. Weir EG, Cowan K, LeBeau P, Borowitz MJ. A limited antibody panel can distinguish B-precursor acute lympho-blastic leukemia from normal B precursors with four color flow cytometry: implications for minimal residual disease detection. Leukemia 1999;13:558–567.

37. Agematsu K. Memory B-cells and CD27. Histol Histopathol 2000;15:573–576.

38. Jacquot S. CD27/CD70 interactions regulate T dependent B-cell differentiation. Immunol Res 2000;21:23–30.

39. Tangye SG, Liu YJ, Aversa G, Philips JH, de Vries JE. Identification of functional human splenic memory B cells by expression of CD148 and CD27. J Exp Med 1998;188:1691–1703.

40. Klein U, Goossens T, Fischer M, et al. Somatic hypermutation in normal and transformed human B cells. Immunol Rev 1998;162:261–280.

41. Klein U, Jajewski K, Kuppers R. Human immunoglobulin (Ig)M+ IgD+ peripheral blood B cells expressing the CD27 cell surface antigen carry somatically mutated variable region genes: CD27 as a general marker for somati-cally mutated (memory) B cells. J Exp Med 1998;188:1679–1689.

42. Klein U, Kuppers R, Jajewski K. Evidence for a large compartment of IgM-expressing memory B cells in humans. Blood 1997;89:1288–1298.

43. Klein U, Rajewsky, Küppers R. Phenotypic and molecular characterization of human peripheral blood B-cell subsets with special reference to N-region addition and J kappa -usage in V B-cell- subsets to identify traces of receptor editing processes. Curr Top Microbiol Immunol 1999;246:141–147.

44. Matutes E, Owusuankomah K, Morilla R, et al. The immunological profile of B-cell disorders and proposal of a scoring system for the diagnosis of CLL. Leukemia 1994;8:1640–1645.

45. Bennet JM, Catovsky D, Daniel MT, et al. Proposals for the classification of chronic (mature) B and T lymphoid leukaemias. J Clin Pathol 1989;42:567–584.

46. Matutes E, Worner I, Sainati L, de Olivera MP, Cayovsky D. Advances in the lymphoproliferative disorders. Review of our experience in the study of over 1000 cases. Biol Clin Hematol 1989;11:53–62.

47. Matutes E. Immunophenotype of the chronic lymphoproliferative disorders. Haematologica 1998;83(suppl): 193–198.

48. Matutes E, Morilla R, Owusu-Ankomah K, et al. The immunophenotype of hairy-cell leukemia (HCL) –Proposal for a scoring system to distinguish HCL from B-cell disorders with hairy or villous lymphocytes. Leuk Lymph 1994;14:57–61.

49. Trentin L, Zambello R, Sancetta R, et al. B lymphocytes from patients with chronic lymphoproliferative disorders are equipped with different costimulatory molecules. Cancer Res 1997;57:4940–4947.

50. Deneys V, Michaux L, Leveugle P, et al. Atypical lymphocytic leukemia and mantle cell lymphoma immunologically very close: flow cytometric distinction by use of CD20 and CD54 expression. Leukemia 2001;15:1458–1465.

51. Moreau E, Matutes E, a'Hern RP, et al. Improvement of the chronic lymphocytic leukemia scoring system with the monoclonal antibody SN8 (CD79b). Am J Clin Pathol 2000;108:378–382.

52. Braylan RC, Orfao A, Borowitz MJ, Davis BH. Optimal number of reagents required to evaluate hematolymphoid neoplasias: Results of an International Consensus Meeting. Cytometry 2001;46:23–27.

53. Catovsky D. Chronic lymphoproliferative disorders. Curr Opin Oncol 1995;7:3–11.

54. Melo JV, Catovsky D, Galton DAG. The relationship between chronic lymphocytic leukemia and prolymphocytic leukaemia. I. Clinical and laboratory features of 300 patients and characterization of an intermediate group. Br J Haematol 1986;63:377–387.

55. Orfao A, Gonzalez M, San Miguel JF, et al. Clinical and immunological findings in large B-cell chronic lymphocytic leukemia. Clin Immunol Immunopahol 1988;46:177–185.

56. Marotta G, Raspadori D, Sestigiani C, Scalia G, Biqazzi C, Lauria F. Expression of the CD11c antigen in B-cell chronic lymphoproliferative disorders. Leuk Lymph 2000;37:145–149.

57. Melo JV, Catovsky D, Galton DA. The relationship between chronic lymphocytic leukaemia and prolymphocytic leukaemia. II. Patterns of evolution of "prolymphocytoid" transformation. Br J Haematol 1986;64:77–86.

58. Melo JV, Wardle J, Chetty M, et al. The relationship between chronic lymphocytic leukaemia and prolymphocytic leukaemia. III. Evaluation of cell size by morphology and volume measurements. Br J Haematol 1986;84:469–478.

59. Bouroncle BA, Wiseman BK, Doan CA. Leukemic reticuloendotheliosis. Blood 1958;13:609–615.

60. Bouroncle BA. Leukemic reticuloendotheliosis (Hairy-cell leukemia). Blood 1979;53:412–436.

61. Bouroncle BA. Clínica, biología y formas variantes de tricoleucemia. In: Lopez Borrasca, et al. Enciclopedia de Hematologia Iberoamericana (EHIA). Universidad de Salamanca, Salamanca, 1992.

62. Frassoldati A, Lamparelli T, Federico M, et al. Hairy cell leukemia: a clinical review based on 725 cases of the Italian Cooperative Group (ICGHCL). Leuk Lymph1994;13:307–316.

63. Troussard X, Maloisel F, Flandrin G. Hairy cell leukemia. What is new forty years after the first description? Hematol Cell Ther 1998;40:139–148.

64. Polliack A. Hairy cell leukemia and allied chronic lymphoid leukemias: current knowledge and new therapeutic options. Leuk Lymph 1997;26:41–51.

65. Rozman C, Montserrat E. Chronic lymphocytic leukemia. N Engl J Med 1995;333:1052–1057.

66. Ahmad E, Garcia D, Davis BH. Clinical utility od CD23 and FMC7 antigen coexistent expression in B-cell lymphoproliferative disorder subclassification. Cytometry 2002;50:1–7.

67. Melo JV, San Miguel JF, Moss VE, Catovsky D. The membrane phenotype of hairy cells: a study with monoclonal antibodies. Semin Oncol 1984;11:381–385.

68. Bain BJ, Catovsky D. The leukaemic phase of non-Hodgkin's lymphoma. J Clin Pathol 1995;48:189–193.

69. Lopez-Guillermo A, Cabanillas F, McLaughlin P, et al. Molecular response assessed by PCR is the most important factor predicting failure-free survival in indolent follicular lymphoma: update of the MDACC series. Ann Oncol 2000;11(suppl 1):137–140.

70. Almasri NM, Iturraspe JA, Braylan RC. CD10 expression in follicular lymphoma and large cell lymphoma is different from that of reactive lymph node follicles. Arch Pathol Lab Med 1998;122:539–544.

71. Cao J, Vescio RA, Rettig MB, et al. A CD10-positive subset of malignant cells is identified in multiple myeloma using PCR with patient-specific immunoglobulin gene primers. Leukemia 1995;9:1948–1953.

72. San Miguel JF, Gonzalez M, Gascon A, et al. Immunophenotypic heterogeneity of multiple myeloma: influence on the biology and clinical course of the disease. Castellano-Leones (Spain) Cooperative Group for the Study of Monoclonal Gammapathies. Br J Haematol 1991;77:185–190.

73. Bellido M, Rubiol E, Ubeda J, et al. Flow cytometry using the monoclonal antibody CD10-PE/Cy5 is a useful tool to identify follicular lymphoma cells. Eur J Haematol 2001;66:100–106.

74. Sun Y, Wyatt RT, Bigley A, Krontiris TG. Expression and replication timing patterns of wildtype and translocated BCL2 genes. Genomics 2001;73:161–170.

75. Cornfield DB, Mitchell DM, Almasri NM, et al.: Follicular lymphoma can be distinguished from benign follicular hyperplasia by flow cytometry using simultaneous staining of cytoplasmic bcl-2 and cell surface CD20. Am J Clin Pathol 2000;114:258–263.

76. Rodriguez J, McLaughlin P, Fayad L, et al. Follicular large cell lymphoma: long-term follow-up of 62 patients treated between 1973-1981. Ann Oncol 2000;11:1551–1556.

77. Weisenburger D, Armitage JO. Mantle cell lymphoma: an entity comes of age. Blood 1996;87:4483–4494.

78. Kurtin PJ. Mantle cell lymphoma. Adv Anat Patholo 1998;5:376–398.

79. Elnenaei MO, Jadayer DM, Matutes E, et al. Cyclin D1 by flow cytometry as a useful tool in the diagnosis of B-cell maligancies. Leuk Res 2001;25:115–123.

80. Matutes E, Morilla R, Owusu-Ankomah K, Houlihan A, Catovsky D. The immunophenotype of splenic lymphoma with villous lymphocytes and its relevance to the differential diagnosis with other B-cell disorders. Blood 1994; 83:1558–1562.

81. Catovsky D, Matutes E. Splenic lymphoma with circulating villous lymphocytes/splenic marginal-zone lymphoma. Semin Hematol 1999;36:148–154.

82. Trourssard X, Valensi F, Duchayne E, et al. Splenic lymphoma with villous lymphocytes: clinical presentation, biology and prognostic factors in a series of 100 patients. Br J Haematol 1996;93:731–736.

83. Kramer PA, Oosterhuis WP, Vankammen E, et al. A patient with a variant form of hairy-cell leukemia. Nether J Med 1993;43:262–268.

84. Matutes E, Meeus P, Mc Lennan K, Catovsky D. The significance of minimal residual disease in hairy cell leukaemia treated with deoxycoformycin: a long-term follow-up study. Br J Haematol 1997;98:375–387.

85. Bossuyt X, Bogaerts A, Schiettekatte G, Blanckaert N. Serum protein electrophoresis and immunofixation by a semiautomated electrophoresis system. Clin Chem 1998;44:944–949.

86. Iida S, Rao P, Nallasivam P, et al. The t(9;14) (p13;q32) chromosomal translocation associated with lympho-plasmacytic lymphoma involves the PAX-5 gene. Blood 1996;88:4110–4117.

87. Jacob MC, Agrawal S, Chaperot L, et al. Quantification of cellular adhesion molecules on malignant B cells from non-Hodgkin's lymphoma. Leukemia 1999;13:1428–1433.

88. Czader M, Porwit A, Tani E, Ost A, Mazur J, Auer G. DNA image cytometry and the expression of proliferative markers (proliferating cell nuclear antigen and Ki67) in non-Hodgkin's lymphomas. Mod Pathol 1995;8:51–58.

89. Winter JN, Andersen J, Variakojis D, et al. Prognostic implications of ploidy and proliferative activity in the diffuse, aggresive non-Hodgkin's lymphomas. Blood 1996;88:3919–3125.

90. Subira D, Castañon S, Aceituno E, et al. Flow cytometric analysis of cerebrospinal fluid samples and its utility in routine clinical practice. Am J Clin Pathol 2002;117:952–958.

91. Cabezudo E, Matutes E, Ramrattan M, Morilla R, Catovsky D. Analysis of residual disease in chronic lymphocytic leukemia by flow cytometry. Leukemia 1997;11:1909–1914.

92. Lenormand B, Bizet M, Fruchart C, et al. Residual disease in B-cell chronic lymphocytic leukemia patients and prognostic value. Leukemia 1994;8:1019–1026.

93. Garcia-Vela A, Delgado I, Benito L, et al. CD79b expression in B cell chronic lymphocytic leukemia: its implication for minimal residual disease detection. Leukemia 1999;13:1501–1505.

94. Ocqueteau M, Orfao A, Garcia R, San Miguel JF. Detection of monoclonality in bone marrow plasma cells by flow cytometry: limitations for minimal residual disease detection. Br J Haematol 1996;93:251–252.

95. Terol MJ, Lopez-Guillermo A, Bosh F, et al. Expression of beta-integrin adhesion molecules in non-Hodgkin's lymphoma: correlation with clinical and evolutive features. J Clin Oncol 1999;17:1869–1875.

96. Keating MJ. Chronic lymphocytic leukemia. Semin Oncol 1999;26:107–114.

IV   CLINICAL ASPECTS: *PROGNOSIS*

10 Staging of Chronic Lymphocytic Leukemia

Kanti R. Rai, MD and Niraj Gupta, MD

1. INTRODUCTION

Chronic lymphocytic leukemia (CLL) is characterized by a heterogeneous natural history. Some patients have an indolent clinical course and live for 10–20 yr without any major problems from CLL, whereas others have a rapid downhill course and succumb to their disease within 2–3 yr after the diagnosis. Approximately half of the CLL patients have a disease course somewhere in between the two extremes. It is extremely important for the clinician to be able to distinguish prospectively patients who would have a benign clinical course from those likely to have an aggressive course and poor outcome, so that subsequent appropriate therapeutic interventions can be carefully planned. Clinical staging systems allow us to categorize patients into different stages and thus help in predicting the course of the disease and survival outlook with a reasonable certainty. Moreover, stratification of the patients according to stage enables investigators to design and conduct clinical trials evaluating the efficacy of new therapeutic strategies.

2. HISTORICAL PERSPECTIVE

In 1966, Boggs et al. *(1)* from Wintrobe's group in Salt Lake City, published a detailed analysis of the factors influencing the duration of survival in CLL. They observed that patients with a survival of less than 5 yr had more severe extent of the disease at diagnosis, compared with, patients with an overall survival of more than 5 yr. Soon after, in 1967, Galton *(2)* published his classification of CLL into four groups based solely on the presence of enlargement of the lymph nodes and/or spleen. He also noted that in patients not receiving any cytotoxic therapy the rate of increase of lymphocyte count was inversely related to survival. In 1967, Dameshek *(3)* proposed a staging system classifying patients into four categories based on the presenting symptoms and the extent of abnormal findings on physical examination and laboratory evaluation. He noted a correlation between these stages and prognosis in CLL patients. Both Galton and Dameshek, independently of each other, postulated that CLL was a disease associated with progressive accumulation of functionally and immunologically incompetent lymphocytes. In 1973, the next major study on the clinical course of CLL was published by Hansen *(4)*, giving a detailed review of case histories of 189 patients. Hansen also reported that the presence of more evidence of disease at the time of diagnosis was associated with a shorter survival, thus confirming the findings of previous investigators. However, a simplified, well-structured staging system for CLL was still lacking.

From: *Contemporary Hematology*
Chronic Lymphocytic Leukemia: Molecular Genetics, Biology, Diagnosis, and Management
Edited by: G. B. Faguet © Humana Press Inc., Totowa, NJ

Table 1
Staging System of Rai

Risk category	Rai stage	Features
Low[a]	0	Lymphocytosis only (in blood and marrow)
Intermediate[a]	I	Lymphocytosis plus enlarged nodes
	II	Lymphocytosis plus enlarged spleen or liver with or without enlarged nodes
High[a]	III	Lymphocytosis plus anemia (Hb < 11g/dL) with or without enlarged nodes, liver, spleen
	IV	Lymphocytosis plus thrombocytopenia (platelets < 100,000/μL with or without enlarged nodes, liver, spleen

[a] Modified Rai stage.

3. STAGING SYSTEMS

3.1. Rai et al.

In 1975, my colleagues and I (KRR) proposed a system of clinical staging, stratifying CLL patients into five stages (5) (Table 1). The criteria of our staging system were based on Galton and Dameshek's postulate that CLL is characterized by a continuous accumulation of immunologically inert lymphocytes; thus, with increasing tumor burden, clinical disease would progress from observable enlarged lymphoid masses, with relatively preserved marrow function in early stages, to severely impaired marrow reserve as the disease progresses. Our staging system soon gained wide acceptance among clinicians, as well as clinical investigators worldwide, as it relied on readily measurable clinical and laboratory parameters.

3.1.1. MODIFIED RAI STAGING

The validity and usefulness of the Rai staging system in predicting survival outlook was subsequently confirmed by several investigators from around the world (6–8). However, it was gradually recognized that having to stratify patients into five different stages made it a little difficult and laborious to design prospective therapeutic clinical trials. In 1987, we suggested that the five clinical stages in the original Rai system could to be reduced to three, in recognition of the fact that there were essentially three and not five distinct survival patterns in the actuarial survival curves in our original report (Fig. 1) (9). Thus, in the modified Rai staging system, patients were categorized as low risk (Rai stage 0), intermediate risk (Rai stages I and II) and high risk (Rai stages III and IV) (Table 1). The National Cancer Institute-Sponsored Working Group also recommends using the modified Rai staging system for prospective clinical studies because of its simplicity and ease of use (10).

3.2. Binet et al.

Binet et al. (11) recognized the need for a staging system with fewer stages than in the Rai schema and proposed another CLL staging system (originally in 1977 and revised in 1981; Table 2). Binet's system divided patients into three stages. Stage C included patients with anemia (hemoglobin <10 g/dL) or thrombocytopenia (platelet count <100,000/μL) or both. All the remaining (non-stage C) patients were subdivided on the basis of whether they had three or more areas of lymphoid enlargement (stage B), or only two or fewer areas of lymphoid enlargement (stage A). The five lymphoid areas considered in this system are cervical, axillary, inguinal (unilateral or bilateral, single node or multiple nodes), spleen, and liver. Binet et al subsequently validated the usefulness of their staging system in a large series of patients.

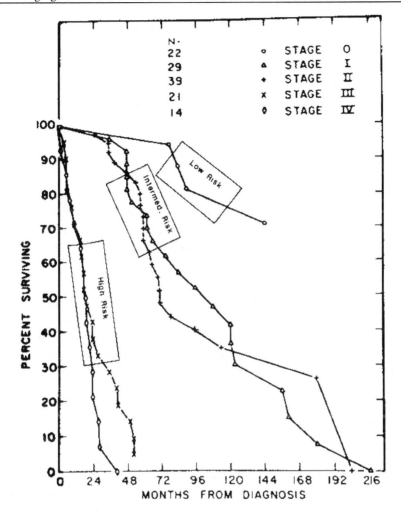

Fig.1. Three-stage modified Rai staging system. (Adapted from ref. 5.)

Table 2
Staging System of Binet et al. and the International Workshop on CLL (IWCLL)

Clinical stage	Features
A	No anemia or thrombocytopenia and fewer than three areas of lymphoid enlargement A (0), A (I) or A (II)[a]
B	No anemia or thrombocytopenia, with three or more involved areas. B (I) or B (II)[a]
C	Anemia and/or thrombocytopenia regardless of the number of areas of lymphoid enlargement C (III) or C (IV)[a]

[a] IWCLL-recommended Rai-Binet integrated staging system.

3.3. Other Staging Systems

Over the years, several other staging systems for CLL have also been proposed *(12–18)*. Each system has been tested in a large series of patients and has been found to be valid. However, in current practice, only the Rai or Binet systems are used by clinicians and researchers. Brief descriptions of some of the other notable staging systems is provided below.

3.3.1. INTERNATIONAL WORKSHOP ON CLL

In 1980, the International Workshop on CLL (IWCLL) recommended an integrated Rai-Binet staging system, in which each Binet group is further defined by using the Rai stage in roman numerals in parentheses, e.g., A (0) or A (I), B (I), or B (II), and so on (Table 2). The IWCLL noted that within each of the three groups in the Binet system, there might be subsets of patients with distinct a biological and natural history not otherwise appreciated. However, most investigators and physicians find this integrated system cumbersome and follow either Rai or Binet.

3.3.2. TOTAL TUMOR MASS SCORING SYSTEM

In 1981, Jaksic and Vitale *(13)*, proposed a unique method of estimating the total tumor mass (TTM) in CLL and formulated a scoring system to be used for staging. TTM was defined as the sum of (a) the square root of the absolute lymphocyte count/μL, (b) diameter of the largest lymph node (in cm), and (c) enlargement of the spleen below the costal margin (in cm). They observed that the median survival was more than 101 mo, when the TTM was less than 9.0 and 39 mo when the TTM was greater than 9.0.

3.3.3. MANDELLI ET AL.

Mandelli et al. *(14)* analyzed a large series of patients and suggested four independent criteria for poor prognosis in CLL: (1) absolute lymphocyte count greater than 60,000/μL, (2) hemoglobin less than 11 g/dL, (3) number of sites of lymph nodes greater than 2 cm (cervical, axillary, inguinal. and others) or spleen enlarged more than 3 cm below the costal margin, and (4) liver enlarged more than 3 cm below the costal margin. Patients were divided into four stages: stage I, patients with none of the aforementioned criteria; stage II, presence of any one of these four criteria; stage III, presence of any two of the four criteria; and stage IV, presence of any three or all of the four criteria listed above. They observed an excellent correlation of this staging system with survival, with median survival after 7 yr of follow-up being 59 and 32 mo for stages I and II and for stages III and IV, respectively.

3.3.4. LEE ET AL.

In 1987, Lee et al. *(15)*, from the M.D. Anderson Medical Center, identified the following poor prognostic features for CLL: (1) age more than 60 yr, (2) serum alkaline phosphatase greater than 80 U/dL, (3) serum uric acid greater than 7.0 mg/dL, (4) serum lactate dehydrogenase (LDH) greater than 325 U/dL, and (5) presence of external lymphadenopathy. Patients were divided into three categories; (a) low risk, LDH less than 325 U/dL and the presence of one of the prognostic features mentioned above; (b) intermediate risk, LDH less than 325 U/dL and two to three poor prognostic features listed above or LDH more than 325 U/dL with one poor prognostic feature; and (c) high risk, LDH greater than 325 U/dL and the presence of two poor prognostic features or all of the aforementioned poor prognostic features. The median survival times were 10, 6, and 2 yr for low-, intermediate-, and high-risk groups, respectively.

4. LIMITATIONS OF THE CLINICAL STAGING SYSTEMS

4.1. Clinical Staging and Prognosis of Individual Patients

Both the Rai and the Binet system fail to differentiate prospectively patients within a clinical stage in whom the disease would remain quiescent and who would have an indolent course from those likely to have a rapid progression of the disease with an aggressive clinical course.

Over the years, several other clinical, hematological, and laboratory parameters, as well as immunophenotypic and cytogenetic characteristics, have been evaluated in large numbers of patients in an attempt to determine whether the clinical course of the disease could be predicted more precisely and the accuracy of the clinical stages be improved. These prognostic factors are discussed in detail elsewhere in this textbook. However, many of these variables do not predict progression of the disease and add little to the information provided by the clinical stage. We briefly discuss two promising, newly discovered independent prognostic variables in CLL.

4.1.1. CYTOGENETICS

Genomic aberrations in CLL are much more common than originally thought. Döhner et al. (19), using fluorescent in situ hybridization (FISH), observed that about 80% of the CLL patients had one or more chromosomal abnormalities, in contrast to the previously reported incidence of 40–50% with conventional banding analysis. They noted that the most common aberration was chromosome 13q deletion, followed by 11q deletion, trisomy 12q, and 17p deletion. Cytogenetic abnormalities in CLL patients also serve as an independent predictor for disease progression and overall survival (19). Patients with 11q and 17p deletions have a poor clinical outcome, compared with those who have 13q deletions as the sole aberration, trisomy 12, and normal karyotype. Moreover, patients with poor-risk cytogenetic abnormalities (11q and 17p deletion) present with advanced disease at diagnosis.

4.1.2. MUTATIONAL STATUS OF IgV GENES

In 1999, both Damle et al. (20) and Hamblin et al. (21) simultaneously, but independently of each other, suggested that CLL has two distinct subsets: a pregerminal subset, arising from the pregerminal "virgin" B-lymphocytes with unmutated IgV genes, and a postgerminal subset, arising from the memory B-lymphocytes with mutated IgV genes. The mutational status of IgV genes has been shown to be an independent variable predictor of disease outcome. Patients who have mutated IgV genes have a superior overall disease outcome, compared with those who have unmutated IgV genes. Some researchers have also reported that the expression of CD-38 correlates with the presence of unmutated genes and thus confers an unfavorable disease outcome (20).

4.1.2.1. Correlation Between IgV Mutations and Karyotypic Abnormalities. Döhner et al. (22) also analyzed 211 CLL patients in their series on the mutational status of IgV genes. They observed a significant correlation between the mutational status of IgV genes and the occurrence of specific genomic aberrations. Patients with 13q as the sole aberration, predicting favorable outcome, also had a higher incidence of mutated IgV genes; and the patients with unfavorable cytogenetic abnormalities, like 17p and 11q deletions, had a higher incidence of unmutated IgV genes. Thus, cytogenetic evaluation and mutational status of IgV genes provide complementary prognostic information.

4.2. Clinical Staging and Immune Cytopenias

Patients with anemia and/or thrombocytopenia of immune origin, rather than secondary to marrow infiltration by CLL B-lymphocytes, were not considered a separate prognostic group in any of the staging systems. It has been suggested by some investigators that CLL patients who have anemia and/or thrombocytopenia of immune origin seem to have a better clinical outcome, compared with those who have anemia and/or thrombocytopenia owing to bone marrow infiltration *(23,24)*. Data from a large number of patients would be required to reach a definitive conclusion. Some investigators have suggested classifying these patients as stage C or Rai stage III or IV, *immune (25)*.

5. STAGING WORKUP

Both the modified Rai and the Binet staging systems are based on simple clinical and laboratory parameters and thus only require the following: complete physical examination (looking for lymphadenopathy, hepatomegaly, and splenomegaly) and a complete blood count for absolute lymphocyte count, hemoglobin levels, and platelet count (*see* Part III, on diagnosis).

5.1. Is Bone Marrow Aspiration and Biopsy Required for Staging?

Neither the Rai nor the Binet staging system requires evaluation of the bone marrow. However, bone marrow aspiration and biopsy could be useful in delineating the cause (autoimmune vs nonimmune) of anemia and/or thrombocytopenia, assessing response to therapy, and recognizing complications of CLL, like pure red cell aplasia. In addition, histology of the marrow provides important prognostic information *(26,27)*.

5.2. Is Radiological Evaluation to Assess Lymphoid *Enlargement Required for Staging?*

In both the Rai and the Binet staging systems, lymphoid enlargement (lymphadenopathy and hepatosplenomegaly) was assessed by a physical examination. Lymph nodes, spleen, and liver were considered to be enlarged if they were clinically palpable. Moreover, the patients were not stratified according to the size of lymph nodes, liver, or spleen. It is unknown whether identifying patients with subclinical (not appreciated on physical examination) lymphadenopathy and or hepatosplenomegaly using imaging studies would have any impact on the natural history of the disease. Hence, the routine use of radiological investigations (computed tomography scan of the chest/abdomen/pelvis, radionuclide scan of liver/spleen, and so on) solely for the staging purposes cannot be recommended.

6. CONCLUSIONS

Ever since, Turk's *(28)* attempt to classify lymphoid malignancies, exactly a century ago, there has been significant progress in our ability to predict prospectively the prognosis of in CLL with a high level of accuracy. The challenge now is to identify patients prospectively, especially in the low- and intermediate-risk categories, who are likely to have an indolent course and those more likely to have aggressive disease. In the last decade, various laboratory, molecular, and cytogenetic parameters have been reported to be important independent predictors of disease progression and survival; however, the numbers of patients evaluated and the numbers of studies confirming the prognostic importance of these individual variables are relatively small. Larger cooperative trials are needed to establish firmly the prognostic significance of these newly identified variables. Integration of some of these novel, significant prognostic variables into the present clinical staging systems would help us to form a comprehensive and accurate description of the clinical behavior of the disease.

REFERENCES

1. Boggs DR, Sofferman SA, Wintrobe MM, et al. Factors influencing the duration of survival of patients with chronic lymphocytic leukemia. Am J Med 1966;40:243–254.
2. Galton DAG. The pathogenesis of chronic lymphocytic leukemia. Can Med J 1967;94:1005–1010.
3. Dameshek W. Chronic lymphocytic leukemia—an accumulative disease of immunologically incompetent lymphocytes. Blood 1967;29:566–584.
4. Hansen MM. Chronic lymphocytic leukemia: clinical studies based on 189 cases followed for a long time. Scand J Haematol 1973;18(suppl):3–286.
5. Rai KR, Sawitsky A, Cronkite EP, et al. Clinical staging of chronic lymphocytic leukemia. Blood 1975;46:219–234.
6. Skinnider LF, Tan L, Schmidt J, et al. Chronic lymphocytic leukemia: a review of 745 cases and assessment of clinical staging. Cancer 1982;50:2951–2955.
7. Santoro A, Musumeci R, Rilke F, et al. Clinical classification and survival in chronic lymphocytic leukemia. Tumori 1979;65:39–49.
8. Phillips EA, Kempin S, Passe S, Mike V, Clarkson B. Prognostic factors in chronic lymphocytic leukemia and their implicatons for therapy. Clin Hematol 1977;6:203–222.
9. Rai KR. A critical analysis of staging in CLL. In: Gale RP, Rai KR, eds. CLL Recent Progress and Future Directions, vol. 59. UCLA Symposia on Molecular and Cellular Biology, Alan R. Liss, New York, 1987, p. 253.
10. Cheson BC, Bennet JM, Rai KR, et al. Guidelines for clinical protocols for chronic lymphocytic leukemia: recommendations of the National Cancer Institute-sponsored working group. Am J Hematol 1988;29:152.
11. Binet JL, Auduier A, Dighiero G, et al. A new prognostic classification of chronic lymphocytic leukemia derived from a multivariate survival analysis. Cancer 1981;48:198–206.
12. International Workshop on CLL (IWCLL). Chronic lymphocytic leukemia: Proposal for a revised prognostic staging system. Br J Haematol 1981;48:365–367.
13. Jaksic B, Vitale B. Total tumour mass score (TTM). A new parameter in chronic lymphocytic leukemia. Br J Haematol 1981;49:405–413.
14. Mandelli F, DeRossi G, Mancini P, et al. Prognosis in chronic lymphocytic leukemia: A retrospective multicenteric study from the GIMEMA Group. J Clin Oncol 1987;5:398–406.
15. Lee JS, Dixon DO, Kantarjian HP, et al. Prognosis of chronic lymphocytic leukemia: Multivariate regression analysis of 325 untreated patients . Blood 1987;6:929–936.
16. Baccarani M, Cavo M, Gobbi M, et al. Staging of chronic lymphocytic leukemia. Blood 1982;59:1191–1196.
17. Rundles RW, Moore JO. Chronic lymphocytic leukemia. Cancer 1978;42:941–945.
18. Paolino W, Infelise V, Levis A, et al. Adenosplenomegaly and prognosis in uncomplicated chronic lymphocytic leukemia. A study of 362 cases. Cancer 1984;54:339–346.
19. Dohner H, Stilgenbauer, Benner A, et al. Genomic aberrations and survival in chronic lymphocytic leukemia. N Engl J Med 2000;343:1910–1916.
20. Damle R, Wasil T, Fais F, et al. Ig V genes mutation status and CD-38 expression as novel prognostic indicators in chronic lymphocytic leukemia. Blood 1999;94:1840–1847.
21. Hamblin TJ, Davis Z, Gardiner A, et al. Unmutated Ig V genes are associated with a more aggressive form of chronic lymphocytic leukemia. Blood 1999;94:1848–1854.
22. Krober A, Seiler T, Benner A, et al. V_H mutation status, CD38 expression level, genomic aberrations, and survival in chronic lymphocytic leukemia. Blood 2002;100:1410–1416.
23. Geisler C, Hansen MM. Chronic lymphocytic leukemia: a test of a new proposed staging system. Scand J Haematol 1981;27:279–286.
24. Rubenstein DB, Longo DL. Peripheral destruction of platelets in chronic lymphocytic leukemia: recognition, prognosis and therapeutic implications. Am J Med 1981;71:729–732.
25. Montserrat E, Rozman C. Prognostic factors in chronic lymphocytic leukemia. In: Polliack A, Catovsky D, eds. Chronic Lymphocytic Leukemia, Harwood, London, 1981, pp. 111–122.
26. Montserrat E, Rozman C. Clinico-pathological staging of chronic lymphocytic leukemia. In: Gale RP, Rai KR, eds. Chronic Lymphocytic Leukemia: Recent Progress and Future Directions. Alan R. Liss, New York, 1987, pp. 215–224.
27. Geisler CH, Raflkiaer E, Hansen MM, et al. The bone marrow histological pattern has independent prognostic value in early stage chronic lymphocytic leukemia. Br J Haematol 1986;62:47–54.
28. Turk. Ein System der Lymphomatosen. Wien Klin Wochenschr 1903:16:1073.

11 Prognostic Indicators of Chronic Lymphocytic Leukemia

Francesc Bosch, MD *and Emili Montserrat,* MD

1. INTRODUCTION

Chronic lymphocytic leukemia (CLL) has a variable clinical course. Although the median survival of patients with this form of leukemia is around 10 yr (Fig. 1), in individual patients the prognosis is extremely variable, ranging from a very short to a normal life span. Thus, some CLL patients will have an excellent prognosis and will never require treatment, whereas in others the prognosis is poor and prompt treatment is required. Moreover, a large proportion of patients are now being diagnosed while asymptomatic and at a much younger age than previously. This results in longer overall survival, but it also poses special problems in respect to clinical management *(1,2)*.

Clinical staging systems are the most useful prognostic parameters in CLL *(3,4)* (Table 1). However, they are not accurate enough to identify subgroups of patients with progressive CLL. Moreover, mechanisms causing citopenias are not taken into consideration, and this means that criteria used to define clinical stages do not necessarily parallel tumor mass. Since the introduction of staging systems, there has been a continuous effort to identify new prognostic factors in CLL. Thus, other variables have been investigated in the attempt to add prognostic power to clinical stages. Interestingly, some of these new prognostic variables are emerging from our biological understanding of this disease. However, it is not clear whether the newly identified prognostic parameters will replace classical clinical variables or, rather, will be integrated into a clinicobiological prognostic system. Assessment of prognostic factors should help us to decide whether a CLL patient needs to be treated and what therapeutic approach should be employed. In this chapter, our current knowledge of prognostic factors in CLL patients is reviewed.

2. CLASSICAL PROGNOSTIC FACTORS

2.1. Age

CLL is the most common leukemia of elderly people in Western countries. The incidence of the disease varies greatly with age. Thus, whereas in individuals younger than 30 yr the incidence × 100,000/yr is less than 1, in those older than 80 yr the incidence × 100,000/yr is about 25. As a result of increasing life expectancy in the overall population and the higher incidence of CLL in the elderly, the median age of patients at diagnosis is now 70 yr, compared with 60–65 yr a few decades ago. However, an increasing number of patients (10–20%) are being diagnosed when they are younger than 50 because they have undergone numerous analyses for routine or trivial reasons. Studies analyzing the influence of age on the natural history of CLL as well as the

From: *Contemporary Hematology*
Chronic Lymphocytic Leukemia: Molecular Genetics, Biology, Diagnosis, and Management
Edited by: G. B. Faguet © Humana Press Inc., Totowa, NJ

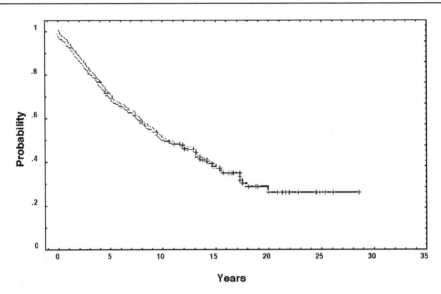

Fig. 1. Overall survival of CLL patients ($N = 820$). Median survival is 10 yr.

Table 1
Binet and Rai Clinical Staging System of CLL

Binet stage		Rai stage			Median
Stage	Characteristics	Stage	Characteristics	Risk	survival (yr)
Binet A	Hb > 10 g/dL, platelets > 100 × 10⁹/L and < 3 lymph node areas involved[a]	Rai 0	Lymphocytosis	Low	>10
Binet B	Hb > 10 g/dL, platelets > 100 × 10⁹/L and ≥ 3 lymph node areas involved[a]	Rai I	Lymphocytosis + lymphadenopathy	Intermediate	5
Binet C	Hb < 10 g/dL or platelets < 100 × 10⁹/L	Rai II	Lymphocytosis + splenomegaly and/or liver enlargment		
		Rai III	Lymphocytosis + Hb < 11.0 g/dL	High	3
		Rai IV	Lymphocytosis + platelets < 100 × 10⁹/L		

[a]Lymph node areas: 1, head and neck (including Waldeyer's ring) (uni- or bilateral); 2, axillar (uni- or bilateral); 3, inguinal (uni- or bilateral); 4, splenomegaly; 5, hepatomegaly.

prognosis of young patients have been conducted in recent years (5,6). Younger and older patients with CLL show similar overall median survival (around 10 yr), but the causes of death are different (6). Younger patients usually die because of the direct effect of the leukemia, whereas some elderly patients die of causes unrelated to the leukemia. In a registry study, however, it was found that CLL shortens life expectancy independently of the age at presentation (7). Rozman et al. (8) compared two cohorts of CLL patients in whom the diagnosis was established between

1960–1979 and 1980–1989, respectively. They showed that the diagnosis in the second group was established at an older age, in both men and women, and at an earlier stage of disease (Binet stage A). Moreover, survival was more than double in the second group and the impact of disease on life expectancy was much lower. These findings indicate that that such differences might be partly caused by changes in the natural history of the disease (8).

Elderly patients have consistently poor prognosis, for reasons that have not been well analyzed. Older individuals have an increased incidence of interacting diseases. This degree of comorbidity (generally not seen in younger populations) has a major impact on survival and on the ability to tolerate treatment. Thus, in some studies, age is an adverse prognostic factor. In fact, unrelated illnesses are an important cause of death in patients older than 70 yr (9). The prevalence of CLL-unrelated competing causes of death is high in patients with early disease (10). Interestingly, Kozvch et al. (11) found that age more than 70 yr was an adverse prognostic feature for patients receiving fludarabine: median survival was 32 mo compared with a median survival of 67 mo in patients aged 60–69 yr.

2.2. Gender

In most series there are more men than women (M/F ratio: 1.5). The impact of gender on prognosis is controversial, with some studies showing no difference in survival according to gender and others demonstrating a better survival for women. The longer life expectancy of women in the general population, as well as the fact that among women the disease tends to present with fewer unfavorable features than in men, might be the most likely explanations for a better survival in women with CLL (12,13).

2.3. Clinical Stage

The clinical staging systems independently developed by Rai et al. (3) and Binet et al. (4) in the early 1980s, which are based on easily obtainable biological and clinical parameters, are extremely useful for assessing prognosis in patients with CLL. These staging systems not only facilitate the treatment of patients according to individual prognosis, but also make it possible to conduct and compare trials based on the risk of disease. Rai's stages were further classified as low (Rai stage 0), intermediate (Rai stages I and II), and high (Rai stages III and IV) risk. The International Workshop on CLL (IWCLL) proposed an integration of the two staging systems, but this did not gain wide acceptance (14). Median survival for Binet stage A is 15 yr, declining to 5 and 3 yr for Binet stages B and C, respectively (Fig. 2A) (15). Median survival for Rai stage 0 is 16 yr, 8 yr for Rai stages I and II, and 3 yr for Rai stages III and IV (Fig. 2B) (15).

Although they are easy to apply and reproducible, staging systems are not devoid of limitations. For example, the mechanisms accounting for cytopenias (i.e, bone marrow infiltration, hypersplenism, autoimmune basis) are not taken into consideration. As a result, patients are classified in an advanced stage independently of the origin of the anemia or thrombocytopenia, although there is some indication that the mechanism of the cytopenia is also a factor in prognosis (16). Most important, perhaps, is the prognostic heterogeneity within each of the clinical stages. Thus, staging systems do not allow identification of individuals in an early stage (40–60% of all patients) who are likely to progress and those in whom the disease will remain stable for many years. This is important since it is possible that patients in an early stage who are likely to progress could benefit from treatment immediately after diagnosis, before progression occurs. Conversely, in some patients presenting in an advanced stage the disease runs an indolent course and for long periods they may not require therapy; the staging systems do not identify these patients either.

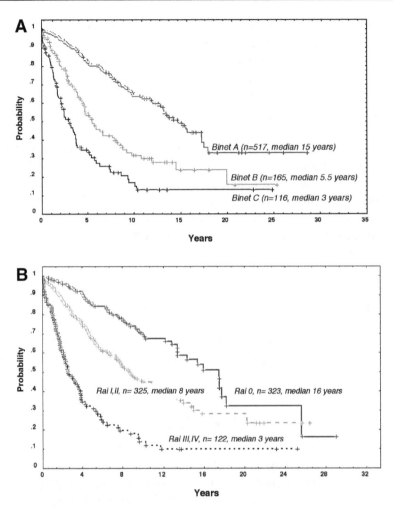

Fig. 2. Survival according to Binet (**A**) and Rai (**B**) stages.

Other classification methods have been proposed in the last two decades. The GIMEMA study group, in a large retrospective analysis of prognostic factors, identified four parameters associated with poor prognosis: lymphocytosis (> 60×10^9/L), anemia (Hb < 10 g/dL), number of enlarged lymph nodes (> 2 cm), or palpable hepatoesplenomegaly (> 3 cm) *(17)*. On the other hand, Jaksic and Vitale *(18)* defined the total tumor mass score, a quantitative staging system based on the clinical assessment of disease involvement within all major compartments.

Although the great majority of CLL patients are diagnosed in an indolent phase, of them 30–40% progress to a more advanced clinical stage and finally die of their leukemia *(15)*. Several efforts have been made to identify subpopulations of CLL patients in an early stage who have a high risk of progressing to a more advanced stages. Han et al. *(19)* coined the term "benign monoclonal lymphocytosis" to describe the clinical course of a small but interesting series of 20 patients whose disease did not show progressive changes during the follow-up time. Oscier et al. *(20)* analyzed their series of Rai stage 0 patients to identify factors predictive of disease progression. Parameters that correlated with an increased risk of disease progression included the initial lymphocyte count, surface immunoglobulin phenotype, and some complex karyotype abnormalities.

Montserrat et al. *(21)* further extended these observations and proposed the term *smoldering CLL* for a subset of stage A patients whose life expectancy was not different from that of an age- and sex-matched control population. Patients with smoldering CLL, which accounts for 30% of all patients with CLL, had a hemoglobin level greater than 13 g/dL, lymphocyte count less than 30×10^9/L, a nondiffuse pattern of BM involvement, and a lymphocyte doubling time (LDT) of less than 12 mo. The French Cooperative Group on CLL analyzed a large, prospective series of stage A CLL, randomized for early vs delayed therapy. This provided a definition of smoldering CLL differing from that of Montserrat et al. through exclusion of LDT and bone marrow (BM) pattern *(22,23)*. Finally, Molica et al. *(24)* demonstrated that whatever criteria were used, all the proposals succeeded in defining a subset of patients with a low rate of progression (about 15% at 5 yr) and long life expectancy (>80% at 10 years).

Recent studies have investigated whether novel prognostic factors may be helpful in the identification of a subset of early-stage CLL patients with high risk of progression. Three serum parameters (β2-microglobulin, serum thymidine kinase, and sCD23) may add prognostic information to the subclassification of patients in stage A *(25–27)*. Moreover, CD38 lymphocyte expression and the presence of somatic mutations of the immunoglobulin gene in early CLL stages have recently been correlated with a high risk of progression *(28,29)*.

How these results translate into the timing of therapy is still a complex issue. A meta-analysis studied 2048 patients with early disease in which immediate therapy with chlorambucil or chlorambucil plus prednisone/prednisolone was compared with deferred therapy using the same agents. The 10-yr survival was not different (44% vs 47%) *(30)*, thus supporting a conservative treatment strategy for patients with early CLL. Nonetheless, this approach should be reconsidered when results of trials based on new treatments become available.

2.4. Bone Marrow Infiltration

BM aspiration and biopsy are useful to evaluate the bulk of the disease and also to ascertain the origin of cytopenias. The prognostic value of bone marrow study has been analyzed by many investigators *(32–39)*. The BM infiltration pattern (i.e., diffuse vs nondiffuse) correlated with clinical stage, disease progression, and survival in some studies *(32–37)* but not in others *(38)*. Whether bone marrow aspirates could replace bone marrow biopsy in the assessment of bone marrow involvement is controversial. In a controlled study. Montserrat et al. *(37)* demonstrated that reproducibility is higher for BM biopsy than for lymphocyte infiltration evaluated in BM smears.

Rozman et al. *(32)* found BM pattern to be the most important prognostic factor in CLL, but patients in their series were basically treated with chlorambucil and other alkylating-based regimens. Since prognostic factors may chane over the time as treatments become more effective, the prognostic importance of the degree of bone marrow infiltration in CLL needs to be reevaluated in patients treated with the newer and more effective regimens. In this regard, Geisler et al. *(38)*, in a prospective multicenter trial, pointed out that relatively intensive (i.e., CHOP) therapy given to most patients at the time of disease progression was the most likely explanation for the lack of prognostic value of BM biopsy in their study. In contrast, Mauro et al. *(36)* found BM pattern and WBC count to be correlated with response and response duration in patients with active disease treated with fludarabine plus prednisone.

In concludion, BM biopsy and aspirate are complementary methods to evaluate not only the degree of BM involvement in CLL but also to gain insight in the mechanisms of cytopenias in this disease. However, BM biopsy is a more reliable method and its serial evaluation provides important information when response to therapy is evaluated.

Finally, BM involvement in CLL patients has been estimated using noninvasive methods. Lecouvet et al. *(40)*, using BM magnetic resonance imaging (MRI), detected BM abnormalities in 7 of 21 (33%) patients with early-stage CLL. Treatment-free interval was significantly shorter in patients with quantitative MRI abnormalities than in those with normal MRI findings. Although these results should be considered preliminary, MRI would make it possible to evaluate BM involvement using a noninvasive method.

2.5. Lymphocyte Morphology

Numerous morphological variants of CLL have been described, although their prognostic significance is controversial. Lymphocyte size, number of prolymphocytes, and the presence of cleaved and/or lymphoplasmocytic cells have all been associated with poor prognosis *(41–43)*. Melo et al. *(41)* showed that CLL cases with an absolute prolymphocyte count of 15×10^9/L or less have "standard-prognostic risk," whereas the survival outlook for the cases with prolymphocytes more than 15×10^9/L was as bad as that for prolymphocytic leukemia (PLL). Such an observation was confirmed by Vallespí et al. *(42)*, who demonstrated that the presence of prolymphocytes and cleaved lymphocytes correlated with a poor prognosis, whereas granular lymphocytes and small-size lymphocytes were related to a good prognosis. Moreover, in a multivariate analysis, only an increased prolymphocyte count retained prognostic significance *(42,43)*.

Two variants of CLL have been recognized in addition to typical CLL by the French-American-British (FAB) Group *(44)*: (1) CLL/PL, which includes cases with more than 10% and less than 55% prolymphocytes; and (2) CLL of mixed cell type, a less well-defined form with pleomorphic lymphocytes but less than 10% prolymphocytes. Criel et al. *(45)* analyzed a group of 390 patients diagnosed with CLL. Cases were subclassified as morphologically typical and atypical CLL according to the criteria of the FAB proposal. Typical CLL cases were mostly diagnosed at a low-risk stage (Binet A/Rai 0), required no immediate treatment, and long expected survival; atypical CLL cases mostly presented at a more advanced risk stage (Binet B/Rai I–II), usually required immediate treatment, and had a shorter expected survival. On the other hand, Oscier et al. *(46)* analyzed 270 patients with Binet stage A CLL looking for adverse prognostic factors. In the multivariate analysis, atypical lymphocyte morphology (i.e., >10% prolymphocytes or >15% lymphocytes with cleaved nuclei or lymphoplasmacytoid cells), more than two karyotypic abnormalities, lymphocyte count more than 30×10^9/L, LDT less than 1 yr, and enlargement of one or more lymph node groups were found to be risks for disease progression. In the univariate analysis, the presence of trisomy 12 also correlated with progressive disease, but this was largely a consequence of the association between trisomy 12 and atypical lymphocyte morphology.

In conclusion, CLL can be subclassified into at least two different subgroups with distinctive clinical features, cytogenetic abnormalities, and different prognoses. The diagnosis of atypical CLL, however, should not be accepted without carefully ruling out the possibility of other chronic lymphoproliferative disorders with leukemic expression.

2.6. Immunodeficiency

CLL patients have an increased risk of developing bacterial infections *(47–49)*. Different reasons have been offered for this infection predisposition, especially the presence of hypogammaglobulinemia. Rozman et al. *(50)* investigated the prognostic significance of gamma-globulin and immunoglobulin levels in chronic lymphocytic leukemia. The survival probability of patients with initial levels of gammaglobulin of less than 700 mg/dL was significantly lower than that of patients with initial levels of 700 mg/dL or more. On the other hand, the worse prognosis observed in patients with low Ig levels did not seem to be necessarily correlated with an excess of severe infections in these patients. In line with this finding, other investigators were unable to demonstrate a relationship between hypogammaglobulinemia and reduced overall survival (51–53).

T-cell immunodeficiency has also been implicated in the increased number of infections and was correlated with prognosis (54–56). Totterman et al. (55) showed that CLL patients had an increase in the absolute number of phenotypically activated, HLA-DR+ CD4+ and CD8+ cells and T suppressor/effector (CD11b+/CD8+) cells, but in more advanced clinical stages a reduced proportion of T-suppressor/effector (CD11b+) cells was shown.

A number of soluble molecules may have an impact on the immune system. Thus, leukemic B-cells, through the elaboration of suppressive cytokines such as transforming growth factor-β (TGF-β) and release of soluble CD27, downregulate the expression of CD40 ligands (CD154), originally expressed by CD4-positive T-cells after immune activation (57–60). Such down-regulation has been considered responsible, at least in part, for the immune deficiency that is acquired in CLL (61). Finally, immunodeficiency has been correlated with the presence of autoimmune phenomena, probably by accumulating anergic self-reactive CD5+ B-cells (62,63).

2.7. Lymphocyte Proliferation and Cell Cycle Regulation

CLL is a human malignancy caused principally by defects that prevent programmed cell death rather than by alterations in cell cycle regulation. In the vast majority of patients, CLL cells are predominantly G_0 quiescent cells that gradually accumulate in the patient's body, not because they are dividing more rapidly than normal, but because they are surviving too long. Several methods have been used to evaluate tumor cell proliferation and to correlate kinetic cellular parameters with clinical features and outcome. One of the first and most useful methods of evaluating cell proliferation is the analysis of lymphocyte doubling time (LDT), defined as the time needed to double the peripheral blood lymphocyte count (64,65). Montserrat et al. (64) analyzed the LDT in 100 untreated patients with CLL. LDT was investigated in relation to clinical stages, bone marrow histological patterns, treatment-free period, and survival. Although it was partially correlated with clinical stages and bone marrow pattern, LDT was shown to have a clear prognostic significance by itself. Thus, whereas an LDT of 12 or fewer months identified a population of patients with poor prognosis, an LDT of higher than 12 mo was indicative of good prognosis, as substantiated by long treatment-free periods and survival. Because of its simplicity, LDT constitutes a largely accepted parameter for assessing the pace of disease development (64,66).

Other methods have been used to correlate tumor cell proliferation with clinical outcome. Cordone et al. (67) analyzed the frequency and clinical significance of Ki-67+ cells in patients with CLL. The percentage and absolute number of Ki-67+ leukemic cells was found to be higher in advanced stages of the disease and also correlated with the proportion of prolymphocytes. Moreover, Ki-67 identified patients with more aggressive forms of CLL and Richter's syndrome, in which all the large lymphoma cells were Ki-67+. On the other hand, Del Giglio et al. (68) focused on the expression of proliferating cell nuclear antigen (PCNA), a 36-Kda nuclear protein, the regulation of which is cell cycle-dependent. In CLL, PCNA levels correlated with cell proliferation, clinical stage, and the LDT. Interestingly, low PCNA levels were predictive of a response to fludarabine. Orfao et al. (69) analyzed the proliferation rate of peripheral blood (PB) lymphocytes from CLL patients, as expressed by the absolute PB S-phase leukocyte count. This parameter was related to other clinical and biological factors. Taken independently, it is also an important variable in predicting early death in CLL (69).

Other molecules related to cell cycle regulation have been studied. Thus, p27^k protein, a cyclin-dependent kinase inhibitor, was studied in B-CLL patients. As expected, increased levels of p27^k protein correlated with LDT *(70)*. Moreover, survival of patients with increased expression of p27 was shorter than in those with low p27^k expression *(70)*. In addition, although overexpression of cyclin D1 is a specific marker of mantle-cell lymphoma *(71,72)*, some sporadic cases with aggressive behavior overexpress cyclin D1 *(73)*.

3. NOVEL PROGNOSTIC FACTORS

3.1. Immunophenotype Characteristics

Immunophenotypic analysis of chronic lymphoproliferative disorders allows an accurate classification of such disorders. Matutes et al. *(74)* analyzed circulating cells from 666 cases, including CLL, PLL, hairy cell leukemia, and others. On the basis of the most common marker profile in CLL [CD5+, CD23+, FMC7–, and weak expression (+/–) of surface immunoglobulin (SIg) and CD22], a scoring system was devised. Considering each marker individually, no single one distinguished CLL from other diseases, although the most reliable were SmIg intensity and FMC7 *(74)*. Moreover, Moreau et al. *(75)* found that the replacement of CD22 by CD79b (SN8) in the original scoring system increased its potential to discriminate between CLL and other B-cell lymphoproliferative diseases. Geisler et al. *(76)* examined 540 cases of CLL using immunofluorescence flow cytometry with a panel of surface membrane markers, including IgM and IgD, the monoclonal antibodies anti-CD3, -5, -20, -21, -22, and -23, as well as anti-FMC7. In a multivariate analysis, and independently of clinical variables, CD23 and IgM intensity proved to be useful prognostic markers in the management of CD5+, B-cell CLL *(76)*.

Other studies attempting to correlate immunophenotype with prognosis have been inconclusive *(77,78)*. In a series of patients with B-cell CLL fulfilling strict immunological criteria, a high CD20 expression significantly correlated with atypical morphology and worse prognosis *(79)*. Thus, quantitative immunophenotyping makes it possible to analyze the biological heterogeneity of disease better, although it is difficult to transfer these results into prognosis *(79)*. Non-B-lineage antigens have been analyzed in several studies, with inconclusive results *(80)*.

3.2. Genetic Abnormalities

Over the years, the correlation between cytogenetic abnormalities and the outcome of patients with CLL has been investigated. The initial studies, performed using conventional cytogenetic techniques, yielded unclear and sometimes controversial results *(81)*. The main reason for this was the difficulty in obtaining enough metaphases for study. With the advent of the fluorescence *in situ* hybridization (FISH) techniques, important progress has been made, and the contribution of cytogenetics to the understanding and prognosis of CLL constitutes one of the most important breakthroughs in the understanding of this disease during the last decade. Thus, patients with del(13q) as a single abnormality have an excellent prognosis (median survival: 133 mo), whereas those with del(11q) or del(17p) have poor survival (median survival: 79 and 32 mo, respectively) *(82)*. The relevance of cytogenetics in CLL relies on a number of facts. Thus, cytogenetics identifies distinct clinical forms of the disease. For example, patients with trisomy 12 tend to present atypical lymphocytes in peripheral blood *(83)*; those with del(11q) are usually young men presenting with tumoral disease that does not respond to therapy; del(17p) is associated with progressive disease and refractoriness to treatment. Moreover, the prognostic significance of cytogenetic abnormalities is independent of other important prognostic variables such as clinical stages. Finally, del(11q) and del(17p) are correlated with poor response to treatment, including

Table 2
Variables Correlating With the Mutational Status of IgV$_H$ Genes

Variable	Unmutated IgV$_H$	Mutated IgV$_H$
Sex predominance	Male	No sex predominance
Stage at diagnosis	Advanced	Early stages
Morphology	Atypical	Typical
CD38 expression	Increased	Diminished
Cytogenetic abnormalities	+12, del(11q), del(17p)	del(13q14)
ZAP-70 expression	High	Low
Treatment response	Poor response	Usually no therapy is needed
Survival	Short	Long

[a] It retains its prognostic influence after autologous stem cell transplantation.

autologous stem cell transplantation (84), and they are prevalent in forms with unmutated IgV genes (85).

Recurrent chromosomal abnormalities have been linked to alterations in the function of putative oncogenes located in the altered region. Therefore, deletions in 17p13 are associated with p53 and deletions of 11q with ATM. For the 13q14 deletion, the most frequent chromosomal abnormality in CLL, few candidate genes have been found (86). Other mechanisms of alteration of tumor suppressor genes such as mutations, deletions, or hypermethylations have been implicated in progression of disease. Thus, abnormalities of p53 (considering deletions, mutations, or dysfunctions) have been correlated with resistance to therapy and bad prognosis (87).

3.3. IgV$_H$ Mutations

CLL has long been considered a homogeneous disease of CD5+B-cells, which are pregerminal cells that have not been exposed to antigenic stimulation. In 1999, two different groups reported an important breakthrough in CLL (29,88). These groups clearly showed that the mutational status of the somatic mutations of the variable region of the immunoglobulin genes (IgV$_H$) correlates with different disease subsets. Thus, those patients with unmutated IgV$_H$ genes have a poorer prognosis than those displaying mutated IgV$_H$ genes. Hamblin et al. (29) analyzed the IgV$_H$ gene sequences of 84 patients with CLL and demonstrated two patterns: 38 (45%) showed 98% sequence homology with the germline IgV$_H$ gene, whereas 46 (55%) showed evidence of somatic mutation. Since somatic mutation takes place in the germinal center, CLL can be either a tumor of pregerminal center B-cells (unmutated) or a tumor of postgerminal center B-cells (mutated).

According to different studies, CLL cases present distinctive clinical features, treatment requirements, and outcome, depending on the mutational status of the IgV$_H$ gene (Table 2). Thus, patients with an unmutated IgV$_H$ gene (mostly men) are more likely to have an advanced stage, progressive disease, atypical morphology, unfavorable cytogenetic findings [i.e., del(11q), del(17p)], need for therapy, and shorter survival irrespective of stage than those presenting with a mutated IgV$_H$ gene. It is of great interest that the prognostic value of the IgV$_H$ mutational status is independent of clinical stage. Thus, patients with stage A CLL have a median survival of 8 yr if they have unmutated B-cells, compared with 25 yr if B-cells are mutated (29). Lin et al. (87) have recently shown that the poor outcome of unmutated cases may be related to p53 dysfunction.

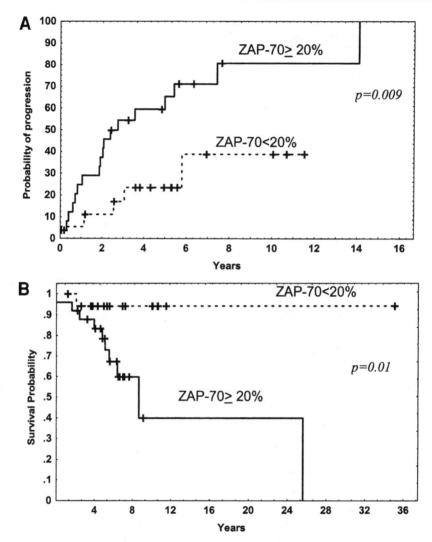

Fig. 3. Prognostic implications of ZAP-70 expression in Binet A patients with CLL. (**A**) Actuarial risk of disease progression in Binet A patients according to the category of ZAP-70 expression. (**B**) Survival curves of Binet A stage patients according to ZAP-70 expression.

Unfortunately, most laboratories are currently unable to isolate and characterize IgV_H gene sequences, and, even if the technique is available, it is quite costly and time-consuming. Damle et al. *(88)* first suggested a correlation between CD38 expression on the surface of neoplastic lymphocytes and IgV_H mutational status: CD38+ $\geq$ 30%, unmutated IgV_H genes; CD38+ < 30%, mutated IgV_H genes. Nevertheless, the value of CD38 as a surrogate for the IgV_H mutation is controversial *(89,90)*. It is worth emphasizing, however, that CD38 expression has prognostic importance by itself. Recently, Hamblin et al. *(28)* have reported that CD38 expression and IgV_H mutational status are independent prognostic variables and that CD38 expression may vary during the course of the disease. In this study based on 145 patients it was found that the two assays (IgV_H mutations, CD38 expression) gave discordant results in 42 patients (28.3%) and that in 10 of 41 patients CD38 expression varied over time *(28)*.

Table 3
Parameters With Prognostic Significance in CLL

	Risk	
Parameter	Low	High
Classical		
Clinical stage		
Binet	A	B, C
Rai	0	I, II, III, IV
Bone marrow infiltration		
Biopsy	Nondiffuse pattern	Diffuse pattern
Aspirate	≤80% lymphocytes	>80% lymphocytes
WBC count $(\times 10^9/L)^a$	≤50	>50
Prolymphocytes in peripheral blood $(\%)^a$	≤10	>10
Lymphocyte doubling time[a]	<12 mo	>12 mo
Novel		
Serum markers[b]	Normal	Increased
Cytogenetics	Normal	del(11q)
	del(13q) isolated	del(17p)
CD38 expression	≤30%	>30%
IgV$_H$ genes	Mutated	Unmutated
ZAP-70 expression	Low	High

[a] Continuous variables.
[b] Lactate dehydrogenase, β2 microglobulin, thymidine kinase, CD23, and others.

3.4. ZAP-70 Expression

Investigations using DNA microarrays *(91)* have shown that CLL cells exhibit a characteristic gene expression profile in which a small subset of genes, including ZAP-70, IM1286077, and C-type lectin, correlates with the mutational status of IgV$_H$ genes *(91,92)*. ZAP-70, a member of the Syk/ZAP-70 protein tyrosine kinase family, is normally expresed in T cells and NK cells and plays a critical role in the initiation of T-cell signalling *(93,94)*. Crespo et al. *(95)* and Wiestner et al. *(96)* demonstrated that among patients with CLL, expression of ZAP-70, as detected by flow-cytometric analysis or RT-PCR, correlated with IgV$_H$ mutational status, disease progression, and survival. Thus, ZAP-70 expression analysis is able to identify a subgroup of patients in Binet A stage with adverse prognosis (Fig. 3). As opposed to CD38 expression, ZAP-70 expression does not change over the time. Also ZAP-70 can be studies by cytofluorometry, which makes of this marker a more convenient parameter than IgV$_H$ mutations. For these reasons, ZAP-70 expression analysis should be included in the diagnositc workup of patients with CLL *(95)*.

4. CONCLUSIONS

The clinical staging systems independently developed by Rai et al. *(3)* and Binet et al. *(4)* in the early 1980s, based on easily obtainable biological and clinical parameters, are extremely useful for assessing prognosis in patients with CLL. These staging systems not only facilitate the treatment of patients according to individual prognosis, but also make it possible to conduct and compare trials based on risk of disease. Since their introduction, however, many attempts either to substitute or to modify clinical staging systems have been made. Over the last few years, important biological parameters related to CLL prognosis have been discovered. Whether classical staging systems and other clinical parameters should be substituted or complemented by these biological parameters has not yet been elucidated. If at all possible, the most relevant parameters correlating with prognosis (Table 3) should be evaluated prospectively in trials. Retrospective studies performed on stored tumor samples would also be useful, since these would provide information more rapidly than prospective studies. At the same time, new prognostic factors should be fully standardized. All this should lead to the identification of the most relevant prognostic factors in CLL. Meanwhile, the classical prognostic factors—particularly clinical stages—should continue to be the basis for assessing prognosis, as well as for forming the benchmark against which new prognostic parameters should be measured.

REFERENCES

1. Montserrat E. Classical and new prognostic factors in chronic lymphocytic leukemia: where to now? Hematol J 20002;3:7–9.
2. Caligaris-Cappio F, Hamblin TJ. B-cell chronic lymphocytic leukemia: a bird of a different feather. J Clin Oncol 1999;17:399–408.
3. Rai KR, Sawitsky A, Cronkite EP, Chanana AD, Levy RN, Pasternack BS. Clinical staging of chronic lymphocytic leukemia. Blood 1975;46:219–234.
4. Binet JL, Auquier A, Dighiero G, Chastang C, Piguet H, Goasguen J, et al. A new prognostic classification of chronic lymphocytic leukemia derived from a multivariate survival analysis. Cancer 1981;48:198–206.
5. Montserrat E, Gomis F, Vallespi T, et al. Presenting features and prognosis of chronic lymphocytic leukemia in younger adults. Blood 1991;78:1545–1551.
6. Mauro FR, Foa R, Giannarelli D, et al. Clinical characteristics and outcome of young chronic lymphocytic leukemia patients: a single institution study of 204 cases. Blood 1999;94:448–454.
7. Diehl LF, Karnell LH, Menck HR. The American College of Surgeons Commission on Cancer and the American Cancer Society. The National Cancer Data Base report on age, gender, treatment, and outcomes of patients with chronic lymphocytic leukemia. Cancer 1999;86:2684–2692.
8. Rozman C, Bosch F, Montserrat E. Chronic lymphocytic leukemia: a changing natural history? Leukemia 1997; 11(6):775-778.
9. Catovsky D, Fooks J, Richards S. The UK Medical Research Council CLL trials 1 and 2. Nouv Rev Fr Hematol 1988;30:423–427.
10. Call TG, Phyliky RL, Noel P, Habermann TM, Beard CM, O'Fallon WM, et al. Incidence of chronic lymphocytic leukemia in Olmsted County, Minnesota, 1935 through 1989, with emphasis on changes in initial stage at diagnosis. Mayo Clin Proc 1994;69(4):323–328.
11. Kozuch P, O'Brien S, Kantarjian H, Lerner S, Do K-A, Keating MJ. The M.D. Anderson Cancer Center Experience in CLL patients aged 70 years and older. In: VIIIth International Workshop on CLL, Paris, Programme and Abstract Book, 1999, p. 61.
12. Catovsky D, Fooks J, Richards S. Prognostic factors in chronic lymphocytic leukaemia: the importance of age, sex and response to treatment in survival. A report from the MRC CLL 1 trial. MRC Working Party on Leukaemia in Adults. Br J Haematol 1989;72:141–149.
13. cartwright RA, Gurnet KA, Moorman AV. Sex ratios and the risks of haematological malignancies. Br J Haematol 2002;118:1071–1077.
14. International Workshop on CLL. Chronic lymphocytic leukaemia: proposals for a revised prognostic system. Br J Haematol 1981;48:365–367.
15. Rozman C, Montserrat E. Chronic lymphocytic leukemia. N Engl J Med 1995;333:1052–1057.
16. Mauro FR, Foa R, Cerretti R, et al. Autoimmune hemolytic anemia in chronic lymphocytic leukemia: clinical, therapeutic, and prognostic features. Blood 2000;95:2786–2792.
17. Mandelli F, De Rossi G, Mancini P, et al. Prognosis in chronic lymphocytic leukemia: a retrospective multicentric study from the GIMEMA group. J Clin Oncol 1987;5:398–406.
18. Jaksic B, Vitale B. Total tumour mass score (TTM): a new parameter in chronic lymphocyte leukaemia. Br J Haematol 1981;49:405–413.
19. Han T, Ozer H, Gavigan M, et al. Benign monoclonal B cell lymphocytosis—a benign variant of CLL: clinical, immunologic, phenotypic, and cytogenetic studies in 20 patients. Blood 1984;64:244–252.

20. Oscier DG, Stevens J, Hamblin TJ, Pickering RM, Fitchett M. Prognostic factors in stage AO B-cell chronic lymphocytic leukaemia. Br J Haematol 1990;76:348–351.

21. Montserrat E, Vinolas N, Reverter JC, Rozman C. Natural history of chronic lymphocytic leukemia: on the progression and progression and prognosis of early clinical stages. Nouv Rev Fr Hematol 1988;30:359–361.

22. French Cooperative Group on Chronic Lymphocytic Leukemia. Natural history of stage A chronic lymphocytic leukemia untreated patients. Br J Haematol 1990;76:45–57.

23. French Cooperative Group on Chronic Lymphocytic Leukemia. Effects of chlorambucil and therapeutic decision in initial forms of chronic lymphocytic leukemia (stage A): results of a randomized clinical trial on 612 patients. Blood 1990;75:1414–1421.

24. Molica S. Progression and survival studies in early chronic lymphocytic leukemia. Blood 1991;78:895–899.

25. Keating M, Lerner S, Kantarjian H, Freireich EJ, O'Brien S. The serum β2-microglobulin level is more powerful than stage in predicting response and survival in chronic lymphocytic leukemia. Blood 1995;86(suppl 1):606a.

26. Sarfati M, Chevret S, Chastang C, et al. Prognostic importance of serum soluble CD23 level in chronic lymphocytic leukemia. Blood 1996;88:4259–4264.

27. Hallek M, Langenmayer I, Nerl C, et al. Elevated serum thymidine kinase levels identify a subgroup at high risk of disease progression in early, nonsmoldering chronic lymphocytic leukemia. Blood 1999;93:1732–1737.

28. Hamblin TJ, Orchard JA, Ibbotson RE, et al. CD38 expression and immunoglobulin variable region mutations are independent prognostic variables in chronic lymphocytic leukemia, but CD38 expression may vary during the course of the disease. Blood 2002;99:1023–1029.

29. Hamblin TJ, Davis Z, Gardiner A, Oscier DG, Stevenson FK. Unmutated Ig V(H) genes are associated with a more aggressive form of chronic lymphocytic leukemia. Blood 1999;94:1848–1854.

30. Chemotherapeutic options in chronic lymphocytic leukemia: a meta-analysis of the randomized trials. CLL Trialists' Collaborative Group. J Natl Cancer Inst 1999;91:861–868.

31. Cheson B, Bennett JM, Grever MR, et al. National Cancer Institute Sponsored Working Group guidelines for chronic lymphocytic leukemia: Revised guidelines for diagnosis and treatment. Blood 1996;87:4990–4997.

32. Rozman C, Montserrat E, Rodriguez-Fernandez JM, et al. Bone marrow histologic pattern—the best single prognostic parameter in chronic lymphocytic leukemia: a multivariate survival analysis of 329 cases. Blood 1984;64:642–648.

33. Pangalis GA, Boussoditis VA, Kiitas C. B-chronic lymphocytic leukemia. Disases progression in 150 untreated stage A and B patients as predicted by bone marrow patterns. Nouv Rev Fr Hematol 1988;30:373–375.

34. Han T, Minowa M, Bloom ML, Samadori N, Sandberg AA, Henderson ES. Bone marrow infiltration patterns and their prognostic significance in chronic lymphocytic leukemia: correlation with clinical, immunologic, phenotypic, and cytogenetic data. J Clin Oncol 1984;2:562–570.

35. Desablens B, Claisse JF, Piprot-Choffat C, Gontier MF. Prognostic value of bone marrow biopsy in chronic lymphocytic leukemia. Nouv Rev Fr Hematol 1989;31:179–182.

36. Mauro FR, De Rossi G, Burgio VL, et al. Prognostic value of bone marrow histology in chronic lymphocytic leukemia. A study of 335 untreated cases from a single institution. Haematologica 1994;79(4):334–341.

37. Montserrat E, Villamor N, Reverter JC, et al. Bone marrow assessment in B-cell chronic lymphocytic leukaemia: aspirate or biopsy? A comparative study in 258 patients. Br J Haematol 1996;93:111–116.

38. Geisler CH, Hou-Jensen K, Jensen OM, et al. The bone-marrow infiltration pattern in B-cell chronic lymphocytic leukemia is not an important prognostic factor. Danish CLL Study Group. Eur J Haematol 1996;57:292–300.

39. Molica S, Tucci L, Levato D, Docimo C. Clinical and prognostic evaluation of bone marrow infiltration (biopsy versus aspirate) in early chronic lymphocytic leukemia. A single center study. Haematologica 1997;82:286–290.

40. Lecouvet FE, Van de Bergh B, Micahux L, et al. Early chronic lymphocytic leukemia: prognostic value of quantitative bone marrow MR imaging findings and correlation with hematologic variables. Radiology 1997;204:813–818.

41. Melo JV, Catovsky D, Gregory WM, Galton DA. The relationship between chronic lymphocytic leukaemia and prolymphocytic leukaemia. IV. Analysis of survival and prognostic features. Br J Haematol 1987;65:23–29.

42. Vallespi T, Montserrat E, Sanz MA. Chronic lymphocytic leukaemia: prognostic value of lymphocyte morphological subtypes. A multivariate survival analysis in 146 patients. Br J Haematol 1991;77:478–485.

43. Molica S, Alberti A. Investigation of nuclear clefts as a prognostic parameter in chronic lymphocytic leukemia. Eur J Haematol 1988;41:62–65.

44. Bennett JM, Catovsky D, Daniel MT, et al. Proposals for the classification of chronic (mature) B and T lymphoid leukaemias. French-American-British (FAB) Cooperative Group. J Clin Pathol 1989;42:567–584.

45. Criel A, Verhoef G, Vlietinck R, et al. Further characterization of morphologically defined typical and atypical CLL: a clinical, immunophenotypic, cytogenetic and prognostic study on 390 cases. Br J Haematol 1997;97:383–391.

46. Oscier DG, Matutes E, Copplestone A, et al. Atypical lymphocyte morphology: an adverse prognostic factor for disease progression in stage A CLL independent of trisomy 12. Br J Haematol 1997;98:934–939.

47. Sampalo A, Brieva JA. Humoral immunodeficiency in chronic lymphocytic leukemia: role of CCD95/CD95L in tumoral damage and escape. Leuk Lymphoma 2002;43:881–884.

48. Molica S. Infections in chronic lymphocytic leukemia: risk factors, and impact on survival, and treatment. Leuk Lymphoma 1994;13:203–214.

49. Perkins JG, Flynn JM, Howard RS, Byrd JC. Frequency and type of serious infections in fludarabine-refractory B- cell chronic lymphocytic leukemia and small lymphocytic lymphoma. Cancer 2002;94:2033–2039.

50. Rozman C, Montserrat E, Vinolas N. Serum immunoglobulins in B-chronic lymphocytic leukemia. Natural history and prognostic significance. Cancer 1988;61:279–283.

51. Lee JS, Dixon DO, Kantarjian HM, Keating MJ, Talpaz M. Prognosis of chronic lymphocytic leukemia: a multivariate regression analysis of 325 untreated patients. Blood 1987;69:929–936.

52. Mandelli F, De Rossi G, Mancini P, et al. Prognosis in chronic lymphocytic leukemia: a retrospective multicentric study from the GIMEMA group. J Clin Oncol 1987;5:398–406.

53. Orfao A, Gonzalez M, San Miguel JF, et al. B-cell chronic lymphocytic leukaemia: prognostic value of the immunophenotype and the clinico-haematological features. Am J Hematol 1989;31:26–31.

54. Foa R, Catovsky D, Brozovic M, et al. Clinical staging and immunological findings in chronic lymphocytic leukemia. Cancer 1979;44:483–487.

55. Totterman TH, Carlsson M, Simonsson B, Bengtsson M, Nilsson K. T-cell activation and subset patterns are altered in B-CLL and correlate with the stage of the disease. Blood 1989;74:786–792.

56. Apostolopoulos A, Symeonidis A, Zoumbos N. Prognostic significance of immune function parameters in patients with chronic lymphocytic leukaemia. Eur J Haematol 1990;44:39–44.

57. Lotz M, Ranheim E, Kipps TJ. Transforming growth factor beta as endogenous growth inhibitor of chronic lymphocytic leukemia B cells. J Exp Med 1994;179:999–1004.

58. Lagneaux L, Delforge A, Bron D, Massy M, Bernier M, Stryckmans P. Heterogenous response of B lymphocytes to transforming growth factor- beta in B-cell chronic lymphocytic leukaemia: correlation with the expression of TGF-beta receptors. Br J Haematol 1997;97:612–620.

59. Ranheim EA, Cantwell MJ, Kipps TJ. Expression of CD27 and its ligand, CD70, on chronic lymphocytic leukemia B cells. Blood 1995;85:3556–3565.

60. Kato K, Cantwell MJ, Sharma S, Kipps TJ. Gene transfer of CD40-ligand induces autologous immune recognition of chronic lymphocytic leukemia B cells. J Clin Invest 1998;101:1133–1141.

61. Grewal IS, Flavell RA. The CD40 ligand. At the center of the immune universe? Immunol Res 1997;16:59–70.

62. Caligaris-Cappio F. Cellular interactions, immunodeficiency and autoimmunity in CLL. Hematol Cell Ther 2000; 42:21–25.

63. Arkwright PD, Abinun M, Cant AJ. Autoimmunity in human primary immunodeficiency diseases. Blood 2002; 99:2694–2702.

64. Montserrat E, Sanchez-Bisono J, Vinolas N, Rozman C. Lymphocyte doubling time in chronic lymphocytic leukaemia: analysis of its prognostic significance. Br J Haematol 1986;62:567–575.

65. Molica S, Alberti A. Prognostic value of the lymphocyte doubling time in chronic lymphocytic leukemia. Cancer 1987;60:2712–2716.

66. Molica S, Reverter JC, Alberti A, Montserrat E. Timing of diagnosis and lymphocyte accumulation patterns in chronic lymphocytic leukemia: analysis of their clinical significance. Eur J Haematol 1990;44:277–281.

67. Cordone I, Matutes E, Catovsky D. Monoclonal antibody Ki-67 identifies B and T cells in cycle in chronic lymphocytic leukemia: correlation with disease activity. Leukemia 1992;6:902–906.

68. Del Giglio A, O'Brien S, Ford RJ, Jr., et al. Proliferating cell nuclear antigen (PCNA) expression in chronic lymphocytic leukemia (CLL). Leuk Lymphoma 1993;10:265–271.

69. Orfao A, Ciudad J, Gonzalez M, et al. Prognostic value of S-phase white blood cell count in B-cell chronic lymphocytic leukemia. Leukemia 1992;6:47–51.

70. Vrhovac R, Delmer A, Tang R, Marie JP, Zittoun R, Ajchenbaum-Cymbalista F. Prognostic significance of the cell cycle inhibitor p27Kip1 in chronic B-cell lymphocytic leukemia. Blood 1998;91:4694–4700.

71. Bosch F, Jares P, Campo E, et al. PRAD-1/cyclin D1 gene overexpression in chronic lymphoproliferative disorders: a highly specific marker of mantle cell lymphoma. Blood 1994;84:2726–2732.

72. Bosch F, Lopez-Guillermo A, Campo E, et al. Mantle cell lymphoma: presenting features, response to therapy, and prognostic factors. Cancer 1998;82:567–575.

73. Levy V, Ugo V, Delmer A, et al. Cyclin D1 overexpression allows identification of an aggressive subset of leukemic lymphoproliferative disorder. Leukemia 1999;13:1343–1351.

74. Matutes E, Owusu-Ankomah K, Morilla R, et al. The immunological profile of B-cell disorders and proposal of a scoring system for the diagnosis of CLL. Leukemia 1994;8:1640–1645.

75. Moreau EJ, Matutes E, A'Hern RP, et al. Improvement of the chronic lymphocytic leukemia scoring system with the monoclonal antibody SN8 (CD79b). Am J Clin Pathol 1997;108:378–382.

76. Geisler CH, Larsen JK, Hansen NE, et al. Prognostic importance of flow cytometric immunophenotyping of 540 consecutive patients with B-cell chronic lymphocytic leukemia. Blood 1991;78:1795–1802.

77. Orfao A, Gonzalez M, San Miguel JF, et al. B-cell chronic lymphocytic leukaemia: prognostic value of the immunophenotype and the clinico-haematological features. Am J Hematol 1989;31:26–31.

78. Newman RA, Peterson B, Davey FR, et al. Phenotypic markers and BCL-1 gene rearrangements in B-cell chronic lymphocytic leukemia: a Cancer and Leukemia Group B study. Blood 1993;82:1239–1246.

79. Molica S, Levato D, Dattilo A, Mannella A. Clinico-prognostic relevance of quantitative immunophenotyping in B- cell chronic lymphocytic leukemia with emphasis on the expression of CD20 antigen and surface immunoglobulins. Eur J Haematol 1998;60:47–52.

80. Tassies D, Montserrat E, Reverter JC, Villamor N, Rovira M, Rozman C. Myelomonocytic antigens in B-cell chronic lymphocytic leukemia. Leuk Res 1995;19:841–848.

81. Juliusson G, Oscier DG, Fitchett M, et al. Prognostic subgroups in B-cell chronic lymphocytic leukemia defined by specific chromosomal abnormalities. N Engl J Med 1990;323:720–724.

82. Dohner H, Stilgenbauer S, Benner A, et al. Genomic aberrations and survival in chronic lymphocytic leukemia. N Engl J Med 2000;343:1910–1916.

83. Oscier DG, Matutes E, Copplestone A, et al. Atypical lymphocyte morphology: an adverse prognostic factor for disease progression in stage A CLL independent of trisomy 12. Br J Haematol 1997;98:934–939.

84. Lange A, Ritgen M, Brüggeman M, Schmitz N, Kneba M, Dreger P. Unmutated VH Gene Status Retains Its Adverse Prognostic Influence after Autologous Stem Cell Transplantation (SCT) for Chronic Lymphocytic Leukemia (CLL). Blood 2001;98(suppl 1):3574a.

85. Stilgenbauer S, Bullinger L, Lichter P, Dohner H. Genetics of chronic lymphocytic leukemia: genomic aberrations and V(H) gene mutation status in pathogenesis and clinical course. Leukemia 2002;16:993–1007.

86. Migliazza A, Bosch F, Komatsu H, et al. Nucleotide sequence, transcription map, and mutation analysis of the 13q14 chromosomal region deleted in B-cell chronic lymphocytic leukemia. Blood 2001;97:2098–2104.

87. Lin K, Sherrington PD, Dennis M, Matrai Z, Cawley JC, Pettitt AR. Relationship between p53 dysfunction, CD38 expression and IgVH mutation in chronic lymphocytic leukemia. Blood 2002;100:1404–1409.

88. Damle RN, Wasil T, Fais F, et al. Ig V gene mutation status and CD38 expression as novel prognostic indicators in chronic lymphocytic leukemia. Blood 1999;94:1840–1847.

89. Del Poeta G, Maurillo L, Venditti A, et al. Clinical significance of CD38 expression in chronic lymphocytic leukemia. Blood 2001;98:2633–2639.

90. Ibrahim S, Keating M, Do KA, et al. CD38 expression as an important prognostic factor in B-cell chronic lymphocytic leukemia. Blood 2001;98:181–186.

91. Rosenwald A, Alizadeh AA, Widhopf G, et al. Relation of gene expression phenotype to immunological mutation genotype in B cell chronic lymphcytic leukemia. J Exp Med 2001;194:1639–1647.

92. Chen L, Widhopf G, Huynh L, et al. Expression of ZAP-70 is associated with increased B-cell receptor signaling in chronic lymphocytic leukemia. Blood 2002;100:4609–4614.

93. Chan AC, Irving BA, Fraser JD, Weiss A. The zeta chain is associated with a tyrosine kinase and upon T-cell antigen receptor stimulation associates with ZAP-70, a 70-kDa tyrosine phosphoprotein. Proc Natl Acad Sci USA 1991;88:9166–9170.

94. Chan AC, Iwashima M, Turck CW, Weiss A. ZAP-70: a 70 kd protein-tyrosine kinase that associates with the TCR zeta chain. Cell 1992;71:649–662.

95. Crespo M, Bosch F, Villamor N, et al. ZAP-70 expression as a surrogate for immunoglobulin-variable-region mutations in chronic lymphocytic leukemia. N Engl J Med 2003;348:1764–1775.

96. Wiestner A, Rosenwald A, Barry TS, et al. ZAP-70 expression identifies a chronic lymphocytic leukemia subtype with unmutated immunoglobulin genes, inferior clinical outcome, and distinct gene expression profile. Blood 2003;in press.

V CLINICAL ASPECTS: *TREATMENT*

12   Guidelines for Clinical Management of CLL

Guillaume Dighiero, MD, PhD

1. INTRODUCTION

B-cell chronic lymphocytic leukemia (B-CLL), the most common form of leukemia in Western countries, results from the relentless accumulation of small, mature, slowly dividing, monoclonal B-lymphocytes *(1)*. Affected patients are always adults: the median age at diagnosis is 64 yr. B-CLL cells are characterized by coexpression of the pan-B-cell markers CD5 and CD23, negativity for CD22 and FMC7 molecules, and low expression of the B-cell receptor surface Ig and Ig-associated molecule CD79b *(2–4)*.

The possibility that genetic or familial factors may predispose to CLL is suggested by multiple reports of familial clustering, with first-degree relatives exhibiting a two- to sevenfold excess risk over the general population *(5,6)*. Unlike acute leukemia and chronic granulocytic leukemia, CLL has not been associated with prior irradiation, and only a few reports suggest specific environmental predisposing factors *(6)*. The low incidence of CLL among individuals of Japanese origin, including those who migrated to Hawaii, has been used to support the view that genetic influences play a stronger role than environmental factors in the pathogenesis of the disease *(6)*. The nature of the genetic predisposition, however, remains unknown. No consistent chromosomal or proto-oncogene abnormality has been found in CLL, and the number of cases reporting common chromosomal and human lymphocyte antigen (HLA) phenotypes among affected siblings is small *(1)*.

CLL is usually recognized first by the patient's primary care physician. Since the disease is far from uniform, decisions about therapy are often difficult. In addition, the mechanism of disease initiation and progression remains largely an enigma, and the growing characteristics of the clonal population result from an unbalanced complex of proliferation and apoptosis. In clinical terms, about one-third of patients never require treatment and have a long survival; in another third an initial indolent phase is followed by progression of the disease; and in the remaining have aggressive disease requiring immediate treatment is present at the outset.

The development of the Rai *(7)* and Binet *(8)* staging systems has allowed the division of CLL patients with into three prognostic groups: good, intermediate, and poor (Table 1). Binet's good prognosis group (stage A) includes twice as many patients as Rai's (stage 0), whereas the opposite applies to patients with an intermediate prognosis (Binet stage B or Rai stages I and II). These differences can affect the design of clinical trials.

2. PRIMARY TREATMENT DECISIONS

Once the diagnosis of CLL has been made, the treating physician is faced with the decision of not only how to treat the patient, but when to initiate therapy. Criteria for initiating treatment may be quite different between clinical practice and clinical trial conduct. A subset of patients are

From: *Contemporary Hematology*
Chronic Lymphocytic Leukemia: Molecular Genetics, Biology, Diagnosis, and Management
Edited by: G. B. Faguet © Humana Press Inc., Totowa, NJ

Table 1
Rai and Binet Staging Systems

Prognosis	Staging systems	Criteria	% of patients	Median survival	CLL-related death (%)	Treatment decision
Good	Rai 0	Lymphocytosis alone; Hb ≥ 11 g/dL and platelets ≥ 100 × 10^9/L	31	10-yr survival 59%	27	Wait and watch until progression
	Binet A	Lymphocytosis, Hb ≥ 10 g/dL and platelets ≥ 100 × 10^9/L; more than three lymphoid areas (1) enlarged[a]	63	10-yr survival 51%	31	Wait and watch until progression
Intermediate	Rai I + II	Lymphocytosis, Hb ≥ 11 g/dL and platelets ≥ 100 × 10^9/L; lymphadenopathy (stage I), spleen and/or liver enlarged; nodes may or may not be enlarged (stage II)	61	96 mo		Treatment if progressive disease
	Binet B	Lymphocytosis, Hb ≥ 10 g/dL and platelets ≥ 100 × 10^9/L; three or more areas enlarged	30	81 mo	>80	Treatment in most cases
Poor	Rai III + IV	Lymphocytosis, hemoglobin < 110 g/L (stage III), platelets < 100 × 10^9/L (stage IV), organomegaly may or may not be present	8	63 mo	>80	Treatment in most cases
	Binet C	Lyphocytosis, platelets < 100 × 10^9/L; anemia and organomegaly may or may not be present	7	60 mo	>80	Treatment in most cases

[a]Enlarged lymphoid areas considered are cervical, axillary, and inguina areas, whether unilateral or bilateral, spleen, and liver.

considered to have smoldering CLL; they predominate among those with Rai stage 0 or Binet stage A. The two staging systems have improved the identification of patients who need immediate treatment, and there is consensus based on long-term randomized trials that treatment can be appropriately deferred for most of these patients. However, there is increasing evidence that some of these patients rapidly progress to aggressive disease, and early identification constitutes an important aim. By contrast, there is consensus that most patients in Binet stage B or C, or Rai stage III or IV, and patients with Rai stages I or II with progressive disease whose life expectancy does not exceed 7 yr should be considered for early treatment. Although most such patients require treatment at presentation, some can still be monitored without therapy until they exhibit evidence of progressive or symptomatic disease, and early identification of these patients constitutes an important goal. On this basis we discuss the treatment for indolent and aggressive forms of CLL.

2.1. Treatment of Indolent CLL

It is not clear whether early therapy benefits patients with indolent CLL. This form of the disease includes patients with a median age of 64 yr displaying a survival greater than 10 yr. In indolent CLL, Chlorambucil (CB) given daily or intermittently, alone or combined with corticosteroids, is the most commonly used drug. It often provides a period of relief from any symptoms, even in advanced disease. However, there has been much uncertainty as to whether such chemotherapy should be started immediately or whether this therapy could be appropriately deferred until required for the relief of symptoms. Several randomized trials have been activated to address this question.

The French Cooperative Group in CLL performed two long-term trials (CLL-80 and CLL-85) in stage A patients addressing this question (9,10). In the CLL-80 trial (mean follow-up >11 yr), early therapy with CB using a daily continuous schedule (dCB), was compared with a watch and wait policy, whereas in the CLL-85 trial (mean follow-up > 6 yr) CB given in an intermittent schedule associated with prednisone (CBPr) was compared with a watching policy. The CLL-80 and -85 trials included, respectively, 609 and 926 previously untreated CLL stage A patients randomized according to a first intention to treat basis between no treatment (CLL-80, 308 patients; CLL-85, 466 patients) or dCB (CLL-80, 301 patients) or CBPr (CLL-85, 460 patients). Endpoints were overall survival, treatment response, and disease progression. No benefit for early treatment was observed in either trial: relative risk of death = 1.14; $p = 0.23$ [confidence interval (CI): 0.92–1.41] for CLL-80 and relative risk of death = 0.96; $p = 0.74$ (CI: 0.75–1.23) for CLL-85). In the CLL-80 and -85 trials, 76 and 70% of patients, respectively, responded to therapy.

Although a benefit of CB in slowing disease progression was observed, no effect on overall survival was found. In the abstention group from the CLL-80 trial, 49% of patients did not evolve and did not need any therapy after a follow-up of more than 11 yr. However, 31% of stage A patients died of causes related to disease, 43% progressed to stages B and C, and 53% required treatment during evolution. Similar results were observed for Rai stage 0 patients (27% of CLL-related deaths and 42% required subsequent treatment), which includes half as many patients as stage A (Table 2). When patients were segregated according to the French stages A' and A", no demonstrable benefit could be observed for early treatment. Although some of these A' and A" patients may have a different survival from each other there is no evidence that it is better to treat one group and not the other.

All together, these results indicate that neither of the two CB schedules prolonged survival in these patients. Since deferring therapy until it is required because of disease progression to stages B or C does not compromise survival, initial therapy could have been appropriately deferred for

Table 2
Long-Term Evolution of Rai and Binet Good-Prognosis Patients

Stage	% of patients	10-yr survival (%)	% of patients without evolution	% of CLL-related deaths	% of patients evolving to B or C	% of patients receiving treatment
0	31	59	57	27	32	43
A	65	51	47	31	41	53

this low-risk stage A group; this group constitutes almost two-thirds of patients with CLL and has a median age at diagnosis of 64 yr and an expected survival of more than 10 yr, which is close to the life expectancy of a normal population matched for sex and age *(9,10)*. In addition, deferring therapy until disease progression demands it has been shown not to compromise survival *(10)*.

The establishment of the International Workshop on CLL (IWCLL) allowed results to be shared. To answer the question further of whether early therapy with CB is better than deferring treatment for stage A CLL patients, a number of series were pooled *(14)*: the 78 Medical Research Council (MRC)-CLL1 trial (78 patients), the 84 MRC-CLL2 (239 patients) *(11)*, the 76 Cancer and Leukemia Group B (CALGB) (45 patients) *(12)*, the French Cooperative Trials 80 (609 patients) and 85 (926 patients) *(9,10)*, and the Program for the Study and Treatment of Hemato-logical Diseases (PETHEMA, 157 patients) *(13)*. The additive results of treatment comparison for all deaths suggest that in terms of survival there is definately no evidence that treating patients immediately with standard CB treatments prolongs survival *(10,14)*. Because more than 50% of these early-stage patients more than 50% may die of other causes, data for patients who died of something that was definitely not CLL were censored. Again, this analysis clearly showed that early treatment was unable to prolong survival in indolent CLL.

Although these results demonstrate that CB given in classical schedules fails to influence survival in indolent CLL, it has been proposed that high-dose continuous CB influences CLL survival. The International Society for Chemo- and Immunotherapy (IGCI) CLL-01 trial *(15)* compared the classical intermittent CB plus prednisone schedule with high-dose CB (15 mg fixed dose daily to either complete remission or toxicity or to a maximum of 6 mo). A significant difference in response, which was also translated into a survival difference in favor of high-dose CB, was observed, although these results need to be further confirmed.

These results also suggest that although the Rai and Binet staging systems have succeeded in identifying patients with a favorable prognosis (Rai stage 0 and Binet stage A), about 30% of these patients still die of causes related to CLL and about 50% of them require treatment during the course of disease *(10)*. Thus, early identification of patients who will not evolve, i.e., a definition of smoldering CLL, is an important goal so we can therapeutic strategies better.

2.2. Treatment of Smoldering CLL

The French group proposed a classification that segregated stage A into A' and A" *(11,15,23)*. Criteria for A' were hemoglobin level higher than 120 g/L and lymphocyte count lower than 30,000/mm³; and for A" they were hemoglobin under 120 g/L and/or lymphocyte count higher than 30,000/mm³. The survival of these two groups was clearly different, with a 5-yr survival of 82% in the A' group and 62% in the A" group. Interestingly, the survival of the A' group was very close to that of a sex- and age-matched French population *(9,10,16)*.

In a further step, the 609 patients included in the CLL-80 trial were classified according to Binet stage A, the further stages A' and A", stage 0, as well as Montserrat's proposal (17) to define smoldering CLL. A' accounted for 80% of stage A, smoldering CLL according to Montserrat accounted for 58%, and stage 0 accounted for 48%. Five-year survival rates were, respectively, 87, 88, and 89% for these three groups of patients, and 5-yr freedom of disease progression rates were, respectively, 75, 80, and 84% *(16)*. In addition, the long-term results of the CLL-80 trials showed that death related to CLL was observed in 27% of Rai stage 0 patients (including 40% of stage A patients) and 29% of A' patients (including 80% of stage A patients). Therapy was required for 43% of patients in Rai stage 0 and for 51% of A' patients *(10)*. Although the choice between different proposals remains arbitrary, a definition of smoldering CLL appears to be feasible. Whatever the definition used, survival rates of patients are close to those of the normal population. However, about 10% of patients with smoldering CLL will progress to stage C within 5 yr; more than 25% of these patients will die from CLL, and 50% of these patients will need treatment. These results further emphasize the need for a better understanding both of the mechanisms involved in surveillance of the leukemic population and of the cause of this disease, which hopefully should allow the development of new therapeutic and effective approaches.

Neither the Rai nor the Binet staging system can predict which patients among the good prognosis group will shift into progressive disease, and the present modifications of these staging systems (aiming at early identification) also fail to predict evolution adequately (10). Either we are still lacking adequate prognostic markers, or evolution to a more aggressive disease may result from occurrence of a second (unpredictable) malignant hit.

To address this question, we have studied the long-term evolution of patients included in the abstention arms of the CLL-80 and -85 trials from the French Cooperative Group on CLL. Table 3 depicts progression to stages B and C and treatment requirement for stage A patients included in the abstention arm. In more than two-thirds of patients who progressed to more aggressive stages or treatment requirement such evolution occurred during the first 3 yr, which could indicate (at least for these patients) that evolution is a consequence of the presence of a previously unidentified prognostic factor. However, the one-third of patients for whom evolution occurs following the initial 3 yr, must be considered; for at least some patients, a second malignant hit could be involved. Table 4 depicts the different clinical and hematological parameters that could significantly predict subsequent treatment requirement. Although higher tumor mass, as expressed by increased lymphocytosis, splenomegaly, and lymph node involvement, could help in predicting treatment requirement, the initial presence of these parameters does not result in further treatment prescription for one-third of these patients.

Unfortunately, with the exception of clinicohematological staging systems, i.e., the Rai and Binet classifications, most of the prognostic factors so far described have been assessed only in retrospective studies and with heterogeneous cohorts of patients in terms of prognostic factors and prescribed treatments.

Serum levels of β2-microglobulin and lactate dehydrogenase (LDH) can help predict disease activity (18). However, although these factors can help to predict disease progression, as shown in Table 5, they do not provide better information in survival terms than the A' and A" substaging. Soluble CD23 in serum results from cleavage of membrane CD23 and provides a highly quantitative and reproducible method to gain insight into CD23 expression. Very high levels of the soluble form are found in CLL and appear to be closely related to clinical stage, overall survival, and disease activity. Interestingly, in stage A patients, high soluble CD23 levels, whether observed at baseline or during the course of the disease, predict a high probability of short-term progression (19). Therefore, monitoring soluble CD23 levels in CLL could be a valuable tool in helping physicians to delineate patients who should be treated promptly. Again, soluble CD23 levels clearly predict disease progression but do not predict survival better than the A' and A" substaging (20).

The level of serum thymidine kinase (TK) in CLL has been shown to increase according to disease stage and to predict shortened survival. Moreover, in patients with indolent disease (i.e., Binet stage A or Rai stage 0), increase in serum TK anticipates the manifestations of disease progression for several months and then allows us to forecast transition from smoldering disease to a more aggressive course (21). Studies comparing TK levels and survival of A' and A" patients have not been reported. Recognition of these abnormalities at diagnosis is therefore of considerable potential interest, as they could better predict short-term progression in patients with early-

Table 3
Progression to Stages B and C or Switch to Treatment (Tt switch) for Stage A Patients Initially Randomized in the Abstention Arm of CLL-80 and CLL-85 Trials From the French Cooperative Group

Time (mo)	CLL-80 (308 patients)		CLL-85 (466 patients)	
	A to C (%)	Tt switch (%)	A to C (%)	Tt switch (%)
<12	15/4.9	36/11.7	23/5.0	50/10.7
<24	28/9.1	64/20.8	53/11.9	114/24.4
<36	40/13.3	97/31.6	63/13.5	146/31.3
<48	50/16.5	112/36.5	69/14.8	165/35.6
<60	55/18.1	125/40.7	79/17.0	180/38.8
<72	57/18.7	135/43.9	82/17.6	187/40.3
<84	57/18.7	138/44.9	83/17.8	191/41.2
>84 <132	61/19.8	158/54.6		
Total	61/19.8	158/54.6	83/17.8	191/41.2

Table 4
CLL-80, Stage A, Abstention Arm: Variables Predicting Treatment Requirement

Variable	Total (no.) (n = 308)	Treated (%) (n = 158)	Untreated (%) (n = 150)	p-value
Lymphocytosis < 30 × 10^9/L	262	52	48	
Lymphocytosis > 30 × 10^9/L	46	61	39	0.001
Splenomegaly yes	40	65	35	0.0095
Involved areas				
0	130	42	58	
1	110	55	45	
2	68	70	30	0.0001
Stage				
0	127	43	57	
1	129	58	42	
2 + 3	52	65	35	0.0001
Stage A'	246	51	49	
Stage A"	62	60	40	0.0001

Table 5
Comparison Between A', A", Substaging and Lactate Dehydrogenase (LDH) and β2-Microglobulin Levels

Parameter	Factors[a]				
	0	1	2	1 or 2	A'
No. of patients	151	57	10	67	176
Survival by yr (%)[b]					
3	98	87	47	81	96
5	95	71	31	66	91
7	88	53	0	45	84

[a] Cutoff values were < 1.25 N for LDH and < 3 mg for β2-microglobulin. 0 factor, normal values for bath; 1 factor, increased values of 1; 2 factors, increased values of both.
[b] Survival was according to CLL-related deaths.

stage of CLL, which would allow the physician to plan treatment more precisely. However, recent reports have emphasized that the presence in the leukemic B-cells of some cytogenetic abnormalities (22) or the mutational profile of IgV genes or the expression of the CD38 marker (23–26) are better predictors of rapid progression and survival. Patients with del(11q) or del(17p) progress rapidly, respond poorly to therapy, and have short survival. In contrast, those with normal cytogenetics or isolated del(13q) have a good prognosis (22). However, to detect cytogenetic abnormalities, fluorescence in situ hybridization (FISH) techniques, which are expensive and not widely available, are required.

Since the vast majority of CLL B-cells coexpress membrane IgM and IgD and this phenotype is characteristic of normal naive B-cells, it has been proposed that the normal counterpart of leukemic cells may be mantle-zone B-cells assumed to correspond to naive B-cells expressing unmutated V genes. However, more than half of CLL cases harbor somatic mutations of V_H genes (23), as if they had matured in a lymphoid follicle. These recent results suggest that there are two types of CLL: one that arises from relatively less differentiated (immunologically naive) B-cells with unmutated heavy chain genes, and has a poor prognosis, and another that evolves from more differentiated B-cells (memory B-cells) with somatically mutated heavy chain genes and has a good prognosis (23–26). However, recent data derived from gene expression profiling analysis failed to distinguish unmutated and mutated cases clearly, favoring the view that all cases of CLL have a common cell origin and/or a common mechanism of malignant transformation (27,28). Since the ability to sequence IgV genes is not available in most laboratories, a valid and easily performed surrogate assay is desirable. Since CD38 surface expression is predictive of a worse prognosis, Damle et al. (24) suggested that CD38 determination might be a useful alternative In this regard, there is some correlation between the expression of the CD38 antigen on neoplastic lymphocytes and IgV_H gene mutations, but this is far from absolute. Interestingly, CD38 expression appears to have prognostic value by itself.

It is unclear whether patients with Binet stage A or Rai indolent forms whose leukemic B-cells express unmutated V genes or deleterious chromosomal abnormalities like del(11q) deletion or del(17p) would benefit from early treatment. This possibility should be tested in a prospective clinical trial. By contrast, there is consensus that most patients displaying advanced CLL forms (i.e., Binet stage B or C, or Rai stage III or IV or progressive Rai stage I or II) whose life expectancy does not exceed 7 yr should be considered for early treatment (9).

2.3. Treatment of Advanced CLL

Early treatment is prescribed for most patients with advanced forms of CLL, including (1) classical chemotherapeutic regimens, (2) purine analogs, (3) monoclonal antibodies, (4) autologous or allogeneic bone marrow transplantation, and (5) other treatments.

2.3.1. CLASSICAL CHEMOTHERAPEUTIC REGIMENS

CB alone or associated with corticosteroids using a daily or intermittent schedule has been traditionally used to treat CLL. Ten randomized trials (14), involving 2035 patients mostly with Binet stage B or C or following the Rai staging system in some, compared CB with polychemotherapy regimens [cyclophosphamide, oncovin, and prednisone (COP) in four, cyclophosphamide, hydroxydaunomycin, oncovin, and prednisone (ChOP) in five, and CB plus epirubicin in the remaining one]. The CLL-80 trial from the French Cooperative Group compared daily continuous CB with 12 monthly COP regimens (one each during the first 6 mo and one every 3 mo during 18 mo) in 291 previously untreated stage B patients. Long-term results from this trial failed to demonstrate any benefit in response and survival using the COP regimen compared with

CB *(29)*. Similar results were observed in an MRC trial in which 234 patients were randomly allocated to receive CB or COP *(30)*. In addition, a Spanish trial (58 patients) *(31)* and an Eastern Cooperative Oncology Group trial (99 patients) *(32)* compared intermittent CB associated with prednisone with the COP regimen and failed to find any difference in terms of survival.

Five different trials compared the ChOP regimen with CB in advanced symptomatic CLL patients (Binet stages B and/or C and Rai stages III and IV) and failed to find differences in terms of survival, although better responses, which did not translate into survival advantage, were observed for the ChOP regimen in all these trials *(33–37)*. Only the International Society for Chemo-Immunotherapy (ISCI) trial found a significant difference in response, which also translated into a survival advantage favoring high-dose CB *(37)*. However, these results have not yet been reproduced and need to be confirmed. In the CL-L80 trial, the French Cooperative Group on CLL randomized 70 stage C patients between COP and ChOP (COP plus doxorubicin 25 mg/m^2 iv d 1) *(38–40)*. Median survival was 22 mo with COP and 62 mo with ChOP, supporting a beneficial effect of low-dose doxorubicin for stage C patients. However, Jaksic et al. *(37)* recently found a better overall response in "advanced CLL" with high dose CLB when compared with ChOP, and the Eastern Cooperative Oncology Group has reported a median survival of 49 mo in stage C patients treated by chlorambucil + prednisone (CLB + PRD) or COP, which did not significantly differ from the survival observed in the CLL-80 ChOP arm of the French Cooperative Trial *(32)*. The ChOP regimen has been compared with CLB + PRD in advanced CLL in randomized trials by the Danish and Swedish groups, and no survival difference could be found *(35,36)*. Although higher responses with ChOP were observed in all these trials, they failed to translate into survival advantage.

To analyze the interest of ChOP compared with standard treatments, data from these different groups were pooled for meta-analysis study *(14)*. These series had long follow-ups and included advanced stage patients not always defined by the same staging system. Although the initial trial from the French Cooperative Group as well as other groups employing anthracycline-containing regimens generated the hypothesis that ChOP was a better treatment, the following trials have not supported it. Overall, the pooling of the data does not show evidence that ChOP actually prolongs survival compared with standard treatment. When excluding deaths not caused by CLL, ChOP might be better, but definitely not significantly. Since the French study was confined to stage C patients, analysis within subgroups was also carried out, and again there was no evidence of a different effect. Although the French trial was correctly designed and carried out and its statistical significance is clear, meta-analysis studies did not confirm these initial results. Alternatively, the possibility exists that the higher dose of cyclophosphamide used in the French ChOP study compared with classical ChOP could have an influence on these results. Recent results from the CLL-90 study, in which this schedule was found to be superior to the classical cyclophosphamide, adriamycin, and cisplatin (CAP) regimen *(41)*, might favor this view.

In nonrandomized trials, others combinations have given results generally identical to those obtained with CLB, including mechlorethamine, oncovin, procarbazine, and prednisone (MOPP) *(42)*, vincristine, BCNU, cyclophosphamide, melphalan, and prednisone (M2) *(43)*, CAP *(33)*, cyclophosphmide, adriamycin, cytosine-arabinoside, vincristine, and prednisone (POACH) *(34)*.

2.3.2. Purine Analogs

During the late 1980s, purine analogs emerged as major drugs in CLL and generated tremendous interest *(44–49)*. They were first used in progressive and refractory CLL patients. Long-term, single-institution nonrandomized studies indicate that fludarabine (FDB), alone or associated with prednisone, is able to induce 30% of true clinical, hematological, and bone marrow biopsy-confirmed complete remission, as well as an overall response rate of about 78%, whereas resistance to FDB is observed in 22% *(48)*. Once complete remission is obtained, the median time to progression is around 30 mo. The vast majority of patients appear to be relapsing, but there is a small subset of 10–15% long-term responders; recurrence can also be anticipated for them. The median survival of these patients is close to 5 yr, which is no different from previous reports in CLL. In regard to relapsing patients, about 60% of these can be rescued with FDB, although the expected duration of response is on the order of 15 mo, compared with 30 mo for initial responders *(48)*. Overall, these results indicate that FDB as a single agent or combined with corticosteroids is not curative. The association with corticosteroids is probably disadvantageous *(47)*.

Among the agents tested so far in combination with FDB, cyclophosphamide has led to the most impressive results, with overall response rates of up to 90% and a complete remission rate around 40% in previously untreated patients *(48,50–52)* and as salvage treatment *(53,54)*. However, the superiority of this combination over FDB alone has not been validated through a randomized trial. The French Cooperative Group on CLL has recently completed a phase II trial of oral FDB and cyclophosphamide in previously untreated B-CLL patients. The preliminary results of this study support the high activity of this combination *(52)*.

The historical series of the Scripps clinic experience on the use of 2-chloro-deoxyadenosine (CDA) in the treatment of alkylator failure CLL showed that 4% of these patients obtained a complete remission and 50% a partial remission, for an overall response rate of 54% *(55)*. In previously untreated patients, an overall response rate of 85% and a 60% complete remission rate were observed *(56)*. When the different nonrandomized studies were pooled ($N = 102$), 37% obtained a complete remission using the National Cancer Institute (NCI) criteria *(57)*, and 39% obtained partial response *(56)*. Overall, CDA has potent activity in CLL. Myelosuppression and infection are the major toxicities; the long-term impact on progression-free and overall survival remains to be elucidated. Determination of the relative effectiveness of CDA compared with FDB for front-line therapy of CLL will ultimately require a randomized study. These initial results derived from nonrandomized trials seem to be indicating that purine analogs may play an important role in CLL treatment, either in front-line therapy or in salvage therapy.

To define whether these drugs are able to improve survival in CLL, two randomized trials compared FDB to anthracyclin-containing regimens *(41,58)*, two compared FDB with CB using a classical schedule *(56,57)*, and compared FDB with high-dose CB. A European trial *(58)* compared FDB therapy with the CAP regimen for treatment of CLL in a randomized, multicenter prospective trial, including 100 previously untreated stage B + C patients and 96 pretreated patients with CB or similar nonanthracycline-containing regimens. Patients were randomly assigned to six courses of either FDB (25 mg/m^2/d on d 1–5) or CAP (cyclophosphamide 750 mg/m^2/d and doxorubicin 50 mg/m^2/d on d 1, and prednisone 40 mg/m^2/d on d 1–5). Remission rates were significantly higher after FDB than after CAP, with overall response rates of 60 and 44%, respectively ($p = 0.023$). A higher response rate to fludarabine was observed in both untreated (71 vs 60%, $p = 0.26$) and pretreated (48 vs 27%, $p = 0.036$) patients, although the difference was statistically significant only in pretreated cases. In the latter group, remission duration and survival did not differ between treatment groups with a median remission duration of 324 d after FDB and 179 d after CAP ($p = 0.22$) and median survival times of 728 d and 731 d, respectively. In untreated cases, on the other hand, FDB induced significantly longer remissions than CAP ($p < 0.001$), although this difference did not translate into survival advantage. Treatment-associated side effects consisted in both regimens were predominantly myelosuppression and in particular granulocytopenia. CAP-treated patients had a higher frequency and severity of nausea and vomiting (25 vs 5%, $p < 0.001$) and alopecia (65 vs 2%, $p < 0.001$). These results indicate that FDB compared favorably with CAP in terms of response, although this difference did not induce a survival improvement.

In 1990, the French Cooperative Group (41) activated a trial in which previously untreated patients with stage B or C CLL were randomly allocated to receive six monthly courses of either FDB 25 mg/m^2 iv daily for 5 d or cyclophosphamide 750 mg/m^2 iv on d 1, doxorubicin 50 mg/m^2 iv on d 1 and prednisone 40 mg/m^2 orally on d 1–5 (CAP) or to the mini-ChOP regimen previously used by this group, consisting of iv vincristin 1 mg/m^2 and doxorubicin 25 mg/m^2 on d 1, plus cyclophosphamide 300 mg/m^2 and prednisone 40 mg/m^2 given orally on d 1–5. Endpoints were treatment response, overall survival and tolerance. From June 1, 1990 to April 15, 1998, 938 patients (651 stage B and 287 stage C) were randomized in 73 centers. Compared with ChOP and FDB, CAP induced lower overall remission rates (58.2%; ChOP, 71.5%; FDB; 71.1%; $p < 0.0001$ for each), including lower clinical remission rates (CAP, 15.2%; ChOP, 29.6%; FDB, 40.1%; $p = 0.003$).

On the basis of these results (observed in a previous interim analysis held in September 1996), it was decided to discontinue accrual in this group. As expected, median survival was better for stage B (81 mo) than for stage C patients (60 mo). Causes of death were related to CLL in 75% of cases, and overall survival did not differ among the three arms (67, 70, and 69 mo in the ChOP, CAP, and FDB groups, respectively). Incidences of infections ($< 5\%$) and autoimmune hemolytic anemia ($< 2\%$) during the six courses were similar in the randomized groups, whereas FDB, compared with ChOP and CAP, induced more frequent protracted thrombocytopenia ($p = 0.003$) and less frequent nausea/vomiting ($p = 0.003$) and hair loss ($p < 0.0001$). For patients with stage B and C CLL, first-line FDB and ChOP regimens both provided similar overall survival and response rates at closing and better results than CAP. However, there was an increase in clinical remission rate and a trend toward a better tolerance of FDB over ChOP that may influence the choice between these regimens as front-line treatments in patients with CLL (41).

In a randomized study, Rai et al. aimed to compare FDB and CB for patients with previously untreated CLL with active disease (59). Eligible patients were all high-risk or those intermediate-risk patients who had active disease and all were previously untreated, with a performance status of less than 3. Between October 1990 and December 1994, 544 previously untreated CLL patients with active disease were randomized to receive FDB (25 mg/m^2 iv daily for 5 d) or CB (40 mg/m^2 po on d 1) or a combination of FDB + CB (20 mg/m^2 of each drug) q4 wk for up to 12 mo. Nonresponders or responders in FDB-alone and CB-alone arms whose CLL progressed within 6 mo of treatment were crossed over to the other arm. Survival analysis for this report was based on 385 patients.

A significantly higher overall response rate of 70% was obtained among 167 evaluable patients on FDB [27% complete response (CR) + 43% partial response (PR)] compared with 45% (3% CR + 42% PR) among 173 patients on CB ($p = 0.0001$). Among 119 patients on FDB + CB, 65% overall responses were noted (25% CR + 40% PR). Response duration following FDB was significantly longer than with CB: 117 patients with either CR or PR on FDB had a median duration of response of 32 mo vs 18 mo among 73 patients on CB ($p = 0.0002$). Similarly, the median progression-free survival (time from study entry to disease progression or death from any cause) was 27 mo for patients receiving FDB vs 17 mo for patients on CB ($p < 0.0001$). With a median follow-up of 30 mo, there was no difference in the overall survival ($p = 0.49$), although this comparison is complicated by the crossover design of the study. An estimated 62% of patients on both arms survived for at least 4 yr. Seventy-four patients initially treated with CB received FDB, with only 29 crossovers from FDB to CB. Both drugs were well tolerated, with similar toxicity profiles, except for a 20% grade 3 + grade 4 leukopenia with FDB vs 7% with CB ($p =$ 0.001). However, toxicities were significantly worse for the combination arm, which displayed 42 and 45% thrombocytopenia and neutropenia of grade 3 and grade 4 level and approximately twice the frequency of serious grade 3 and 4 infections than the individual one-arm protocols. These results caused the combination arm to be stopped somewhat sooner than the total protocol.

An Italian trial *(60)* compared FDB using classical schedule to intermittent CB associated with prednisone in 150 advanced CLL patients. Response rates were very close in both arms, possibly because this study was employing CB at higher dosage than in the American trial. Response duration was longer in the FDB arm, and toxicity was comparable.

The European Organization for Research and Treatment of Cancer (EORTC) started a randomized trial aiming to compare high-dose continuous CB (10 mg/m^2) with FDB at classical dosage (25 mg/m^2 on d 1–5 every 3 wk). This treatment was administered for 18 wk *(61)*. Eighty-four patients have been enrolled so far in this trial, and response evaluation was available for 74 patients with a median follow-up of 33 mo. Response rates, overall survival, and progression-free survival were comparable in both arms. The German CLL Study Group *(51)* compared (in younger patients resistant to alkylating agents) high-dose CB (0.2 mg/kg/d) given continuously for 6 mo with FDB (25 mg/m^2 on d 1–3 every 28 d) plus cyclophosphamide (250 mg/m^2 on d 1–3 every 28 d). A higher response rate (88 vs 67%) and lower toxicity was observed for the association of FDB and cyclophosphamide.

The Polish Leukemia Study Group *(62)* compared CDA plus prednisone (CDA at 0.12 mg/kg/d and prednisone at 30 mg/m^2 during five consecutive days each month) with a classical intermittent CB plus prednisone schedule, in 229 previously untreated advanced CLL patients. Although the CDA-containing regimen obtained a significantly higher response rate (86% overall response vs 59% for the CB-containing regimen; $p < 0.002$), again, better response did not translate into survival advantage.

2.3.3. MONOCLONAL ANTIBODIES

The humanized monoclonal antibody Campath 1H (alemtuzumab) directed against the CD52 antigen has shown important activity against B-CLL cells. CD52 is abundantly expressed on the surface of virtually all peripheral B- and T-lymphocytes, on monocytes but not granulocytes, red blood cells, and on platelets. The mechanism of action described for Campath 1H is the ability to induce cell lysis using host effector mechanisms such as complement fixation and antibody-dependent cell cytotoxicity (ADCC) and a direct effect through the induction of apoptosis (reviewed in refs. *63* and *64*). Several studies showed the effectiveness of Campath 1H in patients with either previously untreated or relapsed/refractory B-CLL patients *(65,66)*. Clearing of blood lymphoid tumor cells was observed in virtually all patients, and clearing of bone marrow B-CLL cells was seen in 30–40% of previously treated patients and up to 70% of naive patients. However, only a minority of patients had a complete response in regard to the lymph node component of the disease.

Campath 1H has been tested as consolidation therapy after chemotherapy in a short series of six patients with relapsed B-CLL; partial to complete response was seen in five patients *(67)*. This finding suggests that Campath 1H may be effective in eliminating residual disease after conventional chemotherapy. In these trials, Campath 1H was usually applied at a dose of 30 mg iv three times a week for a maximum of 12 wk. Premedication with diphenhydramine and acetaminophen as well as prophylaxis against opportunistic infections is required. The main toxicities were mild infusion-related side effects such as rigor, fever, nausea, vomiting, rash, and fatigue, which mostly occurred during the first week of therapy. About half of the patients with previously treated CLL developed transient thrombocytopenia, neutropenia, or infections, which were severe [World Health Organization (WHO) grade 3 and 4] in approx 20% *(68)*. These results suggest that the best indication for Campath would be as a treatment for CLL patients without bulky tumoral disease or for residual disease. They also indicate that Campath is effective as a second-line therapy in patients refractory to alkylant drugs and purine analogs. Interestingly, this drug can be also subcutaneously scheduled *(69)*.

Owing to the weak expression of CD20 by CLL B-cells and to initial poor results in CD5+ lymphocytic lymphoma *(70)*, anti-CD20 antibody has been less evaluated in CLL. Because of these data, rituximab was expected to play an adjuvant role after a debulking treatment, for example, as an in vivo purging agent before stem cell collection and transplantation, or as a potentiator of chemotherapy with FDB and cyclophosphamide. However, phase I/II studies with anti-CD20 in CLL have shown that the drug could be active at least on blood lymphocytosis, but either at very high doses, or with a three weekly schedule and then at a high cost *(71,72)*. Radio-labeled anti-CD20 antibodies (yttrium 90 or iodine 131), currently being investigated in low-grade lymphoma, have been less explored in CLL *(73)*. Two limitations to its use are anticipated: a consummation of the product both by blood lymphocytes, which have to be reduced with other drugs first, and, given its constant lymphocyte infiltration, by bone marrow irradiation related to the targeting of the radiolabeled drug. As expected, preliminary trials in lymphoma have confirmed hematological toxicity, with a risk of myelodysplastic syndromes, especially in patients previously treated with alkylating drugs. Finally, recent work from the M.D. Anderson Cancer Center, has shown that the association of FDB, rituximab, and Campath is able to achieve a significant number of complete remissions, including complete molecular remissions *(74)*.

2.3.4. AUTOLOGOUS AND ALLOGENEIC BONE MARROW TRANSPLANTATION

The rationale for intensive treatment is based on the speculation that increasing the quality of response should provide a longer time to progression interval and the assumption that it is the best way to increase overall survival. Moreover, allogenic transplant has been demonstrated to cure some patients through the graft vs leukemia effect.

Myeloablative treatments followed by autologous or allogenic stem cell rescue were first proposed as palliation intent for patients with advanced disease that was resistant or relapsing after standard treatments *(75–80)*. A large European retrospective survey of stem cell transplantation in CLL has recently summarized the available data and outcome from 413 patients *(79)*. Despite great differences in previous treatments, patient selection, source and treatment of stem cells, conditioning regimens, age, and status at transplantation, these data suggest that autologous stem cell transplantation compares favorably with allogenic transplantation in terms of treatment-related toxicity, mortality, and overall survival. Results of the autotransplantation procedure are better when performed soon in the course of the disease (< 36 mo) and when peripheral stem cells are used; cell manipulation, either positive (CD34) or negative (B-cell purging), does not translate into improved survival. However, a lower incidence of relapse is observed with allotransplants, suggesting a graft vs leukemia allogenic effect and the possibility that some of these patients might have achieved cure *(79)*.

Autologous stem cell transplantation (ASCT) has also been investigated in younger patients with refractory/relapsed B-CLL or in first remission, leading to high response rate and prolonged progression-free survival *(79–81)*. Although it has been suggested that previous treatment with FDB could impair the harvest of peripheral stem cells, ASCT could be performed in most patients after fludarabine therapy *(79)*. Performed early in first remission, ASCT has showed promising results, with an impressive rate of complete response at the molecular level *(25)*. Through assessment of the residual disease after the transplant procedure with sensitive clone-specific methods, it has been shown that patients who became polymerase chain reaction (PCR) negative after transplantation (either allogenic or autologous) experienced long-term disease-free survival *(81,82)*, whereas the persistence or recurrence of the clone-specific signal predicted relapse *(81,82)*. Since only patients demonstrating chemosensitivity are selected for a transplant program and since these patients are known by their long-term outcome, the place of ASCT in front-line treatment of younger B-CLL patients should be prospectively investigated. PCR negaitivity in residual disease has been obtained for the first time in CLL, which constitutes an important step in the strategy leading to cure *(81)*. The time has come to evaluate more precisely the place of intensive treatment, either as part of the initial strategy (especially in "young" patients) or as salvage treatment for poor responders after first-line treatment. In this setting, first-line chemotherapy preceding intensive treatment should combine a maximal antitumor effect and a low stem cell toxicity to avoid difficulties of stem cell collection.

Stem cell allotransplantation in CLL is often limited by the patient's age and donor availability *(75–77)*. Only 10% of patients with advanced stage CLL, and fulfilling the eligibility for this treatment, actually undergo allotransplantation *(97)*. The procedure is associated with a high treatment-related mortality (40%) and a 20% relapse rate at 3 yr. Quality of life after allotransplantation is often a matter of concern. Some groups have developed an alternative method using less toxic, non myeloablative regimens *(83,84)*, which has been proposed in patients with CLL until they are 65–70 yr old *(85)*. This perspective deserves further study.

Another approach toward eliminating residual disease is postremission treatment with monoclonal antibodies like Campath or anti-CD20. Both have been demonstrated by clone-specific molecular probes to induce complete molecular remission following an initial chemotherapy regimen. In the case of anti-CD20, a higher response rate could be achieved by increasing either the dose *(71)* or the frequency of administration *(72)* of rituximab.

3. ANCILLARY TREATMENTS

3.1. Radiotherapy

Radiotherapy, administred as either P32 *(86)*, as total body irradiation *(87)*, extracorporal irradiation of blood *(88)*, or thymic irradiation *(89)*, was found to be effective in a few patients, but severe myelosuppression is a frequent sequel to this treatment. Splenic irradiation has been used more often, mainly in patients with massive splenomegaly, when splenectomy was difficult and the patient had associated autoimmune cytopenias. Recently, the UK MRC observed a better survival for patients treated bywith splenic irradiation as compared with CLB or CLB + PRD, in two randomized trials, but this difference was not significant *(12)*. Finally, irradiation of large lymph nodes may be used in patients who are resistant to chemotherapy.

3.2. Splenectomy

The main indications for splenectomy are corticosteroid-resistant or -dependent autoimmune hemolytic anemia or thrombocytopenia and massive painful splenomegaly. Although several groups have reported that splenectomy may be an efficient treatment in CLL *(90–92)*, this has not been demonstrated in randomized studies.

3.3. Intravenous Immunoglobulins

The fact that hypogammaglobulinemia was the major cause of the increased infectious risk in CLL prompted the use of intravenous immmunoglobulins to prevent infection. In a double-blind randomized study, intravenous immunoglobulins (400 mg/kg body weight given every 3 wk) reduced the incidence of bacterial infections by 50% (96). However, the number of severe bacterial infections and viral infections was unaffected, and survival was not modified. In addition, because intravenous immunoglobulins are expensive, their role in preventing infection in routine practice for CLL patients is a matter of debate. In general, infections should be treated with broad-spectrum antibiotics, and intravenous immunoglobulins should be limited to patients with severe hypogammaglobulinemia displaying frequent infectious complications.

4. NEW THERAPIES

4.1. Anti-Idiotypic Vaccines

Since all major chemotherapeutic treatments in CLL induce good responses but are unable to effect a cure, one of the major questions that needs to be answered is whether there is a place for immunotherapeutic approaches like anti-idiotypic vaccines. Since each B-cell undergoes a unique, characteristic, rearrangement and since malignant B-cell hemopathies are characterized by clonal expansion of a clone displaying a unique rearrangement, idiotype constitutes a privileged tumor antigen. One of the aims of tumor immunotherapy is the induction of CD8 cytotoxic T-lymphocytes. Although, trials of idiotype vaccination have not been reported in CLL, interesting results were reported in the case of lymphoma patients (93).

4.2. Gene Therapy

To improve the immunosuppression associated with CLL, Kipps et al. (94) have designed an elegant gene transfer procedure, using an adenovirus as a vector to transfect CD40 L (CD154) into CLL B cells, in order to elicit an antileukemia effect in vitro. This trial is presently under evaluation; whatever the results, it points in the direction of targeting cell–cell regulation defects as a basis of treatment innovative strategies.

4.3. New Drugs

Many new drugs are presently under study for CLL treatment. The agents currently considered to be the most promising include those that induce apoptosis (506U78, clofarabine, retinoids, arsenicals); those that interfere with cell cycling (flavopiridol, UCN-01, rapamycin) or tumor-associated angiogenesis (thalidomide, SU5416, SU6668); and those that inhibit protein kinase C inhibition (Bryostatin) and the proteasome (PS-134), among others (reviewed in ref. 95).

5. CONCLUSIONS

Once the diagnosis of CLL has been substantiated the treating physician must decide not only how to treat the patient, but when to initiate therapy (reviewed in ref. 97). In a subset of patients, smoldering CLL is diagnosied, mostly among those with Rai stage 0 or Binet stage A. Identification of patients who need immediate treatment has been improved by the two staging systems. On the basis of long-term randomized trials, immediate treatment can be appropriately deferred for most of these patients (in the absence of cure) (10,11,14). However, there is increasing evidence that some of these patients rapidly progress to aggressive disease, and early identification constitutes an important aim. About 30% of these patients will progress to more advanced stages or require treatment within 3 yr after diagnosis (10). Most of them should correspond to stages A or 0, displaying unmutated V_H genes or deletereous chromosomal abnormalities in chromosomes 11 or 17 (22–26). It is unclear whether patients with Binet stage A or Rai indolent forms whose leukemic B-cells have these abnormalities would benefit from early treatment. (This possibility should be tested in a prospective clinical trial.) By contrast, there is consensus that most patients with Binet stage B or C, or Rai stage III or IV, as well as patients with Rai stages I or II with progressive disease whose life expectancy does not exceed 7 yr, should be considered for early treatment (86). Although most of these patients require treatment at presentation, some patients can still be monitored without therapy until they exhibit evidence of progressive or symptomatic disease; early identification of these patients also constitutes an important goal.

CB is the best tolerated and least expensive drug (86). FDB and other purine analogs like 2-CDA are the best single agents in CLL since they yield better response rates (41,48,55,57–62). Long-term randomized trials have compared FDB with CB and ChOP or CAP regimens (41,58–61). Higher response rates and longer durations of remission and progression-free survival are found with FDB than with CB (58,60). Nevertheless, neither FDB nor CB prolonged survival. When FDB was compared with ChOP and CAP, rates of response and progression free-survival were roughly similar for mini-ChOP and FDB, and better than the rates for CAP (41,58). None of these treatments can cure CLL. In addition, a meta-analysis of 10 randomized trials involving 2035 patients with advanced CLL compared CB with several combination chemotherapy regimens; in none of these trials did improvement in response rates translate into improved survival (14). The lack of improvement in survival despite superior response rates has been observed with other chronic lymphoid malignancies and could be owing to subsequent treatment or the failure of the treatment to eliminate all malignant cells.

Another interesting point emerging from the comparison of historical with modern series of patients is the observation of a consistent prolongation of median survival time. For stage C patients, our group of previously untreated patients displayed a median survival of 2 yr (8). It is of interest that the same survival patterns were observed in initial Rai (7) and Hansen (98) series, compared with present results, indicating a survival close to 60 mo for these patients in most series. For stage B patients, results from initial French Cooperative Group trials (29) showed a median survival of 58 mo, whereas in the more recent trial of this same group (41), survival was 81 mo. The availability of new drugs like purine analogs, polychemotherapy, or even intensive therapy regimens able to salvage patients failing to respond to initial therapy may probably explain at least in part this improvement of overall survival in CLL patients.

In recent years, monoclonal antibodies like anti-CD52 (Campath) and anti-CD20 [rituximab (Mabthera)] emerged as major drugs in CLL and generated a tremendous interest. Campath is an anti-CD52 monoclonal antibody (63–69), and Campath studies in CLL have mainly been conducted in patients previously treated with FDB or alkylating agents or untreated patients. The most striking effect observed in these studies is a constant reduction of abnormal blood lymphocytosis, which normalizes in 97–100% of patients, usually in less than 4 wk. The response was also assessed by the disappearance of CD5/CD19 coexpressing cells from blood in most of patients tested with immunophenotyping; in some of them, the clonal signal could no longer be detected by PCR analysis (67). These impressive results unfortunately extend less frequently to other sites of lymphoid infiltration, mostly lymph nodes, so that complete responses rates range from 0 to 5% in previously treated patients to 33% in untreated ones. A large tumor burden in lymph nodes predicts a poor response rate. These results suggest that the best indication for

Campath in front-line therapy would be as a treatment of CLL patients without bulky tumoral disease or for residual disease.

Because of the weak expression of CD20 by CLL B-cells and the initial poor results in CD5+ lymphocytic lymphoma, anti-CD20 antibody has been less evaluated in CLL. Considering these data, rituximab was expected to play an adjuvant role after a debulking treatment, for example, as an in vivo purging agent before stem cell collection and transplantation, or as a potentiator of chemotherapy with Fludarabine and cyclophosphamide. However, phase I/II studies with anti-CD20 in CLL have shown that the drug could be active at least on blood lymphocytosis, but either at very high doses, or with a three weekly schedule and then at a high cost *(71,72)*. Radiolabeled anti-CD20 antibodies (yttrium 90 or iodine 131), currently being investigated in low-grade lymphoma, have been less investigated in CLL *(73)*. Two limitations to its use are anticipated: a consummation of the product both by blood lymphocytes, which have to be reduced with other drugs first, and, given its constant lymphocyte infiltration, by bone marrow irradiation related to the targeting of the radiolabeled drug. As expected, preliminary trials in lymphoma have confirmed hematological toxicity, with a risk of myelodysplastic syndromes, especially in patients previously treated with alkylating drugs *(10)*.

As concerns toxicity, purine analogs cause more myelosuppression and reductions in CD4 lymphocytes than CB, and they cost more than combination chemotherapy *(41,48,59)*. Alopecia, vomiting, diarrhea, and cardiac toxicity are problems with combination chemotherapy, which, like FDB, requires intravenous administration *(41,58)*. Tolerance to Campath is usually limited to rigors and fever during the first injections *(65–67)*. Hematological toxicity is not observed, both in vitro and in vivo, and stem cell collection for autografting was successful in most of the patients treated. However, a prolonged lymphocytopenia and the possibility of opportunistic infections exist with this drug *(66)*. Although anti-CD20 antibodies are usually well tolerated, serious adverse effects, sometimes lethal, have been rarely recorded in patients exhibiting high lymphocyte counts *(99–101)*.

Evaluations of treatments called intensification procedures, which aim for a complete molecular remission (no evidence of molecular markers of the malignant clone after treatment), are in progress. They include purine analogs with or without other drugs followed by autologous bone marrow transplantation or monoclonal antibodies (e.g., Campath or anti-CD20), or both. Some patients have entered a sustained molecular remission with such intense treatments, but it is unknown whether the treatment cures the disease or just delays a relapse. Conventional allogeneic bone-marrow transplantation can probably be curative in some cases, but only 10% of patients with CLL are eligible for this treatment, which has a 40% mortality rate. Allogeneic bone marrow transplantation, in which the patient's marrow is not ablated by high-dose chemotherapy, is another option under evaluation. Randomized trials of these strategies are time-consuming and expensive, but essential.

Meanwhile, what should physicians do for patients with CLL? Patients with stage A (or stage 0) need only observation. Young stage A or stage 0 and indolent stage I and II patients could be considered for early treatment in the context of clinical trials, if they display unmutated V genes or deleterious chromosomal abnormalities. Most patients in Binet stage B or C, and progressive Rai stage I and II, and Rai stage III and IV should be considered for early treatment. Young patients (< 65 yr?), for whom a cure is possible in principle, should participate in a randomized trial of one of the aggressive new strategies. For an older patient, or one with considerable comorbidity, the aim should be palliation. For this we prefer CB. For patients who do not fit either category, therapeutic decisions vary. Some physicians prefer to start with CB and switch to mini-ChOP or purine analogs if there is no response, whereas other physicians initiate treatment with FDB.

Treatment of CLL is generally palliative in intent. Patients who have relapsed may be followed without therapy until they experience disease-related symptoms or progressive disease, with deterioration of blood counts, discomfort from lymphadenopathy or hepatosplenomegaly, recurrent infections, or associated autoimmune disorders. FDB is the best option for patients refractory to alkylating agents *(41,48,58,59)*, and we recommend mini-ChOP *(41)* or Campath *(66)* for patients who are refractory to FDB. Recent data suggest that in selected patients allogeneic bone marrow transplantation or high-dose chemotherapy with autologous stem cell support may be reasonable treatment options, particularly in the context of a clinical research protocol. We believe that, depending on age and coexisting diseases, intensification procedures are justified for these patients.

REFERENCES

1. Dighiero G, Travade P, Chevret S, Fenaux P, Chastang C, Binet JL. B-cell chronic lymphocytic leukemia: present status and future directions. French Cooperative Group on CLL. Blood 1991;78:1901–1914.
2. Matutes E, Owusu-Ankomah K, Morilla R, et al. The immunological profile of B-cell disorders and proposal of a scoring system for the diagnosis of CLL. Leukemia 1994;8:1640–1645.
3. Zomas AP, Matutes E, Morilla R, Owusu-Ankomah K, Seon BK, Catovsky D. Expression of the immunoglobulin-associated protein B29 in B cell disorders with the monoclonal antibody SN8 (CD79b). Leukemia 1996;10:1966–1970.
4. Ternynck T, Dighiero G, Follezou J, Binet JL. Comparison of normal and CLL lymphocyte surface Ig determinants using peroxidase-labeled antibodies. I. Detection and quantitation of light chain determinants. Blood 1974;43:789–795.
5. Conley CL, Misiti J, Laster AJ. Genetic factors predisposing to chronic lymphocytic leukemia and to autoimmune disease. Medicine 1980;59:323–334.
6. Linet MS, Van Natta ML, Brookmeyer R, et al. Familial cancer history and chronic lymphocytic leukemia. A case-control study. Am J Epidemiol 1989;130:655–664.
7. Rai KR, Sawitsky A, Cronkite EP, Chanana AD, Levy RN, Pasternack BS. Clinical staging of chronic lymphocytic leukemia. Blood 1975;46:219–234.
8. Binet JL, Auquier A, Dighiero G, et al. A new prognostic classification of chronic lymphocytic leukemia derived from a multivariate survival analysis. Cancer 1981;48:198–206.
9. French Cooperative Group on Chronic Lymphocytic Leukemia. Effects of chlorambucil and therapeutic decision in initial forms of chronic lymphocytic leukemia (stage A): results of a randomized clinical trial on 612 patients. Blood 1990;75:1414–1421.
10. Dighiero G, Maloum K, Desablens B, et al. Chlorambucil in indolent chronic lymphocytic leukemia. French Cooperative Group on Chronic Lymphocytic Leukemia. N Eng J Med 1998;338:1506–1514.
11. Catovsky D, Fooks J, Richards S. The UK Medical Research Council CLL trials 1 and 2. Nouv Rev Fr Hematol 1988;30:423–427.
12. Shustik C, Mick R, Silver R, Sawitsky A, Rai K, Shapiro L. Treatment of early chronic lymphocytic leukemia: intermittent chlorambucil versus observation. Hematol Oncol 1988;6:7–12.
13. Spanish Cooperative Group Pethema. Treatment of chronic lymphocytic leukemia: a preliminary report of Spanish (Pethema) trials. Leuk Lymphoma 1991;5:89–91.
14. CLL Trialists' Collaborative Group. Chemotherapeutic options in chronic lymphocytic leukemia: a meta-analysis of the randomized trials. CLL Trialists' Collaborative Group. J Natl Cancer Inst 1999;91:861–868.
15. Jaksic B, Brugiatelli M. High dose continuous chlorambucil vs intermittent chlorambucil plus prednisone for treatment of B-CLL—IGCI CLL-01 trial. Nouv Rev Fr Hematol 1988;30:437–442.
16. French Cooperative Group on Chronic Lymphocytic Leukaemia. Natural history of stage A chronic lymphocytic leukaemia untreated patients. Br J Haematol 1990;76:45–57.
17. Montserrat E, Vinolas N, Reverter JC, Rozman C. Natural history of chronic lymphocytic leukemia: on the progression and prognosis of early clinical stages. Nouv Rev Fr Hematol 1988;30:359–361.
18. Keating MJ, Lerner S, Kantarjian H, Freireich EJ, O'Brien S. The serum beta2-microglobulin (beta2M) level is more powerful than stage in predicting response and survival in chronic lymphocytic leukemia (CLL). Blood 1998;86:606a.

19. Sarfati M, Bron D, Lagneaux L, Fonteyn C, Frost H, Delespesse G. Elevation of IgE-binding factors in serum of patients with B cell-derived chronic lymphocytic leukemia. Blood 1988; 71:94–98.

20. Léotard S. Etude de la valeur pronostique du CD23 soluble dans la leucémie Lymphnoeud Chronique chez des patients en stade A, non traités. Comparaison avec la béta2-microglobuline, l'albumine et la LDH. Thëse pour le diplúme d'état de Docteur en Pharmacie. Université de Paris Sud, 1998.

21. Hallek M, Langenmayer I, Nerl C, et al. Elevated serum thymidine kinase levels identify a subgroup at high risk of disease progression in early , nonsmoldering chronic lymphocytic leukemia. Blood 1999;93(5): 1732–1737.

22. Dohner H, Stilgebauer S, Benner A, et al. Genomic aberrations and survival in chronic lymphocytic leukemia. N Engl J Med 2000;343(26):1910–1916.

23. Schroeder HW, Jr., Dighiero G. The pathogenesis of chronic lymphocytic leukemia: analysis of the antibody repertoire. Immunol Today 1994;15:288–294.

24. Damle RN, Wasil T, Fais F, et al. Immunoglobulin V gene mutation status and CD38 expression as novel prognostic indicators in chronic lymphocytic leukemia. Blood 1999;94:1840–1848.

25. Hamblin TJ, Davis Z, Oscier DG, Stevenson FK. Unmutated immunoglobulin VH genes are associated with a more aggressive form of chronic lymphocytic leukemia. Blood 1999;94:1848–1855.

26. Maloum K, Pritsch O, Magnac C, et al. Expression of unmutated VH genes is a detrimental prognostic factor in chronic lymphocytic leukemia. Blood, 2000;96:377–379.

27. Klein U, Tu Y, Stolovitzky GA, et al. Gene expression profiling of B cell chronic lymphocytic leukemia reveals a homogeneous phenotype related to memory B cells. J Exp Med 2001;194:1625–1638.

28. Rosenwald A, Alizadeh AA, Widhopf G, et al. Relation of gene expression phenotype to immunoglobulin mutation genotype in B cell chronic lymphocytic leukemia. J Exp Med 2001;194:1639–1647.

29. French Cooperative Group on Chronic Lymphocytic Leukemia. A randomized clinical trial of chlorambucil versus COP in stage B chronic lymphocytic leukemia. Blood 1990;75:1422–1425.

30. Catovsky D, Hamblin T, Richards S. Preliminary results of UK MRC trial in chronic lymphocytic leukemia-CLL3. In: Proceedings of the 27th Congress of the International Society of Haematology (ISH-EHA). Br J Haematol 1998;102:278, abstract O-114.

31. Montserrat E, Alcala A, Parody R, et al. Treatment of chronic lymphocytic leukemia in advanced stages. A randomized trial comparing chlorambucil plus prednisone versus cyclophosphamide, vincristine, and prednisone. Cancer 1985;56:2369–2375.

32. Raphael B, Andersen JW, Silber R, et al. Comparison of chlorambucil and prednisone versus cyclophosphamide, vincristine, and prednisone as initial treatment for chronic lymphocytic leukemia: long-term follow-up of an Eastern Cooperative Oncology Group randomized clinical trial. J Clin Oncol 1991;9:770–776.

33. Hester JP, Gehan EA. Cytoxan, adriamycin, prednisone (CAP) chemotherapy for chronic lymphocytic leukemia (abstract). Proc Am Soc Clin Oncol 1978;19:214.

34. Keating MJ, Scouros M, Murphy S, Kantarjian H, Hester J, McCredie KB, Hersh EM, Freireich EJ. Multiple agent chemotherapy (POACH) in previously treated and untreated patients with chronic lymphocytic leukemia. Leukemia 1988;2:157–164.

35. Hansen MM, Andersen E, Birgens H, Christensen BE, Christensen TG, Geisler C. CHOP versus chlorambucil + prednisolone in chronic lymphocytic leukemia. Leuk Lymphoma 1991;(Suppl 4):97–100.

36. Kimby E, Mellstedt H. Chlorambucil/prednisolone versus CHOP in symtomatic chronic lymphocytic leukemia of B-cell type. Leuk Lymphoma 1991;(suppl 4):93–96.

37. Jaksic B, Brugiatelli M, Krc I, et al. High dose chlorambucil versus Binet's modified cyclophosphamide, doxorubicin, vincristine, and prednisone regimen in the treatment of patients with advanced B-cell chronic lymphocytic leukemia. Results of an international multicenter randomized trial. International Society for Chemo-Immunotherapy, Vienna. Cancer 1997;79:2107–2114.

38. French Cooperative Group on Chronic Lymphocytic Leukaemia. Effectiveness of "CHOP" regimen in advanced untreated chronic lymphocytic leukaemia. Lancet 1986;1:1346–1349.

39. French Cooperative Group on Chronic Lymphocytic Leukaemia. Long-term results of the CHOP regimen in stage C chronic lymphocytic leukaemia. Br J Haematol 1989;73:334–340.

40. French Cooperative Group on CLL. Is the CHOP regimen a good treatment for advanced CLL? Results from two randomized clinical trials. French Cooperative Group on Chronic Lymphocytic Leukemia. Leuk Lymphoma 1994;13:449–456.

41. Leporrier M, Chevret S, Cazin B, et al. Randomized comparison of fludarabine, CAP, and ChOP in 938 previously untreated stage B and C chronic lymphocytic leukemia patients. Blood 2001;98:2319–2325.

42. Binet JL, Leporrier M, Dighiero G, et al. A clinical staging system for chronic lymphocytic leukemia. Prognostic significance. Cancer 1977;40:855–864.
43. Kempin S, Lee BJd, Thaler HT, et al. Combination chemotherapy of advanced chronic lymphocytic leukemia: the M-2 protocol (vincristine, BCNU, cyclophosphamide, melphalan, and prednisone). Blood 1982;60:1110–1121.
44. Grever MR, Kopecky KJ, Coltman CA, et al. Fludarabine monophosphate: a potentially useful agent in chronic lymphocytic leukemia. Nouv Rev Fr Hematol 1988;30:457–459.
45. Piro LD, Carrera CJ, Beutler E, Carson DA. 2-Chlorodeoxyadenosine: an effective new agent for the treatment of chronic lymphocytic leukemia. Blood 1988;72:1069–1073.
46. Keating MJ, Kantarjian H, Talpaz M, et al. Fludarabine: a new agent with major activity against chronic lymphocytic leukemia. Blood 1989;74:19–25.
47. O'Brien S, Kantarjian H, Beran M, et al. Results of fludarabine and prednisone therapy in 264 patients with chronic lymphocytic leukemia with multivariate analysis-derived prognostic model for response to treatment [see comments]. Blood 1993;82:1695–1700.
48. Keating MJ, O'Brien S, Lerner S, et al. Long-term follow-up of patients with chronic lymphocytic leukemia (CLL) receiving fludarabine regimens as initial therapy. Blood 1998;92:1165–1171.
49. Byrd JC, Rai KR, Sausville EA, Grever MR. Old and new therapies in chronic lymphocytic leukemia: now is the time for a reassessment of therapeutic goals. Semin Oncol 1998;25:65–74.
50. O'Brien SM, Kantarjian HM, Cortes J, et al . Results of the fludarabine and cyclophosphamide combination regimen in chronic lymphocytic leukemia. J Clin Oncol. 2001;19:1414–1420.
51. Hallek M, Schmitt B, Wilhelm M, et al. Fludarabine plus cyclophosphamide is an efficient treatment for advanced chronic lymphocytic leukaemia (CLL): results of a phase II. Br J Haematol. 2001;114(2):342–348.
52. Cazin B, Maloum K, Divine M, et al.. Oral fludarabine and cyclophosphamide in previously CLL Data on 59 patients (abstract). Blood 2001;98 (Suppl 1):3214a.
53. Frewin R, Turner D, Tighe M, et al. Combination therapy with fludarabine and cyclophosphamide as salvage treatment in lymphoproliferative disorders. Br J Haematol. 1999;104:612–613.
54. Flinn IW, Byrd JC, Morrison C, et al. Fludarabine and cyclophosphamide with filgrastim support in patients with previously untreated indolent lymphoid malignancies. Blood 2000;96:71–75.
55. Saven A, Piro LD. 2-Chlorodeoxyadenosine: a potent antimetabolite with major activity in the treatment of indolent lymphoproliferative disorders. Hematol Cell Ther 1996;38:S93–101.
56. Saven A, Lemon RH, Kosty M, Beutler E, Piro LD. 2-Chlorodeoxyadenosine activity in patients with untreated chronic lymphocytic leukemia. J Clin Oncol 1995;13:570–574.
57. Cheson BD, Bennett JM, Grever M, et al. National Cancer Institute-sponsored Working Group guidelines for chronic lymphocytic leukemia: revised guidelines for diagnosis and treatment. Blood 1996;87:4990–4997.
58. The French Cooperative Group on CLL, Johnson S, Smith AG, Loffler H, et al. Multicentre prospective randomised trial of fludarabine versus cyclophosphamide, doxorubicin, and prednisone (CAP) for treatment of advanced-stage chronic lymphocytic leukaemia. Lancet 1996; 347:1432–1438.
59. Rai KR, Peterson BL, Appelbaum FR, et al. Fludarabine compared with chlorambucil as primary therapy for chronic lymphocytic leukemia, N Engl J Med 2000;343:1750–1757.
60. Spriano M, Chiurazzi F, Liso V, Mazza P, Molica S, Gobbi M. Multicentre prospective randomized trial of fludarabine versu chlorambucil and prednisone in previously untreated patients with active B-CLL (abstract). In: Proceedings of the International Workshop on CLL. Paris, October 1999, p. 86.
61. Jaksic B, Delmer A, Brugiatelli M, et al. Interim analysis of a randomised EORTC study comparing high dose chlorambucil (HD-CLB) vs fludarabine (FAMP) in untreated B-cell chronic lymphocytic leukaemia (CLL). Hematol Cell Ther 1997; 39:S87.
62. Robak T, Blonski JZ, Kasznicki M, et al. Cladribine with prednisone versus chlorambucil with prednisone as first-line therapy in chronic lymphocytic leukemia: report of a prospective, randomized, multicenter trial. Blood 2000;96:2723–2729.
63. Riechmann L, Clark M, Waldmann H, Winter G. Reshaping human antibodies for therapy. Nature 1988;332:323–327.
64. Flynn JM, Byrd JC. Campath-1H monoclonal antibody therapy. Cur Opin Immunol 2000;12:574–581.
65. Osterborg A, Fassas AS, Anagnostopoulos A, et al. Humanized CD52 monoclonal antibody Campath-1H as first-line treatment in chronic lymphocytic leukaemia. Br J Haematol 1996;93:151–153.
66. Osterborg A, Dyer MJ, Bunjes D, et al. Phase II multicenter study of human CD52 antibody in previously treated chronic lymphocytic leukemia. European Study Group of CAMPATH-1H Treatment in Chronic Lymphocytic Leukemia. J Clin Oncol 1997;15:1567–1574.

67. Dyer MJ, Kelsey SM, Mackay HJ, et al. In vivo "purging" of residual disease in CLL with Campath-1H. Br J Haematol 1997;97:669–672.
68. Gilleece MH, Dexter TM. Effect of campath-1H antibody on human hematopoietic progenitors in vitro. Blood 1993;82:807–812.
69. Bowen AL, Zomas A, Emmett E, Matutes E, Dyer MJ, Catovsky D. Subcutaneous Campath-1H in fludarabine-resistant/relapsed chronic lymphocytic leukemia. Br J Haematol 1997;96:617–619.
70. Grillo-Lopez AJ, Hedrick E, Rashford M, Benyunes M. Rituximab: ongoing and future clinical development (review). Semin Oncol 2002;29 (suppl 2):105–112.
71. O'Brien SM, Kantarjian H, Thomas DA, et al. Rituximab dose-escalation trial in chronic lymphocytic leukemia. J Clin Oncol 2001;19:2165–2170.
72. Byrd JC, Murphy T, Howard RS, et al. Rituximab using a thrice weekly dosing schedule in B-cell chronic lymphocytic leukemia and small lymphocytic lymphoma demonstrates clinical activity and acceptable toxicity. J Clin Oncol 2001;19:2153–2164.
73. Kaminski MS, Estes J, Zasadny KR, et al. Radioimmunotherapy with iodine (131)I tositumomab for relapsed or refractory B-cell non-Hodgkin lymphoma: updated results and long-term follow-up of the University of Michigan experience. Blood 2000;96:1259–1266.
74. Rai KR, Dohner H, Keating MJ, Montserrat E. Chronic lymphocytic leukemia: case-based session. Hematology (Am Soc Hematol Educ Program) 2001;Jan:140–156.
75. Michallet M, Corront B, Hollard D, et al. Allogeneic bone marrow transplantation in chronic lymphocytic leukemia: 17 cases. Report from the EBMTG, Bone Marrow Transplant 1991;7:275–279.
76. Rabinowe SN, Soiffer RJ, Gribben JG, et al. Autologous and allogeneic bone marrow transplantation for poor prognosis patients with B-cell chronic lymphocytic leukemia. Blood. 1993;82:1366–1376.
77. Khouri IF, Keating MJ, Vriesendorp HM. Autologous and allogeneic bone marrow transplantation for chronic lymphocytic leukemia: preliminary results. J Clin Oncol 1994;12:748–758.
78. Michallet M, Archimbaud E, Bandini G, et al. HLA-identical sibling bone marrow transplantation in younger patients with chronic lymphocytic leukemia. European Group for Blood and Marrow Transplantation and the International Bone Marrow Transplant Registry. Ann Intern Med 1996;124:311–315.
79. Michallet M, Thiebaut A, Dreger P, et al. Peripheral blood stem cell (PBSC) mobilization and transplantation after fludarabine therapy in chronic lymphocytic leukaemia (CLL): a report of the European Blood and Marrow Transplantation (EBMT) CLL subcommittee on behalf of the EBMT Chronic Leukaemias Working Party (CLWP). Br J Haematol 2000;108:595–601.
80. Dreger P, von Neuhoff N, Kuse R, et al. Early stem cell transplantation for chronic lymphocytic leukaemia: a chance for cure? Br J Cancer 1998;77:2291–2297.
81. Provan D, Bartlett-Pandite L, Zwicky C, et al. Eradication of polymerase chain reaction-detectable chronic lymphocytic leukemia cells is associated with improved outcome after bone marrow tranplantation. Blood 1996; 88:2228–2235.
82. Sutton L, Maloum K, Gonzalez H, et al. Autologous hematopoietic stem cell transplantation as salvage treatment for advanced B cell chronic lymphocytic leukemia. Leukemia 1998;12:1699–1707.
83. Giralt S, Estey E, Albitar M, et al. Engraftment of allogenic hematopoietic progenitor cells with purine analog-containing chemotherapy: harnessing graft versus leukemia without myeloablative therapy. Blood 1997;89:4531–4536.
84. Slavin S, Nagler A, Naparstek E, et al. Nonmyeloablative stem cell transplantation and cell therapy as an alternative to conventional bone marrow transplantation xith lethal cytoreduction for the treatment of malignant and non malignant hematologic diseases. Blood 1998;91:756–763.
85. Khouri IF, Keating M, Korbling M, Pet al. Transplant-lite: induction of graft-versus-malignancy using fludarabine-based nonablative chemotherapy and allogeneic blood progenitor-cell transplantation as treatment for lymphoid malignancies. J Clin Oncol 1998;16:2817–2824.
86. Lawrence JH, Low-Beer BVA, Carpender JWJ. Chronic lymphatic leukemia: study of 100 patients with radio-active phosphorus. JAMA 1949;140:585.
87. Johnson RE: Total body irradiation of chronic lymphocytic leukemia. Cancer 1976;37:2691.
88. Chanana AD, Cronkite EP, Rai KR: The role of extracorporeal irradiation of blood in the treatment of leukemia. Int J Radiat Oncol Biol Phys 1976;1:539–548.
89. Richards F, Spurr CL, Ferree C, Blake DD, Raben M: The control of chronic lymphocytic leukemia with mediastinal irradiation. Am J Med 1978;64:947–954.
90. Ferrant A, Michaux JL, Sokal G. Splenectomy in advanced chronic lymphocytic leukemia. Cancer 1986;58: 2130–2696.

91. Stein RS, Weikert D, Reynols V Greer JP, Flexner JM: Splenectomy for end-stage chronic lymphocytic leukemia. Cancer 1987;59:1815–1818.

92. Delpero JR, Mouvenaeghel G, Gastaut JA, et al. Splenectomy for hypersplenism in chronic lymphocytic leukemia and malignant non-Hodgkin's lymphoma. Br J Surg 1990;77:443–449.

93. Hsu FJ, Caspar CB, Czerwinski D, et al. Tumor-specific idiotype vaccines in the treatment of patients with B-cell lymphoma—long-term results of a clinical trial. Blood 1997;89:3129–3135.

94. Kipps TJ. Future strategies toward the cure of indolent B-cell malignancies. Molecular genetic approaches. Semin Hematol 1999;36:3–8.

95. Cheson BD. Emerging therapies and future directions in chronic lymphocytic leukaemia-chemotherapy. Hematol Cell Ther 2000;42(1):41–47.

96. Cooperative Group for the Study of Immunoglobulin in Chronic Lymphocytic Leukemia. Intravenous immunoglobulin for the prevention of infection in chronic lymphocytic leukemia. A randomized control trial. N Engl J Med 1988;319:902–907.

97. Dighiero G, Binet JL. When and how to treat chronic lymphocytic leukemia. N Engl J Med 2000;343:1799–1802.

98. Hansen MM. Chronic lymphocytic leukaemia. Clinical studies based on 189 cases followed for a long time. Scand J Haematol 1973;(suppl 18):3–286.

99. Lim LC, Koh LP, Tan P. Fatal cytokine release syndrome with chimeric anti-CD20 monoclonal antibody rituximab in a 71-year-old patient with chronic lymphocytic leukemia. J Clin Oncol 1999;17:1962–1963.

100. Yang H, Rosove MH, Figlin RA. Tumor lysis syndrome occurring after the administration of rituximab in lymphoproliferative disorders: high-grade non-Hodgkin's lymphoma and chronic lymphocytic leukemia. Am J Hematol 1999;62:247–250.

101. Winkler U, Jensen M, Manzke O, Schulz H, Diehl B, Engert A. Cytokine-release syndrome in patients with B-cell chronic lymphocytic leukemia and high lymphocyte counts after treatment with an anti-CD20 monoclonal antibody (rituximab, IDEC-C2B8). Blood 1999;94:2217–2224.

13 Chemotherapy of Chronic Lymphocytic Leukemia

Alessandra Ferrajoli, MD, Michael J. Keating, MB, BS, and Susan M. O'Brien, MD

1. INTRODUCTION

Chronic lymphocytic leukemia (CLL) is the most common form of adult leukemia in the United States and Europe and accounts for approx 25% of all leukemias in those regions. Patients with CLL are often asymptomatic at presentation, and the disease is discovered on routine examination. The course of the disease is heterogeneous: a subset of patients will have indolent disease, may never require therapy, and may eventually die of unrelated causes; another subset will have aggressive disease and will survive for only a few years despite treatment. In most patients, the disease will have an intermediate clinical behavior, with slowly increasing leukocytosis and progressive lymphadenopathy and organomegaly, and patients will require treatment at some point. (More details on the epidemiology and clinical presentation of CLL are described in other chapters of this textbook).

Major advances in the treatment of CLL have taken place in the past two decades. Traditionally, the goal of treatment for patients with CLL has been palliation, which was easily achievable with oral alkylating agents such as chlorambucil. With more effective therapies and achievement of complete remission, the goal of treatment in the 21st century is shifting toward cure. The focus of current treatment strategies is not just remission, but attainment of molecular remission: not only elimination of visible disease but eradication of the malignant clone.

In this chapter, we describe the use of alkylating agents, alone or in combination with other agents, purine analogs and purine analogs-based combinations, and newer treatment approaches including monoclonal antibodies.

2. ALKYLATING AGENTS

2.1. Chlorambucil

The most frequently used chemotherapeutic agent in CLL is chlorambucil. It is given orally, is easily absorbed from the gastrointestinal tract, and is well tolerated and inexpensive. Two commonly used schedules of chlorambucil are 0.1 mg/kg daily or 0.4–1 mg/kg, with the total dose given over 1–3 d every 3–4 wk.

Even though chlorambucil has been used for more than four decades, the optimal dose, duration of treatment, and timing of retreatment have not been established. The available information on

From: *Contemporary Hematology*
Chronic Lymphocytic Leukemia: Molecular Genetics, Biology, Diagnosis, and Management
Edited by: G. B. Faguet © Humana Press Inc., Totowa, NJ

response rate and toxicity has been derived from clinical trials in which chlorambucil represented the "standard treatment" or the study was designed to answer other questions such as whether to intervene with treatment early or late in the disease course. An example of this is the large randomized trial conducted by the French Cooperative Group on CLL comparing chlorambucil (0.1 mg/kg daily) vs observation in patients with indolent CLL. This trial addressed the question of whether early treatment with chlorambucil benefited patients with indolent CLL. Chlorambucil was able to produce high response rates in patients with indolent CLL (complete responses in 45% of the patients and partial responses in 31%), but early treatment intervention did not result in improved survival *(1)*.

In 1999, the CLL Trialists' Collaborative Group published a meta-analysis of randomized clinical trials addressing early intervention with chlorambucil. Data from more than 2000 patients enrolled in six different trials were reviewed. The results confirmed the lack of survival benefit with chlorambucil in patients with early-stage CLL *(2)*.

A large randomized trial comparing chlorambucil (40 mg/m^2 orally every 28 d) and fludarabine (25 mg/m^2 iv daily for 5 d every 28 d) was recently published *(3)*. In this study, 193 patients with previously untreated CLL received chlorambucil for a maximum of 12 cycles. The overall response rate to chlorambucil was 37% (complete responses were obtained in 4% of the patients and partial responses in 33%). The response rate obtained in this study was significantly lower than that observed in the French Cooperative Group study of patients with indolent disease *(1)*; this can be explained by differences in the patient populations (indolent vs more advanced disease) and by the different response criteria utilized by the two studies. [The study by Dighiero et al. *(1)* did not require bone marrow evaluation at time of response, whereas the study published by Rai et al. *(3)* utilized the stricter National Cancer Institute-Working Group (NCI-WG) criteria for response; Table 1 shows the NCI-WG criteria.] Overall survival was comparable with single-agent chlorambucil and single-agent fludarabine.

Chlorambucil used at higher doses appears to have superior activity. High-dose chlorambucil (induction with 15 mg daily until complete response or for up to 6 mo, followed by maintenance with 5–15 mg twice a week) was compared with a modified cyclophosphamide, doxorubicin, vincristine, and prednisone (CHOP) regimen in patients with advanced or progressive CLL. The overall response rates were 89.5% with high-dose chlorambucil and 75% with the modified CHOP regimen, and the median survival durations were 68 and 47 mo, respectively *(4)*.

The most common side effect of chlorambucil treatment is myelosuppression, which can be ameliorated by dose modification. Chlorambucil has been reported to be associated with an increased incidence of second cancers (skin, breast, and colon), especially when patients were treated on a daily schedule *(1)*. Secondary acute leukemias have been observed in patients with CLL treated with chlorambucil, but at a much lower incidence than that seen in patients treated for polycythemia vera or when chlorambucil was used as an immunosuppressant in rheumatological disorders *(5–7)*. Because of its tolerability and ease of administration, chlorambucil remains a viable treatment choice for elderly patients and whenever palliation is the goal of treatment.

2.2. Chlorambucil and Prednisone

Chlorambucil is frequently combined with prednisone (30–100 mg/m^2 orally) and prescribed on an intermittent schedule, such as five consecutive days of treatment every 2–4 wk. Based on data from a small subset of patients, the combination was thought to be more effective than chlorambucil alone; when compared in clinical trials, no differences in response rates or overall

Table 1
National Cancer Institute-Working Group Criteria for Response in CLL

Criterion	Value
Complete response	
Physical examination	Normal
Symptoms	None
Lymphocytes	$<4 \times 10^3/\mu L$
Neutrophils	$>1.5 \times 10^3/\mu L$
Platelets	$>100 \times 10^3/\mu L$
Hemoglobin	>11 g/dL
Bone marrow lymphocytes	<30%
Bone marrow biopsy	No nodules or infiltrates
Nodular partial response	Complete resonse with bone marrow nodules or infiltrates
Partial response	
Physical examination (nodes, liver, spleen)	>50% decrease
Plus 1	
Neutrophils	$>1.5 \times 10^3/\mu L$
Platelets	$>100 \times 10^3/\mu L$ or 50% improvement
Hemoglobin	>11 g/dL
Duration of complete or partial response	>2 mo
Progressive disease	
Physical examination (nodes, liver, spleen)	>50% increase or new sites
Circulating lymphocytes	>50% increase
Other	Richter's syndrome
Stable disease	All others

survive were reported, and the use of corticosteroids was associated with an increased incidence of infections (1,2,8–10). At present, the major indication for corticosteroid use in CLL is the management of autoimmune hemolytic anemia or thrombocytopenia.

2.3. Cyclophosphamide

Cyclophosphamide is an alternative to chlorambucil and is usually reserved for patients with CLL who are refractory to or not able to tolerate chlorambucil. Cyclophosphamide has not been evaluated extensively as a single agent against CLL; the largest experience has been in combination regimens with vincristine and prednisone (COP or CVP) or CHOP (see Subheading 2.4. for details). The dose of cyclophosphamide commonly used in CLL is 1–2 g/m² every 3–4 wk.

2.4. Alkylating Agent-Based Combination Chemotherapy

Various alkylating agent-based drug combinations have been used in CLL, mainly in patients with advanced-stage disease. Frequently used combination regimens include COP (or CVP) and CHOP. The results of the largest alkylator-based combination studies are shown in Table 2.

The French Cooperative Group compared the COP (CVP) regimen with chlorambucil in patients with Binet stage B disease and found similar times to disease progression and overall survival (11).

Table 2
Large Randomized Studies of Alkylating Agent-Based Combination Chemotherapy
in Previously Untreated CLL

Regimen	Entry period	No. of patients	CR (%)	PR (%)	Survival (mo)
COP vs Chl *(11)*	1980–1984	291	28/20	41/46	57/58
COP vs Chl-PRD *(12)*	1980–1983	122	23/25	59/47	45/56
ChOP vs Chl-PRD *(14)*	1985–1990	287	24/14	46/38	ND
ChOP vs Chl-PRD *(15)*	1982–1988	113	ND	ND	50/46
ChOP vs Chl-PRD *(16)*	1984–1989	157	67/29	19/53	ND
ChOP vs HD-Chl *(4)*	1987–1993	228	30/60	42/28	47/68

COP, cyclophosphamide, vincristine, and prednisone; CHOP, cyclophosphamide, doxorubicin, vincristine, prednisone; Chl, chlorambucil; PRD, prednisone; CR, complete remission; PR, partial remission; ND, no difference; HD, high dose. ChOP, Binet modified CHOP (doxorubicin 25 mg/m^2).

The Eastern Cooperative Oncology Group compared COP with chlorambucil and prednisone in patients with advanced CLL *(12)*. Patients treated with COP had a median survival of 3.9 yr, and patients treated with chlorambucil and prednisone had a median survival of 4.8 yr.

In another study conducted by the French Cooperative Group, patients with advanced disease (Binet stage C) were randomized to receive either COP or the modified CHOP regimen (cyclophosphamide given orally at 300 mg/m^2 on d 1–5 and doxorubicin given at 25 mg/m^2) *(13)*. The group treated with the modified CHOP regimen had longer median survival (4.5 yr). The superiority of the modified CHOP regimen was clear in this study, but patients in the COP arm had an unusually poor outcome, with a median survival of only 2 yr.

In a subsequent clinical trial coordinated by the French Cooperative Group, patients with Binet stage B disease were randomized to receive either intermittent chlorambucil and prednisone or the modified CHOP regimen *(14)*. The complete response rate was superior with CHOP, but there was no difference in survival between the two groups.

Two large European trials compared standard-dose CHOP with chlorambucil and prednisone. In the study conducted by the Lymphoma Group of Central Sweden in 113 patients with symptomatic CLL, CHOP produced a higher complete response rate; no survival advantage was seen *(15)*. In a multicenter study conducted in Denmark, 157 patients with Binet stage B or C disease were treated with standard-dose CHOP or intermittent chlorambucil and prednisone. Similar to the Swedish study, patients treated with the CHOP regimen had a higher rate of complete response, but no difference in survival was observed *(16)*. In both studies patients treated with the CHOP regimen developed myelosuppression and required dose reduction.

The intense combination treatment of carmustine (BCNU), cyclophosphamide, vincristine, melphalan, and prednisone (the M-2 protocol) was investigated in patients with advanced CLL. Kempin et al. *(17)* reported a high response rate (81% overall responses) and a median survival of 47 mo. However, these encouraging results were not reproduced in a similar study published a few years later *(18)*.

Alkylating agent-based combination chemotherapy, particularly with the inclusion of an anthracycline, appear to be more toxic and does not offer a significant advantage in previously untreated patients with CLL compared with single-agent chlorambucil.

Among patients with CLL who have relapsed or are refractory to therapy with chlorambucil, combination chemotherapy produces responses in about one-third.

Keating et al. *(19)* obtained responses (complete and partial) in 26% of previously treated patients with the multiagent regimen POACH (cyclophosphamide, Adriamycin, cytosine-arabinoside, vincristine, and prednisone); the median survival was 15 mo. Similarly, the M-2 protocol produced responses in 35% of previously treated patients, with a median survival of 15 mo *(17)*. Thus, responses are attainable with alkylating agent-based combination chemotherapy in patients who have failed prior treatment, but the responses are of short duration and have little impact on survival. The better results obtained with purine analogs and purine analog-based combinations have made these regimens more attractive than traditional alkylating agent-based combinations; they are described in Subheading 3.

3. PURINE ANALOGS

Since the early 1980s, numerous studies have been conducted with purine analogs in CLL. Of the three purine analogs (fludarabine, pentostatin, and cladribine), fludarabine has been the most extensively studied.

3.1. Pentostatin

Pentostatin (2'-deoxycoformycin) was the first purine analog to be tested in clinical trials. This agent inhibits the enzyme adenosine deaminase, and its development was based on the observations that children with severe combined immunodeficiency lack adenosine deaminase and that lymphocytes are rich in the enzyme. Pentostatin at a dose of 4 mg/m^2 weekly or every 2 wk induced responses in 5 of 28 patients with advanced CLL refractory to alkylating agents in the initial study by Grever at al. *(20)*. These results were confirmed in a phase II study by the Cancer and Leukemia Group B, in which pentostatin 4 mg/m^2 weekly for 3 wk and then every 2 wk produced complete responses in 3% and partial responses in 23% of patients *(21)*.

A common side effect of all nucleoside analogs is immunosuppression; infections occurred in up to one-third of patients treated with pentostatin *(22)*. Myelosuppression, nausea and vomiting, rash, mucositis, and, less commonly, neurotoxicity have also been observed in patients with CLL treated with pentostatin *(23,24)*.

Although single-agent pentostatin appeared to have less activity in CLL than other purine analogs (vide *see* just above), there is significant interest in using this agent in combination because it is regarded as less myelosuppressive. Two clinical studies evaluating the combination of pentostatin and an alkylating agent recently started; one combines pentostatin and chlorambucil with the support of granulocyte/macrophage colony-stimulating factor *(25)*, and the other is evaluating the efficacy of pentostatin and cyclophosphamide *(26)*. The combination of pentostatin and the monoclonal antibody rituximab is also being evaluated in a phase II multicenter study *(27)*.

3.2. Cladribine

Cladribine [2-chlorodeoxyadenosine (2-CdA)] is an adenosine deaminase-resistant purine analog; it is activated within the cell to chlorodeoxyadenosine triphosphate. In vitro, 2-CdA is toxic to lymphocytes. The exact mechanism of action is unknown, but induction of apoptosis appears to be important for its effect on nonreplicating cells *(28)*.

In the initial study of 2-CdA reported by Piro et al. *(29)*, an overall response rate of 22% was seen among 18 patients with CLL. In this study, 2-CdA was administered as a continuous infusion for 7 d at a dose of 0.5–0.2 mg/kg/d. Several other studies confirmed the activity of 2-CdA in CLL, with overall response rates as high as 80% in previously untreated patients and as low as 20% in previously treated patients with more advanced disease *(30–35)*.

In patients refractory to fludarabine, treatment with 2-CdA was not effective. Despite an initial positive report, subsequent studies showed that 2-CdA produced a low response rate in this patient population, and a high incidence of infectious complications was noted *(36–38)*.

2-CdA is usually given as continuous infusion for 5–7 d at a dose of 0.12 mg/kg/d, but similar results have been obtained with 2-h daily infusions for 5–7 d and with subcutaneous and oral administration *(31,32)*. Multiple courses of 2-CdA are required to achieve a maximal response in CLL. The most relevant toxicities are immunosuppression and myelosuppression.

3.3. Fludarabine

Fludarabine monophosphate (2-fluoro-ara-AMP) is the purine analog with the most clinical activity in CLL. Fludarabine is water-soluble and is relatively resistant to adenosine deaminase; it is rapidly dephosphorylated to F-ara-A after intravenous administration, enters the cells by a carrier-mediated transport system, and undergoes intracellular rephosphorylation to its active metabolite, 2-fluoro-arabinofuranosyl-adenosine-triphosphate (F-ara-ATP), by the rate-limiting enzyme deoxycytidine kinase *(39)*. F-ara-ATP inhibits DNA and RNA synthesis and affects DNA repair, but the exact mechanism of cytotoxicity in quiescent cells, such as malignant lymphocytes, is not known. The activity of F-ara-ATP in CLL could be mediated by the induction of apoptosis *(28,40)*.

Fludarabine was introduced into clinical trials in the early 1980s; the first results using this agent to treat CLL were published in 1988 by Grever et al. *(41)*. In this study, 32 patients with advanced stage CLL were treated at a dose of 20 mg/m^2 daily for five consecutive days; the complete remission rate was 3%, with an overall response rate of 12% *(41)*. Keating et al. *(42)* treated 68 patients with relapsed or refractory CLL with fludarabine 25–30 mg/m^2 daily for 5 d. The complete remission rate was 15%, and the overall response rate was 44%.

Since the first positive reports, fludarabine has been used extensively in the management of patients with relapsed or refractory CLL. At the University of Texas M.D. Anderson Cancer Center, a series of studies was conducted with fludarabine: a 5-d schedule at a dose of 30 mg/m^2, a 3-d schedule at a dose of 30 mg/m^2, a combination of fludarabine (30 mg/m^2 for 5 d) and prednisone, and fludarabine given once a week at a dose of 30 mg/m^2. The response rate with the 3-d schedule of fludarabine was slightly less than that observed with the 5-d regimen (overall response rate 46% vs 59%); the 3-d schedule produced less immunosuppression *(43)*. O'Brien et al. *(44)* reported the results in 169 patients treated with fludarabine and prednisone: the overall response rate was 52%, and the median duration of response was 22 mo. These results were similar to those obtained with the 5-d schedule of single-agent fludarabine, but the incidence of opportunistic infections was increased with the combination of fludarabine and prednisone *(44)*. The once-a-week schedule had a lower overall response rate (24%) in 46 previously treated patients compared with the 5- and 3-d schedules *(45)*. Survival correlated with response to treatment in the above studies. The most durable responses were observed in patients who obtained a complete response and in patients with less prior treatment.

A retrospective analysis of previously treated patients who received single-agent fludarabine as salvage therapy showed that response rates were higher in patients with early-stage disease, minimal prior therapy, age less than 70 yr and normal serum albumin levels *(44,46)*.

Table 3
Large Randomized Studies of Fludarabine in Previously Untreated CLL

Regimen	Entry period	No. of patients	CR (%)	PR (%)	Survival (mo)
F vs 1ChOP vs CAP *(50)*	1990–1998	938	40/15/30	31/43/42	69/70/67
F vs CAP *(48)*	1990–1992	100	23/17	48/43	NA
F vs Chl *(3)*	1990–1994	509	20/4	43/33	66/56

F, fludarabine; ChOP, Binet modified CHOP (doxorubicin 25 mg/m^2); CAP, cyclophosphamide, doxorubicine, and prednisone; CHOP, cyclophosphamide, doxorubicin, vincristine, and prednisone; Chl, chlorambucil; CR, complete remission; PR, partial remission; NA, not available.

Sorensen et al. *(47)* reported the outcome of 724 patients with relapsed or alkylating agent-refractory CLL treated with fludarabine. The overall response rate was 32%, the median duration of response was 13.1 mo, and the overall survival was 12.6 mo.

The French Cooperative Group conducted a randomised trial of fludarabine vs cyclophosphamide, doxorubicin, and prednisone (CAP) in 96 previously treated patients. Patients treated with fludarabine had a higher overall response rate and higher complete response rate than patients treated with CAP (48% and 13% vs 27% and 6%, respectively). There were no differences between the two treatment groups in median response duration and median survival *(48)*.

Fludarabine has also been evaluated as front-line therapy for CLL. Keating et al. *(49)* observed an overall response rate of 80% and a complete remission rate of 37% in 35 patients; the median response duration was 33 mo. The addition of prednisone to fludarabine did not improve the response rate in previously untreated patients *(44)*.

Front-line treatment with fludarabine has been compared with alkylating agent-based therapy in randomized clinical trials (Table 3). The French Cooperative Group assigned 100 patients with advanced CLL to receive treatment with fludarabine or the anthracycline-containing alkylating agent-based regimen CAP. The overall response rates and complete response rates were 71 and 23%, respectively, among the 52 patients who received fludarabine and 60 and 17%, among the 48 patients treated with CAP. Treatment with fludarabine induced significantly longer remissions than CAP, and this translated into a trend toward overall longer survival *(48)*.

The French Cooperative Group compared fludarabine and two anthracycline-containing alkylating agent-based regimens: CAP and modified CHOP for initial treatment of CLL. In all, 938 patients were entered on the study, and 924 were evaluable for response. Among the 336 patients treated with fludarabine, the overall response rate was 71%, and the complete response rate was 40%. Among the 237 patients treated with CAP, the overall response rate was 58%, and the complete response rate was 15%. The modified CHOP regimen produced an overall response rate of 71% and a complete response rate of 30% in 351 patients. Fludarabine treatment produced a higher rate of complete remission and was better tolerated than the modified CHOP; both fludarabine and ChOP produced higher overall response rates than CAP. The median survival was similar in the three arms (69, 67, and 70 mo for fludarabine, modified CHOP, and CAP, respectively) *(50)*.

A large Intergroup trial compared fludarabine with chlorambucil or a combination of the two agents as front-line treatment for CLL. Over 500 patients were treated among the three arms. Fludarabine produced an overall response rate of 63% and a complete response rate of 20%

compared with an overall response rate of 37% and a complete response rate of only 4% with chlorambucil. Fludarabine plus chlorambucil resulted in an overall response rate of 61%; this arm of the study was terminated early because of excessive toxicity. Fludarabine was superior to chlorambucil in terms of median duration of remission and median progression-free survival, but overall survival was not significantly different between the two treatment arms (66 vs 56 mo). Crossover was allowed for lack of response or early relapse: 79 patients received fludarabine after failing chlorambucil, and 46% of them had a complete or partial remission; only 7% of the 29 patients who received chlorambucil after failing fludarabine responded (3). A higher rate of serious infections was observed in the combination arm. There was a trend toward a higher rate of bacterial infections with fludarabine compared with chlorambucil, although the incidence of such infections was low in both arms. Fludarabine was associated with an increased incidence of viral reactivation (51).

The most common toxicities with fludarabine treatment are immunosuppression, myelo-suppression, and resultant infection (52,53). The immunosuppression may be prolonged, but infections are uncommon in patients in remission (54). Tumor lysis syndrome is a rare compli-cation of fludarabine treatment, as well as of alkylating agents and fludarabine-based combina-tions (55). The association of fludarabine treatment and the development of hemolytic anemia has been reported, but a causal relationship has not been proved (56).

An oral formulation of fludarabine has been developed with a bioavailability of 55%; pharma-cokinetic studies have demonstrated that a once-daily dose oral of 40 mg/m^{2}is equivalent to the standard intravenous dose of 25 mg/m^2 (57). A multicenter trial using oral fludarabine in patients who had received prior chlorambucil was conducted in Europe. Among 78 evaluable patients, the overall response rate was 51%, and complete remissions were obtained in 18% (58). The optimal treatment duration was six cycles; as seen with the intravenous formulation, responses rates with oral fludarabine were higher in patients with early-stage disease. The oral formulation had a toxicity profile similar to that of the parental formulation, with a mild increase in gastrointestinal adverse events.

3.4. Purine Analog-Based Combination Chemotherapy

Fludarabine has produced high overall response rates when used as initial therapy of CLL and has shown greater activity than chlorambucil. However, most responses are partial, with only a minority of patients achieving a complete response. This has led to the use of fludarabine in combination with other agents to improve efficacy.

3.4.1. Fludarabine and Doxorubicin or Mitoxantrone

The combination of fludarabine and doxorubicin with or without prednisone was investigated in 30 patients with previously treated CLL, most of whom had received prior fludarabine. This combination was active, with an overall response rate of 55%, but complete remissions were seen in only 3% of patients (59).

The combination of fludarabine and mitoxantrone was given to 53 previously treated patients with CLL. Complete and partial responses were observed, but, despite its significant activity in low grade lymphoma, this combination did not appear to be more effective than fludarabine alone in the treatment of CLL (60,61).

3.4.2. Fludarabine and Alkylating Agents

The combination of fludarabine with alkylating agents is under investigation, based on prom-ising in vitro findings. The incubation of lymphocytes from patients with CLL with activated cyclophosphamide produced DNA interstrand crosslinks that were efficiently repaired in 6–8 h; in the presence of fludarabine, this repair mechanism was inhibited, and 80% of the DNA interstrand crosslinks were still detected 24 h later (61,62).

Two small phase I studies of the combination of fludarabine and chlorambucil were conducted by Elias et al. (63) and Weiss et al. (64). Both demonstrated clinical activity, but the treatment was limited by significant myelosuppression, especially thrombocytopenia. Another study reported on continuous-infusion cisplatin (although not a classical alkylating agent, this drug also produces DNA crosslinks) and fludarabine plus cytarabine in 26 patients. Patients had received extensive prior treatment for CLL, and most of them were refractory to fludarabine. Responses were seen in 19% of the patients, myelosuppression was reported in more than half of the patients treated, and a high incidence of infectious complications was noted (65).

3.4.2.1. Fludarabine and Cyclophosphamide. The combination of fludarabine, at a dose of 30 mg/m^2 given daily for 3 d, and cyclophosphamide at doses between 300 and 500 mg/m^2 daily for 3 d was investigated in 128 patients by O'Brien et al. (66). The initial dose of cyclophosphamide was 500 mg/m^2, but this was reduced to 300 mg/m^2 because of excessive myelosuppression. Remission rates differed according to disease status at the beginning of treatment. The overall response rates were 88% for patients who had not received prior treatment, 85 and 80% for patients who had received prior treatment with alkylating agents and fludarabine, respectively, and 39% for patients who were refractory to fludarabine; complete response rates were 34, 15, 12, and 3%, respectively. The most significant side effects were myelosuppression and infections. Remission durations appeared to be longer than those seen in comparable patients treated with single agent fludarabine.

Flinn et al. (67) gave cyclophosphamide, 600 mg/m^2, on the first day and fludarabine, 20 mg/ m^2 daily for 5 d, followed by filgastrin, 5 µg/kg/sc daily, to 60 patients with previously untreated lymphoid malignancies. This study included 17 patients with CLL; all 17 responded, with 47% of them achieving a complete remission and 53% achieving a partial response. Hematological toxicity was mild with the filgastrin support (67).

A multicenter study using fludarabine, 30 mg/m^2 daily for 3 d, and cyclophosphamide, 250 mg/ m^2 daily for 3 d, in 32 patients with CLL was conducted by Hallek et al. (68). The overall response rates were 86% in the previously untreated patients and 94% in the previously treated patients, and the complete response rates were 21 and 11%, respectively. Myelosuppression and infections were again reported with this combination treatment.

3.4.3.2. Fludarabine, Cyclophosphamide, and Rituximab. Rituximab is a chimeric antibody targeting CD20 that has significant activity in the treatment of non-Hodgkin's lymphoma (69). Rituximab has been studied as a single agent in CLL in both previously treated and untreated patients. Nguyen et al. (70) treated 15 patients with resistant/relapsed CLL with rituximab at 375 mg/m^2 weekly for 4 wk; a marked decrease in the number of circulating leukemia cells was observed, but none of the patients achieved a response. In a recently reported study by the German Chronic Lymphocytic Leukemia Study Group (71), rituximab at the standard dose of 375 mg/m^2 weekly for 4 consecutive wk was given to patients with CLL who had received prior treatment. No complete responses and a partial response of 25% were seen in the 28 evaluable patients. Rituximab was given at higher doses (500 mg/m^2 to 2250 mg/ m^2) to 40 previously treated patients with CLL; a response rate of 36% was observed, with a higher response rate at the higher doses, and no complete remissions were observed (72). Similar results were obtained by Byrd et al. (73) when rituximab was given at the standard dose (375 mg/m^2) but three times a week for 4 wk. The overall response rate in 26 previously treated patients with CLL was 46%, none of the patients achieved a complete response.

Rituximab has shown greater activity when it was investigated in chemotherapy-naïve patients. Rituximab at 375 mg/m^2 weekly for 4 wk produced partial responses in 8 of 14 (57%) patients with CLL who had not received prior treatment *(74)*. Thomas et al. *(75)* reported an overall response rate of 83% and a complete response rate of 17% in patients with early-stage CLL treated with 8 wk of standard dose rituximab.

The first infusion of rituximab in patients with CLL has been associated with fever and chills and less commonly, nausa, vomiting, hypotension, and dyspnea. In some patients a cytokine-release syndrome has been observed and is associated with an increase in plasma levels of tumor necrosis factor-α, interleukin-6, and interleukin-8. Fractionating the first dose of rituximab may attenuate its severity *(73,76)*. Tumor lysis syndrome has rarely been reported following rituximab administration *(77)*.

Despite rituximab's modest single-agent activity in CLL, the combination of this antibody with chemotherapy appears to be a promising strategy. A combination of fludarabine, cyclophosphamide, and rituximab is being studied in patients with CLL. Fludarabine is given at a dose of 25 mg/m^2 and cyclophosphamide at a dose of 250 mg/m^2 for three consecutive days; rituximab is given on the first day of each cycle. The rituximab dose is 375 mg/m^2 in the first cycle and 500 mg/m^2 in the subsequent cycles. Patients receive up to six cycles of treatment. The results of this ongoing study were recently updated: among 136 previously treated patients, the overall response rate was 71%, the complete response rate was 21%, and documentation of molecular remission by undetectable Ig rearrangements on polymerase chain reaction analysis was obtained in 5 of 13 patients who achieved a complete response *(78)*. The treatment was well tolerated; first-infusion side effects were noted and were rare in subsequent cycles. Mild gastrointestinal toxicity and moderate myelosuppression and immunosuppression were also seen.

The same three-agent regimen is under investigation in chemotherapy-naïve patients. Wierda et al. *(79)* reported results in 135 patients; the overall response rate was 95%, complete responses were seen in 63%, and molecular remissions were demonstrated in 31 of 55 patients who had bone marrow examined for the presence of Ig rearrangements by polymerase chain reaction analysis. Grade 3–4 neutropenia, but not thrombocytopenia, appeared to be more frequent with the three-drug regimen compared with the use of the same chemotherapy without rituximab. Median follow-up is less than 2 yr; most patients have not relapsed, and median time to progression is not yet known. These preliminary results suggest that this combination is the most active regimen reported so far in the treatment of CLL 79.

3.4.3.3. Fludarabine and Rituximab. The Cancer and Leukemia Group B (CALGB) conducted a randomized trial of fludarabine (25 mg/m^2, d 1–5) given monthly for 6 mo followed 2 mo later by rituximab (375 mg/m^2) given weekly for 4 wk compared to concomitant fludarabine and rituximab (fludarabine 25 mg/m^2, d 1–5 monthly for 6 mo and rituximab 375 mg/m^2 given on d 1 and 4 of the first cycle, than monthly on d 1 of fludarabine). Byrd et al. *(80)* recently reported results in 104 patients; the overall response rate was 90% in the arm with concomitant treatment and 77% in the arm with sequential treatment; complete responses were 47 and 28%, respectively. Neutropenia was more common in patients treated with concomitant fludarabine and rituximab. First infusion reactions were more severe in the concomitant fludarabine and rituximab arm of the study and could be overcome by using a stepped-up dosing of rituximab (50 mg/m^2 on d 1, 325 mg/m^2 on d 3, and 375 mg/m^2 on d 5).

4. OTHER TREATMENT STRATEGIES AND FUTURE DIRECTIONS

This chapter focuses on chemotherapy, only one of the treatment strategies available for CLL. Promising results have been obtained with the use of monoclonal antibodies such as Campath 1H.

Nonmyeloablative allogeneic stem cell bone marrow transplantation has been explored, with encouraging responses and reduced toxicity, enabling older patients to undergo this treatment modality. New biological agents such as the bcl-2 antisense and the proteasome inhibitor PS-341 are in the early phases of clinical trials, and treatment with autologous DNA vaccine is also being investigated. Details regarding these treatment strategies are discussed in other chapters of this textbook.

5. CONCLUSIONS

Great progress has been made in our knowledge of the pathophysiology and treatment of CLL in the past two decades. Purine analogs, especially fludarabine, have been shown to be powerful agents against CLL, and the combination of fludarabine, cyclophosphamide, and rituximab has shown a very high rate of complete remission. The direction for future treatments will be to continue to improve the quality of response and to effect disease eradication at the molecular level. The most successful strategy has not yet been defined but will probably involve a combination of cytotoxic chemotherapy and immunotherapy.

REFERENCES

1. Dighiero G, Maloum K, Desablens B, et al. Chlorambucil in indolent chronic lymphocytic leukemia. French Cooperative Group on Chronic Lymphocytic Leukemia. N Engl J Med 1998;338:1506–1514.
2. Chemotherapeutic options in chronic lymphocytic leukemia: a meta- analysis of the randomized trials. CLL Trialists' Collaborative Group. J Natl Cancer Inst 1999;91:861–868.
3. Rai KR, Peterson BL, Appelbaum FR, et al. Fludarabine compared with chlorambucil as primary therapy for chronic lymphocytic leukemia. N Engl J Med 2000;343:1750–1757.
4. Jaksic B, Brugiatelli M, Krc I, et al. High dose chlorambucil versus Binet's modified cyclophosphamide, doxorubicin, vincristine, and prednisone regimen in the treatment of patients with advanced B-cell chronic lymphocytic leukemia. Results of an international multicenter randomized trial. International Society for Chemo-Immunotherapy, Vienna. Cancer 1997;79:2107–2114.
5. Berk PD, Goldberg JD, Silverstein MN, et al. Increased incidence of acute leukemia in polycythemia vera associated with chlorambucil therapy. N Engl J Med 1981;304:441–447.
6. Dedrick RL, Morrison PF. Carcinogenic potency of alkylating agents in rodents and humans. Cancer Res 1992; 52:2464–2467.
7. Patapanian H, Graham S, Sambrook PN, et al. The oncogenicity of chlorambucil in rheumatoid arthritis. Br J Rheumatol 1988;27:44–47.
8. Han T, Ezdinli EZ, Shimaoka K, Desai DV. Chlorambucil vs. combined chlorambucil-corticosteroid therapy in chronic lymphocytic leukemia. Cancer 1973;31:502–508.
9. Catovsky DRS, Fooks J, Hamblin TJ. CLL trials in the United Kingdom. The Medical Research Council Trials 1, 2 and 3. Leuk Lymphoma 1991;(suppl):105–112.
10. Pethema SCG. Treatment of chronic lymphocytic leukemia: a preliminary report of Spanish (Pethema) trials. Leuk Lymphoma 1991;(suppl):89–91.
11. A randomized clinical trial of chlorambucil versus COP in stage B chronic lymphocytic leukemia. The French Cooperative Group on Chronic Lymphocytic Leukemia. Blood 1990;75:1422–1425.
12. Raphael B, Andersen JW, Silber R, et al. Comparison of chlorambucil and prednisone versus cyclophosphamide, vincristine, and prednisone as initial treatment for chronic lymphocytic leukemia: long-term follow-up of an Eastern Cooperative Oncology Group randomized clinical trial. J Clin Oncol 1991;9:770–776.
13. Long-term results of the CHOP regimen in stage C chronic lymphocytic leukaemia. French Cooperative Group on Chronic Lymphocytic Leukaemia. Br J Haematol 1989;73:334–340.
14. Is the CHOP regimen a good treatment for advanced CLL? Results from two randomized clinical trials. French Cooperative Group on Chronic Lymphocytic Leukemia. Leuk Lymphoma 1994;13:449–456.
15. Kimby E MH. Chlorambucil/prednisone versus CHOP in symptomatic chronic lymphocytic leukemias of B-cell type. A randomozed trial. Leuk Lymphoma 1991;(suppl):93–96.
16. Hansen MM, Birgens H, Christensen BE, et al. CHOP versus chlorambucil + prednisone in chronic lymphocytic leukemia. Leuk Lymphoma 1991;(suppl):97–100.

17. Kempin S, Lee BJ 3rd, Thaler HT, et al. Combination chemotherapy of advanced chronic lymphocytic leukemia: the M-2 protocol (vincristine, BCNU, cyclophosphamide, melphalan, and prednisone). Blood 1982;60: 1110–1121.
18. Case DC, Jr., Porensky RS, Fanning JP. Combination chemotherapy with the M-2 protocol (BCNU, cyclophosphamide, vincristine, melphalan, and prednisone) for chronic lymphocytic leukemia (stages III and IV). Oncology 1985;42:350–353.
19. Keating MJ, Scouros M, Murphy S, et al. Multiple agent chemotherapy (POACH) in previously treated and untreated patients with chronic lymphocytic leukemia. Leukemia 1988;2:157–164.
20. Grever MR, Leiby JM, Kraut EH, et al. Low-dose deoxycoformycin in lymphoid malignancy. J Clin Oncol 1985; 3:1196–1201.
21. Dillman RO, Mick R, McIntyre OR. Pentostatin in chronic lymphocytic leukemia: a phase II trial of Cancer and Leukemia Group B. J Clin Oncol 1989;7:433–438.
22. Vose JM, Cabanillas F, O'Brien S, Dang N, Drapkin R, Foss F. Infectious complications of pentostatin therapy. Oncology (Huntingt) 2000;14:41–42.
23. Keating MJ, O'Brien S, Kantarjian H, et al. Nucleoside analogs in treatment of chronic lymphocytic leukemia. Leuk Lymphoma 1993;10:139–145.
24. Cheson BD, Vena DA, Barrett J, Freidlin B. Second malignancies as a consequence of nucleoside analog therapy for chronic lymphoid leukemias. J Clin Oncol 1999;17:2454–2460.
25. Waselenko JK, Grever MR, Beer M, Lucas MA, Byrd JC. Pentostatin (Nipent) and chlorambucil with granulocyte-macrophage colony-stimulating factor support for patients with previously untreated, treated, and fludarabine-refractory B-cell chronic lymphocytic leukemia. Semin Oncol 2000;27:44–51.
26. Weiss MA. A phase I and II study of pentostatin (Nipent) with cyclophosphamide for previously treated patients with chronic lymphocytic leukemia. Semin Oncol 2000;27:41–43.
27. Drapkin R. Pentostatin and rituximab in the treatment of patients with B-cell malignancies. Oncology (Huntingt) 2000;14:25–29.
28. Robertson LE, Chubb S, Meyn RE, et al. Induction of apoptotic cell death in chronic lymphocytic leukemia by 2-chloro-2'-deoxyadenosine and 9-beta-D-arabinosyl-2-fluoroadenine. Blood 1993;81:143–50.
29. Piro LD, Carrera CJ, Beutler E, Carson DA. 2-Chlorodeoxyadenosine: an effective new agent for the treatment of chronic lymphocytic leukemia. Blood 1988;72:1069–1073.
30. Juliusson G, Liliemark J. High complete remission rate from 2-chloro-2'-deoxyadenosine in previously treated patients with B-cell chronic lymphocytic leukemia: response predicted by rapid decrease of blood lymphocyte count. J Clin Oncol 1993;11:679–689.
31. Robak T, Blasinka-Morawiec M, Krykowski E, et al. Intermittent 2-hour intravenous infusions of 2-chloro-deoxyadenosine in the treatment of 110 patients with refractory or previously untreated B- cell chronic lymphocytic leukemia. Leuk Lymphoma 1996;22:509–514.
32. Juliusson G, Christiansen I, Hansen MM, et al. Oral cladribine as primary therapy for patients with B-cell chronic lymphocytic leukemia. J Clin Oncol 1996;14:2160–2166.
33. Rai KR. Cladribine for the treatment of hairy cell leukemia and chronic lymphocytic leukemia. Semin Oncol 1998;25:19–22.
34. Robak T, Blonski JZ, Urbanska-Rys H, Blasinska-Morawiec M, Skotnicki AB. 2-Chlorodeoxyadenosine (Cladribine) in the treatment of patients with chronic lymphocytic leukemia 55 years old and younger. Leukemia 1999;13:518–523.
35. Robak T, Blonski JZ, Kasznicki M, et al. Cladribine with or without prednisone in the treatment of previously treated and untreated B-cell chronic lymphocytic leukaemia - updated results of the multicentre study of 378 patients. Br J Haematol 2000;108:357–368.
36. Juliusson G, Elmhorn-Rosenborg A, Liliemark J. Response to 2-chlorodeoxyadenosine in patients with B-cell chronic lymphocytic leukemia resistant to fludarabine. N Engl J Med 1992;327:1056–1061.
37. O'Brien S, Kantarjian H, Estey E, et al. Lack of effect of 2-chlorodeoxyadenosine therapy in patients with chronic lymphocytic leukemia refractory to fludarabine therapy. N Engl J Med 1994;330:319–322.
38. Saven A, Lemon RH, Piro LD. 2-Chlorodeoxyadenosine for patients with B-cell chronic lymphocytic leukemia resistant to fludarabine. N Engl J Med 1993;328:812–813.
39. Plunkett W, Gandhi V, Huang P, et al. Fludarabine: pharmacokinetics, mechanisms of action, and rationales for combination therapies. Semin Oncol 1993;20:2–12.
40. Huang P, Sandoval A, Van Den Neste E, Keating MJ, Plunkett W. Inhibition of RNA transcription: a biochemical mechanism of action against chronic lymphocytic leukemia cells by fludarabine. Leukemia 2000;14:1405–1413.

41. Grever MR, Kopecky KJ, Coltman CA, et al. Fludarabine monophosphate: a potentially useful agent in chronic lymphocytic leukemia. Nouv Rev Fr Hematol 1988;30:457–459.
42. Keating MJ, Kantarjian H, Talpaz M, et al. Fludarabine: a new agent with major activity against chronic lymphocytic leukemia. Blood 1989;74:19–25.
43. Robertson LE, O'Brien S, Kantarjian H, et al. A 3-day schedule of fludarabine in previously treated chronic lymphocytic leukemia. Leukemia 1995;9:1444–1449.
44. O'Brien S, Kantarjian H, Beran M, et al. Results of fludarabine and prednisone therapy in 264 patients with chronic lymphocytic leukemia with multivariate analysis-derived prognostic model for response to treatment. Blood 1993;82:1695–1700.
45. Kemena A, O'Brien S, Kantarjian H, et al. Phase II clinical trial of fludarabine in chronic lymphocytic leukemia on a weekly low-dose schedule. Leuk Lymphoma 1993;10:187–193.
46. Keating MJ, Smith TL, Lerner S, et al. Prediction of prognosis following fludarabine used as secondary therapy for chronic lymphocytic leukemia. Leuk Lymphoma 2000;37:71–85.
47. Sorensen JM, Vena DA, Fallavollita A, Chun HG, Cheson BD. Treatment of refractory chronic lymphocytic leukemia with fludarabine phosphate via the group C protocol mechanism of the National Cancer Institute: five-year follow-up report. J Clin Oncol 1997;15:458–465.
48. Johnson S, Smith AG, Loffler H, et al. Multicentre prospective randomised trial of fludarabine versus cyclophosphamide, doxorubicin, and prednisone (CAP) for treatment of advanced-stage chronic lymphocytic leukaemia. The French Cooperative Group on CLL. Lancet 1996;347:1432–1438.
49. Keating MJ, O'Brien S, Lerner S, et al. Long-term follow-up of patients with chronic lymphocytic leukemia (CLL) receiving fludarabine regimens as initial therapy. Blood 1998;92:1165–1171.
50. Leporrier M, Chevret S, Cazin B, et al. Randomized comparison of fludarabine, CAP, and ChOP in 938 previously untreated stage B and C chronic lymphocytic leukemia patients. Blood 2001;98:2319–2325.
51. Morrison VA, Rai KR, Peterson BL, et al. Impact of therapy With chlorambucil, fludarabine, or fludarabine plus chlorambucil on infections in patients with chronic lymphocytic leukemia: Intergroup Study Cancer and Leukemia Group B 9011. J Clin Oncol 2001;19:3611–3621.
52. Cheson BD. Infectious and immunosuppressive complications of purine analog therapy. J Clin Oncol 1995;13: 2431–2448.
53. Cheson BD, Vena DA, Foss FM, Sorensen JM. Neurotoxicity of purine analogs: a review. J Clin Oncol 1994;12: 2216–2228.
54. Anaissie EJ, Kontoyiannis DP, O'Brien S, et al. Infections in patients with chronic lymphocytic leukemia treated with fludarabine. Ann Intern Med 1998;129:559–566.
55. Cheson BD, Frame JN, Vena D, Quashu N, Sorensen JM. Tumor lysis syndrome: an uncommon complication of fludarabine therapy of chronic lymphocytic leukemia. J Clin Oncol 1998;16:2313–2320.
56. Myint H, Copplestone JA, Orchard J, et al. Fludarabine-related autoimmune haemolytic anaemia in patients with chronic lymphocytic leukaemia. Br J Haematol 1995;91:341–344.
57. Foran JM, Oscier D, Orchard J, et al. Pharmacokinetic study of single doses of oral fludarabine phosphate in patients with "low-grade" non-Hodgkin's lymphoma and B-cell chronic lymphocytic leukemia. J Clin Oncol 1999;17:1574–1579.
58. Boogaerts MA, Van Hoof A, Catovsky D, et al. Activity of oral fludarabine phosphate in previously treated chronic lymphocytic leukemia. J Clin Oncol 2001;19:4252–4258.
59. Robertson LE, O'Brien S, Kantarjian H, et al. Fludarabine plus doxorubicin in previously treated chronic lymphocytic leukemia. Leukemia 1995;9:943–945.
60. O'Brien S. Clinical challenges in chronic lymphocytic leukemia. Semin Hematol 1998;35:22–26.
61. Bellosillo B, Villamor N, Colomer D, Pons G, Montserrat E, Gil J. In vitro evaluation of fludarabine in combination with cyclophosphamide and/or mitoxantrone in B-cell chronic lymphocytic leukemia. Blood 1999;94:2836–28343.
62. Koehl U LL, Nowak B, Ruiz van Haperen V, Kornhuber D, Schwabe D, O'Brien S, Keating M, Plunkett W, Yang LW. Fludarabine and cyclophosphamide: synergistic cytotoxicity associated with inhibition of interstrand cross-link removal. Proc Am Assoc Cancer Res 1997;38:10.
63. Elias L, Stock-Novack D, Head DR, et al. A phase I trial of combination fludarabine monophosphate and chlorambucil in chronic lymphocytic leukemia: a Southwest Oncology Group study. Leukemia 1993;7: 361–365.
64. Weiss M, Spiess T, Berman E, Kempin S. Concomitant administration of chlorambucil limits dose intensity of fludarabine in previously treated patients with chronic lymphocytic leukemia. Leukemia 1994;8:1290–1293.

65. Giles FJ, O'Brien SM, Santini V, et al. Sequential cis-platinum and fludarabine with or without arabinosyl cytosine in patients failing prior fludarabine therapy for chronic lymphocytic leukemia: a phase II study. Leuk Lymphoma 1999;36:57–65.

66. O'Brien SM, Kantarjian HM, Cortes J, et al. Results of the fludarabine and cyclophosphamide combination regimen in chronic lymphocytic leukemia. J Clin Oncol 2001;19:1414–1420.

67. Flinn IW, Byrd JC, Morrison C, et al. Fludarabine and cyclophosphamide with filgrastim support in patients with previously untreated indolent lymphoid malignancies. Blood 2000;96:71–75.

68. Hallek M, Schmitt B, Wilhelm M, et al. Fludarabine plus cyclophosphamide is an efficient treatment for advanced chronic lymphocytic leukaemia (CLL): results of a phase II study of the German CLL Study Group. Br J Haematol 2001;114:342–348.

69. McLaughlin P, Grillo-Lopez AJ, Link BK, et al. Rituximab chimeric anti-CD20 monoclonal antibody therapy for relapsed indolent lymphoma: half of patients respond to a four-dose treatment program. J Clin Oncol 1998;16:2825–2833.

70. Nguyen DT, Amess JA, Doughty H, Hendry L, Diamond LW. IDEC-C2B8 anti-CD20 (rituximab) immuno-therapy in patients with low-grade non-Hodgkin's lymphoma and lymphoproliferative disorders: evaluation of response on 48 patients. Eur J Haematol 1999;62:76–82.

71. Huhn D, von Schilling C, Wilhelm M, et al. Rituximab therapy of patients with B-cell chronic lymphocytic leukemia. Blood 2001;98:1326–1331.

72. O'Brien SM, Thomas D, Freireich EJ, Andreeff M, Giles FJ, Keating MJ. Rituxan has significant activity in patients with CLL. Blood 1999;94;603a.

73. Byrd JC, Murphy T, Howard RS, et al. Rituximab using a thrice weekly dosing schedule in B-cell chronic lymphocytic leukemia and small lymphocytic lymphoma demonstrates clinical activity and acceptable toxicity. J Clin Oncol 2001;19:2153–2164.

74. Hainsworth JD, Burris HA, 3rd, Morrissey LH, et al. Rituximab monoclonal antibody as initial systemic therapy for patients with low-grade non-Hodgkin lymphoma. Blood 2000;95:3052–306.

75. Thomas DA O'Brien S, Giles FJ, et al. Single agent rituxan in early stage chronic lymphocytic leukemia (CLL). Blood 2001;98:364a.

76. Winkler U, Jensen M, Manzke O, Schulz H, Diehl V, Engert A. Cytokine-release syndrome in patients with B-cell chronic lymphocytic leukemia and high lymphocyte counts after treatment with an anti-CD20 monoclonal antibody (rituximab, IDEC-C2B8). Blood 1999;94:2217–2224.

77. Yang H, Rosove MH, Figlin RA. Tumor lysis syndrome occurring after the administration of rituximab in lymphoproliferative disorders: high-grade non-Hodgkin's lymphoma and chronic lymphocytic leukemia. Am J Hematol 1999;62:247–250.

78. Garcia Manero G, O'Brien S, Cortes J, et al. Update of results of the combination of fludarabine, cyclophospha-mide and rituxan for previously treated patients with chronic lymphocytic leukemia (CLL). Blood 2001;98:633a.

79. Wierda W, O'Brien S, Albitar M, et al. Combined fludarabine, cyclophosphamide, and rituximab achieves a high complete remission rate as initial treatment for chronic lymphocytic leukemia (CLL). Blood 2001;98:771a.

80. Byrd JC, Peterson BL, Morrison VA, et al. Randomized phase 2 study of fludarabine with concurrent versus sequential treatment with rituximab in symptomatic, untreated patients with B-cell chronic lymphocytic leukemia: results from Cancer and Leukemia Group B 9712 (CALGB 9712). Blood 2003;101:6–14.

14 Autologous and Allogeneic Transplantations for Chronic Lymphocytic Leukemia

Mauricette Michallet, MD, PhD

1. INTRODUCTION

Survival in B-cell chronic lymphocytic leukemia (CLL) is poor if one of the following risk factors is present: advanced stage, short lymphocyte doubling time, unfavorable cytogenetics, CD38 marker, or unmutated status of the variable region of the immunoglobulin heavy chain gene *(1–4)*. The use of intensive myeloablative therapy followed by autologous or allogeneic stem cell transplantation (SCT) for CLL has greatly increased over the last few years *(5–13)*. As the safety and efficacy of autotransplantation rely on supportive care, improvements in peripheral blood stem cell (PBSC) mobilization and the cytotoxic therapy administered can induce long-lasting clinical and molecular remissions *(8,9,13–15)*. The mortality of the procedure could be further reduced and should be well below 10% *(8,9)*, but recently, in most series, a continuous increase in molecular relapses has been observed after autotransplantation. In allogeneic settings, the graft-vs-leukemia (GVL) activity should be responsible for very substantial disease control *(16,17)* and seems to cure a subset of poor-risk patients but at the price of an excessively high treatment-related mortality (TRM) *(13)*. The recent development of a nonmyeloablative conditioning regimen followed by donor lymphocyte infusion (DLI) may help to improve the tolerability of allogeneic SCT in patients with CLL *(18–27)*. Nevertheless, several issues in SCT for CLL remain unsettled, and all data concerning this settings are important in an attempt to build a therapeutic strategy for CLL including conventional chemotherapy, serotherapy, autotransplantation, and a standard or reduced-intensity conditioning regimen followed by a related or unrelated allotransplantation.

2. AUTOTRANSPLANTATION IN CLL

2.1. Retrospective Analysis

Autografting for patients with CLL has increased significantly over the past few years, with 482 cases in the European Blood and Marrow Transplant (EBMT) database and a growing number of published single-center series *(7–9,13,14)*. Owing to improvements in supportive therapy, the mortality of the procedure is low and was well below 10%, but in most series a steady decline of the event-free survival curve has been observed because of relapses occurring up to 5 yr after transplantation, and it is still not clear whether autografting can be curative. Two important pilot

From: *Contemporary Hematology*
Chronic Lymphocytic Leukemia: Molecular Genetics, Biology, Diagnosis, and Management
Edited by: G. B. Faguet © Humana Press Inc., Totowa, NJ

studies carried out in Germany and England have effectively shown an important molecular remission rate after autotransplantation, but these two studies also found an increasing number of molecular relapse during the follow-up after transplantation. Nevertheless, owing to the low toxicity of the procedure, the outcome of autografted patients is characterized by overall survival figures of more than 75% at 3 yr post-transplant, which is generally better than that after allotransplantation, at least in the early post-transplantation years.

The largest single-center series of patients treated with autologous SCT for CLL has been reported by the Dana-Farber Cancer Center (28). One hundred and fifty-two patients with advanced CLL underwent intensive therapy including total body irradiation (TBI) and cyclophosphamide followed by reinfusion of autologous bone marrow (BM) purged with anti-B-cell monoclonal antibodies and complement. There were eight treatment-related deaths (5%). With a median follow-up of about 30 mo, only 14 patients have relapsed, but an important number of patients (63 of 136 evaluable patients) showed persistent disease at the molecular level. It was shown in this study that there was a correlation between relapse after transplantation and (1) the importance of B-cell depletion and (2) persistent negativity of polymerase chain reaction (PCR) results. At the University of Kiel (29), 93 patients with poor-risk CLL received autotransplants, 90 (97%) were reinfused with purged autologous stem cell grafts (CD34+B–/CD34+) following preparation with TBI/cyclophosphamide. The median number of CD34+ mobilized was 4.7 × 10^6/kg (range, 1.7–28.9). Engraftment led to prompt neutrophil recovery greater than 0.5 g/L after a median of 10 d (range, 8–16 d) and platelets over 20 g/L after a median of 11 d (range, 8–40 d), and the median length of hospitalization was 15 d (range, 10–50 d). The TRM was 5% (range, 1–9%), the overall survival was 92% (range, 84–100%) at 42 mo, and the progression-free survival 87% at 24 mo and 60% at 36 mo. A high percentage of molecular relapse was observed, 22% at 24 mo and 80% at 36 mo after transplantation. A significant impact of cytogenetics on molecular relapse rate after transplantation was also observed, with a great number of relapses in patients with the 11q– abnormality.

The EBMT has recently updated data on the outcome of 482 autologous transplants (autoT) from the EBMT registry (13) (Table 1). There were 381 men (79%) and 101 women (21%), with a median age of 50 yr (range, 22–66 yr). The median interval between diagnosis and transplantation was 26 mo (range, 4–215 mo). At diagnosis, 68% of the patients studied were in Binet stages B or C. Thirty-five percent of patients had received one conventional line of therapy, 37% two lines, and 28% three lines before autoT. These lines included fludarabine for 126 of 482 patients (26%); 40 of 482 patients (8%) had received chlorambucil-containing treatment and 72 of 482 patients (15%) a combination of cyclophosphamide, vincristine, adriamycin, and prednisone (CHOP).

At transplantation, 413 patients were evaluated for response to therapy: 129 of 413 (31%) were in complete remission (CR), 223 of 413 (54%) were in partial remission (PR), and 61 of 413 (15%) were in progressive disease (PD). Three hundred and eighty-three patients (80%) received PBSCs. From 170 patients, the PBSCs were mobilized by either chemotherapy alone (4%), by granulocyte colony-stimulating factor (G-CSF) (11%) or, more frequently, by combining chemotherapy and G-CSF (85%). Sixty-nine patients (14%) received BM as the hematopoietic stem cell source, and 30 patients received BM and PBSCs (6%). In addition, 200 of 437 evaluated patients (46%) received a purged graft after negative or positive selection. For the conditioning regimen, 258 of 456 patients (57%) received a TBI-containing regimen. After autoT, 440 of 452 patients (97%) were engrafted [within 12 d (range, 1–119 d), achieving 0.5 g/L neutrophils, and within 20 d (range, 4–1098 d), achieving platelets greater than 50 g/L].

Table 1
General Characteristics of the CLL Population
Receiving Transplants Between 1994 and 2000

Parameter	AutoT [no. (%)]	AlloT [no. (%)]
Patients		
Total	482	209
Female	381 (79)	163 (78)
Male	101 (21)	46 (22)
Median age	50 yr	42 yr
Range	22–66	22–64
Interval from diagnosis to transplantation (mo)	(n = 467)	(n = 205)
≤ 36 mo	279 (60)	84 (41)
> 36 mo	188 (40)	121 (59)
Median	26 mo	45 mo
Range	4–215 mo	5–198 mo
Stage at diagnosis (Binet)	(n = 146)	(n = 46)
A	46 (32)	11 (24)
B	68 (46)	24 (52)
C	32 (22)	11 (24)
No. of therapeutic lines	(n = 216)	(n = 86)
1	75 (35)	19 (22)
2	81 (37)	24 (28)
3	60 (28)	43 (50)
Fludarabine		
Yes	126 (26)	44 (21)
No	356 (74)	165 (79)
CHOP		
Yes	72 (15)	32 (15)
No	410 (85)	177 (85)
Chlorambucil		
Yes	40 (8)	30 (14)
No	442 (92)	179 (86)
Status at transplantation	(n = 413)	(n = 172)
CR	129 (31)	19 (11)
PR	223 (54)	78 (45)
PD	61 (15)	75 (44)
Source of stem cell		
PB	383 (80)	115 (55)
BM	69 (14)	90 (43)
BM + PB	30 (6)	4 (2)
TBI	(n = 456)	(n = 194)
Yes	258 (57)	125 (64)
No	198 (43)	69 (36)

AutoT, autotransplantation; AlloT, allotransplantation; PR, partial remission; CR, complete remission; PD, progressive disease; PB, peripheral blood; BM, bone marrow; TBI, total body irradiation; CHOP, cyclophosphamide, vincristine, Adriamycin, and prednisone.

We evaluated 347 patients for disease response: 279 (80%) achieved a CR, 41 (12%) achieved a PR, and 227 (8%) were in stable disease or had progressed. Univariate analysis showed that the projected 3-yr survival was 79% (SE = 3%). At 42 mo after autoT, 75% of patients were still alive. The projected 3-yr TRM was 11% (SE = 2%), and the risk of relapse at 3 yr was 40% (SE = 4%). After autoT, the risk of relapse increased over time and was higher at 60 mo than at 20 mo after transplantation.

Using log-rank comparisons, we found no significant association between survival and gender or age of recipient. Even though it concerned only a small subset of patients were involved, we found a significant association between survival and stage at diagnosis, with worse survival for stage C patients. In addition, we found a significant association between survival and (1) short interval (≤36 mo) between diagnosis and transplantation ($p < 0.01$); (2) status of the disease before transplantation, in favor of CR ($p < 0.01$); (3) number of lines of conventional therapies, in favor of one line ($p = 0.01$); and (4) conditioning regimen, in favor of TBI ($p < 0.01$). Finally, we also showed a trend in favor of PBPCs as the source of stem cells ($p = 0.08$).

The multivariate analysis considered age and gender of recipient, year of transplantation, type of transplant, interval between diagnosis and transplantation, fludarabine, and CHOP before transplantation, disease status before transplantation, and TBI during conditioning. The results of multivariate analysis demonstrated a significant association between survival and (1) short interval between diagnosis and transplantation [>36 mo vs ≤ 36 mo: hazard ratio (HR) = 2.58] (Fig. 1); (2) CR before transplantation (PR vs CR/PD vs CR: HR = 2.37/HR = 6); and (3) TBI-containing regimen (HR = 0.35).

In an analysis from the International Bone Marrow Transplant Registry (IBMT), Esteve et al. *(14)* demonstrated similar results for 124 autologous transplantations: 87% CRs after transplantation, TRM of 6%, overall survival of 63 ± 7%, and risk of relapse at 68 ± 9%, which was significantly higher than after allogeneic transplantation (23 ± 13%, $p < 0.001$). In a multivariate analysis, the author demonstrated a significant relation between survival and number of therapeutic lines, disease status, stage before transplantation, percentage of lymphocytes in the marrow, and interval between diagnosis and transplantation.

The Medical Research Council has been conducting a pilot study *(30)* of autografting in CLL since 1996. They entered 119 patients and information is available on 59 patients who have undergone autoT. Concerning PBSCs mobilization, 16 patients had an insufficient number of CD34+ cells after mobilization, 15 were remobilized, and 8 had a true failure of mobilization. The median number of CD34+ cells mobilized after cyclophosphamide and GCSF was 2.7×10^6/kg (range, 0–6). Of these, 78% became PCR-negative for IgH CDR-III rearrangements after autografting. All patients who were in morphological CR at the time of autograft were PCR-negative after transplantation, and only 5 of 29 of these patients have had a molecular relapse. This study also found an increasing number of molecular relapses during the follow-up after transplantation (Fig. 2). Nevertheless, survival was excellent in the transplantation patients, with a projected overall survival of over 80% at 3 yr. The TRM was about 3%.

Although a number of single-center or multi-center SCT studies have been performed or are currently under way, the impact of autologous SCT on the prognosis of CLL is still unclear. To determine the real place of autoT in CLL, we now urgently need a large randomized trial for selected patients.

2.2. Myeloablative Regimens

Although encouraging results have been observed after high-dose chemotherapy alone followed by autologous SCT, in the vast majority of published data on SCT for CLL, the

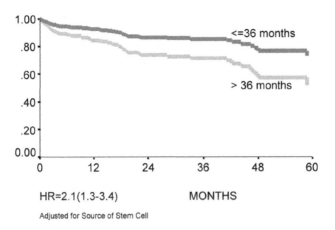

Fig. 1. Autologous transplants in CLL survival: effect of interval diagnosis-transplant (adjusted for source of stem cell). Data from EBMT database.

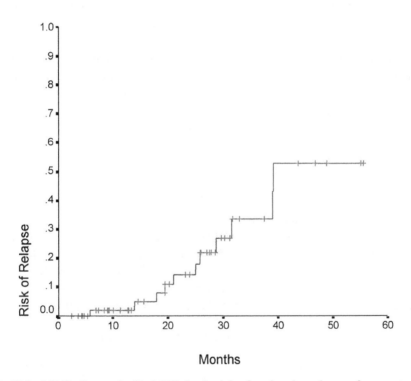

Fig. 2. CLL. MRC pilot study (D. Millighan): risk of molecular relapse after autotransplantation.

myeloablative regimen included TBI because CLL cells are highly sensitive to irradiation. On the other hand, from the results of conventional therapy, it is unlikely that cytotoxic drugs alone can eradicate CLL *(31,32)*. A retrospective analysis from the EBMT *(13)* also suggested that TBI-based regimens were superior to chemotherapy, although selection bias could not be discounted as a cause for the difference. Thus, TBI/cyclophosphamide still appears to be the gold standard for autografting of patients with CLL, although regimens employing high-dose chemotherapy alone may have similar efficacy.

2.3. Stem-Cell Source and PBSCs Mobilization

Because of their favorable engraftment kinetics, mobilized PBPCs have now replaced BM as the principal source of stem cells. A variety of G-CSF-based mobilization regimens are currently in use. Very preliminary data indicate that the mobilisation efficacy of more intensive protocols such as the Dexa-BEAM regimen appears to be somewhat better than that of classical cyclophosphamide plus G-CSF combinations (8). This superior stem cell yield, however, is at the expense of increased toxicity and cost.

We have performed a retrospective European survey of PBSC mobilization (33) in patients who have received fludarabine before transplantation. We did not observe any mobilization problems, with a median of 4.29×10^4/kg colony-forming units-granulocyte/macrophage (CFU-GM) and 2.2×10^6/kg CD34+ cells. Variables that may influence mobilization efficacy were stage, time from diagnosis, extent of pretreatment (fludarabine alone: 6.3×10^6 vs 1.9×10^6 fludarabine + other chemotherapy), number of courses of fludarabine [<6 cures: 1.9×10^6 vs $\geq$ 6 cures: 2.6×10^6 $(p = 0.02)$] and interval between the last course of fludarabine and the start of mobilization [<2 mo: 1.5×10^6 $\geq$2mo: 4.8×10^6 $(p = 0.02)$]. In France, we recently performed a study of PBSC mobilization after treatment combined with fludarabine and cyclophosphamide per os. Thirty-eight patients were analyzed, and 51 mobilizations were achieved. Twenty mobilizations were not performed because of insufficient CD34+ cells, and 31 mobilizations were followed by 46 apheresis procedures. Seventeen apheresis procedures were done more than 200 d after the last course of fludarabine/cyclophosphamide. The authors observed seven failures, in five cases the CD34+ cells number was less than 2×10^6 and in five cases more than 2×10^6. In total, in 55% of the cases, mobilization was not possible, in 10% we obtained $0-1 \times 10^6$ CD34+ cells, either $1-2 \times 10^6$ CD34+ cells, or $2-3 \times 10^6$ CD34+ cells and in 15% more than 3×10^6 CD34+.

2.4. Purging

The technique for ex vivo B-cell depletion from stem cell grafts has been further refined during recent years (34). With modern CD34+ cell selection devices such as Isolex 300i or Clinimacs, it is possible to eliminate 3–4 logs of CLL cells from fresh leukapheresis products. Purging efficacy can be further increased by incorporating a negative B-cell depletion step into the procedure (35). This maneuver also allows the elimination of presumptive CD34+ CLL cells. In spite of sophisticated purging technologies, there is still uncertainty about the clinical benefit.

3. ALLOTRANSPLANTATION IN CLL

Although allotransplantation adds immunotherapeutic effects to the cytotoxic effects and might thus be curative, its use in patients with CLL has been difficult and contentious, partly because many patients with CLL are older and/or have indolent disease, which does not justify aggressive treatment. Even in experienced centers, the treatment-related mortality (TRM) of allogeneic SCT in patients with CLL has been reported to be as high as 36% (6,7,10,11). A recent update of the EBMT database comprising 209 allografted patients with CLL showed a TRM of 40% at 36 mo after transplantation, which is much greater than after standard indications such as acute leukemia or chronic myeloid leukemia (5,13). The causes of these discouraging results are not completely clear, but patient age, selection of poor risk patients with advanced disease and extensive pretreatment, and the CLL-associated incompetence of the immune system may all contribute to the high TRM observed. The recent development of conditioning regimens with reduced intensity may help to improve the tolerability of allogenic SCT in patients with CLL *(25,36)*. The information available to date is too limited to justify the investigation of allografting for CLL in a large phase III multicenter study.

The EBMT has recently updated data on the outcome of 209 allogeneic transplants from their registry *(13)* (Table 1). There were 163 men (78%) and 46 women (22%), with a median age of 42 yr (range, 22–64 yr). The median interval between diagnosis and transplantation was 45 mo (range, 5–198 mo) and at diagnosis, 76% of patients studied were in stages B or C; 22% of patients had received one conventional line of therapy, 28% two lines, and 50% three lines. These lines included fludarabine for 44 of 209 patients (21%), chlorambucil in 30 of 209 patients (14%), and 32 of 209 (15%) received ChOP. At transplantation, 172 patients were evaluated for response to therapy: 19 of 172 patients (11%) were in CR, 78 of 172 (45%) in PR, and 75 of 172 (44%) in PD. Ninety patients (43%) received BM, 115 PBSCs (55%), and 4 BM and PBPCs (2%). One hundred and sixty-six patients (83%) received an allotransplant from HLA-identical sibling donors, 6 from syngeneic donors (3%), 16 (8%) from matched and mismatched related donors, and 12 (6%) from unrelated donors. For pretransplantation conditioning, 125 of 194 patients (64%) received a TBI-containing regimen and for graft-vs-host disease (GVHD) prophylaxis, 38 of 171 patients (22%) received a T-depleted graft.

After alloT, 183 of 197 patients (93%) were engrafted [within 16 d (range, 0–100 d), achieving 0.5 g/L neutrophils and 25 d (range, 0–214 d), achieving platelets > 50 g/L]. Sixty-five patients (34%) out of 190 who were evaluable developed acute GVHD of grade 2 or higher, and 47 patients (49%) out of 95 who were evaluable developed chronic GVHD (28 limited and 19 extensive). After transplantation, 141 patients were evaluated for disease response: 101 patients (72%) achieved a CR, 19 patients (13%) a PR, and 21 patients (15%) were in stable disease or progressed. Univariate analysis showed that the projected 3-yr survival was 55% (SE = 5%), which was significantly worse than after autoT [79% (SE = 3%); (p < 0.01)] (Fig. 3). At 5 mo after alloT, 75% of patients were still alive. The projected 3-yr TRM was 40% (SE = 5%), which was significantly worse than after autoT [11% (SE = 3%); (p < 0.01)] and the risk of relapse at 3 yr was 27% (SE = 7%) (Fig. 4).

Using log-rank comparisons, we found no significant association between survival and gender or age of recipient. Even though it concerned only a small subset of patients, we found a significant association between survival and stage at diagnosis, with worse survival for stage C patients. Regarding conventional therapy before transplantation, we could not prove any survival difference after alloT and autoT between patients treated with ChOP and others. After alloT, we found a significant association between survival and fludarabine (p = 0.03), survival and chlorambucil (p = 0.02) given before transplantation. Finally, we showed a significant association between survival and stem cell source in favor of PBPCs (p = 0.05). The results of multivariate analysis using the same parameters as after autoT demonstrated a significant association between survival and (1) fludarabine (HR = 0.48) (Fig. 5) and (2) year of transplantation (HR = 0.87).

In an analysis from the IBMT registry, Esteve et al. *(14)* demonstrated similar results for 46 allogeneic transplantations with 70% CR after transplantation, a TRM of 28%, an overall survival of 56 ± 7%, and a risk of relapse of 23 ± 13%. In a multivariate analysis, the authors showed a significant association between survival and disease status, stage before transplantation, and chemosensitivity.

In a retrospective analysis from EBMT registry, Dreger et al. *(36)* showed that 72 patients were transplanted after a reduced conditioning regimen for CLL in Europe. The median age was 54 yr (range, 37–65 yr) and the interval between diagnosis and transplantation was 49 mo (range, 8–

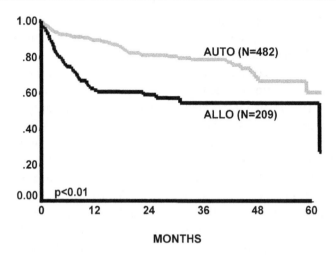

Fig. 3. Survival in CLL transplantations. Data from EBMT.

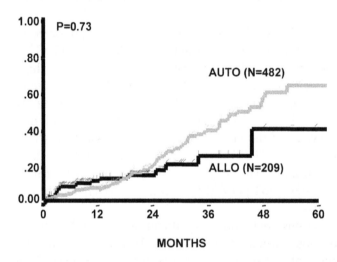

Fig. 4. Risk of relapse in CLL transplantation. Data from EBMT database.

146 mo). The status at transplant was 3 patients in stage A, 21 patients in stage B, and 46 patients in stage C; all patients were treated before transplantation with a median of three therapeutic lines, 79% received fludarabine, 68% had a short lynmphocyte doubling time, 73% had a high initial lymphocyte count, and 13% were previously autotransplanted. Most of the patients (65/72) received PBSCs as grafts from HLA-identical donors (59/72) and fludarabine associated with an alkylating agent (70%). With this strategy, it takes time to achieve a complete donor chimerism and a disease response (Figs. 6 and 7). The cumulative incidence of acute GVHD higher than grade II was 31% (15% for grades III and IV), and that of chronic GVHD was 51%. The probability of overall survival was 74% (range, 31–87%), the risk of relapse at 2 yr was 27% (range, 14–40%), with a median follow-up of 12 mo (range, 1–37 mo). There was a significant association between TRM and GVHD of grade II or higher ($p = 0.005$) and TBI used during the conditioning ($p = 0.05$); there was also a significant association between relapse and disease status ($p = 0.001$),

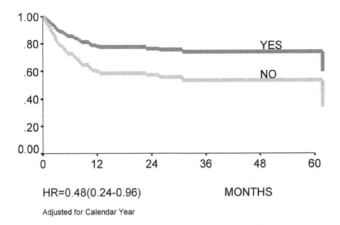

HR=0.48(0.24-0.96)   MONTHS

Adjusted for Calendar Year

Fig. 5. Allogeneic transplants for CLL survival: effect of fludarabine given (adjusted for calandar year). Data from EBMT database.

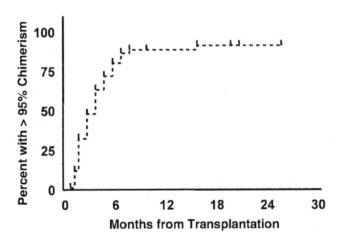

Fig. 6. Allotransplantations after reduced conditioning regimens for CLL (P. Dreger): time to >95% chimerism. Data from EBMT database.

nongenoidentical donor ($p = 0.003$), short lymphocyte doubling time ($p = 0.07$), and stage C ($p = 0.07$).

4. DISCUSSION

CLL will not affect life expectancy, although the disease is incurable with conventional treatment. However, in patients with advanced-stage disease or with adverse prognostic factors, survival time is considerably reduced (1–4,37–40). The prognostic factors are the same in younger and older patients (2). The disease can be treated with conventional chemotherapy (31,41–49), but most of the responses observed with different regimens are partial remission.

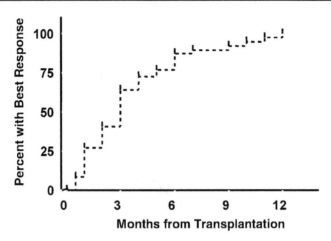

Fig. 7. Allotransplantations after reduced conditioning regimens for CLL (P. Dreger): time to best response. Data from EBMT database.

More recently, fludarabine *(50–56)*, 2-chlorodeoxyadenosine, and deoxycoformycin *(57–60)* have been shown to achieve complete remission in previously treated CLL patients, and randomized comparisons between fludarabine and other regimens *(61)* have demonstrated that fludarabine produces more complete responses but is without benefit in terms of overall survival. The median time to progression for responders to fludarabine was 31 mo, and for refractory patients the median survival was only 48 wk *(32)*. Some interesting results were observed with the association of fludarabine and other agents *(62,63)* or after using Campath-1H *(64)*. Nevertheless, all these therapeutic approaches have not yet cured CLL, hence the consideration of innovative dose-intensive therapies.

Allotransplantation adds immunotherapeutic effects to cytotoxic effects and may thus be a curative treatment for CLL, as we and other authors have demonstrated *(5,6,7,13)*. Moreover, the sensitivity to donor lymphocyte infusions suggests an important role of the GVL effect for the success of alloT *(13,14,16,17)*. Nevertheless, even in highly experienced centers, the TRM has been reported to be as high as 30–40% *(5–7,13)*, which is clearly higher than after alloT for standard indications *(65)*. The causes of these discouraging results are not completely clear, but patient age, selection of poor-risk patients with advanced disease and extensive pretreatment, and the CLL-associated incompetence of the immune system may all contribute to the high TRM observed. The demonstration in this disease of the GVL effect *(16,17)* and, in parallel, the recent development of conditioning regimens with reduced intensity *(18,25–27,36)* may help to make it possible to propose allogeneic SCT to a larger number of CLL patients, even older patients. TRM after a reduced intensity regimen is much lower than after a myeloablative-conditioning regimen *(21–23,36)*.

In contrast to allogeneic transplantation, the number of autotransplantations for CLL has dramatically increased over the past few years *(13,66)*. Because of mobilization of PBSCs and other improvements in supportive therapy, the mortality of the procedure is now well below 10%. High-dose radiochemotherapy followed by autologous SCT can induce or maintain long-term complete remissions at the molecular level, as has been shown in various studies *(8,9)*. With this strategy, it was demonstrated that the persistence of the tumor-specific PCR signal after autografting is strongly predictive for subsequent disease recurrence, whereas patients achieving molecular remission are not at risk for short-term relapse *(28)*. In the vast majority of published stem cell transplantations for CLL, the myeloablative regimen included TBI. The rationale behind this is that CLL cells—like other indolent lymphatic neoplasms—are sensitive to irradiation. Thus, TBI/cyclophosphamide still appears to be the gold standard for autografting of patients with CLL, and we have demonstrated the significantly favorable impact of a TBI-containing regimen on outcome after autotransplantation. Two other parameters significantly influenced outcome after autotransplantation: being in CR or very good PR before transplantation and having a short interval between diagnosis and autotransplantation.

Although the outcome of patients after autotransplantation is characterized by an 3-yr overall survival of more than 75% and thus is generally better than that after allotransplantation, in most series, a steady decline of the event-free survival curve was observed owing to continuous relapses occurring up to 5 yr after transplantation, and it is still not clear whether autografting can be curative in at least certain subsets of patients with CLL. In spite of sophisticated purging technologies *(34,35)*, only a little information on the clinical benefit of ex vivo B-cell depletion is available, meaning that clear-cut evidence for the usefulness of purging of CLL autografts is still lacking. Because of their favorable engraftment kinetics, mobilized PBPCs have now replaced bone marrow as the principal source of stem cells for autotransplantation *(65)*. Very preliminary data indicate that the mobilization efficacy of more intensive protocols such as the Dexa-BEAM regimen appears better than classic cyclophosphamide plus G-CSF combinations *(8)*, but many other variables could influence PBSC mobilization in this disease *(29,33)*.

In conclusion, hematopoietic stem cell transplantations could be proposed in CLL, but we need more prospective studies to determine the real place of allotransplantation, particularly after reduced-intensity conditioning and timing of autotransplantation throughout the history of the disease. In the light of all observed results, we would nevertheless make the following recommendations for SCT in CLL: (1) fludarabine should be used during therapy before allotransplantation and pilot studies should be developed of allotransplantations after reduced-intensity conditioning regimen; (2) a TBI-containing conditioning regimen should be used before autotransplantation; (3) the interval between CLL diagnosis and autotransplantation should be short; and *(4)* patients should be in CR or very good PR before autotransplantation.

REFERENCES

1. Döhner H, Stilgenbauer S, Döhner K, Bentz M, Lichter P. Chromosome aberrations in B-cell chronic lymphocytic leukemia: reassessment based on molecular cytogenetic analysis. J Mol Med 1999;77:266.
2. Mauro FR, Foa R, Giannarelli D, et al. Clinical characteristics and outcome of young chronic lymphocytic leukemia patients: a single institution study of 204 cases. Blood 1999;94:448.
3. Damle RN, Wasil T, Fais F, et al. Ig V gene mutation status and CD38 expression as novel prognostic indicators in chronic lymphocytic leukemia. Blood 1999;94:1840.
4. Hamblin TJ, Davis Z, Gardiner A, Oscier DG, Stevenson FK. Unmutated Ig V_H genes are associated with a more aggressive form of chronic lymphocytic leukemia. Blood 1999;94:1848.
5. Michallet M, Archimbaud E, Rowlings PA, et al. HLA-identical sibling bone marrow transplants for chronic lymphocytic leukemia. Ann Intern Med 1996;124:311.
6. Khouri I, Przepiorka D, van BK, et al. Allogeneic blood or marrow transplantation for chronic lymphocytic leukaemia: timing of transplantation and potential effect of fludarabine on acute graft-versus-host disease. Br J Haematol 1997;97:466.
7. Rabinowe SN, Soiffier RJ, Gribben J et al. Autologous and allogeneic bone marrow transplantation for poor prognosis patients with B-cell chronic leukemia. Blood 1993;4:1366.
8. Dreger P, von Neuhoff N, Kuse R, et al. Early stem cell transplantation for chronic lymphocytic leukaemia: a chance for cure? Br J Cancer 1998;77: 2291.

9. Milligan DW, Davies FE, Morgan GJ, et al. Fludarabine followed by stem cell autografting for younger patients with CLL: preliminary results from the MRC pilot study. Bone Marrow Transplant 1999;23(suppl 1):S53.

10. Pavletic S, Khouri I, King R, et al. HLA-matched unrelated donor (MUD) bone marrow transplantation for B-cell chronic lymphocytic leukemia (results from the CLL Working Group, National Marrow Donor Program) [abstract]. Proc ASCO 2000;19:4a.

11. Pavletic ZS, Arrowsmith ER, Bierman PJ, et al. Outcome of allogeneic stem cell transplantation for B cell chronic lymphocytic leukemia. Bone Marrow Transplant 2000;25:717.

12. Esteve J, Villamor N, Colomer D, et al. Different significance of minimal residual disease after autologous and allogeneic stem cell transplantation for chronic lymphocytic leukemia: prognostic and therapeutic implications. Blood 2001;98(suppl 1).

13. Michallet M, van Biezen A, Bandini G, et al. Analysis of prognostic factors on the outcome of autologous and allogeneic stem cell transplantation for chronic lymphocytic leukemia. Blood 2001;98:859a.

14. Esteve J, Montserrat E, Dreger P, et al. Stem cell transplantation (SCT) for chronic lymphocytic leukemia (CLL): outcome and prognostic factors after autologous and allogeneic transplants. [abstract]. Blood 2001;98(suppl 1):482a.

15. Van Biesen K, Keralavarma B, Devine S, Stock. Allogeneic and autologous transplantation for chronic lymphocytic leukemia. Leukemia 2001,15:1317.

16. Mehta J, Powles R, Singhal S, Iveson T, Treleaven J, Catovsky D. Clinical and hematologic response of chronic lymphocytic and prolymphocytic leukemia persisting after allogeneic bone marrow transplantation with the onset of acute graft-versus-host disease: possible role of graft-versus-leukemia. Bone Marrow Transplant 1996;17:371.

17. Rondon G, Giralt S, Huh Y, et al. Graft-versus-leukemia effect after allogeneic bone marrow transplantation for chronic lymphocytic leukemia. Bone Marrow Transplant 1996;18:669.

18. McSweeney PA, Niederwieser D, Shizuru JA, et al. Hematopoietic cell transplantation in older patients with hematologic malignancies: replacing high-dose cytotoxic therapy with graft-versus-tumor effects. Blood 2001;97:3390.

19. Schetelig J, Held TK, Bornhäuser M, et al. Nonmyeloablative allogeneic stem cell transplantation in chronic lymphocytic leukemia from related and unrelated donors [abstract]. Blood 2000;96 (suppl 1):200a.

20. Mackinnon S. Who may benefit from donor leucocyte infusions after allogeneic stem cell transplantation? Br J Haematol 2000;110:12.

21. Martino R, Caballero MD, Canals C, et al. Allogeneic peripheral blood stem cell transplantation with reduced-intensity conditioning: results of a prospective multicentre study. Br J Haematol 2001;115:653.

22. Corradini P, Tarella C, Olivieri A, et al. Reduced-intensity conditioning followed by allografting of hematopoietic cells can produce clinical and molecular remissions in patients with poor-risk hematologic malignancies. Blood 2002;99:75.

23. Perez-Simon JA, Kottaridis P, Martino R, et al. Reduced-intensity conditioning with or without CAMPATH-1: comparison between two prospective studies in patients with lymphoproliferative disorders [abstract]. Blood 2001;98:743a.

24. Dreger P, Glass B, Seyfarth B, et al. Reduced-intensity allogeneic stem cell transplantation as salvage treatment for patients with indolent lymphoma after failure of autologous SCT. Bone Marrow Transplant 2000;26:1361.

25. Khouri IF, Keating M, Korbling M, et al. Transplant-lite: induction of graft-versus-malignancy using fludarabine-based nonablative chemotherapy and allogeneic blood progenitor-cell transplantation as treatment for lymphoid malignancies. J Clin Oncol 1998;16:2817.

26. Slavin S, Nagler A, Naparstek E, et al. Nonmyeloablative stem cell transplantation and cell therapy as an alternative to conventional bone marrow transplantation with lethal cytoreduction for the treatment of malignant and nonmalignant hematologic diseases. Blood 1998;91:756.

27. Childs R, Clave E, Contentin N, et al. Engraftment kinetics after nonmyeloablative allogeneic peripheral blood stem cell transplantation: full donor T-cell chimerism precedes alloimmune responses. Blood 1999;94:3234.

28. Provan D, Bartlett-Pandite L, Zwicky C et al. Eradication of PCR detectable chronic lymphocytic cells is associated with improved outcome after bone marrow transplanation. Blood 1996;88:2228.

29. Dreger P, von Neuhoff N, Sonnen R, et al: Factors determining feasibility and outcome of autologous stem cell transplantation for CLL. Ann Oncol 1999;10(suppl 3):72.

30. Milligan DW, Davies FE, Morgan GJ et al. Fludarabine followed by stem cell autografting for younger patients with CLL: preliminaryresults from MRC pilot study. Bone Marrow Transplant 1999;23(suppl 1):S53.

31. French Cooperative Group on Chronic Lymphocytic Leukemia. Effectiveness of CHOP regimen in advanced untreated chronic lymphocytic leukemia. Lancet 1986;1:1346.

32. Keating MJ, O'Brien S, Lerner S, et al. Long-term follow-up of patients with chronic lymphocytic leukemia (CLL) receiving fludarabine regimens as initial therapy. Blood 1998;92:1165.

33. Michallet M, Apperley J. Peripheral blood progenitor cell mobilisation and transplantation after fludarabine therapy in chronic lymphocytic leukemia in Europe. Bone Marrow Transplant 1997;19(suppl 1):S146.

34. Scime R, Indovina A, Santoro A, et al. PBSC mobilization, collection and positive selection in patients with chronic lymphocytic leukemia. Bone Marrow Transplant 1998;22:1159.

35. Paulus U, Schmitz N, Viehmann K, et al: Combined positive/negative selection for highly effective purging of PBPC grafts: towards clinical application in patients with B-CLL. Bone Marrow Transplant 1997;20:415.

36. Dreger P, Van Biezen A, Brand R, et al. Allogeneic stem cell transplantation (SCT) for chronic lymphocytic leukemia (CLL) using intensity-reduced conditioning: a survey of the European Blood and Marrow Transplant Group (EBMT). Blood 2001;98:3095a.

37. Baccarani L, Cavo M, Gobbi M, Lauria F, Tura S. Staging of chronic lymphocytic leukemia. Blood 1982;591191.

38. Montserrat E, Sanchez-Bisono J, Vinolas N, Rozman C. Lymphocyte doubling time in chronic lymphocytic leukemia: analysis of its prognostic significance. Br J Haematol 1986;62:567.

39. Molica S, Alberti A. Prognostic value of lymphocyte doubling time in chronic lymphocytic leukemia. Cancer 1987;60:567.

40. Keating MJ, Lerner S, Kantarjian H, Freireich EJ, O'Brien S. The serum $\beta 2$ microglobulin level is more powerful than stage in predicting response and survival in chronic lymphocytic leukemia. Blood 1995;86(suppl 1):606a.

41. Sawitsky A, Rai KR, Glidewell O, et al. Comparison of daily versus intermittent chlorambucil and prednisone therapy in the treatment of patients with chronic lymphocytic leukemia. Blood 1977;50:1049.

42. Knospe WH, Loeb V, Huguley CM, et al. Bi-weekly chlorambucil of chronic lymphocytic leukemia. Cancer 1974;33:555.

43. Keller JW, Knospe WH, Raney M, et al. Treatment of chronic lymphocytic leukemia using chlorambucil and prednisone with or without cycle-active consolidation chemotherapy. Cancer 1986;58:1185.

44. Montserrat E, Alcala A, Parody R, et al. Treatment of chronic lymphocytic leukemia in advanced stages—a randomized trial comparing chlorambucil plus prednisone versus cyclophosphamide, vincristine and prednisone. Cancer 1985;56:2369.

45. Raphael B, Andersen JW, Silber R, et al. Comparison of chlorambucil and prednisone as initial treatment for chronic lymphocytic leukemia. Long-term follow-up of an Eastern Cooperative Oncology Group randomized clinical trial. J Clin Oncol 1991;9:770.

46. French Cooperative Group on Chronic Lymphocytic Leukemia. Is the CHOP regimen a good treatment for advanced CLL? Results from two randomized clinical trials. Leuk Lymphoma 1994;13:449.

47. Keating MJ, Scouros M, Murphy S, et al. Multiple agent chemotherapy (POACH) in previously treated and untreated patients with chronic lymphocytic leukemia. Leukemia 1988;2:391.

48. Keating MJ, Hester JP, McCredie KB, et al. Long-term results of CAP therapy in chronic lymphocytic leukemia. Leuk Lymphoma 1990;2:391.

49. Kempin S, Lee BJ III, Thaler HT, et al. Combination chemotherapy of advanced chronic lymphocytic leukemia: the M-2 protocol (vincristine, BCNU, cyclophosphamide, melphalan and prednisone). Blood 1982;60:1110.

50. Keating MJ, Kantarjian MJ, O'Brien S, et al. Fludarabine: a new agent with marked cytoreductive activity in untreated chronic lymphocytic leukaemia. J Clin Oncol 1991;9:44.

51. O'Brien S, Kantarjian H, Beran M, et al. Results of fludarabine and prednisone therapy in 264 patients with chronic lymphocytic leukemia with multivariate analysis-derived prognostic model for response to treatment. Blood 1993;82:1695.

52. Robertson LE, O'Brien S, Kantarjian H, et al. A 3-day schedule of fludarabine in previously treated chronic lymphocytic leukemia. Leukemia 1995;9:1444.

53. Hiddemann W, Rottmann R, Woermann B, et al. Treatment of advanced chronic lymphocytic leukemia by fludarabine—results of a clinical phase II study. Ann Hematol 1991;63:1.

54. Montserrat E, Lopez-Lorenzo JL, Manso F, et al. Fludarabine in resistant or relapsing B-cell chronic lymphocytic leukemia—The Spanish Group experience. Leuk Lymphoma 1996;21:467.

55. Gjedde SB, Hansen MM. Salvage therapy with fludarabine in patients with progressive B-chronic lymphocytic leukemia. Leuk Lymphoma 1996;21:317.

56. Puccio CA, Mittelman A, Lichtman SM, et al. A loading dose/continuous infusion schedule of fludarabine phosphate in chronic lymphocytic leukemia. J Clin Oncol 1991;9:1562.

57. Juliusson G, Elmhorn-Rosenborg A, Liliemark J. Response to 2-chlorodeoxyadenosine in patients with B-cell chronic lymphocytic leukemia resistant to fludarabine. N Engl J Med 1992;327:1056.

58. Saven A, Carrera CJ, Carson DA, et al. 2–Chlorodeoxyadenosine treatment of refractory chronic lymphocytic leukemia. Leuk Lymphoma 1991;5(suppl 1):133.

59. Dillman RO, Mick R, McIntyre OR. Pentostatin in chronic lymphocytic leukemia: a phase II trial of Cancer and Leukemia Group B. J Clin Oncol 1989;7:433.

60. Saven A, Lemon RH , Kosty M, Beutler E, Piro LD. 2-Chlorodeoxydeadenosine activity in patients with untreated chronic lymphocytic leukemia. J Clin Oncol 1995;13:570.

61. Leporrier M, Chevret S, Cazin B, et al. Randomized comparison of fludarabine, CAP, and CHOP in 938 previously untreated stage B and C chronic lymphocytic leukemia patients. Blood 2001;98:2319.

62. Cazin B, Maloum K, Divine M, et al (French Cooperative Group for CLL). Oral fludarabine and cyclophospha-mide in previously untreated CLL: preliminary data on 59 patients. Blood 2001;98:3214a.

63. Bellosillo B, Villamor N, Colomer D, Pons G, Montserrat E, Gil J. In vitro evaluation of fludarabine in combination with cyclophosphamide and/or mitoxantrone in B-cell chronic lymphocytic leukaemia. Blood 1999;94:2836.

64. Kennedy B, Rawstron A, Carter C, et al. Campath-1H and fludarabine in combination are highly active in refrac-tory chronic lymphocytic leukemia. Blood 2002;99:2245.

65. Gratwohl A, Passweg J, Baldomero H, et al. Blood and marrow transplantation activity in Europe 1996. European Group for Blood and Marrow Transplantation (EBMT). Bone Marrow Transplant 1998;22:227.

66. Gribben JG, Neuberg D, Soiffer RJ, et al: Autologous versus allogeneic bone marrow transplantation for patients with poor prognosis CLL. Blood 1998;92:322a.

15 Monoclonal Antibody Therapy in Chronic Lymphocytic Leukemia

Thomas S. Lin, MD, PhD, Margaret S. Lucas, PA, and John C. Byrd, MD

1. INTRODUCTION

1.1. Monoclonal Antibodies

Monoclonal antibodies have played an increasingly important role in the therapy of hematological malignancies over the past several years. Monoclonal antibodies offer the potential of targeted therapy with minimal toxicity to normal cells, and clinical studies over the past decade have demonstrated the feasibility, safety, and clinical efficacy of such treatments. Monoclonal antibodies are now used to treat diseases as diverse as acute myelogenous leukemia, diffuse large B-cell non-Hodgkin's lymphoma (NHL), and mycosis fungoides *(1–3)*. Monoclonal antibodies have had the greatest impact, however, on the treatment of indolent B-cell lymphoproliferative disorders such as follicle center NHL and chronic lymphocytic leukemia (CLL) *(4–7)*.

1.2. Chronic Lymphocytic Leukemia

Indolent B-cell lymphoproliferative disorders such as CLL are ideal targets for monoclonal antibody therapies. Although CLL responds to cytotoxic chemotherapy, only a proportion of patients achieve complete remission (CR), and treatment is palliative. For many years, therapy for CLL consisted of oral alkylating agents (such as chlorambucil) and combination chemotherapeutic regimens, such as cyclophosphamide, vincristine, and prednisone (CVP) *(8–10)*. In recent years the purine analog fludarabine and fludarabine-containing combination regimens have shown significant clinical efficacy in relapsed and previously untreated CLL *(11–18)*. Despite improved response rates and durations of response, however, these new regimens are not curative. The failure of traditional cytotoxic agents to cure CLL, as well as other indolent B-cell lymphoproliferative disorders, may result from these diseases' indolent nature, as well as intrinsic resistance mechanisms to chemotherapy. Only a small fraction of CLL cells undergo growth and division at one time. Cytotoxic chemotherapeutic agents often act only against actively dividing cells undergoing transcription and DNA replication and are ineffective against resting cells. Fludarabine, which acts against both dividing and nondividing cells, is an exception to this rule.

The inherent resistance of CLL and other indolent B-cell lymphoproliferative disorders to chemotherapy arises from the defective apoptosis of these malignancies. Unlike acute leuke-

From: *Contemporary Hematology*
Chronic Lymphocytic Leukemia: Molecular Genetics, Biology, Diagnosis, and Management
Edited by: G. B. Faguet © Humana Press Inc., Totowa, NJ

mias or aggressive lymphomas, which are characterized by uncontrolled growth and a high proliferative index, CLL arises from cellular defects in programmed cell death. Anti-apoptotic proteins such as Bcl-2, Mcl-1, and X-linked inactivator of apoptosis (XIAP) are overexpressed in CLL, and high levels of Mcl-1 may be associated with failure to achieve CR after initial therapy with fludarabine *(19)*. Although antibody-dependent cellular cytotoxicity (ADCC) and complement-dependent cytotoxicity (CDC) have been implicated as potential mechanisms of action *(20,21)*, evidence also indicates that monoclonal antibodies exert their anticancer effects in CLL, at least in part, by inducing apoptosis *(22,23)*. Thus, monoclonal antibodies act directly against the cellular defects in apoptosis that give rise to CLL. However, the success of monoclonal antibodies in CLL may depend on the use of multiple mechanisms of action to eliminate tumor cells.

1.3. Introduction of Monoclonal Antibodies Into Clinical Practice

Several problems have limited the successful introduction of monoclonal antibody therapies into clinical practice. These obstacles include (1) identification of tumor-specific antigens, (2) antigen surface density, (3) antibody production, (4) internalization of antigen or antigen-antibody complex, (5) antigenicity of the antibody resulting in host sensitization, (6) infusion toxicity from host humoral response, and (7) delivery of antibody to bulky tumors. An ideal antigen should be expressed at relatively high density on tumor cells, but not on most normal cells, and should not undergo shedding, internalization, or other modification. B-cell malignancies each express a unique immunoglobulin (Ig) idiotype (Id), which is generated by recombination of the genetic sequences for variable Ig light and heavy chains. Each clonal B-cell lymphoproliferative disorder produces a unique Id protein, and thus Id would be the ideal antigen for monoclonal antibody therapy. Early studies of immunotherapy focused on monoclonal antibodies directed against tumor-specific idiotype (anti-Id MAbs). These studies yielded promising results, and several patients with NHL achieved long-lasting remissions *(24–28)*. However, relapse was common and was often accompanied by genetic mutation of the Id protein *(29–31)*. Whereas anti-Id MAb therapy was tested primarily in patients with indolent B-cell NHL, anti-Id MAb therapy was given to several patients with CLL *(32–34)*. In these case reports, individual patients with CLL received anti-Id MAb, with transient responses in two of three patients; immune deficiency was felt to contribute to the lack of response in the third patient *(34)*.

Despite the theoretical advantages of using anti-Id MAb, identification of an individual patient's Id protein sequence and generation of an individualized anti-Id MAb are not feasible on a large scale with current available technology. Id vaccines may be an alternative approach if the immune deficiency of CLL can be overcome to allow generation of a primary and persistent secondary immune response. Id vaccines, which have shown promise in B-cell NHL, are now entering clinical trials in CLL. Development of monoclonal antibodies has become focused on the use of antigens specific for tumors, as opposed to patient-specific antigens, to allow broad therapeutic applicability of each monoclonal antibody. Monoclonal antibodies generated against several such antigens in CLL are reviewed in this chapter.

1.4. "Humanization" of Monoclonal Antibodies

Initial studies of monoclonal antibody therapies were complicated by significant infusion-related toxicity owing to host recognition of xenotropic sequences in the murine monoclonal antibodies. The formation of human anti-mouse antibodies (HAMAs) limited the clinical utility of initial monoclonal antibodies, and patients also developed serum sickness *(35,36)*. However, recombinant DNA technology has allowed the generation of chimeric and "humanized" murine monoclonal IgG antibodies in which murine sequences have been replaced with the human Fc fragment. It is now technologically possible to generate humanized IgG molecules whose Fab portions contain only the murine sequences necessary to recognize the tumor-specific antigen of interest. These chimeric and humanized antibodies have proved to be less immunogenic, resulting in reduced infusion-related toxicity *(37–39)*. In addition, incorporation of the human Fc fragment allows activation of patients' host immune systems through induction of ADCC and CDC. Thus, recombinant DNA technology has allowed the production of monoclonal antibodies that are better tolerated by patients and more effective clinically. Although technical problems must be addressed with each new individual monoclonal antibody, several antibodies have entered clinical practice or are undergoing active clinical investigation in CLL.

1.5. Radioisotope-Conjugated Monoclonal Antibodies

There is currently great interest in the use of radioisotope-conjugated antibodies to deliver radiotherapy directly to targeted cells. CLL cells are sensitive to radiotherapy, and splenic irradiation has been used as palliative therapy in CLL patients with splenomegaly *(40–42)*. However, most work to date in this field has focused on indolent and aggressive NHL. A preliminary report recently indicated that the ^{131}I-labeled anti-CD20 antibody tositumomab (Bexxar®) is effective in previously treated patients with advanced CLL *(43)*. To date, no clinical data are available regarding the use of the ^{90}Y-labeled anti-CD20 antibody ibritumomab (Zevalin®) in the treatment of CLL. However, several technical limitations make it doubtful that radioisotope-conjugated antibodies will have a significant impact in the nontransplant therapy of CLL. These limitations include the high degree to which CLL cells infiltrate the blood, bone marrow, and spleen. The effectiveness of radioimmunotherapy is predicated on the ability to deliver targeted radiation therapy to a single or several sites of concentrated tumor cells. In addition to toxicity from delivery of radioisotope directly to an individual cell, each cell is subjected to emitted radiation from delivery of radioisotope-conjugated antibodies to neighboring cells. The tendency of CLL to involve the bone marrow heavily raises substantial concern that marrow toxicity or myelodysplasia may result from exposure of neighboring normal hematopoietic stem cells to harmful radiation. This concern was confirmed by the aforementioned study, in which myelosuppression was the dose-limiting toxicity and was related to the total body dose of radiation *(43)*. Thus, radioimmunotherapy may have a limited role in the treatment of CLL patients with significant bone marrow disease.

1.6. Summary

Monoclonal antibody therapy in CLL is an active area of laboratory and clinical research. Advances in recombinant DNA techniques have made it possible to generate monoclonal antibodies against many potential tumor-specific antigens, and the promise of directed monoclonal antibody therapy is rapidly being realized in many hematologic malignancies. Despite these rapid advances, significant research must be performed to identify new monoclonal antibodies and incorporate monoclonal antibodies into clinical therapy. In particular, the development of new antibodies against different cell surface antigens and the optimal use of current monoclonal antibodies in combination chemotherapy regimens are two active areas of investigation. This chapter will review current monoclonal antibody therapies for CLL and provide a brief overview of areas of active, ongoing investigation.

2. MONOCLONAL ANTIBODIES

2.1. Rituximab

2.1.1. PRECLINICAL STUDIES

Rituximab (Rituxan®, IDEC-C2B8), a chimeric murine-derived monoclonal antibody that recognizes the CD20 antigen found on the surface of normal and malignant B-cells, is the best studied and most widely used monoclonal antibody in CLL and indolent B-cell NHL. CD20 is thought to be a calcium channel that interacts with the B-cell immunoglobulin receptor complex *(44,45)*. CD20 is an excellent target; CD20 is expressed in 90–100% of CLL and B-cell NHL, and it is thought that the antigen is not internalized or shed. However, recent data indicate that significant levels of soluble CD20 can be detected in the sera of patients with CLL and B-cell NHL; in addition, higher levels of soluble CD20 correlate with poorer survival *(46,47)*.

In vitro and in vivo data indicate that rituximab depletes CLL cells by several mechanisms. Rituximab induces both ADCC and CDC, and caspase 3 activation and induction of apoptosis play an important role in the action of rituximab *(20–23)*. In addition, rituximab induces calcium influx, which contributes to maturation arrest and apoptosis. In preliminary studies from our laboratory, rituximab induced apoptosis in vitro within 4 h; this induction was independent of complement but required crosslinking with anti-Fcγ antibody. Preliminary data from our laboratory also indicated that Mcl-1 and XIAP are overexpressed in patients who fail to respond to rituximab (ms. submitted). Complement activation may be important, as increased expression of the complement inhibitors CD55 and CD59 resulted in resistance to rituximab in NHL cell lines and CLL cells *(21,48)*. Blocking both CD55 and CD59 resulted in a five- to sixfold increase in rituximab-induced cell lysis of poorly responding CLL samples, although CD55 and CD59 levels did not predict complement susceptibility *(48)*. Thus, rituximab may exert its anticancer effects through more than one mechanism of action.

2.1.2. CLINICAL STUDIES

Phase I clinical studies in indolent B-cell NHL established a dose of 375 mg/m^2 given by iv infusion weekly for 4 doses, although the length of treatment was empirically established. In the pivotal phase II trial in 166 patients with relapsed or refractory indolent B-cell NHL or CLL, an overall response rate (ORR) of 48% was seen (6% CR), with a median response duration of 12 mo *(6)*. On basis of this trial, the Food and Drug Administration (FDA) granted approval for the clinical marketing of rituximab. Subsequent analysis of the pivotal study showed that patients with indolent (grade I and II) follicle center B-cell NHL had an ORR of 60%, whereas only 4 of 30 patients with small lymphocytic lymphoma (SLL)/CLL (13%) responded to therapy. The same dosing schedule in a British study of 48 patients achieved only a single partial remission (PR) in 10 patients with relapsed or refractory SLL/CLL (10%), although the ORR was only 27% in patients with follicular lymphoma *(49)*. Similarly, only 1 PR was seen in nine evaluable patients with fludarabine-refractory CLL (11%), although seven patients had stable disease *(50)*. A small study in seven patients with refractory or relapsed CLL showed a striking, but transient, reduction (median 93%) in peripheral lymphocyte count, but little activity against nodal disease was observed *(51)*. Recently, the German CLL Study Group reported its experience with weekly rituximab in 28 patients with previously treated CLL. Seven patients (25%) achieved PR with a median duration of 20 wk. Forty-five percent of patients experienced at least a 50% reduction of peripheral lymphocyte count lasting for 4 wk or longer *(5)*.

Thus, weekly rituximab appears to have limited activity in CLL, and the antibody is more effective in reducing peripheral lymphocyte count than in clearing bone marrow or lymphaden-

Table 1
Selected Phase II Trials of Weekly Rituximab in CLL/SLL

Study	No. of doses	Prior therapy	No. of evaluable patients	Response rate (ORR, %)
McLaughlin et al., 1998 (6)	4	Yes	30	13
Nguyen et al., 1999 (49)	4	Yes	10	10
Winkler et al., 1999 (50)	4	Yes	9	11
Ladetto et al., 2000 (51)	4	Yes	7	0
Huhn et al., 2001 (5)	4	Yes	28	25
Hainsworth et al., 2000 (54)	4	No	22	64
Hainsworth et al., 2001 (56)	4	No	56	44
Thomas et al., 2001 (57)	8	No	21	90

CLL, chronic lymphocytic leukemia; SLL, small lymphocytic lymphoma; ORR, overall response rate.

opathy. The preferential response of peripheral lymphocyte count may be due to increased CD20 expression on circulating CLL cells, compared with bone marrow cells. Quantitative flow cytometry showed that B-CLL cells bound an average of 9050 anti-CD20 molecules, compared with only 4070 molecules for bone marrow CLL cells and 3950 molecules for lymph node cells (52). This increased binding of rituximab to circulating CLL cells in peripheral blood may explain the ability of rituximab to reduce peripheral lymphocytosis. In addition, stromal cells in bone marrow and lymph nodes may provide an additional survival advantage to CLL cells in these environments over circulating CLL cells.

Limited clinical data suggest that weekly rituximab may be more effective in previously untreated SLL/CLL (53–57). Fourteen of 22 patients with untreated SLL/CLL (64%) responded to 4 weekly doses of rituximab 375 mg/m^2, and the ORR was similar to that seen in untreated follicular NHL patients (58%) (53). This study was expanded, and patients with stable or responsive disease also received maintenance therapy with rituximab, given by 4 weekly doses of 375 mg/m^2 every 6 mo for up to 4 courses. Fifty-six of 70 enrolled patients were evaluable, and an ORR of 44% (9% CR) was observed, with 44% additional patients experiencing stable disease (56). Although the increased ORR in untreated CLL/SLL patients is encouraging, the small percentage of patients achieving CR indicates that single-agent rituximab will not produce long-term survival in CLL. A recent study of 8 weekly doses of rituximab 375 mg/m^2 in 31 untreated, early-stage CLL patients (21 evaluable) with β2-microglobulin levels of 2.0 mg/dL or more showed an ORR of 90% (19% CR, 19% nodular PR) (57). The results of clinical trials using weekly dosing of rituximab in CLL are summarized in Table 1.

2.1.3. LIMITATIONS OF WEEKLY RITUXIMAB IN CLL

Several theories may explain the inferior clinical activity of weekly rituximab in CLL, compared with its effectiveness in indolent follicle center NHL. First, CLL/SLL cells express lower CD20 density than follicle center NHL cells, thereby decreasing the number of target antigen sites and the amount of antibody delivered to individual tumor cells. In an analysis of 70 patients with chronic B-cell leukemias and 17 normal donors, normal B-lymphocytes expressed approx 94,000 CD20 molecules per cell. Whereas other chronic B-cell leukemias such as mantle cell lymphoma and hairy cell leukemia expressed between 123,000 and 312,000 CD20 molecules per cell, CLL cells expressed only 65,000 CD20 molecules per cell *(58)*. However, a recent analysis of CD20 expression and clinical response in 10 patients with CLL did not identify a correlation *(59)*.

A second, and more plausible, explanation is that the large intravascular burden from circulating CLL cells may alter rituximab's pharmacokinetics and result in accelerated clearance of antibody from plasma. Lower trough concentrations of rituximab are seen in CLL patients who do not respond to therapy, and the importance of serum rituximab levels was previously documented in follicular NHL *(60,61)*. Whereas detectable plasma levels of rituximab can be observed for more than 6 mo after therapy in follicular NHL, serum concentrations of the antibody decrease more rapidly after treatment in CLL. In addition, the recent discovery of soluble CD20 in the serum of CLL patients suggests that free CD20, derived from cell membrane fragments (remnants of smudge cells) or, less likely, shed antigen, may contribute to rapid clearance of rituximab, although a relationship between soluble CD20 levels and response to rituximab has not been demonstrated *(47)*. Finally, intrinsic mechanisms of resistance, such as overexpression of the anti-apoptotic proteins Bcl-2, Mcl-1, and XIAP, probably explain the common resistance of CLL to rituximab and cytotoxic chemotherapy.

2.1.4. Dosing Schedule Considerations in CLL

Two different clinical strategies have been pursued to overcome these pharmacokinetic and pharmacodynamic obstacles. In a single-institution study of high-dose rituximab, 50 patients with previously treated CLL ($n = 40$) or other B-cell leukemia ($n = 10$) received weekly rituximab dose-escalated to 2250 mg/m^2 *(62,63)*. The ORR was 40%, but no CLL patient achieved CR. However, a statistically significant dose-response relationship was observed; 22% of patients treated with 500–850 mg/m^2 responded, compared with 75% of patients treated with 2250 mg/m^2. ORR was 36% for CLL and 60% for other B-cell leukemias. Median response duration was 8 mo. Eight of 12 patients (67%) developed grade 2 toxicity at 2,250 mg/m^2, primarily manifested as fatigue, although no grade 3 or 4 toxicity was seen. In an alternative approach, 33 patients with relapsed or refractory SLL/CLL received thrice weekly rituximab for 4 wk *(4)*. Patients received 100 mg over 4 h on the first day of therapy and 375 mg/m^2 thereafter. This stepped up dosing approach was designed to minimize infusion-related toxicity. The ORR was 45% (3% CR), and the median response duration was 10 mo. Thirteen patients developed transient infusion-related toxicity that appeared to be related to cytokine release [tumor necrosis factor-α (TNF-α), interferon-γ (IFN-γ), interleukin-8 (IL-8), and IL-6] and that resolved by the third infusion. Thus, both dose escalation and thrice weekly dosing improve the response rate in SLL/CLL and define a role for rituximab in the therapy of relapsed CLL. Although dose escalation and thrice weekly dosing yield few complete responses, it is important to remember that no therapeutic agent achieves a significant CR rate in relapsed or refractory CLL.

2.1.5. Upfront Therapy in Previously Untreated Patients

Recent data indicate that rituximab is effective as upfront therapy for previously untreated early-stage CLL patients with increased risk of progression. Thirty-one patients with Rai stage 0–II CLL with β2-microglobulin levels of 2.0 mg/dL or more (median 3.6), without other indications for therapy, received rituximab 375 mg/m^2 weekly for 8 doses. The ORR was 90%, but only 19% of patients achieved CR *(57)*. The clinical significance of these results is unclear, and it remains to be seen whether time to progression or long-term survival will be affected by early treatment with weekly rituximab. Additionally, Although CLL clearly responds to rituximab, the overwhelming majority of responses in all trials using single-agent rituximab have been PRs, even in previously untreated patients with limited disease. Thus, rituximab as a single agent is unlikely to alter long-term survival significantly in CLL patients.

2.1.6. Toxicity

Infusion-related side effects constitute the most common toxicity of rituximab, although these side effects are generally manageable, particularly with use of a stepped up dosing schedule. Patients can develop transient hypoxemia, dyspnea, and hypotension, which are partly because of inflammatory cytokine release. Although initial studies suggested that patients with lymphocyte counts greater than 50,000/mL may be at greatest risk of this cytokine release syndrome, recent studies of large patient numbers have not substantiated this finding. TNF-α and IL-6 peak at 90 min after the start of infusion, and the rise in cytokines is accompanied by fever, chills, hypotension, and nausea *(50)*. These side effects are usually most severe with the first rituximab infusion and resolve by the third infusion in the thrice weekly dosing schedule *(4)*. An uncommon but potentially severe toxicity is tumor lysis syndrome, which generally affects patients with high numbers of circulating CLL cells *(64,65)*. Patients at risk should receive prophylactic allopurinol, hydration, and careful observation, and it may be necessary to administer the first dose of rituximab in an in-patient setting if the risk of tumor lysis is sufficiently high. However, patients who develop tumor lysis syndrome after the first dose of rituximab can safely receive subsequent doses, especially after the number of circulating CLL cells is reduced *(64)*. Other side effects are minimal and should not affect administration of this antibody. Rare toxicities that can, however, be serious include skin toxicity, pure red cell aplasia, and hepatitis B reactivation.

2.1.7. Combination Therapy

There is currently interest in combining monoclonal antibody therapy with cytotoxic chemotherapy in the treatment of hematological malignancies, and several studies have looked specifically at rituximab. Given the very low CR rates in CLL/SLL in response to single-agent rituximab, combination with traditional cytotoxic drugs or other monoclonal antibodies may be necessary to impact long-term survival in CLL significantly. Several completed clinical trials have addressed the potential role of rituximab in combination regimens against B-cell lymphoid malignancies, including CLL *(2,66–69)*. The results of these studies are summarized in Table 2. Rituximab has been successfully combined with fludarabine in both NHL and CLL *(70–72)*. Concurrent administration of these two agents in a randomized phase II Cancer and Leukemia Group B (CALGB) trial in previously untreated CLL patients yielded a higher CR rate (48%) than did sequential administration (38%) *(70)*. Patients received standard fludarabine 25 mg/ m^2 d 1–5 every 4 wk for 6 cycles. Patients were randomized to receive concurrent rituximab 375 mg/m^2 on d 1 of each cycle, with an additional d 4 dose during cycle 1, or sequential rituximab 375 mg/m^2 weekly for 4 doses beginning 2 mo after completion of fludarabine. A recent update of this CALGB study indicated a statistically significant difference in CR rate, with concurrent and sequential therapy achieving 47% CR and 28% CR, respectively *(71)*.

A multicenter European phase II study of fludarabine and rituximab in 29 evaluable patients with CLL achieved an ORR of 90% (CR 34%). Patients received fludarabine 25 mg/m^2 on d 1–5 every 4 wk for 4 cycles, as well as rituximab 375 mg/m^2 every 4 wk for 4 doses, beginning on d 1 of cycle 3 of fludarabine. Overall and complete response rates were similar in previously treated (ORR 91%, CR 45%) and untreated patients (ORR 89%, CR 28%). Fifteen patients developed a total of 29 infections, and one patient died of cerebral hemorrhage resulting from prolonged thrombocytopenia *(73)*. A similar combination regimen of 6 cycles of fludarabine,

Table 2
Combination Regimens With Concurrent Rituximab in CLL/SLL

Study	Prior therapy	Rituximab dose (mg/m^2)	No. of cycles	Other agents	No. of evaluable patients	ORR (%) (CR)
Byrd et al., 2001 (70)	Yes	375 q4wk	6	Flu	51	90 (47)
Schulz et al., 2001 (73)	Yes	375 q4wk	4	Flu	29	90 (34)
Garcia-Manero et al., 2001 (74)	Yes	500 q4wk	6	Flu/Cy	102	73 (23)
Wierda et al., 2001 (75)	No	500 q4wk	6	Flu/Cy	79	95 (66)

CLL, chronic lymphocytic leukemia; SLL, small lymphocytic lymphoma; Flu, flydarabine; Cy, cycloposphamide; ORR, overall response rate.

cyclophosphamide, and rituximab has also shown promise in a single-institution study. One hundred two evaluable patients received fludarabine 25 mg/m^2 and cyclophosphamide 250 mg/ m^2 on d 2–4 of cycle 1 and on d 1–3 of cycles 2–6, in addition to rituximab 375 mg/m^2 on d 1 of cycle 1 and 500 mg/m^2 on d 1 of cycles 2–6. The ORR was 73% (CR 23%), and 5 of 13 patients in CR achieved molecular remission (74). The same authors administered this regimen to 79 previously untreated CLL patients with symptomatic disease requiring initiation of therapy by National Cancer Institute (NCI) criteria. The ORR was 95%, and 66% of patients achieved CR (75). Molecular remissions were observed in 22 of 37 tested patients who achieved CR (59%); 8 of 11 tested patients remained in molecular remission 6–12 mo after treatment. The major toxicities of this regimen were grade 4 neutropenia and infection, which occurred in 20% and 17%, respectively, of treatment cycles.

Finally, a report recently described the use of an aggressive regimen containing fludarabine and rituximab as upfront, cytoreductive therapy for untreated patients with CLL, with the intent of pursuing autologous stem cell transplantation. Thirteen patients, with a median age of 47 yr, received fludarabine 25 mg/m^2 on d 1–3, cyclophosphamide 200 mg/m^2 on d 1–3, and mitoxantrone 10 mg/m^2 on d 1 every 4 wk for 4–6 cycles, followed by rituximab 375 mg/m^2 weekly for 4 doses. All patients responded (ORR 100%, CR 77%), and four patients (31%) achieved a molecular remission (76). The ability of this regimen to induce complete hematological and molecular remissions is promising, although patients have not been followed long enough to determine whether these initial remissions will be durable.

2.1.8. RADIOISOTOPE CONJUGATES OF ANTI-CD20

Anti-CD20 monoclonal antibody has been conjugated to the radioisotopes yttrium-90 [^{90}Y-ibritumomab (Zevalin)] and iodine-131 [^{131}I-tositumomab (Bexxar)]. Several published clinical trials have demonstrated the efficacy of Zevalin and Bexxar in indolent B-cell NHL, particularly follicle center grade I and II NHL (77–83). The results of these trials in indolent B-cell NHL have been extensively reviewed elsewhere and will not be discussed in this chapter. There has been some reluctance to use Zevalin and Bexxar in patients with SLL/CLL, primarily owing to concern regarding potential myelotoxicity resulting from bystander radiation in patients with significant marrow involvement. However, a preliminary report recently indicated that Bexxar is effective in previously treated patients with advanced CLL. Eleven patients with heavily pretreated CLL received a total body dose of 35–55 cGy in this phase I dose escalation study; three patients (27%)

achieved PR, and six patients (55%) had stable disease *(43)*. As expected, myelosuppression was the dose limiting toxicity and was related to the total body dose of radiation. Thus, although CLL cells are sensitive to radiation, myelotoxicity limits the use of Zevalin and Bexxar in patients with significant marrow involvement. However, these radioisotope conjugates may be more effective than rituximab in patients with bulky lymphadenopathy, given their ability to deliver radiation to surrounding SLL/CLL cells. Future studies of Zevalin and Bexxar in SLL/CLL should focus on patients with primarily bulky nodal disease, as well as in sequential combination regimens with agents such as Campath 1H, which effectively eliminates blood and bone marrow CLL disease but is generally ineffective in bulky nodal disease.

2.1.9. SUMMARY

Rituximab, the most thoroughly tested and best tolerated monoclonal antibody in hematological malignancies, has clinical activity in CLL, especially when given thrice weekly. However, further studies of rituximab-containing combination regimens are necessary, as single-agent rituximab, like all other agents, is unlikely to alter long-term survival in CLL significantly. Although most studies to date have combined rituximab with traditional cytotoxic agents, several trials are now examining the use of rituximab with only monoclonal antibodies. These trials will be discussed in the following sections.

2.2. Campath 1H

2.2.1. PRECLINICAL STUDIES

Campath 1H (alemtuzumab) is a humanized anti-CD52 monoclonal antibody that is extremely effective in fixing complement and depleting normal lymphocytes and lymphoma cells *(84–86)*. CD52 is a 21–28 kD glycopeptide expressed on the surface of more than 95% of human lymphocytes, monocytes, and macrophages *(87–89)*. CD52 is expressed on a small subpopulation of granulocytes, but CD52 expression has not been detected on erythrocytes, platelets, or bone marrow stem cells. CD52 is expressed on all CLL cells and indolent B-cell NHL cells *(90,91)*. CD52 is not shed, internalized, or modulated. Although its physiological function is unknown, crosslinking of CD52 on B-cell and T-cell lymphoma cell lines resulted in growth inhibition *(89)*. Despite its small size, antibody binding of the CD52 antigen elicits profound complement activation and ADCC. These properties all made CD52 an attractive target for antibody-directed immunotherapy. However, the ubiquitous expression of CD52 on normal lymphocytes and monocytes correctly predicted for the increased hematological and immune toxicity of Campath 1H, which results in an increased incidence of infectious complications.

Laboratory data from our institution indicated that Campath 1H acts in vivo by inducing programmed cell death. In vivo blood samples showed a 19–92% reduction in expression of the anti-apoptotic protein Bcl-2 in six of eight patients undergoing Campath 1H therapy *(61)*. Expression of the anti-apoptotic proteins Mcl-1 and XIAP was also downmodulated in response to Campath-1H treatment. In addition, activation of caspase 3 and cleavage of the DNA repair enzyme poly(ADP-ribose) polymerase (PARP) were observed, suggesting that induction of apoptosis may be an important mechanism of action of Campath 1H *(61)*.

2.2.2. CLINICAL TRIALS

Phase I studies established a dose of 30 mg iv three times a week for 4–12 wk. Because Campath 1H induces more infusion toxicity than does rituximab, clinical practice is to give Campath 1H using stepped up dosing to diminish initial infusion toxicity. Three milligrams on d 1, 10 mg on

Table 3
Selected Phase II Trials of Thrice Weekly Campath 1H in CLL/SLL

Study	No. of weeks	Route	Prior therapy	No. of evaluable patients	ORR (%) (CR)
Osterborg et al., 1997 (7)	12	iv	Yes	29	42 (4)
Ferrajoli et al., 2001 (97)	4	iv	Yes	41	26 (5)
Rai et al., 2001 (96)	12	iv	Yes	136	40 (7)
Keating et al., 2002 (94)	12	iv	Yes	92	33 (2)
Lundin et al., 2001 (98)	18	sc	No	38	87

CLL, chronic lymphocytic leukemia; SLL, small lymphocytic lymphoma; ORR, overall response rate; CR, complete response.

d 2, and 30 mg on d 3 are administered when initiating therapy. Data from several trials have documented the efficacy of Campath 1H in CLL (7,92–95). The results of these studies are summarized in Table 3. A multicenter, European phase II study of 29 recurrent and refractory CLL patients, treated with Campath 1H 30 mg thrice weekly for up to 12 wk, demonstrated an ORR of 42%, although only one patient (4%) achieved CR (7). Although Campath 1H cleared CLL cells from the peripheral blood in 97% of patients, the antibody was less effective at eliminating marrow (36%) and, in particular, nodal disease (7%).

The pivotal trial in 92 heavily pretreated, fludarabine-refractory CLL patients treated with a similar regimen showed an intent-to-treat ORR of 33%, although only 2% of patients achieved CR (93,94). Projected median time to progression exceeded 9 mo, the median follow-up time of the study, and 71% of responders remained in remission at the time of the report. Median peripheral blood CLL count decreased by more than 99.9%. Whereas 74% of all patients with nodal disease responded, with 27% experiencing resolution of their adenopathy, patients with bulky lymph nodes did significantly poorer. Whereas 90% of patients with lymph nodes measuring 2 cm or less responded, with 64% achieving resolution of their adenopathy, only 59% of patients with lymph nodes greater than 5 cm responded, with no patients enjoying resolution of their adenopathy. All patients were placed on prophylactic antibacterial and antiviral agents, and toxicity was manageable, in contrast to previous trials of Campath 1H. However, patients with poor performance status did markedly worse than patients with no or minimal symptoms from their disease. As a result of this pivotal CAM211 study, Campath 1H was recently approved for the treatment of fludarabine-refractory CLL in the United States.

The activity of Campath 1H in CLL was confirmed by a multi-institutional study in 136 patients with fludarabine-refractory B-CLL who received Campath 1H 30 mg thrice weekly for up to 12 wk on a compassionate basis (96). The ORR was 40% (CR 7%), and the median progression-free and overall survivals of responders were 7.3 and 13.4 mo, respectively. Similarly, in a recent single institution study, 41 patients with relapsed B-CLL and 1 patient with T-CLL were treated with Campath 1H 30 mg iv thrice weekly for 4 wk (97). Two patients with B-CLL achieved CR (5%), and nine patients achieved PR (21%), for an ORR of 26%. Interestingly, 7 of 12 patients with B-cell or T-cell prolymphocytic leukemia (B- or T-PLL) responded (3 CR, 4 PR; ORR 58%). Although Campath 1H was more effective at eliminating disease in peripheral blood (CR 36%, PR 36%) and bone marrow (CR 41%, PR 28%) than in lymph nodes (CR 23%, PR 13%), a greater response in nodal disease was seen in this study than in previous trials using Campath 1H. Although Campath 1H is effective therapy in previously treated patients with CLL, the antibody is less effective against bulky lymphadenopathy than it is against peripheral blood or bone marrow disease.

2.2.3. UPFRONT THERAPY IN PREVIOUSLY UNTREATED PATIENTS

A recent report documented the results of a phase II clinical trial in 41 previously untreated patients with CLL. Patients received a prolonged course of Campath 1H 30 mg by sc administration three times a week for up to 18 wk. Except for transient grade I–II fever, first-dose reactions were minimal. ORR was 87% in the 38 patients who received at least 2 wk of treatment, and the intent-to-treat ORR was 81% (98). Campath 1H was most effective at clearing disease from peripheral blood (CR 95%), but bone marrow (CR 45%, PR 34%) and nodal disease (ORR 87%) also responded to therapy. Interestingly, some patients who achieved CR in the bone marrow required the full 18 wk of therapy to do so, suggesting that prolonged administration of Campath 1H may be necessary to clear CLL from bone marrow. The median time to treatment failure had not been reached at the time of study report (18+ mo). These results confirmed that sc administration of Campath 1H is feasible, as had been initially shown in trials in rheumatoid arthritis, and indicate that longer courses of Campath 1H may produce ORR and CR rates similar to those observed with fludarabine. However, sc administration of Campath 1H is currently not approved for CLL by the Food and Drug Administration (FDA).

2.2.4. CORRELATION OF CD52 EXPRESSION WITH CLINICAL RESPONSE

The greater activity of Campath 1H in T-PLL may be caused by increased expression of CD52 on T-PLL cells. Quantitative flow cytometry was used to measure CD52 expression in 24 B-CLL patients, 21 T-PLL patients, and 12 normal volunteers (99). Interestingly, CD52 expression was significantly higher on normal T-lymphocytes than on normal B-lymphocytes, and T-PLL cells expressed higher levels of CD52 than did B-CLL cells. In addition, CD52 expression was slightly higher in patients who responded to Campath 1H. These results suggest that the likelihood of clinical response to Campath 1H may be related to the level of CD52 expression.

2.2.5. INFECTIOUS COMPLICATIONS

Infections constitute the major complication of Campath 1H therapy (84,100,101). All 50 previously treated indolent NHL patients in a multicenter European study developed profound lymphopenia. Opportunistic infections and bacterial septicemia occurred in 14 and 18% of patients, respectively, and 6% of patients died of infectious complications (102). Infections occurred in 55% of patients (27% grade 3–4) in the pivotal CAM211 study, and 13% developed septicemia (94). Although Campath 1H also inhibits B-cells, CD8+ T-cells, natural killer (NK) cells, and monocytes, the antibody's most profound effects are on CD4+ T-lymphocytes (103–105). Treatment with a course of 5–10 daily iv infusions of Campath 1H resulted in almost complete depletion of lymphocytes, but repopulation of lymphocyte subsets occurred with varying kinetics. NK cells and monocytes recovered to normal levels within 1–2 mo, whereas B-cell numbers returned to normal within 5 mo. However, CD8+ T-cells returned to 50% of pretreatment levels by 2 mo but did not increase further, and CD4+ T-cells never reached 20% of pretreatment levels despite 18 mo of follow-up (103).

Paroxysmal nocturnal hemoglobinuria (PNH)-like T-cells emerge during or immediately after Campath 1H treatment in many patients. These PNH-like cells cannot synthesize glycosylphosphatidylinositol (GPI) anchor glycans and, therefore, lack GPI-linked surface proteins, including CD52. As a result, these cells are resistant to CD52-mediated killing. Preliminary studies by one group demonstrated that, even though they lack GPI-linked proteins, these PNH-like T-cells are functional immune effector cells *(106)*. This finding may explain why the great majority of severe opportunistic infections that occur with Campath 1H are observed during active Campath 1H therapy rather than after treatment.

Lymphocyte recovery may depend on the dosing schedule, as the absolute CD4+ T-cell count reached a nadir of 2/µL by wk 4 but increased to 84/µL by wk 12 in the CAM211 trial *(94)*. In an analysis of 42 refractory CLL patients (median CD3+ T-cell count 1900/µL) treated with Campath 1H, extreme lymphopenia of less than 30/µL was seen in all patients after a median of 2 wk of therapy. At a median follow-up of 14 mo, the median CD3+ T-cell count recovered to 930/µL and the median CD4+ T-cell count to 320/µL *(106)*. Recently, Campath 1H was found to deplete CD52+ myeloid peripheral blood dendritic cells, resulting in inhibition of the stimulatory activity of peripheral blood mononuclear cells (PBMCs) in allogeneic mixed lymphocyte reactions. Depletion of CD52+ dendritic cells also inhibited the ability of PBMCs to present antigen to purified CD4+ T-lymphocytes *(107)*. This effect has been hypothesized to explain the low rate of graft-vs-host-disease (GVHD) in allogeneic stem cell transplants using Campath 1H *(108,109)*.

This prolonged inhibition of T-lymphocyte and dendritic cell function probably will limit the clinical use of Campath 1H, particularly in the setting of combination regimens with other immunosuppressive agents such as fludarabine. It is imperative that patients receiving Campath 1H be placed on adequate prophylaxis for *Pneumocystis carinii* pneumonia (PCP) and varicella zoster virus (VZV). In addition, patients should also be monitored for cytomegalovirus (CMV) reactivation. With these prophylactic measures, Campath 1H can be administered safely and with acceptable toxicity.

2.2.6. INFUSION TOXICITY

Infusion-related toxicity occurred in 93% of patients in the CAM211 study, although most reactions were grade 1 or 2. Rigors (90% overall, 14% grade 3), fever (85% overall, 17% grade 3, 3% grade 4), and nausea (53%) were the most infusion-related toxicities *(94)*. Similar rates of rigors (71%), fevers (65%), and nausea (45%) were reported in the multicenter study of 136 B-CLL patients, and almost all infusion toxicities were grade 1 or 2 *(96)*. As has been previously described, most toxicity was observed with the first Campath 1H infusion *(94)*. This first-dose cytokine release syndrome involves TNF-α, IFN-γ, and IL-6 *(110)*. TNF-α levels increase by more than 1000-fold after Campath 1H infusion, and TNF-α has been postulated to be the most important cytokine in this syndrome *(111,112)*. In vitro models demonstrate that ligation of the low-affinity Fc receptor for IgG, FcγR, on NK cells results in release of TNF-α and suggest that this pathway may play a role in inducing infusion toxicity to Campath 1H *(110)*.

2.2.7. HEMATOLOGICAL TOXICITY

Hematological toxicity has been observed in phase II studies of Campath 1H. The multi-institutional trial in 136 B-CLL patients noted 26% neutropenia (22% grade 3 or 4), 35% thrombocytopenia (23% grade 3 or 4), and 21% anemia (11% grade 3) *(96)*. In contrast to infusion toxicity, which is predominantly grade 1 or 2, many patients who develop cytopenias develop more severe grade 3 or 4 toxicity, including severe or life-threatening infections. Although patients may find infusion toxicities such as fever, rigors, and nausea to be more bothersome and uncomfortable, cytopenias and infectious complications constitute the medically serious toxicities of Campath 1H. These toxicities result from ubiquitous expression of CD52 on many hematopoietic cells and are clinically manageable with careful monitoring of peripheral blood counts. Growth factor support with granulocyte/macrophage colony-stimulating factor (GM-CSF) should be avoided, as GM-CSF worsens infusion-related toxicity, by nonspecific immune activation and induction of TNF-α without significantly improving granulocyte recovery (111). The use of G-CSF in this setting is under study.

2.2.8. COMBINATION THERAPY

Until recently, there were few data regarding the use of Campath 1H in combination therapy regimens. Laboratory evidence from our institution indicates that Campath 1H acts through similar apoptotic pathways as fludarabine and may synergize with fludarabine in vivo (61). Preliminary clinical evidence in five CLL patients, refractory to fludarabine alone and Campath 1H alone, suggests that such synergy exists. Fludarabine was given at a dose of 25 mg/m^2 iv for 3–5 d, and Campath 1H was given at 30 mg iv three times weekly for 8–16 wk. Two patients (40%) achieved a CR, and two (40%) achieved a PR; flow cytometric analysis could not detect residual CLL cells in the two CR patients. Patients received prophylactic cotrimoxazole and acyclovir, and no serious adverse events were noted (113).

Two recent reports suggest that the combination of Campath 1H and rituximab can be given safely and may have clinical activity in patients with relapsed CLL. Nine patients received rituximab 375 mg/m^2 during wk 1 and 3–5, in combination with Campath 1H 3, 10, or 30 mg thrice weekly during wk 2–5 in a single-institution phase I dose escalation study (114). Toxicity was acceptable, with no opportunistic infections or treatment-related deaths. Eight patients (89%) experienced significant reduction in absolute lymphocyte count, with a median decrease of 95%, but no objective responses by NCI criteria were seen. Another single-institution study administered rituximab, 375 mg/m^2 weekly for 4 doses, with Campath 1H 30 mg on d 3 and 5 of each week, to 25 patients with previously treated indolent B-cell lymphoproliferative disorders (115). Fourteen patients with CLL and seven patients with CLL/PLL were evaluable for response. Ten of 21 patients with CLL and CLL/PLL achieved a response (48%) by NCI criteria, with a median time to progression of 6 mo, although only a single patient achieved a CR (5%). Similar to results observed with single-agent Campath 1H, a higher response rate was seen in peripheral blood (95% ORR) than in bone marrow (28%) or nodal disease (67%). Fever and rigors (69%) were the most common toxicity, and 54% of patients developed infection.

2.2.9. SUMMARY

Because of the ubiquitous expression of CD52 on lymphocytes and monocytes, Campath 1H causes significantly more hematological and immune toxicity than does rituximab. However, infectious complications are manageable with adequate antibiotic prophylaxis. Most patients receiving Campath 1H experience infusion toxicity, but toxicity is manageable with a "stepped up" dosing schedule. In addition, infusion toxicity usually diminishes as therapy progresses. Campath 1H has clinical activity in CLL, and the antibody demonstrates particular efficacy in T-PLL, a disorder for which few current therapies exist. Campath 1H demonstrates greatest activity against CLL cells in blood, although prolonged therapy may be able to achieve CR in bone marrow. The antibody is less effective against nodal disease; responses, although common, are almost exclusively PR. Further studies of Campath 1H, especially in combination with cytotoxic agents or other monoclonal antibodies, are warranted.

2.3. Hu1D10

2.3.1. PRECLINICAL STUDIES

Hu1D10 (apolizumab, Remitogen®) is a humanized murine IgG monoclonal antibody whose antigenic epitope is a polymorphic determinant on the MHC class II HLA-DR β-chain (116). The

1D10 epitope is a variant of the HLA-DR β-chain and is not shed or downregulated by antibody binding *(117)*. The 1D10 antigen is present on normal and malignant B-lymphocytes, dendritic cells, macrophages, and some activated T-lymphocytes. The 1D10 antigen is expressed in 50% of acute lymphocytic leukemias, 50% of diffuse large cell NHLs, 50–70% of follicular center cell NHLs, and 80–90% of CLLs *(118)*. Expression is uniformly strong in tumors that are ID10-positive. The secondary structure of the β-chain is important for recognition of the epitope, but N-linked glycosylation does not appear to be involved in antigen recognition. The 1D10 antigen is similar, but not identical, to the Lym-1 epitope on HLA-DR.

Hu1D10 induces both ADCC and CDC, and Hu1D10 is more effective at mediating ADCC than murine 1D10 in standard chromium release assays (116). Hu1D10 also induces apoptosis, induces changes in intracellular calcium concentrations, and increases tyrosine phosphorylation in 1D10-positive cells. Data indicate that apoptosis occurs by a caspase-independent pathway. Preliminary in vitro data from our laboratory demonstrated maximal induction of apoptosis after incubation with 10 μg/mL Hu1D10 and goat anti-human Fc antibody, and apoptosis occurred in the absence of complement or effector cells *(118)*. Incubation with Hu1D10 alone did not induce apoptosis, and further experiments with anti-Fcγ and F(ab')2 secondary F(ab')2 fragments provided further evidence that Fc-specific binding is necessary for apoptosis. Pharmacokinetic data obtained in rhesus monkeys indicated a significantly shorter half-life in 1D10+ animals (2.6 d) than in 1D10- animals (8.4 d), with a 2.6-fold lower area under the curve (AUC). A rapid decline in serum Hu1D10 concentration was seen in 1D10+ animals, probably because of a large antigen sink and development of anti-Hu1D10 antibodies. Preliminary pharmacokinetic data in humans indicate a median serum half-life of approximately 11 d, although profound interpatient variability was observed.

2.3.2. Clinical Studies

An initial phase I study in 20 patients with NHL demonstrated that Hu1D10 can be given safely at doses that show potential clinical efficacy *(119)*. Patients received weekly doses ranging from 0.15 to 5 mg/kg, and a regimen giving the drug on 5 consecutive d was also examined. As is the case with other monoclonal antibody therapies, infusion-related toxicity was common but manageable. Observed side effects included fever, chills, nausea, vomiting, rash, flushing, and hypotension, but most toxicities were grade 1 or 2. Hu1D10 showed exciting clinical promise in this phase I trial; four of eight patients with follicular lymphoma achieved clinical response (1 CR, 3 PR), with a median time to response of 106 d. A recent report summarized preliminary results of a phase II multicenter study in patients with relapsed or refractory indolent B-cell lymphoproliferative disorders. Twenty-one patients have received Hu1D10 0.5 or 1.5 mg/kg weekly for 4 doses, including five patients with SLL *(120)*. Therapy has been well tolerated, although no response data have been reported. We are currently conducting a phase I dose escalation study of thrice weekly Hu1D10 in patients with relapsed CLL; initial results have been promising *(121)*.

2.3.3. Summary

Hu1D10 is a promising monoclonal antibody that is being evaluated in ongoing clinical trials. Antigen expression appears to be more uniform than CD20 expression, and 80–90% of CLL cells express 1D10. Hu1D10 administration appears to be safe, and preliminary data indicate that 3–6 mo may be necessary to see maximal response to the antibody. Although there is little information on Hu1D10's clinical efficacy in CLL, an ongoing phase I and subsequently planned phase II study will address this question.

3. RADIOLABELED MONOCLONAL ANTIBODIES

3.1. ^{131}I-Lym-1

Whereas monoclonal antibodies such as rituximab and Campath 1H rely on host immune mechanisms such as CDC and ADCC to kill tumor cells, radioimmunotherapy uses the antigen specificity of a monoclonal antibody to deliver targeted radiation therapy to tumor cells. The monoclonal antibody Lym-1 recognizes an antigenic determinant on HLA-DR, near the 1D10 epitope. However, the epitopes of the two antibodies are distinct. Initial studies in human tumor cell lines demonstrated that Lym-1 stained B-cell leukemia and lymphoma cell lines but did not react with cells of T-cell, myeloid, or erythroid lineage. Approximately 8% of normal circulating peripheral blood lymphocytes stained for Lym-1 by flow cytometry. Forty percent of B-CLL samples were positive for Lym-1, whereas T lymphocytes and T-cell lymphomas were negative by both immunoperoxidase stains and flow cytometry. Thus, Lym-1 specifically recognizes B-cell malignancies but reacts with fewer than 40% of B-CLL samples.

Lym-1 has been conjugated to ^{131}I in order to effect targeted delivery of this radioactive isotope to tumor cells of B-cell origin. Although ^{131}I-Lym-1 has been tested primarily in patients with advanced NHL, the antibody has been given to several patients with B-CLL. Twenty-five patients with previously treated, advanced B-NHL and five patients with relapsed B-CLL were treated with fractionated, low-dose ^{131}I-Lym-1, with a goal of 300 mCi per patient (122). Thirty percent of patients developed HAMAs, but only three patients had therapy interrupted as a result. Four of the five CLL patients responded (80%). The same group also reported that patients who responded to ^{131}I-Lym-1 therapy enjoyed improved survival (84 vs 22 wk) (123). Radiation dosimetry studies revealed a lower tumor radiation dose and a higher liver radiation exposure in CLL patients, compared with NHL patients, resulting in a lower therapeutic index for patients with CLL (124). Toxicity was acceptable, and the dose-limiting toxicity was thrombocytopenia (125).

3.2. ^{90}Y-T101 and Other Anti-CD5 Antibodies

CD5 (T1, Leu-1), a mature T-cell marker that is also expressed in CLL, is the ligand for CD72, which is expressed on all B-lymphocytes. Evidence suggests that CD5 stimulates splenic B-cell activation and proliferation through its interaction with CD72 on splenic B-lymphocytes (126). Interestingly, in vitro studies showed that crosslinking of CD5 on resting B-lymphocytes, but not on T-lymphocytes, led to apoptosis (127–129). The T101 monoclonal antibody, which recognizes CD5, has been conjugated to ^{90}Y in order to increase its activity against tumor cells. Preclinical studies in human leukemia CEM cells demonstrated that T101 is internalized slowly and undergoes little lysosomal degradation. Instead, T101 undergoes recycling to the cell surface, thus providing a possible explanation for the unmodified antibody's low anti-cancer efficacy (130). Thus, conjugation to a radioisotope was necessary to increase the clinical activity of T101.

In a phase I study, two patients with CLL and eight patients with cutaneous T-cell lymphoma (CTCL) were treated with 5 or 10 mCi of ^{90}Y-T101 (131). Therapy was complicated by development of HAMAs after 1 cycle in 9 of 10 patients. Even though only one patient received a second cycle of therapy, both CLL patients and three CTCL patients achieved PR (50%) with a median response duration of 23 wk. However, significant hematological toxicity was observed, with T-cell and B-cell suppression lasting for 2–3 wk and more than 5 wk, respectively.

Finally, the anti-CD5 monoclonal antibody OKT1 has been conjugated to saporin-6 (SAP), a plant ribosome-inactivating protein. Fresh CLL cells from 31 patients were exposed in vitro to OKT1-SAP. OKT1-SAP inhibited CLL proliferation in 90% of patients; this inhibition was dose-dependent, with a 50% inhibitory concentration (IC_{50}) of 4–7 nM (132).

4. TOXIN-CONJUGATED MONOCLONAL ANTIBODIES (IMMUNOTOXINS)

4.1. LMB-2

An alternative approach to radioimmunotherapy is conjugation of a monoclonal antibody to a toxin. The antibody delivers the toxin to the tumor cell, which is killed by action of the toxin. LMB-2 [anti-Tac(Fv)-PE38] is a recombinant immunotoxin derived by fusion of the variable Fv portion of the anti-CD25 monoclonal antibody anti-Tac to a truncated form of *Pseudomonas* exotoxin A *(133)*. CD25 (Tac) is the β-chain of the high-affinity IL-2 receptor and is expressed on the cell surface of T-cell malignancies, including T-CLL *(134,135)*. LMB-2 induced major responses, including one CR, in four of four patients with refractory hairy cell leukemia in an initial phase I clinical study, demonstrating that Fv-based agents can be effective clinically *(133)*. In a phase I dose escalation trial, 35 patients with CD25+ lymphomas and leukemias received LMB-2 at dose levels ranging from 2 to 63 µg/kg iv every other day for 3 doses; the maximum tolerated dose was 40 µg/kg *(136)*. One patient with CLL achieved PR, and 7 other patients with other diseases also responded (1 CR, 6 PR). Recently, in vitro studies of DSP30, an immunostimulatory phosphorothioate oligodeoxynucleotide, demonstrated that DSP30 increased CD25 expression in 14 of 15 CLL samples. More importantly, DSP30 increased the cytotoxicity of LMB-2 in 12 of 13 CLL samples *(137)*. These results indicate that immunomodulatory molecules can increase expression of target antigens on CLL cells and thereby increase activity of monoclonal antibodies against CLL cells. The use of such molecules to increase the antitumor activity of monoclonal antibody therapy is an area of active research.

4.2. hLL2 and BL22

CD22 (Leu-14), the ligand for CD45RO, is expressed on normal B-lymphocytes and B-cell malignancies including CLL; CD22 is recognized by the murine IgG2 monoclonal antibody LL2 (138). Humanized anti-CD22 (hLL2, epratuzumab) is undergoing phase I/II clinical trials in indolent B-cell NHL, and studies in CLL are being planned *(139,140)*. Preclinical in vitro studies demonstrated that LL2 was rapidly internalized after binding to Raji lymphoma cells, eventually undergoing lysosomal degradation *(141)*. To take advantage of this rapid internalization and degradation, LL2 has been conjugated to radioisotopes and biological effectors. LL2 has been conjugated to both ^{131}I and ^{90}Y. An initial phase I clinical study with ^{131}I-LL2 revealed no acute toxicities, and two of five evaluable patients achieved PR. However, grade IV marrow toxicity was observed in three of seven patients who received total doses of 50 mCi, and three of eight patients who received at least two injections developed HAMA *(142)*. Subsequent clinical trials of ^{131}I-LL2 in relapsed NHL have demonstrated promising activity, with three of seven patients achieving PR in one study, and 7 of 21 patients (5 CR, 2 PR) responding in another trial *(143,144)*. Two recent reports described the preliminary results of clinical trials of ^{90}Y-hLL2. In one of the reports, 18 patients with indolent B-cell lymphoproliferative disorders received 2–4 weekly infusions of 2.5 or 5.0 mCi ^{90}Y-hLL2; 7 responses were seen, although the single CLL patient did not respond *(145)*. In the second study 20 evaluable patients with recurrent B-cell NHL received ^{131}I-hLL2 (13 patients) or ^{90}Y-hLL2 (7 patients). Myelosuppression was the primary toxicity, and ^{90}Y-hLL2 appeared to exhibit more favorable tumor dosimetry than ^{131}I-hLL2 *(146)*.

LL2 has also been conjugated to biological effectors. BL22 [RFB4(dsFv)-PE38] is a recombinant immunotoxin generated by fusion of the variable Fv portion of the anti-CD22 monoclonal antibody RFB4 to a truncated form of *Pseudomonas* exotoxin A. In ex vivo experiments with fresh tumor cells from 28 patients with B-cell malignancies, including CLL and follicle center

NHL, BL22 was cytotoxic to cells of 25 patients (89%), indicating the potential clinical use of this immunotoxin (147). A recent report documented the efficacy of BL22 in 16 patients with cladribine-resistant hairy cell leukemia (148). Eleven patients achieved CR (69%), and two patients attained PR (13%). In addition, LL2 has been conjugated to onconase, an amphibian ribonuclease. In preclinical studies, exposure to LL2-onconase was lethal to human Daudi lymphoma cells. LL2-onconase was tolerable to mice and increased the life span of SCID mice inoculated with Daudi lymphoma cells (149). Although the results of in vitro and animal studies have been intriguing, there are no data regarding the safety or efficacy of LL2-onconase in humans. Even though there are no data on the use of LL2 or its radioisotope or immunotoxin conjugates in CLL, studies of hLL2 are warranted, given preclinical evidence of activity against CLL cells (147).

4.3. Anti-B4

CD19 (B4, Leu-12) is expressed on pre-B- and B-lymphocytes. In preclinical studies, the anti-CD19 monoclonal antibody HD37 was conjugated to the ribosome-inactivating protein SAP. HD37-SAP inhibited DNA synthesis in fresh CLL cells and was able to exert greater than a 2-log kill in B-NHL cells (150). HD37 has been conjugated to a deglycosylated ricin A chain and tested in patients with NHL, although no CLL patients were enrolled in the phase I trial (151). Anti-B4 was conjugated to blocked ricin to generate an immunotoxin (anti-B4-bR), which was administered by 7-d continuous iv infusion to 34 patients with relapsed or refractory B-cell neoplasms in a phase I clinical trial, including 4 patients with CLL. Five clinical responses (two CR, three PR) were observed, in addition to 11 transient responses (152). The same authors also administered anti-B4-bR by 5 consecutive daily bolus infusions to 25 patients with refractory B-cell neoplasms; three responses (one CR, two PR) were observed (153).

4.4. Anti-CD23

CD23 is another potential target of monoclonal antibody therapy; like CD20 and CD5, CD23 is expressed on the overwhelming majority of CLL cells. A chimeric macaque-derived anti-CD23 antibody, p6G5G1, has been developed (154). Although these antibodies have been developed as possible therapies for asthma and other allergic disorders, the ubiquitous expression of CD23 on CLL cells indicates that preclinical studies of these compounds in CLL should be pursued. Recently, in vitro studies of a humanized anti-CD23 monoclonal antibody, IDEC-152, demonstrated that crosslinked IDEC-152 induced apoptosis in fresh CLL cells from five patients. In addition, IDEC-152-induced apoptosis was enhanced in the presence of fludarabine or rituximab (155). These promising preclinical results indicate that phase I clinical studies should be undertaken.

5. ANTI-CYTOKINE MONOCLONAL ANTIBODIES

5.1. Cytokine Modulation

A growing area of interest in monoclonal antibody research is the use of cytokine modulation to increase the activity of antibody therapies. Cytokine modulation can induce apoptosis and increase activity of host immune effector cells, thereby enhancing the antitumor activity of monoclonal antibodies. There are many ongoing clinical trials of combined immunotherapy with cytokines and monoclonal antibodies in hematological and solid malignancies. Rituximab has been combined with IL-2 and IL-12 in phase I/II clinical trials in B-cell NHL, and initial results have been promising (156–158). An alternative approach to cytokine-based immunotherapy is the development of anticytokine monoclonal antibodies. Such antibodies may be effective as single agents or they may be used as immunomodulators to enhance the efficacy of tumor-targeted antibodies such as rituximab and Campath 1H. Several such antibodies are in preclinical development, and this section will focus on the scientific rationale for use of each of these antibodies.

5.2. Anti-TNF-α

TNF-α stimulates the proliferation of CLL cells *(159,160)*. Serum levels of TNF-α are increased in patients with CLL, and CLL cells produce TNF-α as an autocrine growth regulator *(161,162)*. Two TNF-α antagonists have been approved by the FDA for clinical use: (1) infliximab, a chimeric anti-TNF-α monoclonal antibody; and (2) etanercept, a recombinant soluble TNF-α receptor/Fc fusion protein. Etanercept (Enbrel®) has been approved for use in rheumatoid arthritis *(163,164)*, and there are data supporting its use in the treatment of myelodysplastic syndrome (MDS), myelofibrosis with myeloid metaplasia, and chronic GVHD *(165–167)*. In addition, etanercept is undergoing active clinical study in a number of other malignancies. Infliximab (cA2), which has been approved for use in rheumatoid arthritis and Crohn's disease *(168–170)*, has shown activity in the therapy of steroid-refractory GVHD *(171)*. In addition to neutralizing soluble TNF-α and depriving CLL cells of a vital growth signal, infliximab may also act via binding of transmembrane TNF-α, leading to lysis of TNF-α expressing cells by ADCC and CDC *(172)*. Infliximab is undergoing clinical investigation in several malignancies, and investigation of infliximab and etanercept as potential therapies in CLL, either as single agents or in combination with antibodies such as rituximab, is warranted.

5.3. Anti-Interferon-γ

Another cytokine important in maintaining the survival of CLL cells is IFN-γ. In preclinical laboratory studies, IFN-γ inhibited apoptosis of CLL cells in culture and resulted in prolonged survival. Purified CLL cells synthesized high levels of IFN-γ, indicating an autocrine pathway of tumor cell activation *(173)*. In the same report, 7 of 10 CLL patients demonstrated increased serum levels of IFN-γ, compared with none of 10 healthy control individuals. A later report showed overexpression of IFN-γ receptors by CLL cells, as well as increased numbers of IFN-γ-producing T-lymphocytes in patients with CLL *(174)*. These studies provided in vitro and in vivo evidence of the anti-apoptotic activity of IFN-γ in CLL. Anti-IFN-γ monoclonal antibodies have been administered in clinical trials of rheumatoid arthritis; initial results indicate that these antibodies are safe and have clinical activity *(175)*. Similar to the TNF-α antibodies infliximab and etanercept, the IFN-γ antibodies were developed for treatment of rheumatological disorders but should be investigated in phase I/II clinical trials in CLL.

5.4. Anti-IL-4

Several interleukins inhibit apoptosis of CLL cells and are, therefore, potential targets of pharmacological intervention by interleukin antagonists. IL-4 is one of the best studied of these interleukins. Initial in vitro studies demonstrated that IL-4 inhibits the TNF-α-induced proliferation of CLL cells, leading to interest in IL-4 as a cytokine therapy for CLL *(176,177)*. However, a phase I dose escalation trial of IL-4 in 14 patients with CLL who were in PR after treatment with chemotherapy yielded no responses. In fact, 10 patients (71%) had progressive disease, with a two- to fourfold increase in the blood lymphocyte count, providing in vivo evidence of the anti-apoptotic effects of IL-4 *(178)*. Interestingly, the blood lymphocyte count decreased after cessation of IL-4 therapy in 8 of 12 evaluable patients. These clinical results concurred with more recent in vitro studies, which showed that IL-4 inhibits apoptosis and maintains viability of CLL cells *(179,180)*. In addition, IL-4 conferred greater protection against apoptosis upon CLL cells from previously treated patients than upon tumor cells from untreated patients, suggesting that the anti-apoptotic action of IL-4 may be one mechanism by which CLL becomes resistant to therapy *(179)*. Recent studies revealed that T-lymphocytes from patients with B-CLL secrete IL-4 and protect B-CLL cells from apoptosis *(181,182)*. A further indication of the importance of IL-4 in maintaining CLL viability and growth was shown by the increased expression of mRNA for IL-4 receptor in fresh CLL cells *(182)*. Thus, preclinical and clinical data support clinical trials of IL-4 antagonists as potential therapeutic agents in CLL.

5.5. Anti-IL-8

Another potential cytokine target of monoclonal antibody therapy in CLL is IL-8. In vitro studies demonstrated constitutive secretion of IL-8 by CLL cells; in contrast, several B-cell lines and cells from hairy cell leukemia patients did not express IL-8 *(183)*. The same authors later showed that, although IL-8 did not induce proliferation of CLL cells, IL-8 protected CLL cells against steroid-induced death. IL-8 increased expression of bcl-2 mRNA and protein, and exogenous IL-8 induced overexpression of IL-8 mRNA, suggesting an autocrine role for IL-8 in maintaining CLL cell survival *(184)*. Fully human anti-IL-8 monoclonal antibodies have been synthesized, as well as a polyethylene glycol (PEG)-conjugated form of a humanized anti-IL-8 F(ab')(2) antibody *(185,186)*. Preclinical evidence suggests that further work should be undertaken to determine whether clinical studies with these antibodies should be pursued in CLL.

6. PRACTICAL ASPECTS OF MONOCLONAL ANTIBODY ADMINISTRATION

As monoclonal antibodies become an increasingly important treatment option in CLL, we wish to share our observations on the clinical administration of rituximab and Campath 1H, the two antibody therapies currently approved for CLL. In particular, we wish to emphasize infusion reactions unique to CLL, which are not necessarily observed in NHL or solid tumor patients, as well as practical differences between the administration of rituximab and the use of Campath 1H.

6.1. Predictors of Infusion Toxicity

The spectrum of infusion reactions varies widely among patients; some patients develop very severe infusion reactions, whereas others experience no reaction. It would be useful clinically to be able to identify patients who are predisposed to experience more severe infusion reactions. Although multiple clinical and laboratory parameters have been suggested to predict infusion reaction severity, our experience is that increasing age is the only significant predictor of infusion toxicity with rituximab. A second parameter that should be considered is the patient's performance status (PS). The clinical trials that defined the toxicity and efficacy of monoclonal antibodies were conducted, in general, in patients with Eastern Cooperative Oncology Group (ECOG) PS 0–2. In addition, the pivotal CAM211 study of Campath 1H showed that almost all clinical responses occurred in patients with no or minimal symptoms (ECOG PS 0–1); essentially no responses were observed in patients with ECOG PS 2. Thus, care should be taken before administering antibody therapy, particularly Campath 1H, to CLL patients with poor PS; such patients may experience greater toxicity with less likelihood of clinical benefit.

Unfortunately, there does not appear to be any correlation with severity of infusion toxicity to a prior antibody and severity of infusion reaction to a second monoclonal antibody. Thus, all patients should be observed carefully during the first administration of any monoclonal antibody, regardless of their experience with prior antibodies.

6.2. Differences Between Rituximab and Campath 1H

Each monoclonal antibody currently in clinical use or under study in CLL has a slightly different infusion toxicity profile. Differences between antibodies can be observed in the likelihood, severity, timing, and duration of infusion reactions. In general, infusion reactions to Campath 1H are more common, more severe, and less likely to "extinguish" with subsequent doses of antibody than reactions to rituximab. Although infusion toxicity rarely occurs after the second dose of rituximab, infusion reactions can occur with each dose of Campath 1H or Hu1D10 throughout the entire treatment period in some patients. Rituximab reactions are generally mild, whereas rash, hypotension and dyspnea are seen more frequently with Campath 1H and Hu1D10 and often require more pharmacological intervention. Interestingly, patients receiving Hu1D10 often do not develop reactions until several hours into or after infusion of the antibody. Therefore, the monitoring and management of infusion toxicity should be adapted to the antibody being used, as well as to the individual patient.

6.3. Prophylaxis Against Toxicity

Several premedications should be considered to minimize the likelihood and severity of infusion reactions and infectious complications. Although not seen with antibody therapy in patients with solid tumors or NHL, tumor lysis is an uncommon complication of antibody treatment in CLL patients. Allopurinol should be given for the first 7–10 d of therapy, and patients should increase oral fluid intake the night before treatment. All patients who have previously received fludarabine or who are being treated with Campath 1H should receive prophylaxis for PCP and VZV. We place our patients on Bactrim DS® twice daily MWF and acyclovir 400–800 mg three times daily, and we continue prophylaxis indefinitely in the absence of adverse effects. Patients undergoing antibody therapy for relapsed CLL are often immuno-compromised, owing to hypogammaglobulinemia and prior immunosuppressive therapy. To minimize the likelihood and severity of infusion toxicity, Tylenol® (650 mg), Benadryl® (50 mg iv), and a potent antiemetic (granisetron or ondansetron) are given approx 30 min prior to starting the infusion.

6.4. Stepped Up Dosing

A stepped up dosing schedule, in our experience, minimizes the severity of infusion toxicity to monoclonal antibody therapy. A small dose is given by slow iv infusion the first day, and the dose and infusion rate are then increased in stepwise fashion to target levels. Patients receiving thrice weekly rituximab should receive a 100-mg dose over 4 h (25 mg/h) on the first day of therapy. The second dose should be 375 mg/m^2 over 4 h, and subsequent doses can be administered over 1 h each. Patients receiving Campath 1H should receive 3 mg over 2 h on d 1, with escalation of the dose to 10 mg on d 2 and 30 mg on d 3.

6.5. Management of Infusion Toxicity

Patients should be monitored with vital signs and pulse oximetry at a minimum of every 15–30 min during antibody infusion. A crash cart and ACLS trained staff should be available to respond to severe infusion reactions. If a reaction occurs, the infusion should be stopped immediately and symptoms treated appropriately. Common infusion toxicities (and their management) include hypotension (iv hydration), asymptomatic hypoxemia (supplemental oxygen), wheezing (oxygen and inhaled B2 agonist), and rigors (Demerol). Severe infusion toxicities may require administration of an iv H2 blocker or, if the reaction is life-threatening, hydrocortisone. However, steroids should be avoided unless they are absolutely necessary. After resolution of the

Table 4
Summary of Monoclonal Antibodies Available in CLL/SLL

Antibody	Antigen	Description	Clinical status
IDEC-C2B8 (rituximab)	CD20	Chimeric	FDA approved
Campath 1H (alemtuzumab)	CD52	Chimeric	FDA approved
Hu1D10 (apolizumab, remitogen)	1D10 (HLA-DRβ)	Chimeric	Clinical trials
^{131}I-Lym	Lym-1 (HLA-DRβ)	Radiolabeled	Clinical trials
^{90}Y-T101	CD5	Radiolabeled	Clinical trials
LMB-2 [anti-Tac(Fv)-PE38]	CD25	Immunotoxin	Clinical trials
^{90}Y-hLL2/^{131}I-hLL2	CD22	Radiolabeled	Clinical trials
BL22 [RFB4(dsFv)-PE38]	CD22	Immunotoxin	Clinical trials
Anti-B4-bR	CD19	Immunotoxin	Clinical trials

CLL, chronic lymphocytic leukemia; SLL, small lymphocytic lymphoma; FDA, Food and Drug Administration.

acute toxicity, the antibody infusion should be restarted at a slower rate. When side effects result in prolongation of the infusion time, it may be necessary to repeat doses of Benadryl and Tylenol. Patients should be monitored for at least 60 min after completion of the first antibody infusion, to observe for possible delayed toxicity. Patients with significant thrombocytopenia should undergo a repeat platelet count after antibody infusion, as approx 50% of these patients will develop transient, severe thrombocytopenia. Thrombocytopenic patients who are receiving Campath 1H should be considered for prophylactic platelet transfusions. With both Campath 1H and rituximab, patients will often develop some degree of fatigue during treatment, although most can continue performing daily tasks. Fatigue generally resolves within a few weeks of completing therapy, particularly if the patient has experienced a clinical response.

With subsequent doses, vital sign monitoring may be done less frequently, and patients may be able to leave immediately after completion of the antibody infusion. Patients who tolerate infusions without significant toxicity may have their premedications reduced or eliminated. However, it is important to continue observing patients for infusion reactions, as some patients will develop infusion toxicity to later doses, especially with Campath 1H. Patients should be educated on symptom management and parameters to seek medical attention. Assessment of fevers can be problematic, as patients often develop benign fevers several hours after Campath 1H treatment, yet are often immunosuppressed. Each fever should be managed on a case-by-case basis, depending on the patient's history and the physician's judgment.

7. CONCLUSIONS

Monoclonal antibody therapy for CLL is an area of exciting and active research. Although monoclonal antibodies such as rituximab and Campath 1H have shown great promise in CLL, clinical trials have clearly demonstrated that the use of single-agent monoclonal antibody therapy is unlikely to yield long-term survival. Thus, ongoing clinical studies are examining the optimal use of monoclonal antibodies in combination treatment regimens. Regimens combining monoclonal antibodies with fludarabine and other traditional cytotoxic chemotherapeutic agents have been promising, and several trials are currently studying the use of combination antibody regimens. In addition, studies are investigating newer antibodies such as Hu1D10 and anti-CD22 (LL2, BL22), as well as antibodies conjugated to radioisotopes (^{90}Y, ^{131}I) and toxins (*Pseudomonas* exotoxin A).

Finally, an increasing area of research is cytokine modulation by use of antibodies directed against anti-apoptotic cytokines that maintain the survival of CLL cells. Although such studies are in their infancy, they may eventually to prove to have the most potential. Thus, there are multiple avenues deserving further investigation in the antibody therapy of CLL (Table 4). As more potential antibodies are brought into clinical trials, two key challenges will be (1) identification of the role of each agent and (2) determination of the best combinations of these agents.

Although many monoclonal antibodies being studied in CLL are also in clinical trials in indolent B-cell NHL and other lymphomas, CLL poses unique challenges. The results of the weekly rituximab trials serve as a reminder that agents and dosing schedules effective in B-cell NHL are not necessarily efficacious in CLL; they are similar, but different, diseases. In particular, there has been reluctance to use radioisotope-conjugated antibodies in CLL, owing to concern about marrow toxicity. Thus, it is important to differentiate CLL from follicle center and other indolent B-cell NHL in clinical trials. Hopefully, continued research in this growing, exciting field will yield improved long-term survival for patients with CLL.

REFERENCES

1. Sievers EL, Larson RA, Stadtmauer EA, et al. Efficacy and safety of gemtuzumab ozogamicin in patients with CD33-positive acute myeloid leukemia in first relapse. J Clin Oncol 2001;19:3244–3254.
2. Coiffier B, Lepage E, Briere J, et al. CHOP chemotherapy plus rituximab compared with CHOP alone in elderly patients with diffuse large B-cell lymphoma. N Engl J Med 2002;346:235–242.
3. Olsen E, Duvic M, Frankel A, et al. Pivotal phase III trial of two dose levels of denileukin diftitox for the treatment of cutaneous T-cell lymphoma. J Clin Oncol 2001;19:376–388.
4. Byrd JC, Murphy T, Howard RS, et al. Rituximab using a thrice weekly dosing schedule in B-cell chronic lymphocytic leukemia and small lymphocytic lymphoma demonstrates clinical activity and acceptable toxicity. J Clin Oncol 2001;19:2153–2164.
5. Huhn D, von Schilling C, Wilhelm M, et al. Rituximab therapy of patients with B-cell chronic lymphocytic leukemia. Blood 2001;98:1326–1331.
6. McLaughlin P, Grillo-Lopez AJ, Link BK, et al. Rituximab chimeric anti-CD20 monoclonal antibody therapy for relapsed indolent lymphoma: half of patients respond to a four-dose treatment program. J Clin Oncol 1998; 16:2825–2833.
7. Osterborg A, Dyer MJ, Bunjes D, et al. Phase II multicenter study of human CD52 antibody in previously treated chronic lymphocytic leukemia: European Study Group of CAMPATH-1H Treatment in Chronic Lymphocytic Leukemia. J Clin Oncol 1997;15:1567–1574.
8. Sawitsky A, Rai KR, Glidewell O, Silver RT. Comparison of daily versus intermittent chlorambucil and prednisone therapy in the treatment of patients with chronic lymphocytic leukemia. Blood 1977;50:1049–1059.
9. Montserrat E, Alcala A, Parody R, et al. Treatment of chronic lymphocytic leukemia in advanced stages: a randomized trial comparing chlorambucil plus prednisone versus cyclophosphamide, vincristine, and prednisone. Cancer 1985;56:2369–2375.
10. Raphael B, Andersen JW, Silber R, et al. Comparison of chlorambucil and prednisone versus cyclophosphamide, vincristine, and prednisone as initial treatment for chronic lymphocytic leukemia: long-term follow-up of an Eastern Cooperative Oncology Group randomized clinical trial. J Clin Oncol 1991;9:770–776.
11. Grever MR, Leiby J, Kraut E, et al. A comprehensive phase I and II clinical investigation of fludarabine phosphate. Semin Oncol 1990;17(5 suppl 8):39–48.
12. Keating MJ, Kantarjian H, Talpaz M, et al. Fludarabine: a new agent with major activity against chronic lymphocytic leukemia. Blood 1989;74:19–25.
13. Keating MJ, Kantarjian H, O'Brien S, et al. Fludarabine: a new agent with marked cytoreductive activity in untreated chronic lymphocytic leukemia. J Clin Oncol 1991;9:44–49.
14. Keating MJ, O'Brien S, Kantarjian H, et al. Long-term follow-up of patients with chronic lymphocytic leukemia treated with fludarabine as a single agent. Blood 1993;81:2878–2884.
15. Keating MJ, O'Brien S, Lerner S, et al. Long-term follow-up of patients with chronic lymphocytic leukemia (CLL) receiving fludarabine regimens as initial therapy. Blood 1998;81:1165–1171.

16. Boogaerts MA, Van Hoof A, Catovsky D, et al. Activity of oral fludarabine phosphate in previously treated chronic lymphocytic leukemia. J Clin Oncol 2001;19:4252–4258.

17. Flinn IW, Byrd JC, Morrison C, et al. Fludarabine and cyclophosphamide with filgrastim support in patients with previously untreated indolent lymphoid malignancies. Blood 2000;96:71–75.

18. O'Brien SM, Kantarjian HM, Cortes J, et al. Results of the fludarabine and cyclophosphamide combination regimen in chronic lymphocytic leukemia. J Clin Oncol 2001;19:1414–1420.

19. Kitada S, Andersen J, Akar S, et al. Expression of apoptosis-regulating proteins in chronic lymphocytic leukemia: correlations with in vitro and in vivo chemoresponses. Blood 1998;91:3379–3389.

20. Golay J, Zaffaroni L, Vaccari T, et al. Biologic response of B lymphoma cells to anti-CD20 monoclonal antibody rituximab in vitro: CD55 and CD59 regulate complement-mediated cell lysis. Blood 2000;95:3900–3908.

21. Treon SP, Mitsiades C, Mitsiades N, et al. Tumor cell expression of CD59 is associated with resistance to CD20 serotherapy in patients with B-cell malignancies. J Immunother 2001;24:263–271.

22. Byrd JC, Kitada S, Flinn IW, et al. The mechanism of tumor cell clearance by rituximab in vivo in patients with B-cell chronic lymphocytic leukemia: evidence of caspase activation and apoptosis induction. Blood 2002;99: 1038–1043.

23. Pedersen IM, Buhl AM, Klausen P, Geisler CH, Jurlander J. The chimeric anti-CD20 antibody rituximab induces apoptosis in B-cell chronic lymphocytic leukemia cells through a p38 mitogen activated protein-kinase-dependent mechanism. Blood 2002;99:1314–1319.

24. Miller RA, Maloney DG, Warnke RA, Levy R. Treatment of B-cell lymphoma with monoclonal anti-idiotype antibody. N Engl J Med 1982;306:517–522.

25. Meeker TC, Lowder J, Maloney DG, et al. A clinical trial of anti-idiotype therapy for B cell malignancy. Blood 1985;65:1349–1363.

26. Brown SL, Miller RA, Horning SJ, et al. Treatment of B-cell lymphomas with anti-idiotype antibodies alone and in combination with alpha interferon. Blood 1989;73:651–661.

27. Brown SL, Miller RA, Levy R. Antiidiotype antibody therapy of B-cell lymphoma. Semin Oncol 1989;16:199–210.

28. Maloney DG, Brown S, Czerwinski DK, et al. Monoclonal anti-idiotype antibody therapy of B-cell lymphoma: the addition of a short course of chemotherapy does not interfere with the antitumor effect nor prevent the emergence of idiotype-negative variant cells. Blood 1992;80:1502–1510.

29. Meeker TC, Lowder J, Cleary ML, et al. Emergence of idiotype variants during treatment of B-cell lymphoma with anti-idiotype antibodies. N Engl J Med 1985;312:1658–1665.

30. Cleary ML, Meeker TC, Levy S, et al. Clustering of extensive somatic mutations in the variable region of an immunoglobulin heavy chain gene from a human B cell lymphoma. Cell 1986;44:97–106.

31. Levy S, Mendel E, Kon S, Avnur Z, Levy R. Mutational hot spots in Ig V region genes of human follicular lymphomas. J Exp Med 1988;168:475–489.

32. Allebes WA, Preijers FW, Haanen C, Capel PJ. The development of non-responsiveness to immunotherapy with monoclonal anti-idiotypic antibodies in a patient with B-CLL. Br J Haematol 1988;70:295–300.

33. Allebes W, Knops R, Herold M, Huber C, Haanen C, Capel P. Immunotherapy with monoclonal anti-idiotypic antibodies: tumour reduction and lymphokine production. Leuk Res 1991;15:215–222.

34. Caulfield MJ, Murthy S, Tubbs RR, Sergi J, Bukowksi RM. Treatment of chronic lymphocytic leukemia with an anti-idiotypic monoclonal antibody. Cleve Clin J Med 1989;56:182–188.

35. Scheinberg DA, Straus DJ, Yeh SD, et al. A phase I toxicity, pharmacology, and dosimetry trial of monoclonal antibody OKB7 in patients with non-Hodgkin's lymphoma: effects of tumor burden and antigen expression. J Clin Oncol 1990;8:792–803.

36. Goodman GE, Hellstrom I, Brodzinsky L, et al. Phase I trial of murine monoclonal antibody L6 in breast, colon, ovarian, and lung cancer. J Clin Oncol 1990;8:1083–1092.

37. Maloney DG, Grillo-Lopez AJ, White CA, et al. IDEC-C2B8 (Rituximab) anti-CD20 monoclonal antibody therapy in patients with relapsed low-grade non-Hodgkin's lymphoma. Blood 1997;90:2188–2195.

38. Pegram MD, Lipton A, Hayes DF, et al. Phase II study of receptor-enhanced chemosensitivity using recombinant humanized anti-p185HER2/neu monoclonal antibody plus cisplatin in patients with HER2/neu-overexpressing metastatic breast cancer refractory to chemotherapy treatment. J Clin Oncol 1998;16: 2659–2671.

39. Baselga JM, Tripathy D, Mendelsohn J, et al. Phase II study of weekly intravenous trastuzumab (Herceptin) in patients with HER2/neu-overexpressing metastatic breast cancer. Semin Oncol 1999;26(4 suppl 12):78–83.

40. Paule B, Cosset JM, Le Bourgeois JP. The possible role of radiotherapy in chronic lymphocytic leukaemia: a critical review. Radiother Oncol 1985;4:45–54.

41. Roncadin M, Arcicasa M, Trovo MG, et al. Splenic irradiation in chronic lymphocytic leukemia: a 10-year experience at a single institution. Cancer 1987;60:2624–2628.

42. Guiney MJ, Liew KH, Quong GG, Cooper IA. A study of splenic irradiation in chronic lymphocytic leukemia. Int J Radiat Oncol Biol Phys 1989;16:225–229.

43. Gupta NK, Cao TM, French JN, et al. Pilot study of Bexxar in advanced previously heavily treated refractory chronic lymphocytic leukemia (CLL). Blood 2001;98:290b.

44. Bubien JK, Zhou LJ, Bell PD, Frizzell RA, Tedder TF. Transfection of the CD20 cell surface molecule into ectopic cell types generates a Ca2+ conductance found constitutively in B lymphocytes. J Cell Biol 1993;121: 1121–1132.

45. Leveille C, Al-Daccak R, Mourad W. CD20 is physically and functionally coupled to MHC class II and CD40 on human B cell lines. Eur J Immunol 1999;29:65–74.

46. Vose JM, Giles FJ, Manshouri T, et al. High levels of soluble CD20 (sCD20) in patients with non-Hodgkin's lymphoma (NHL): correlation with clinical behavior and contrast with patients with Hodgkin's disease (HD). Blood 2001;98:767a.

47. Keating MJ, O'Brien S, Albitar M. Emerging information on the use of rituximab in chronic lymphocytic leukemia. Semin Oncol 2002;29(1 suppl 2):70–74.

48. Golay J, Lazzari M, Facchinetti V, et al. CD20 levels determine the in vitro susceptibility to rituximab and complement of B-cell chronic lymphocytic leukemia: further regulation by CD55 and CD59. Blood 2001;98: 3383–3389.

49. Nguyen DT, Amess JA, Doughty H, Hendry L, Diamond LW. IDEC-C2B8 anti-CD20 (rituximab) immuno-therapy in patients with low-grade non-Hodgkin's lymphoma and lymphoproliferative disorders: evaluation of response on 48 patients. Eur J Haematol 1999;62:76–82.

50. Winkler U, Jensen M, Manzke O, Schulz H, Diehl V, Engert A. Cytokine-release syndrome in patients with B-cell chronic lymphocytic leukemia and high lymphocyte counts after treatment with an anti-CD20 monoclonal antibody (rituximab, IDEC-C2B8). Blood 1999;94:2217–2224.

51. Ladetto M, Bergui L, Ricca I, Campana S, Pileri A, Tarella C. Rituximab anti-CD20 monoclonal antibody induces marked but transient reductions of peripheral blood lymphocytes in chronic lymphocytic leukaemia patients. Med Oncol 2000;17:203–210.

52. Huh YO, Keating MJ, Saffer HL, Jilani I, Lerner S, Albitar M. Higher levels of surface CD20 expression on circulating lymphocytes compared with bone marrow and lymph nodes in B-cell chronic lymphocytic leukemia. Am J Clin Pathol 2001;116:437–443.

53. Hainsworth JD, Burris HA, Morrissey LH, et al. Rituximab as initial therapy for patients with low-grade non-Hodgkin's lymphoma (NHL). Proc Amer Soc Clin Oncol 2000;19:46a.

54. Hainsworth JD. Rituximab as first-line systemic therapy for patients with low-grade lymphoma. Semin Oncol 2000;27(6 suppl 12):25-29.

55. Hainsworth JD, Burris HA, Morrissey LH, et al. Rituximab monoclonal antibody as initial systemic therapy for patients with low-grade non-Hodgkin's lymphoma. Blood 2000;95:3052–3056.

56. Hainsworth JD, Litchy S, Burris HA, Greco FA. Rituximab as first-line and maintenance therapy for patients with small lymphocytic lymphoma (SLL) and chronic lymphocytic leukemia (CLL). Blood 2001;98:363a.

57. Thomas DA, O'Brien S, Giles FJ, et al. Single agent rituxan in early stage chronic lymphocytic leukemia (CLL). Blood 2001;98:364a.

58. Ginaldi L, De Martinis M, Matutes E, Farahat N, Morilla R, Catovsky D. Levels of expression of CD19 and CD20 in chronic B cell leukaemias. J Clin Pathol 1998;51:364–369.

59. Perz J, Topaly J, Fruehauf S, Hensel M, Ho AD. Level of CD20 expression and efficacy of rituximab treatment in patients with resistant or relapsing B-cell prolymphocytic leukemia and B-cell chronic lymphocytic leukemia. Leuk Lymphoma 2002;43:149–151.

60. Berinstein NL, Grillo-Lopez AJ, White CA, et al. Association of serum rituximab (IDEC-C2B8) concentration and anti-tumor response in the treatment of recurrent low-grade or follicular non-Hodgkin's lymphoma. Ann Oncol 1998;9:995–1001.

61. Byrd JC. Personal communication. 2001.

62. Keating MJ, O'Brien S. High-dose rituximab therapy in chronic lymphocytic leukemia. Semin Oncol 2000;27(6 suppl 12):86-90.

63. O'Brien SM, Kantarjian H, Thomas DA, et al. Rituximab dose-escalation trial in chronic lymphocytic leukemia. J Clin Oncol 2001;19:2165–2170.

64. Byrd JC, Waselenko JK, Maneatis TJ, et al. Rituximab therapy in hematologic malignancy patients with circulating blood tumor cells: association with increased infusion-related side effects and rapid blood tumor clearance. J Clin Oncol 1999;17:791–795.

65. Jensen M, Winkler U, Manzke O, Diehl V, Engert A. Rapid tumor lysis in a patient with B-cell chronic lymphocytic leukemia and lymphocytosis treated with an anti-CD20 monoclonal antibody (IDEC-C2B8, rituximab). Ann Hematol 1998;77:89–91.

66. Czuczman MS, Grillo-Lopez AJ, White CA, et al. Treatment of patients with low-grade B-cell lymphoma with the combination of chimeric anti-CD20 monoclonal antibody and CHOP chemotherapy. J Clin Oncol 1999;17: 268–276.

67. Keating MJ, O'Brien S, Lerner S, et al. Combination chemo-antibody therapy with fludarabine (F), cyclophosphamide (C) and rituximab (R) achieves a high CR rate in previously untreated chronic lymphocytic leukemia (CLL). Blood 2000;96:514a.

68. McLaughlin P, Hagemeister FB, Rodriguez MA, et al. Safety of fludarabine, mitoxantrone, and dexamethasone combined with rituximab in the treatment of stage IV indolent lymphoma. Semin Oncol 2000;27:37–41.

69. Vose JM, Link BK, Grossbard ML, et al. Phase II study of rituximab in combination with CHOP chemotherapy in patients with previously untreated, aggressive non-Hodgkin's lymphoma. J Clin Oncol 2001;19:389–397.

70. Byrd JC, Peterson BL, Park K, et al. Rituximab added to fludarabine improves response in previously untreated chronic lymphocytic leukemia: preliminary results from CALGB 9712. Proc Am Soc Clin Oncol 2001;20:280a.

71. Byrd JC, Peterson BL, Park K, et al. Concurrent rituximab and fludarabine has a higher complete response rate than sequential treatment in untreated chronic lymphocytic leukemia (CLL) patients: results from CALGB 9712. Blood 2001;98:772a.

72. Czuczman MS, Fallon A, Scarpace A, et al. Phase II study of rituximab in combination with fludarabine in patients (Pts) with low-grade or follicular B-cell lymphoma. Blood 2000;96:729a.

73. Schulz H, Klein SK, Rehwald U, et al. Phase II study of rituximab in combination with fludarabine in patients (pts) with chronic lymphocytic leukemia (CLL). Blood 2001;98:364a.

74. Garcia-Manero G, O'Brien S, Cortes J, et al. Update of results of the combination of fludarabine, cyclophosphamide and rituximab for previously treated patients with chronic lymphocytic leukemia (CLL). Blood 2001; 98:633a.

75. Wierda W, O'Brien S, Albitar M, et al. Combined fludarabine, cyclophosphamide, and rituximab achieves a high complete remission rate as initial treatment for chronic lymphocytic leukemia. Blood 2001;98:771a.

76. Polliack A, Cohen Y, Daas N, et al. Fludarabine (FLU)-containing regimen and rituximab (RI) as primary therapy with curative intent for younger patients with progressive and advanced B-CLL: high rate of initial response including molecular remissions. Blood 2001;98:364a.

77. Kaminski MS, Zasadny KR, Francis IR, et al. Radioimmunotherapy of B-cell lymphoma with [^{131}I]anti-B1 (anti-CD20) antibody. N Engl J Med 1993;329:459–465.

78. Kaminski MS, Zasadny KR, Francis IR, et al. Iodine-131-anti-B1 radioimmunotherapy for B-cell lymphoma. J Clin Oncol 1996;14:1974–1981.

79. Kaminski MS, Zelenetz AD, Press OW, et al. Pivotal study of iodine I^{131} tositumomab for chemotherapy-refractory low-grade or transformed low-grade B-cell non-Hodgkin's lymphomas. J Clin Oncol 2001;19:3918–3928.

80. Press OW, Eary JF, Appelbaum FR, et al. Radiolabeled-antibody therapy of B-cell lymphoma with autologous bone marrow support. N Engl J Med 1993;329:1219–1224.

81. Vose JM, Wahl RL, Saleh M, et al. Multicenter phase II study of iodine-131 tositumomab for chemotherapy-relapsed/refractory low-grade and transformed low-grade B-cell non-Hodgkin's lymphomas. J Clin Oncol 2000;18:1316–1323.

82. Wiseman GA, White CA, Witzig TE, et al. Radioimmunotherapy of relapsed non-Hodgkin's lymphoma with zevalin, a 90Y-labeled anti-CD20 monoclonal antibody. Clin Cancer Res 1999;5(10 suppl):3281s–3286s.

83. Witzig TE, White CA, Wiseman GA, et al. Phase I/II trial of IDEC-Y2B8 radioimmunotherapy for treatment of relapsed or refractory CD20(+) B-cell non-Hodgkin's lymphoma. J Clin Oncol 1999;17:3793–3803.

84. Flynn JM, Byrd JC. Campath-1H monoclonal antibody therapy. Curr Opin Oncol 2000;12:574–581.

85. Hale G, Bright S, Chumbley G, et al. Removal of T cells from bone marrow for transplantation: a monoclonal antilymphocyte antibody that fixes human complement. Blood 1983;62:873–882.

86. Hale G, Dyer MJ, Clark MR, et al. Remission induction in non-Hodgkin lymphoma with reshaped human monoclonal antibody CAMPATH-1H. Lancet 1988;2:1394–1399.

87. Treumann A, Lifely MR, Schneider P, Ferguson MA. Primary structure of CD52. J Biol Chem 1995;270: 6088–6099.
88. Domagala A, Kurpisz M. CD52 antigen: a review. Med Sci Monit 2001;7:325–331.
89. Rowan W, Tite J, Topley P, Brett SJ. Cross-linking of the CAMPATH-1 antigen (CD52) mediates growth inhibition in human B- and T-lymphoma cell lines, and subsequent emergence of CD52-deficient cells. Immunology 1998;95:427–436.
90. Hale G, Swirsky D, Waldmann H, Chan LC. Reactivity of rat monoclonal antibody CAMPATH-1 with human leukaemia cells and its possible application for autologous bone marrow transplantation. Br J Haematol 1985;60:41–48.
91. Salisbury JR, Rapson NT, Codd JD, Rogers MV, Nethersell AB. Immunohistochemical analysis of CDw52 antigen expression in non-Hodgkin's lymphomas. J Clin Pathol 1994;47:313–317.
92. Bowen AL, Zomas A, Emmett E, Matutes E, Dyer MJ, Catovsky D. Subcutaneous CAMPATH-1H in fludarabine-resistant/relapsed chronic lymphocytic and B-prolymphocytic leukaemia. Br J Haematol 1997;96:617–619.
93. Keating MJ, Byrd JC, Rai K, et al. Multicenter study of Campath-1H in patients with chronic lymphocytic leukemia (B-CLL) refractory to fludarabine. Blood 2000;96:722a.
94. Keating MJ, Flinn I, Jain V, et al. Therapeutic role of alemtuzumab (Campath-1H) in patients who have failed fludarabine: results of a large international study. Med Oncol 2002;19(suppl):S21–S26.
95. Osterborg A, Fassas AS, Anagnostopoulos A, Dyer MJ, Catovsky D, Mellstedt H. Humanized CD52 monoclonal antibody Campath-1H as first-line treatment in chronic lymphocytic leukaemia. Br J Haematol 1996;93:151–153.
96. Rai KR, Coutre S, Rizzieri D, Gribben JG, Flinn I, Rabinowe S, et al. Efficacy and safety of alemtuzumab (Campath-1H) in refractory B-CLL patients treated on a compassionate basis. Blood 2001;98:365a.
97. Ferrajoli A, O'Brien SM, Williams ML, Fardel S, Kantarjian H, Keating MJ. Campath-1H in refractory hematological malignancies expressing CD-52: a phase II clinical trial of 68 patients. Blood 2001;98:366a.
98. Lundin J, Kimby E, Bjorkholm M, et al. Phase II study of subcutaneous alemtuzumab (Campath-1H) therapy of patients with previously untreated chronic lymphocytic leukemia (CLL). Blood 2001;98:772a.
99. Ginaldi L, De Martinis M, Matutes E, et al. Levels of expression of CD52 in normal and leukemic B and T cells: correlation with in vivo therapeutic responses to Campath-1H. Leuk Res 1998;22:185–191.
100. Khorana A, Bunn P, McLaughlin P, Vose J, Stewart C, Czuczman MS. A phase II multicenter study of Campath-1H antibody in previously treated patients with nonbulky non-Hodgkin's lymphoma. Leuk Lymphoma 2001;41: 77–87.
101. Tang SC, Hewitt K, Reis MD, Berinstein NL. Immunosuppressive toxicity of CAMPATH1H monoclonal antibody in the treatment of patients with recurrent low grade lymphoma. Leuk Lymphoma 1996;24:93–101.
102. Lundin J, Osterborg A, Brittinger G, et al. CAMPATH-1H monoclonal antibody in therapy for previously treated low-grade non-Hodgkin's lymphoma: a phase II multicenter study. European Study Group of CAMPATH-1H Treatment in Low-Grade Non-Hodgkin's Lymphoma. J Clin Oncol 1998;16:3257–3263.
103. Brett S, Baxter G, Cooper H, Johnston JM, Tite J, Rapson N. Repopulation of blood lymphocyte sub-populations in rheumatoid arthritis patients treated with the depleting humanized monoclonal antibody, CAMPATH-1H. Immunology 1996;88:13–19.
104. Condiotti R, Nagler A. Campath-1G impairs human natural killer (NK) cell-mediated cytotoxicity. Bone Marrow Transplant 1996;18:713–720.
105. Fabian I, Flidel O, Gadish M, Kletter Y, Slavin S, Nagler A. Effects of CAMPATH-1 antibodies on the functional activity of monocytes and polymorphonuclear neutrophils. Exp Hematol 1993;21:1522–1527.
106. Kennedy B, Rawstron A, Richards S, Hillmen P. Campath-1H in CLL: immune reconstitution and viral infections during and after therapy. Blood 2000;96:164a.
107. Buggins AGS, Mufti GJ, Fishlock K, et al. Peripheral blood dendritic cells express CD52 and are depleted in vivo by treatment with Campath-1H. Blood 2001;98:366a.
108. Hale G, Zhang MJ, Bunjes D, et al. Improving the outcome of bone marrow transplantation by using CD52 monoclonal antibodies to prevent graft-versus-host disease and graft rejection. Blood 1998;92:4581–4590.
109. Hale G, Jacobs P, Wood L, et al. CD52 antibodies for prevention of graft-versus-host disease and graft rejection following transplantation of allogeneic peripheral blood stem cells. Bone Marrow Transplant 2000;26:69–76.
110. Wing MG, Moreau T, Greenwood J, et al. Mechanism of first-dose cytokine-release syndrome by CAMPATH 1-H: involvement of CD16 (FcgammaRIII) and CD11a/CD18 (LFA-1) on NK cells. J Clin Invest 1996;98: 2819–2826.
111. Flinn IW, Sickler J, Lucas M, et al. Randomized trial of early versus delayed GM-CSF with Campath-1H: preliminary feasibility and correlative biologic studies results. Blood 2000;96:838a.

112. Pruzanski W, Urowitz MB, Grouix B, Vadas P. Induction of TNF-alpha and proinflammatory secretory phospholipase A2 by intravenous administration of CAMPATH-1H in patients with rheumatoid arthritis. J Rheumatol 1995;22:1816–1819.

113. Kennedy B, Rawstron A, Carter C, Ryan M, Speed K, Hillmen P. Campath-1H with fludarabine: a novel, highly active combination in refractory CLL. Blood 2000;96:289b.

114. Nabhan C, Tallman MS, Riley MB, et al. Phase I study of rituximab and Campath-1H in patients with relapsed or refractory chronic lymphocytic leukemia. Blood 2001;98:365a.

115. Faderl S, Thomas DA, O'Brien S, et al. An exploratory study of the combination of monoclonal antibodies Campath-1H and rituximab in the treatment of CD52- and CD20-positive chronic lymphoid disorders. Blood 2001;98:365a.

116. Kostelny SA, Link BK, Tso JY, et al. Humanization and characterization of the anti-HLA-DR antibody 1D10. Int J Cancer 2001;93:556–565.

117. Gingrich RD, Dahle CE, Hoskins KF, Senneff MJ. Identification and characterization of a new surface membrane antigen found predominantly on malignant B lymphocytes. Blood 1990;75:2375–2387.

118. Byrd JC. Personal communication. 2002.

119. Link BK, Wang HG, Byrd JC, et al. Phase I study of Hu1D10 monoclonal antibody in patients with B-cell lymphoma. Proc Am Soc Clin Oncol 2001;20:284a.

120. Link BK, Kahl B, Czuczman MS, et al. A phase II study of Remitogen (Hu1D10), a humanized monoclonal antibody in patients with relapsed or refractory follicular, small lymphocytic, or marginal zone/MALT B-cell lymphoma. Blood 2001;98:606a.

121. Abhyankar VV, Lucas MS, Stock W, et al. Phase I study of escalated thrice weekly dosing of Hu1D10 in chronic lymphocytic leukemia/small lymphocytic lymphoma (CLL/SLL): minimal toxicity and early observation of in vivo tumor cell apoptosis. Proc Am Soc Clin Oncol 2002;21:268a.

122. DeNardo GL, DeNardo SJ, Lamborn KR, et al. Low-dose, fractionated radioimmunotherapy for B-cell malignancies using 131I-Lym-1 antibody. Cancer Biother Radiopharm 1998;13:239–254.

123. DeNardo GL, Lamborn KR, Goldstein DS, Kroger LA, DeNardo SJ. Increased survival associated with radiolabeled Lym-1 therapy for non-Hodgkin's lymphoma and chronic lymphocytic leukemia. Cancer 1997;80(12 suppl):2706–2711.

124. DeNardo GL, DeNardo SJ, Shen S, et al. Factors affecting ^{131}I-Lym-1 pharmacokinetics and radiation dosimetry in patients with non-Hodgkin's lymphoma and chronic lymphocytic leukemia. J Nucl Med 1999;40:1317–1326.

125. DeNardo GL, O'Donnell RT, Rose LM, Mirick GR, Kroger LA, DeNardo SJ. Milestones in the development of Lym-1 therapy. Hybridoma 1999;18:1–11.

126. Bikah G, Lynd FM, Aruffo AA, Ledbetter JA, Bondada S. A role for CD5 in cognate interactions between T cells and B cells, and identification of a novel ligand for CD5. Int Immunol 1998;10:1185–1196.

127. Pers JO, Jamin C, Le Corre R, Lydyard PM, Youinou P. Ligation of CD5 on resting B cells, but not on resting T cells, results in apoptosis. Eur J Immunol 1998;28:4170–4176.

128. Cioca DP, Kitano K. Apoptosis induction by hypercross-linking of the surface antigen CD5 with anti-CD5 monoclonal antibodies in B cell chronic lymphocytic leukemia. Leukemia 2002;16:335–343.

129. Pers JO, Berthou C, Porakishvili N, et al. CD5-induced apoptosis of B cells in some patients with chronic lymphocytic leukemia. Leukemia 2002;16:44–52.

130. Ravel S, Colombatti M, Casellas P. Internalization and intracellular fate of anti-CD5 monoclonal antibody and anti-CD5 ricin A-chain immunotoxin in human leukemic T cells. Blood 1992;79:1511–1517.

131. Foss FM, Raubitschek A, Mulshine JL, et al. Phase I study of the pharmacokinetics of a radioimmunoconjugate, 90Y-T101, in patients with CD5-expressing leukemia and lymphoma. Clin Cancer Res 1998;4:2691–2700.

132. Siena S, Bregni M, Formosa A, et al. Immunotoxin-mediated inhibition of chronic lymphocytic leukemia cell proliferation in humans. Cancer Res 1989;49:3328–3332.

133. Kreitman RJ, Wilson WH, Robbins D, et al. Responses in refractory hairy cell leukemia to a recombinant immunotoxin. Blood 1999;94:3340–3348.

134. Uchiyama T, Broder S, Waldmann TA. A monoclonal antibody (anti-Tac) reactive with activated and functionally mature human T cells I: production of anti-Tac monoclonal antibody and distribution of Tac (+) cells. J Immunol 1981;126:1393–1397.

135. Uchiyama T, Nelson DL, Fleisher TA, Waldmann TA. A monoclonal antibody (anti-Tac) reactive with activated and functionally mature human T cells II: expression of Tac antigen on activated cytotoxic killer T cells, suppressor cells, and on one of two types of helper T cells. J Immunol 1981;126:1398–1403.

136. Kreitman RJ, Wilson WH, White JD, et al. Phase I trial of recombinant immunotoxin anti-Tac(Fv)-PE38 (LMB-2) in patients with hematologic malignancies. J Clin Oncol 2000;18:1622–1636.

137. Decker T, Hipp S, Kreitman RJ, Pastan I, Peschel C, Licht T. Sensitization of B-cell chronic lymphocytic leukemia cells to recombinant immunotoxin by immunostimulatory phosphorothioate oligodeoxynucleotides. Blood 2002;99:1320–1326.

138. Stein R, Belisle E, Hansen HJ, Goldenberg DM. Epitope specificity of the anti-(B cell lymphoma) monoclonal antibody, LL2. Cancer Immunol Immunother 1993;37:293–298.

139. Leung SO, Shevitz J, Pellegrini MC, et al. Chimerization of LL2, a rapidly internalizing antibody specific for B cell lymphoma. Hybridoma 1994;13:469–476.

140. Leung SO, Goldenberg DM, Dion AS, et al. Construction and characterization of a humanized, internalizing, B-cell (CD22)-specific, leukemia/lymphoma antibody, LL2. Mol Immunol 1995;32:1413–1427.

141. Shih LB, Lu HH, Xuan H, Goldenberg DM. Internalization and intracellular processing of an anti-B-cell lymphoma monoclonal antibody, LL2. Int J Cancer 1994;56:538–545.

142. Goldenberg DM, Horowitz JA, Sharkey RM, et al. Targeting, dosimetry, and radioimmunotherapy of B-cell lymphomas with iodine-131-labeled LL2 monoclonal antibody. J Clin Oncol 1991;9:548–564.

143. Linden O, Tennvall J, Cavallin-Stahl E, et al. Radioimmunotherapy using ^{131}I-labeled anti-CD22 monoclonal antibody (LL2) in patients with previously treated B-cell lymphomas. Clin Cancer Res 1999;5(10 suppl):3287s–3291s.

144. Vose JM, Colcher D, Gobar L, et al. Phase I/II trial of multiple dose [131]Iodine-MAb LL2 (CD22) in patients with recurrent non-Hodgkin's lymphoma. Leuk Lymphoma 2000;38:91–101.

145. Linden O, Tennvall J, Cavallin-Stahl E, et al. Durable response to 90-ytrrium-epratuzumab (hLL2) in B-cell lymphoma failing chemotherapy by using dose-fractionation schedule. Blood 2001;98:602a.

146. Juweid ME, Stadtmauer EA, Hajjar G, et al. Pharmacokinetics, dosimetry, and initial therapeutic results with [131]I- and ([111])In-/^{90}Y-labeled humanized LL2 anti-CD22 monoclonal antibody in patients with relapsed, refractory non-Hodgkin's lymphoma. Clin Cancer Res 1999;5(10 suppl):3292s–3303s.

147. Kreitman RJ, Margulies I, Stetler-Stevenson M, Wang QC, Fitzgerald DJ, Pastan I. Cytotoxic activity of disulfide-stabilized recombinant immunotoxin RFB4(dsFv)-PE38 (BL22) toward fresh malignant cells from patients with B-cell leukemias. Clin Cancer Res 2000;6:1476–1487.

148. Kreitman RJ, Wilson WH, Bergeron K, et al. Efficacy of the anti-CD22 recombinant immunotoxin BL22 in chemotherapy-resistant hairy-cell leukemia. N Engl J Med 2001;345:241–247.

149. Newton DL, Hansen HJ, Mikulski SM, Goldenberg DM, Rybak SM. Potent and specific antitumor effects of an anti-CD22-targeted cytotoxic ribonuclease: potential for the treatment of non-Hodgkin's lymphoma. Blood 2001;97:528–535.

150. Bregni M, Siena S, Formosa A, et al. B-cell restricted saporin immunotoxins: activity against B-cell lines and chronic lymphocytic leukemia cells. Blood 1989;73:753–762.

151. Stone MJ, Sausville EA, Fay JW, et al. A phase I study of bolus versus continuous infusion of the anti-CD19 immunotoxin, IgG-HD37-dgA, in patients with B-cell lymphoma. Blood 1996;88:1188–1197.

152. Grossbard ML, Lambert JM, Goldmacher VS, et al. Anti-B4-blocked ricin: a phase I trial of 7-day continuous infusion in patients with B-cell neoplasms. J Clin Oncol 1993;11:726–737.

153. Grossbard ML, Freedman AS, Ritz J, et al. Serotherapy of B-cell neoplasms with anti-B4-blocked ricin: a phase I trial of daily bolus infusion. Blood 1992;79:576–585.

154. Yabuuchi S, Nakamura T, Kloetzer WS, Reff ME. Anti-CD23 monoclonal antibody inhibits germline Cepsilon transcription in B cells. Int Immunopharmacol 2002;2:453–461.

155. Pathan N, Hopkins M, Saven A, Reff ME, Grint P, Hariharan K. Induction of apoptosis by IDEC-152 (anti-CD23) in chronic lymphocytic leukemia. Leuk Lymphoma 2001;42(suppl 1):133N.

156. Keilholz U, Szelenyi H, Siehl J, Foss HD, Knauf W, Thiel E. Rapid regression of chemotherapy refractory lymphocyte predominant Hodgkin's disease after administration of rituximab (anti CD20 monoclonal antibody) and interleukin-2. Leuk Lymphoma 1999;35:641–642.

157. Friedberg JW, Neuberg DS, Gribben JG, et al. Phase II study of combination immunotherapy with interleukin-2 (IL-2) and rituximab in patients with relapsed or refractory follicular non-Hodgkin's lymphoma (NHL). Blood 2000;96:730a.

158. Ansell SM, Witzig TE, Kurtin PJ, et al. Phase I study of interleukin-12 in combination with rituximab in patients with B-cell non-Hodgkin's lymphoma. Blood 2002;99:67–74.

159. Moberts R, Hoogerbrugge H, van Agthoven T, Lowenberg B, Touw I. Proliferative response of highly purified B chronic lymphocytic leukemia cells in serum free culture to interleukin-2 and tumor necrosis factors alpha and beta. Leuk Res 1989;13:973–980.

160. Digel W, Stefanic M, Schoniger W, et al. Tumor necrosis factor induces proliferation of neoplastic B cells from chronic lymphocytic leukemia. Blood 1989;73:1242–1246.
161. Foa R, Massaia M, Cardona S, et al. Production of tumor necrosis factor-alpha by B-cell chronic lymphocytic leukemia cells: a possible regulatory role of TNF in the progression of the disease. Blood 1990;76:393–400.
162. Mainou-Fowler T, Miller S, Proctor SJ, Dickinson AM. The levels of TNF alpha, IL4 and IL10 production by T-cells in B-cell chronic lymphocytic leukaemia (B-CLL). Leuk Res 2001;25:157–163.
163. Weinblatt ME, Kremer JM, Bankhurst AD, et al. A trial of etanercept, a recombinant tumor necrosis factor receptor:Fc fusion protein, in patients with rheumatoid arthritis receiving methotrexate. N Engl J Med 1999; 340:253–259.
164. Moreland LW, Schiff MH, Baumgartner SW, et al. Etanercept therapy in rheumatoid arthritis: a randomized, controlled trial. Ann Intern Med 1999;130:478–486.
165. Deeg HJ, Gotlib J, Beckham C, et al. Soluble TNF receptor fusion protein (etanercept) for the treatment of myelodysplastic syndrome: a pilot study. Leukemia 2002;16:162–164.
166. Steensma DP, Mesa RA, Li CY, Gray L, Tefferi A. Etanercept, a soluble tumor necrosis factor receptor, palliates constitutional symptoms in patients with myelofibrosis with myeloid metaplasia: results of a pilot study. Blood 2002;99:2252–2254.
167. Chiang KY, Abhyankar S, Bridges K, Godder K, Henslee-Downey JP. Recombinant human tumor necrosis factor receptor fusion protein as complementary treatment for chronic graft-versus-host disease. Transplantation 2002;73:66–667.
168. Elliott MJ, Maini RN, Feldmann M, et al. Randomised double-blind comparison of chimeric monoclonal antibody to tumour necrosis factor alpha (cA2) versus placebo in rheumatoid arthritis. Lancet 1994;344: 1105–1110.
169. Targan SR, Hanauer SB, van Deventer SJ, et al. A short-term study of chimeric monoclonal antibody cA2 to tumor necrosis factor alpha for Crohn's disease: Crohn's Disease cA2 Study Group. N Engl J Med 1997; 337:1029–1035.
170. van Dullemen HM, van Deventer SJ, Hommes DW, et al. Treatment of Crohn's disease with anti-tumor necrosis factor chimeric monoclonal antibody (cA2). Gastroenterology 1995;109:129–135.
171. Kobbe G, Schneider P, Rohr U, et al. Treatment of severe steroid refractory acute graft-versus-host disease with infliximab, a chimeric human/mouse antiTNFalpha antibody. Bone Marrow Transplant 2001;28:47–49.
172. Scallon BJ, Moore MA, Trinh H, Knight DM, Ghrayeb J. Chimeric anti-TNF-alpha monoclonal antibody cA2 binds recombinant transmembrane TNF-alpha and activates immune effector functions. Cytokine 1995;7:251–259.
173. Buschle M, Campana D, Carding SR, Richard C, Hoffbrand AV, Brenner MK. Interferon gamma inhibits apoptotic cell death in B cell chronic lymphocytic leukemia. J Exp Med 1993;177:213–218.
174. Zaki M, Douglas R, Patten N, et al. Disruption of the IFN-gamma cytokine network in chronic lymphocytic leukemia contributes to resistance of leukemic B cells to apoptosis. Leuk Res 2000;24:611–621.
175. Sigidin YA, Loukina GV, Skurkovich B, Skurkovich S. Randomized, double-blind trial of anti-interferon-gamma antibodies in rheumatoid arthritis. Scand J Rheumatol 2001;30:203–207.
176. van Kooten C, Rensink I, Aarden L, van Oers R. Interleukin-4 inhibits both paracrine and autocrine tumor necrosis factor-alpha-induced proliferation of B chronic lymphocytic leukemia cells. Blood 1992;80:1299–1306.
177. van Kooten C, Rensink I, Aarden L, van Oers R. Effect of IL-4 and IL-6 on the proliferation and differentiation of B-chronic lymphocytic leukemia cells. Leukemia 1993;7:618–624.
178. Lundin J, Kimby E, Bergmann L, Karakas T, Mellstedt H, Osterborg A. Interleukin 4 therapy for patients with chronic lymphocytic leukaemia: a phase I/II study. Br J Haematol 2001;112:155–160.
179. Frankfurt OS, Byrnes JJ, Villa L. Protection from apoptotic cell death by interleukin-4 is increased in previously treated chronic lymphocytic leukemia patients. Leuk Res 1997;21:9–16.
180. Pu QQ, Bezwoda WR. Interleukin-4 prevents spontaneous in-vitro apoptosis in chronic lymphatic leukaemia but sensitizes B-CLL cells to melphalan cytotoxicity. Br J Haematol 1997;98:413–417.
181. Kay NE, Han L, Bone N, Williams G. Interleukin 4 content in chronic lymphocytic leukaemia (CLL) B cells and blood CD8+ T cells from B-CLL patients: impact on clonal B-cell apoptosis. Br J Haematol 2001;112:760–767.
182. Mainou-Fowler T, Proctor SJ, Miller S, Dickinson AM. Expression and production of interleukin 4 in B-cell chronic lymphocytic leukaemia. Leuk Lymphoma 2001;42:689–698.
183. di Celle PF, Carbone A, Marchis D, et al. Cytokine gene expression in B-cell chronic lymphocytic leukemia: evidence of constitutive interleukin-8 (IL-8) mRNA expression and secretion of biologically active IL-8 protein. Blood 1994;84:220–228.

184. di Celle PF, Mariani S, Riera L, Stacchini A, Reato G, Foa R. Interleukin-8 induces the accumulation of B-cell chronic lymphocytic leukemia cells by prolonging survival in an autocrine fashion. Blood 1996;87: 4382–4389.

185. Yang XD, Corvalan JR, Wang P, Roy CM, Davis CG. Fully human anti-interleukin-8 monoclonal antibodies: potential therapeutics for the treatment of inflammatory disease states. J Leukoc Biol 1999;66:401–410.

186. Koumenis IL, Shahrokh Z, Leong S, Hsei V, Deforge L, Zapata G. Modulating pharmacokinetics of an interleukin-8 F(ab')(2) by amine-specific PEGylation with preserved bioactivity. Int J Pharm 2000;198:83–95.

16 Immunotoxin Therapy of Chronic Lymphocytic Leukemia

Arthur E. Frankel, MD and Robert J. Kreitman, MD

1. INTRODUCTION

There are approx 8000 new cases of chronic lymphocytic leukemia (CLL) a year in the United States *(1)*. Most patients eventually progress to an advanced stage or develop rapidly progressive disease with a median survival of only 18–36 mo *(2)*. Although allogeneic bone marrow transplantation (including nonmyeloablative conditioning regimens) offers the possibility of long-term remission or cure *(3)*, most patients either lack suitable donors and have comorbidities that prevent such therapy. Monoclonal antibodies, radiolabeled antibody conjugates, and antibody-drug conjugates have been used in CLL and have produced clinical remissions, but most of the responses have been partial and have not been durable. Hence, additional novel agents that may significantly impact on the natural history of this disease are needed. One such class of agents is the immunotoxins consisting of monoclonal antibodies, antibody fragments, or cytokines linked either chemically or genetically to peptide toxins. The antibody or cytokine directs the molecule to the CLL cell surface. The toxin moiety is internalized and translocated to the cytosol, where it enzymatically inactivates protein synthesis inducing programmed cell death. In this review, we discuss the unique biology of the CLL cell that makes it an attractive candidate for immunotoxin therapy. We describe potential CLL cell surface receptors for targeting with immunotoxins as well as the structure and function of selected CLL immunotoxins. Finally, the clinical results of previous and on-going clinical trials with these agents in CLL are analyzed.

2. CLL BIOLOGY

CLL is a clonal malignancy of B-cells. The genetic lesions producing the accumulation of the offspring of this cell are unknown, although abnormalities of chromosomes 12, 13, or 14 have been detected *(4)*. Although the genetics and molecular mechanisms for the transformation are unknown, the CLL cell surface has been extensively characterized. The surface phenotype gives clues to the cell of origin.

The CLL cell expresses most of the membrane antigens present on mature B-cells, but the cell coexpresses the T-cell antigen CD5 and has almost undetectable amounts of monoclonal surface immunoglobulin. The surface immunoglobulins are usually IgM and IgD. The monoclonal immunoglobulin on the cell membrane is a low-affinity, polyreactive autoantibody. The antibody has the heavy chain variable region idiotyp 51p1 and has not undergone the process of somatic hypermutation (which occurs in germinal centers). The low level of surface immuno-

From: *Contemporary Hematology*
Chronic Lymphocytic Leukemia: Molecular Genetics, Biology, Diagnosis, and Management
Edited by: G. B. Faguet © Humana Press Inc., Totowa, NJ

globulin suggests that the B-lymphocyte has been made anergic by interaction with self-antigen. Continued interaction of the surface immunoglobulin with self-antigen may prevent apoptosis. Similar normal B-lymphocytes are present in the mantle zone of secondary lymphoid follicles and, in small numbers, in the peripheral blood *(5)*. The common properties of the rare normal CD5+ B-lymphocytes and CLL cells have led to the hypothesis that CLL cells are transformed mantle zone-based, anergic, self-reactive CD5+ B-cells that produce polyreactive, natural autoantibodies *(6)*.

3. CLL CELL SURFACE RECEPTORS

A number of target molecules are overexpressed on CLL cells, in some or all cases, including the interleukin-4 receptor (IL-4R), 1D10, CD5, CD18, CD19, CD20, CD21, CD22, CD23, CD24, CD25, CD27, CD29, CD38, CD43, CD44, CD45, CD47, CD50, CD52, CD54, CD55, CD59, CD62L, CD70, CD72, and CD102 (Table 1). A truncated form of CD79b that arises by alternative slicing of the CD79b gene with loss of exon 3 is commonly seen. CD22 is weakly expressed. The Na+/H+ antiporter, CD80, and CD86 are absent or poorly expressed. CD11a, CD49c, CD49d, and CD49e are variably expressed. The cell surface phenotype has been characterized by immuno-fluorescent staining with flow cytometry, immunohistochemistry, and immunoblots. Many of these cell surface markers are useful in diagnosis and in explaining some of the clinical findings of patients with CLL.

The coexpression of C5 and CD19 has been used to confirm the diagnosis of CLL *(7)*. Expression of CD23 and CD25 helps to differentiate CLL from mantle cell lymphoma *(8)*. The level of expression of CD38 has been used to predict the clinical course *(9)*. CD55 and CD59 expression may correlate with patient responsiveness to rituximab *(see* Subheading 4. below) *(10)*. The coexpression of CD27 and CD70 may modify accessory cell function and reduce the ability to activate T cells *(11)*. The CD49d-CD29 complex (α4β3) integrin binds to vascular cell adhesion molecule-1 (VCAM-1) on stimulated endothelium in the bone marrow and secondary lymphoid organs *(12)*. This will lead to accumulation of CLL cells at these sites. Integrin binding also has an anti-apoptotic function. The truncated CD79b disrupts normal B-cell receptor structure and function *(13)*.

A number of these surface antigens are poorly expressed on nonhematopoietic tissues and have been developed as targets for monoclonal antibodies or cytokines.

4. MONOCLONAL ANTIBODY-BASED THERAPY OF CLL

4.1. Monoclonal Antibodies

Two humanized monoclonal antibodies to lymphoid differentiation antigens—CD52 and CD20—were tested in CLL patients. Clinical trials recently began for another humanized mono-clonal antibody, Hu1D10. A fourth humanized monoclonal antibody reactive with CD47 is under development. The anti-CD20 and anti-CD52 antibodies showed significant antileukemic activity (Table 2).

The humanized antibody to CD52—Campath 1H, or alemtuzumab—showed a response rate of approximately 80% in untreated patients or 40% in patients who had previously received cytotoxic chemotherapy *(45–49)*. Most of these responses were partial remissions lasting less than 1 yr. Furthermore, clearing of disease was seen in the blood and bone marrow but not lymph node sites. The limited activity in CLL may be owing to low antigen density *(50)*. Side effects included a high rate of infection and a cytokine release syndrome. These complications may be

Table 1

Cell Surface Molecules Found on CLL Cells

Antigen	Properties	Function	Distribution	Ref.
IL-4 receptor	p140α; p64g	B-cell activation	Heme + cross-reaction IL-13R on multiple tissues	14
1D10	Variant HLA-DRb	Apoptosis regulation	B-cells	15
CD5	p67	ITIM co-receptor	Lymphoid (T + B)	16
CD18	p100	β_2-integrin	Heme	17
CD19	p95	ITAM co-receptor	B-cells	18
CD20	p35	B-cell differentiation/proliferation regulation	B-cells	19
CD21	p145	C3d/EBV receptor	B-cells	20
CD22	p150	ITIM co-receptor	B-cells	21
CD23	p45	FcεRII/CD40 binding	Heme + epithelia	22
CD24	p40 2-chain GPI-linked mucin glycoprotein	Adhesion (binds CD62P)	Heme +neurons + muscle + skin + carcinomas	23
CD25	p55	IL-2Rα	Heme	24
CD27	p110 disulfide-linked dimer; member TNFR	Costimulatory with CD70	Lymphoid (T + B)	25
CD29	p130	β_1-integrin	Most animal and plant cells but not red blood cells	26
CD38	p45	NAD glycohydrolase; adhesion; signaling	Heme + epithelia	27
CD43	p145 sialoglycoprotein	Antiadhesive/adhesive	Heme	28
CD44	p85 glycoprotein with multiple splice variants	Receptor hyaluronic acid; adhesion	Heme + epithelia + endothelia	29
CD45	p180-220	Receptor tyrosine phosphatase	Heme	30
CD47	p50 N-linked glycan	Thrombospondin receptor; integrin regulator	Heme + epithelia + endothelia + fibroblasts	31, 32
CD49d	p140	α_4-integrin	Heme	33

(continued)

Table 1 (*continued*)

Antigen	Properties	Function	Distribution	Ref.
CD50	p110	ICAM-3; binds LFA-1; costimulatory	Heme + endothelium	34
CD52	p20 GPI-linked glycoprotein	Unknown	Lymphoid (T + B) + sperm	35, 36
CD54	p100	ICAM-1; binds LFA-1	Heme + endothelium	37
CD55	p70 GPI-linked glycoprotein	DAF; interferes with complement	Heme + endothelium	38
CD59	p19 GPI-linked glycoprotein	MACIF; membrane attack complex inhibition	Heme + endothelium	39
CD62L	p80	LECAM-1; leukocyte-endothelium adhesion	Lymphoid (T + B)	40
CD70	p50/70/90/100/160	Costimulatory with CD27	Lymphoid (T + B)	41
CD72	p43	A CD5 receptor; ITIM co-receptor	B-cells	42
CD79b-truncated	p50	Immunoglobulin antigen receptor-defective	B-cells	13, 43
CD102	p200	ICAM-2; binds LFA-1	Heme + endothelium	44

CLL, chronic lymphocytic leukemia; DAF, decay-accelerating factor; EBV, Epstein-Barr virus; GPI, glycosylphosphatidylinositol; ICAM, intercellular adhesion molecule; IL-2Ra, interleukin-2 receptor a; ITAM, immunoreceptor tyrosine activation motif; ITIM, immunoreceptor tyrosine-based inhibition motif; LECAM, leukocyte endothelium cell adhesion molecule; LFA, leukocyte factor-association antigen; MACIF, membrane attach complex inhibitory factor; NAD, nicotinamide adenine dinucleotide; TNFR, tumor necrosis factor receptor.

Table 2
Monoclonal Antibodies, Radioimmunoconjugates, and Drug Conjugates for Treatment of CLL

Agent	Disease status	Response (%)	Comments	Ref.
Alemtuzumab	Untreated	89	100% response in blood and 32% in nodes; response durations 8+ – 24+ mo; treatment 30 mg ti wk × 18	45
	Relapsed/refractory	42	97% response blood, 36% response of splenomegaly, 7% response in nodes; mean response duration 12 mo	46
	Refractory	33	82% response without adenopathy and 25% with adenopathy; infections in 56% of patients	47
	Refractory	59	10% showed negative minimal residual disease by flow/PCR and remain in remission >2–3 yr	48
	Refractory	20	3% complete remission; 18% fever, chills, hypotension, dyspnea; 24% infections; 12% rash	49
Rituximab	Relapsed/refractory	7	1/15 patients with a partial response to 375 mg/m^2/wk α 4	55
	Relapsed/refractory	39	500 mg/m^2–2000 mg/m2; dose-dependent response; effect on blood, nodes, and organs but less effect on marrow	56
	Relapsed/refractory	46	250–375 mg/m^2 ti wk α 12 doses; 3/27 thrombopenia; poor marrow response; response correlated with CD20 level	57
	Untreated	94	Flud. 25 mg/m^2/cytoxan 250 mg/m^2 d 2–4 + rituximab 375 mg/m^2 d 1 course 1 and 500 mg/m^2 d 1 courses 2–6 qmo	58
	Relapsed/refractory	70	Same combination schedule as above; 17% serious infections or fever; CR 14% vs 57% in above trial	59
^{90}Y-T101	Advanced/refractory	100	1/1 partial response lasting 6 mo; significant bone marrow suppression	66
^{131}I-Lym-1	Advanced	80	4/5 partial remissions and 1/5 complete remission; thrombopenia	67
B43-genistein	Relapsed	0	0/1 response	72

CLL, chronic lymphocytic leukemia; CR, complete response; Flud., fludarabine; PCR, polymerase chain reaction.

caused by the expression of CD52 on all hematopoietic cells including granulocytes and mono-cytes. CD16-positive natural killer cells bind antibody and release tumor necrosis factor-α (TNF-α) and IL-6 *(51–53)*. Based on the promising response rate and evidence of a unique mechanism of programmed cell death in vitro *(54)*, combination protocols with myeloid growth factors or cytotoxic chemotherapy are being started.

The humanized anti-CD20 monoclonal antibody rituximab has been used for treatment of CLL patients *(55–59)*. The response rate was only 12% in relapsed/refractory CLL patients, which may be attributable partly to low CD20 antigen density and low circulating rituximab levels in treated patients *(60,61)*. Further, few responses were seen in the marrow, possibly partly because of anti-apoptotic signals from bone marrow stroma to the CLL stem cells *(62)*. Increasing the dose intensity, by raising the dose or shortening the interval between doses, led to an improvement in response rate to 40%. Combining rituximab with chemotherapy produced a dramatic increase in response rate and in the number of complete remissions; rituximab + chemotherapy may produce a supra-additive cytotoxicity to CLL cells *(63)*.

Hu1D10 is a humanized antibody to the 1D10 antigen. This antigen is a variant HLA-DRb chain. In an on-going phase I study with relapsed non-Hodgkin's lymphoma patients, some partial responses have been seen *(64)*. Extensive phase I/II studies in CLL patients are planned.

Antibody to CD47 induces CLL cell apoptosis *(31)*. Efforts are under way to prepare a human-ized version of this antibody for clinical testing. The anti-CD22 humanized monoclonal antibody epratuzumab has been tested in refractory large cell lymphoma *(65)*. There are no reports of its use in CLL. The weak expression of CD22 on CLL cells may impact on its activity.

4.2. Radiolabeled Monoclonal Antibodies

Radiolabeled antibody conjugates have been prepared with monoclonal antibodies that are reactive with the lymphoid differentiation antigens CD5, CD20, and CD22 and the Lym-1 anti-gen. Only the ^{131}I-labeled Lym-1 and the ^{90}Y-labeled anti-CD5-radiolabeled conjugates have been tested in CLL (Table 2). One B-CLL patient was treated with ^{90}Y-T101 anti-CD5 murine antibody and had a partial response lasting 6 mo *(66)*. Five of five CLL patients receiving a series of injections up to 300 mCi cumulative dose of ^{131}I-Lym 1 antibody had remissions lasting an average of 6 mo *(67)*. Thus, CLL appears to respond to radiolabeled conjugates, but none of the patients treated to date have shown durable complete remissions. The ^{131}I-labeled LL2 anti-CD22 antibody, the ^{90}Y-labeled ibritumomab anti-CD20 antibody, the ^{131}I-labeled tositumomab anti-CD20 antibody, and the ^{67}Cu-labeled Lym-1 antibody have been tested and have shown clinical activity in non-Hodgkin's lymphomas but have not been used for CLL patients *(68–71)*. Radio-labeled antibodies deserve further testing in CLL.

4.3. Antibody Conjugates

4.3.1. GENISTEIN-ANTIBODY CONJUGATE

Genistein, a tyrosine kinase inhibitor, has been linked to the anti-CD19 murine monoclonal antibody B43 *(72)*. B43-genistein was given to one patient with CLL, but no antileukemic effi-cacy was seen. Dose-limiting toxicity was not reached.

4.3.2. IMMUNOTOXINS

4.3.2.1. Toxin Structure-Function. The immunotoxins constitute a novel class of therapeu-tics for CLL, with a distinct mechanism of action and toxicity. They target peptide ligands (monoclonal antibodies, antibody fragments, growth factors, or hormones) covalently attached

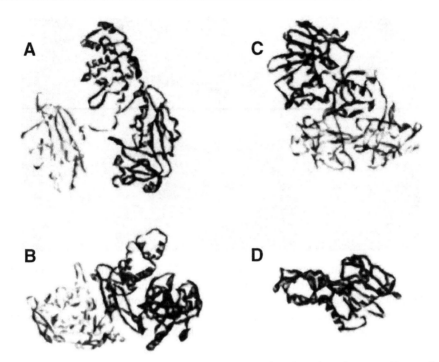

Fig. 1. Toxin three-dimensional structures. All molecules depicted are based on coordinates from Protein Data Bank (PDB) files. The PDB abbreviations are as follows: **(A)** 1ddt, diphtheria toxin; **(B)** 1dma, *Pseudomonas* exotoxin; **(C)** 2aa1, ricin; and **(D)** 1paf, pokeweed antiviral protein. SYBYL molecular modeling software was used to render toxins as shaded ribbons derived from cubic spline fits to the C-α backbone.

to polypeptide toxins. The antibody or other peptide ligand directs the molecule to the tumor cell surface, and the toxin moiety then enters the cell and induces apoptosis by inactivating protein synthesis. Extremely potent catalytic toxins that can kill cells with as few as one molecule per cell are found in plants, bacteria, and fungi. The atomic three-dimensional structures and the genes for a number of toxins used clinically and in the laboratory have been defined (Fig. 1). Many of the peptide toxins have three domains. These include a catalytic domain that enzymatically inactivates protein synthesis, a translocation domain that facilitates the transfer of the catalytic domain to the cytosol, where it can work, and a receptor-binding domain that directs the molecule to the cell surface, and, in some cases, triggers receptor-mediated endocytosis.

Diphtheria toxin (DT), produced by *Corynebacterium diphtheriae*, is a 58-kDa protein. DT is composed of an N-terminal adenosine diphosphate (ADP)-ribosylating catalytic domain, a furin-sensitive RVRR peptide (within a disulfide loop), a hydrophobic middle domain (responsible for translocation of the ADP-ribosylation domain to the cytosol), and a C-terminal cell-binding domain [capable of binding cell-associated heparin-binding epidermal growth factor (EGF)] *(73)*. The N-terminal first 10 amino acid residues of DT may also be required for translocation of the catalytic domain to the cytosol *(107)*. One or more pairs of amphipathic α-helices in the transmembrane middle domain of DT are involved in membrane insertion and channel formation.

Pseudomonas exotoxin (PE) is a product of *Pseudomonas aeruginosa*. It is a 68-kDa protein with an N-terminal domain (which binds the α2-macroglobulin receptor/low-density lipoprotein-like receptor protein), a furin-sensitive RQPRG sequence, a transmembrane domain with

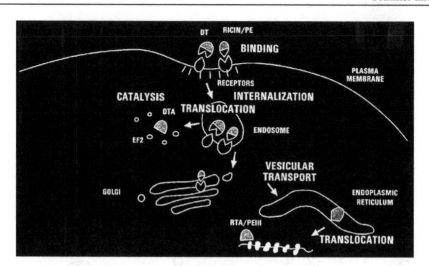

Fig. 2. Mechanisms of cell intoxication by toxins. Toxins bind to cell surface receptors; the complex internalizes to endosomes; the toxin reaches a translocation-competent compartment [endosomes for diphtheria toxin (DT) and endoplasmic reticulum for *Pseudomonas* exotoxin (PE) and ricin); the catalytic domain of the toxin crosses the membrane to the cytosol; cytosolic toxin inactivates protein synthesis. DTA, diphtheria toxin A fragment; PEIII, Pseudomonas exotoxin A; and RTA, ricin toxin A.

amphipathic helices (that participate in membrane translocation), a catalytic domain [which ADP-ribosylates elongation factor-2 (EF2) similar to the DT catalytic fragment], a C-terminal REDLK sequence (with the REDL recognizable by the KDEL receptor), and a C-terminal lysine (sensitive to intracellular carboxy-peptidase) *(74,108,109)*.

Ricin toxin from *Ricinus communis* plant seeds has two separate polypeptide chains linked by a disulfide bond. The B chain (RTB) is a 33-kDa glycoprotein lectin that binds three galactose-terminated oligosaccharides on cell surfaces *(75)*. The A chain (RTA) is a 32-kDa glycoprotein possessing an active site cleft with RNA *N*-glycosidase activity acting on the critical stem-loop structure of rRNA involved in EF2 binding, and a C-terminal membrane insertion signal sequence (ILIPIIALMVY).

Pokeweed antiviral protein (PAP) and saporin (SAP) are type I ribosome-inactivating proteins (RIPs) isolated from the seeds of *Phytolacca americana* and *Saponaria officinalis*, respectively. The three-dimensional structures of these 28-kDa proteins closely resemble RTA, and the proteins have similar enzymatic activity *(76)*.

These proteins intoxicate mammalian cells by a number of discrete steps mediated by different portions of the molecules (Fig. 2). The first step is cell surface binding. DT binds a membrane form of heparin-binding EGF *(77)*. PE binds the α2-macroglobulin low density lipoprotein-like receptor protein *(78)*. Ricin is a lectin with specificity for galactosyl pyranoside groups on cell surface glycoproteins and glycolipids *(79)*. The plant hemitoxins or type I RIPs lack cell-binding domains. The second step is internalization into endosomes. The third step is transfer to a compartment for membrane translocation. In the case of DT, the acidic environment of the endosomes triggers alterations in the structure of the translocation domain of DT *(80)*. In the case of PE and ricin, toxins pass to the trans-reticular Golgi and then travel by retrograde transport through the secretory pathways to the endoplasmic reticulum *(81)*. The fourth step is membrane translocation. The enzymatic domain of DT passes through channels created by the transmembrane domain

(82). In the case of ricin and PE, the enzymatic domain may use pre-existing pores in the endoplasmic reticulum (the translocon) to reach the cytosol. The third and fourth steps taken by type I RIPs are unknown. The final step is inactivation of protein synthesis and apoptosis. Apoptosis facilitates but is not absolutely necessary for cell death *(110).*

We will briefly review the molecular steps in protein synthesis to define the toxin targets better. After the initiation step, an amino-acyl-tRNA residue (Met-tRNA) resides at the ribosomal A site. Later, during protein synthesis, there may be a peptide chain attached to this tRNA. The driving machine for peptide elongation is the transfer of this amino-acyl tRNA or peptidyl-tRNA from the A site to the ribosomal P site. This step is driven by guanosine triphosphate (GTP) and molecular mimicry. EF2 imitates a tRNA-EF1 complex. This complex has a higher affinity for the A site than the amino-acyl or peptidyl-tRNA alone. The peptide-tRNA is driven off the A site to the P site, facilitated by rotational movement between the subunits centered on the A site and replaced by the EF2 itself *(83).* DT and PE enzymatically ADP-ribosylate EF2 at the diphthamide residue located at D575 in domain IV of EF2 *(84).* The catalysis occurs at 100 or more EF2 molecules/min (from a total of about 10^5 EF2 molecules/cell). The chemical change prevents the EF2 domain IV probe, which mimics tRNA, from functioning normally and pushing the tRNA-peptide out of the A site. In addition to the EF2 probe, which displaces the peptidyl-tRNA, there is also the rRNA conformation change, which occurs spontaneously to drive elongation, but which is speeded by other EF2 domains (II–III) in which the GTPase activity modifies structure. Ricin and type I RIPs remove an adenine base (rRNA N-glycosidase activity) from the large rRNA at the S/R stem-loop (S = α-sarcin site and R = ricin site) *(85).* This stem-loop normally switches between two states, which changes overall rRNA and ribosome structure in the large subunit. Once this chemical change occurs (again at 100/min), EF2 can no longer bind properly, and elongation stops. Note that EF2 interacts with the ribosome at two sites, each of which is affected separately by peptide toxins. Once protein synthesis is inhibited, programmed cell death (apoptosis) occurs by unknown signaling pathways.

4.3.2.2. Immunotoxin Synthesis. Important steps for the construction of immunotoxins are to remove normal tissue-binding sites from the toxin and to identify adequately specific ligands. These ligands must also have the property of facilitating internalization of the ligand-receptor complex once bound to the cell surface. Finally, the ligand and toxin must be covalently linked together in such a way that both ligand and non-cell-binding toxin functions are preserved.

Normal tissue binding sites of DT, PE, and ricin can be genetically removed or mutated to reduce normal tissue binding markedly. For DT, this is accomplished by genetically deleting the C-terminal receptor binding domain (amino acids 389–535) to produce DAB_{389} or DT_{388} or by mutating critical amino acid residues in this domain such as CRM107 (S525F). PE is genetically modified by removing domain IA and IB sequences (amino acids 1–252 and 364–380), resulting in PE38, or replacing the four lysines of domain IA with glutamic acids (PE^{Glu4}). The normal ricin tissue-binding domain is the B chain. This can be removed by genetic expression of the A chain alone and by mutating critical residues in the RTB lectin pockets. Ricin can also be manipulated chemically. The ricin can be extracted from the castor beans and purified on matrices; then the ricin is reduced and the RTB is discarded. The RTA can then be further purified from contaminating ricin. Alternatively, ricin can be derivatized to block its lectin sites with oligosaccharides containing a reactive dichlorothiazine group. Since the type I RIPs lack normal tissue-binding sites, no modifications are needed.

The identification of CLL-selective antigens and receptors for targeting is the most difficult step. Some ligands have been chosen for preclinical and clinical development of CLL

Table 3

CLL Immunotoxins

Conjugate	Ligand	Toxin	Linker	Properties (IC 50)	Ref.
RFB4(dsFv)-PE	Anti-CD22 dsFv	PE	Amide	160 pM on CLL cells; active on cells with 350 CD22 sites/cell	86
Anti-CD22-RTA	Anti-CD22 MAb	RTA	SPDP	10,000 pM on CLL cells	87
Anti-Tac(Fv)-PE38	Anti-CD25 sFv	PE	Amide	100 pM; active on cells with only CD25	88
DAB$_{389}$IL-2/DT$_{388}$IL-2	IL-2	DT	Amide	2 pM on HUT102 cells; 1500 pM on CLL cells	89,90
DAB$_{486}$IL-2	IL-2	DT	Amide	100 pM on HUT102 cells; requires IL-2Rα, -b, -g; not tested on CLL	91
DAB389IL-7	IL-7	DT	Amide	1000 pM; requires IL-7Ra, -b, not tested on CLL cells	92
Anti-cCLLa-RTA	Anti-cCLLa MAb	RTA	SPDP	100 pM on CLL cells	93
Anti-CD19-bRicin	Anti-CD19 MAb	bRicin	SMCC	20 pM on Namalwa cells, not tested on CLL cells	94
Anti-CD19-genistein	Anti-CD19 MAb	Genistein	SANPAH	75 nM on B-ALL cell lines; not tested on CLL cells; requires CD19	95
OM124-rRTA	Anti-CD22 MAb	rRTA	SMPT	>10,000 pM on CLL cells; 20 pM with 10 nM monensin	96
OM124/saporin	Anti-CD22 MAb	Saporin	SMPT	70 pM on Daudi cells, not tested on CLL cells	97
T101-RTA	Anti-CD5	RTA	SPDP	>10,000 pM on CLL cells; 10 nM with 50 nM HSA-monensin	98

RTA, ricin toxin A chain; MAb, monoclonal antibody; bRicin, blocked ricin; PE, *Pseudomonas* exotoxin A; IL-2, interleukin-2; PE38, 38-kDa fragment of PE; DAB$_{389}$, 389 N-terminal amino acid residues of diphtheria toxin; DT, diphtheria toxin; sFv, single-chain Fv fragment of MAb; dsFv, disulfide-stabilized sFv; SPDP, 3-(2-pyridyldithio)propionic acid *N*-hydroxysuccinimide ester; HSA, human serum albumin; SMCC, 4-(maleimidomethyl)cyclohexanecarboxylic acid *N*-hydroxysuccinimide ester; pM, picomolar; IL-2R, interleukin-2 receptor; SANPAH, *N*-succinimidyl-6(4'-azido-2'-nitrophenylamino)hexanoate; rRTA, recombinant RTA; SMPT, 4-succinimidyloxylcarbonyl-α-methyl-α-(2-pyridyldithio)-toluene; SPDP, *N*-succinimidyl 3-(2-pyridyldithio) propronate.

Table 4
Clinical Trials of Immunotoxins

Agent	Criteria	Responses (PR + CR)/total	Toxicities	Ref.
T101-RTA	CD5+	0/9	Fever and nausea	98, 99
Anti-CD19-blocked ricin	CD19+	0/5	Transaminasemia, VLS, nausea, headaches	100, 101
DAB$_{486}$IL-2	CD25+ in one of two trials	1/7	Transaminasemia, uremia, proteinuria, fever, chills, bronchospasm	102–104
DAB$_{389}$IL-2	CD25+	2/2	None	Frankel, unpublished data
Anti-Tac(Fv)-PE38	CD25+	1/8	Transaminasemia, fever	105
Anti-CD22(dsFv)-PE38	CD22+	1/1	HUS, VLS, nausea, transaminasemia, myalgias in other patients	106

VLS, vascular leak syndrome with hypoalbuminemia, edema, hypotension, weight gain; PR, partial response; CR, complete response; HUS, hemolytic-uremic syndrome.

309

immunotoxins, even though they are not truly tumor-specific. Instead, all these ligands bind antigens or receptors enriched on CLL cells and not significantly present on vital normal tissues.

Finally, conjugation of the ligand to toxin can be achieved by amide linkage using genetic engineering or by chemical crosslinking using bifunctional reagents such as the thiolating compounds [SPDP, SMPT (*see* Table 3 footnote), and MBS(m-maleidobenzoyl-*N*-hydroxy-succinimide ester)]. The critical tests are as follows: (1) the genetic or chemical modification must not change the functions of the ligand or toxin significantly, and (2) the conjugate must be efficiently internalized from the cell surface. A list of active immunotoxins targeted to CLL cells is shown in Table 3. Some of these have been developed and tested clinically.

4.3.2.3. Clinical Studies of Immunotoxin in CLL. There have been only a few limited pilot studies of immunotoxin therapy for CLL. This is surprising considering the excellent attributes of this disease as a target for immunotoxins. The patients will not mount an immune response against the foreign protein; the leukemic target is easily accessible to the drug in the blood, spleen, marrow, and lymph nodes. The studies are listed in Table 4 and detailed below. The immunotoxins tested to date include anti-CD5-RTA, $DAB_{486}IL2$, $DAB_{389}IL2$ (ONTAK), anti-CD19-blocked ricin, anti-CD25(Fv)-PE38 (LMB-2), and anti-CD22(dsFv)-PE38. In all the trials, only 35 CLL patients have received a variety of immunotoxins. Clinical efficacy was observed only with the fusion proteins containing fragments of the bacterial toxins—diphtheria toxin and *Pseudomonas* exotoxin. The responses were partial remissions and lasted for months. Activity to date has been modest with only rare partial remissions, in most cases. Reasons for the modest activity may be short treatment courses, low doses, dose-limiting vascular or hepatic injury, and, in some cases, poor patient selection with patients included who lacked high antigen density or high-affinity receptors. Nevertheless, more extensive phase II studies are warranted, with adjustment for these variables to define the true activity of these agents in this disease. The observation with rituximab that combination therapies with cytotoxic drugs markedly enhanced the overall and complete remission rate should serve as a guide for immunotoxin development. Like humanized monoclonal antibodies, immunotoxins have a distinct mechanism of action and toxicity profile. Once sufficient numbers of CLL patients are treated on phase I/II trials of immunotoxins, they should be tested in combination with cytotoxic drugs.

REFERENCES

1. Greenlee RT, Murray T, Bolden S, Wingo PA. Cancer statistics 2000. Ca Cancer J Clin 2000;50:7–33.
2. Keating MJ. Chronic lymphocytic leukemia. Sem Oncol 1999;26(suppl 14):107–114.
3. Pavletic ZS, Arrowsmith ER, Bierman PJ, et al. Outcome of allogeneic stem cell transplantation for B cell chronic lymphocytic leukemia. Bone Marrow Transplant 2000;25:717–722.
4. Juliusson G, Merup M. Cytogenetics in chronic lymphocytic leukemia. Sem Oncol 1998;25:19–26.
5. Caligaris-Cappio F. B-chronic lymphocytic leukemia: a malignancy of anti-self B cells. Blood 1996;87:2615–2620.
6. Caligaris-Cappio F, Hamblin TJ. B-cell chronic lymphocytic leukemia: a bird of a different feather. J Clin Oncol 1999;17:399–408.
7. Geisler CH, Larsen JK, Hansen NE, et al. Prognostic importance of flow cytometric immunophenotyping of 540 consecutive patients with B-cell chronic lymphocytic leukemia. Blood 1991;78:1795–1802.
8. Weisenburger DD, Armitage JO. Mantle cell lymphoma—an entity comes of age. Blood 1996;87:4483–4494.
9. Damle RN, Wasil T, Fais F, et al. Immunoglobulin V gene mutation status and CD38 expression as novel prognostic indicators in chronic lymphocytic leukemia. Blood 1999;94:1840–1847.
10. Golay J, Zaffaroni L, Vaccari T, et al. Biologic response of B lymphoma cells to anti-CD20 monoclonal antibody Rituximab in vitro: CD55 and CD59 regulate complement-mediated cell lysis. Blood 2000;95:3900–3908.
11. Ranheim EA, Cantwell MJ, Kipps TJ. Expression of CD27 and its ligand, CD70, on chronic lymphocytic leukemia B cells. Blood 1995;85:3556–3565.

12. Vincent AM, Cawley JC, Burthem J. Integrin function in chronic lymphocytic leukemia. Blood 1996;87: 4780–4788.
13. Hashimoto S, Chiorazzi N, Gregersen PK. Alternative splicing of CD79α (Ig-alpha/mb-1) and CD79β (Ig-beta/B29) RNA transcripts in human B cells. Mol Immunol 1995;32:651–659.
14. Pan PY, Rothman P. IL-4 receptor mutations. Curr Opin Immunol 1999;11:615–620.
15. Link BK, Kostelny SA, Cole MS, Fusselman WP, Tso JY, Weiner GJ. Anti-CD3-based bispecific antibody designed for therapy of human B-cell malignancy can induce T-cell activation by antigen-dependent and antigen-independent mechanisms. Intl J Cancer 1998;77:251–256.
16. Pospisil R, Mage RG. CD5 and other superantigens as 'ticklers' of the B-cell receptor. Immunol Today 1998; 19:106–108.
17. Green LJ, Mould AP, Humphries MJ. The integrin beta subunit. Intl J Biochem Cell Biol 1998;30:179–184.
18. Fujimoto M, Bradney AP, Poe JC, Steeber DA, Tedder TF. Modulation of B lymphocyte antigen receptor signal transduction by a CD19/CD22 regulatory loop. Immunity 1999;11:191–200.
19. Shan D, Ledbetter JA, Press OW. Signaling events involved in anti-CD20-induced apoptosis of malignant human B cells. Cancer Immunol Immunother 2000;48:673–683.
20. Mongini PK, Vilensky MA, Highet PF, Inman JK. The affinity threshold for human B cell activation via the antigen receptor complex is reduced upon co-ligation of the antigen receptor with CD21 (CR2). J Immunol 1997; 159:3782–3791.
21. Tedder TF, Tuscano J, Sato S, Kehrl JH. CD22, a B lymphocyte-specific adhesion molecule that regulates antigen receptor signaling. Ann Rev Immunol 1997;15:481–504.
22. Bonnefoy JY, Lecoanet-Henchoz S, Gauchat JF, et al. Structure and functions of CD23. Intl Rev Immunol 1997; 16:113–128.
23. Aigner S, Sthoeger ZM, Fogel M, et al. CD24, a mucin-type glycoprotein, is a ligand for P-selectin on human tumor cells. Blood 1997;89:3385–3395.
24. Nelson BH, Willerford DM. Biology of the interleukin-2 receptor. Adv Immunol 1998;70:1–81.
25. Agematsu K, Hokibara S, Nagumo H, Komiyama A. CD27: a memory B-cell marker. Immunol Today 2000;21: 204–206.
26. Green LJ, Mould AP, Humphries MJ. The integrin beta subunit. Intl J Biochem Cell Biol 1998;179–184.
27. Konopleva M, Rissling I, Andreeff M. CD38 in hematopoietic malignancies. Chem Immunol 2000;75:189–206.
28. Seveau S, Keller H, Maxfield FR, Piller F, Halbwachs-Mecarelli L. Neutrophil polarity and locomotion are associated with surface redistribution of leukosialin (CD43), an antiadhesive membrane molecule.
29. Bajorath J. Molecular organization, structural features, and ligand binding characteristics of CD44, a highly variable cell surface glycoprotein with multiple functions. Proteins 2000;39:103–111.
30. Justement LB. The role of CD45 in signal transduction. Adv Immunol 1997;66:1–65.
31. Mateo V, Lagneaux L, Bron D, et al. CD47 ligation induces caspase-independent cell death in chronic lympho-cytic leukemia. Nature Med 1999;5:1277–1284.
32. Seiffert M, Cant C, Chen Z, et al. Human signal-regulatory protein is expressed on normal, but not on subsets of leukemic myeloid cells and mediates cellular adhesion involving its counterreceptor CD47. Blood 1999;94: 3633–3643.
33. Hayashida K, Shimaoka Y, Ochi T, Lipsky PE. Rheumatoid arthritis synovial stromal cells inhibit apoptosis and up-regulate Bcl-xL expression by B cells in a CD49/CD29-CD106-dependent mechanism. J Immunol 2000; 164:1110–1116.
34. Berney SM, Schaan T, Alexander JS, et al. ICAM-3 (CD50) cross-linking augments signaling in CD3-activated peripheral human T lymphocytes. J Leukocyte Biol 1999;65:867–874.
35. Focarelli R, Della Giovampaola C, Seraglia R, et al. Biochemical and MALDI analysis of the human sperm antigen gp20, homologue of leukocyte CD52. Biochem Biophys Res Commun 1999;258:639–643.
36. Ginaldi L, De Martinis M, Matutes E, et al. Levels of expression of CD52 in normal and leukemic B and T cells: correlation with in vivo therapeutic responses to Campath-1H. Leukemia Res 1998;22:185–191.
37. Hubbard AK, Rothlein R. Intercellular adhesion molecule-1 (ICAM-1) expression and cell signaling cascades. Free Radical Biol Med 2000;28:1379–1386.
38. Brodbeck WG, Kuttner-Kondo L, Mold C, Medof ME. Structure/function studies of human decay-accelerating factor. Immunology 2000;101:104–111.
39. Qian YM, Qin X, Miwa T, Sun X, Halperin JA, Song WC. Identification and functional characterization of a new gene encoding the mouse terminal complement inhibitor CD59. J Immunol 2000;165:2528–2534.
40. Elangbam CS, Qualls CW, Dahlgren RR. Cell adhesion molecules—update. Vet Pathol 1997;34:61–73.

41. Jacquot S. CD27/CD70 interactions regulate T dependent B cell differentiation. Immunol Res 2000;21:23–30.
42. Adachi T, Wakabayashi C, Nakayama T, Yakura H, Tsubata T. CD72 negatively regulates signaling through the antigen receptor of B cells. J Immunol 2000;164:1223–1229.
43. Gordon MS, Kato RM, Lansigan F, Thompson AA, Wall R, Rawlings DJ. Aberrant B cell receptor signaling from B29 (Igbeta, CD79b) gene mutations of chronic lymphocytic leukemia B cells. Proc Natl Acad Sci USA 2000; 97:5504–5509.
44. Carpenito C, Pyszniak AM, Takei F. ICAM-2 provides a costimulatory signal for T cell stimulation by allogeneic class II MHC. Scand J Immunol 1997;45:248–254.
45. Osterborg A, Fassas AS, Anagnostopoulos A, Dyer MJ, Catovsky D, Mellstedt H. Humanized CD52 mono-clonal antibody Campath-1H as first-line treatment in chronic lymphocytic leukaemia. Br J Haematol 1996; 93:151–153.
46. Osterborg A, Dyer MJ, Bunjes D, et al. Phase II multicenter study of human CD52 antibody in previously treated chronic lymphocytic leukemia. European study group of CAMPATH-1H treatment in chronic lymphocytic leukemia. J Clin Oncol 1997;15:1567–1574.
47. Keating MJ, Byrd J, Rai K, et al. Multicenter study of campath-1H in patients with chronic lymphocytic leukemia (B-CLL) refractory to fludarabine. Blood 1999;94(suppl 1):705a.
48. Kennedy B, Rawstron AC, Evans P, et al. Campath-1H therapy in 29 patients with refractory CLL: true complete remission is an attainable goal. Blood 1999;94(suppl 1):603a.
49. Ferrajoli A, O'Brien S, Kurzrock R, et al. Phase II clinical trial of Campath-1H in refractory hematologic malignancies expresesing the surface antigen CD52. Proc ASCO 2000;19:8a.
50. Ginaldi L, De Martinis M, Matutes E, et al. Levels of expression of CD52 in normal and leukemic B and T cells: correlation with in vivo therapeutic responses to Campath-1H. Leuk Res 1998;22:185–191.
51. Pruzanski W, Urowitz MB, Grouix B, Vadas P. Induction of TNF-alpha and proinflammatory secretory phos-pholipase A2 by intravenous administration of CAMPATH-1H in patients with rheumatoid arthritis. J Rheumatol 1995;22:1816–1819.
52. Moreau T, Coles A, Wing M, et al. Transient increase in symptoms associated with cytokine release in patients with multiple sclerosis. Brain 1996;119:225–237.
53. Wing MG, Moreau T, Greenwood J, et al. Mechanism of first-dose cytokine-release syndrome by CAMPATH-1H: involvement of CD16 (FcgammaRIII) and CD11a/CD18(LFA-1) on NK cells. J Clin Invest 1996;98:2819–2826.
54. Byrd JC, Shinn CA, Jansure J, et al. Campath-1H induces apoptosis in human chronic lymphocytic leukemia cells in vitro independent of complement mediated lysis or Fc receptor ligation. Blood 1999;94(suppl 1):126a.
55. Nguyen DT, Amess JA, Doughty H, Hendry L, Diamond LW. IDEC-C2B8 anti-CD20 (rituximab) immuno-therapy in patients with low-grade non-Hodgkin's lymphoma and lymphoproliferative disorders:evaluation of response on 48 patients. Eur J Haematol 1999;62:76–82.
56. Byrd JC, Grever MR, Davis B, et al. Phase I/II study of thrice weekly rituximab in chronic lymphocytic leukemia (CLL)/small lymphocytic lymphoma (SLL): a feasible and active regimen. Blood 1999;94(suppl 1):704a.
57. O'Brien S, Freireich E, Andreeff M, Lerner S, Keating M. Phase I/II study of rituxan in chronic lymphocytic leukemia (CLL). Blood 1998;92(suppl 1):105a.
58. Keating MJ, O'Brien S, Lerner S, et al. Combination chemo-antibody therapy with fludarabine (F), cytclophosphamide (C) and rituximab (R) achieves a high CR rate in previously untreated chronic lymphocytic leukemia (CLL). Blood 2000;96(suppl 1):514a.
59. Garcia-Manero G, O'Brien S, Cortes J, et al. Combination fludarabine, cyclophosphamide and rituximab for previously treated patients with chronic lymphocytic leukemia (CLL). Blood 2000;96(suppl 1):757a.
60. Ginaldi L, De Martinis M, Matutes E, Farahat N, Morilla R, Catovsky D. Levels of expression of CD19 and CD20 in chronic B cell leukaemias. J Clin Pathol 1998;51:364–369.
61. Berinstein N, Grillo-Lopez A, White CA, et al. Association of serum rituximab concentration and anti-tumor response in the treatment of recurrent low-grade or follicular non-Hodgkin's lymphoma. Ann Oncol 1998;9:1–7.
62. Lagneaux L, Delforge A, Bron D, De Bruyn C, Stryckmans P. Chronic lymphocytic leukemia B cells but not normal B cells are rescued from apoptosis by contact with normal bone marrow stromal cells. Blood 1998;92:2387–2396.
63. Demiden A, Hanna N, Hariharan H. Chimeric anti-CD20 antibody (IDEC-C2B8) is apoptotic and sensitizes drug resistant human B-cell lymphomas and AIDS related lymphomas to the cytotoxic effect of CDDP, VP-16, and toxins. J FASEB 1995;9:206a.
64. Link BK, Wang H, Byrd JC, et al. Phase I trial of humanized 1D10 (Hu1D10) monoclonal antibody targetting class II molecules in patients with relapsed lymphoma. Proc ASCO 2000;19:24a.

65. Leonard JP, Coleman M, Chadburn A, et al. Epratuzumab (HLL2, anti-CD22 humanized monoclonal antibody) is an active and well-tolerated therapy for refractory/relapsed diffuse large B-cell non-Hodgkin's lymphoma (NHL). Blood 2000;96(suppl 1):578a.

66. Foss FM, Raubitscheck A, Mulshine JL, et al. Phase I study of the pharmacokinetics of a radioimmuno-conjugate, 90Y-T101, in patients with CD5-expressing leukemia and lymphoma. Clin Cancer Res 1998;4: 2691–2700.

67. DeNardo GL, Lewis JP, DeNardo SJ, O'Grady LF. Effect of Lym-1 radioimmuno-conjugate on refractory chronic lymphocytic leukemia. Cancer 1994;73:1425–1432.

68. Vose JM, Colcher D, Gobar L, et al. Phase I/II trial of multiple dose 131Iodine-Mab LL2 (CD22) in patients with recurrent non-Hodgkin's lymphoma. Leuk Lymph 2000;38:91–101.

69. Wiseman GA, White CA, Witzig TE, et al. Radioimmunotherapy of relapsed non-Hodgkin's lymphoma with zevalin, a 90Y-labeled anti-CD20 monoclonal antibody. Clin Cancer Res 1999;5(suppl 10):3281s–3286s.

70. Kaminski MS, Estes J, Zasadny KR, et al. Radioimmunotherapy with iodine (131) I tositumomab for relapsed or refractory B-cell non-Hodgkin's lymphoma: updated results and long-term follow-up of the University of Michigan experience. Blood 2000;96:1259–1266.

71. DeNardo GL, Kukis DL, Shen S, DeNardo DA, Meares aCF, DeNardo SJ. 67Cu-versus 131I-labeled Lym-1 antibody: comparative pharmacokinetics and dosimetry in patients with non-Hodgkin's lymphoma. Clin Cancer Res 1999;5:533–541.

72. Uckun FM, Messinger Y, Chen CL, et al. Treatment of therapy-refractory B-lineage acute lymphoblastic leukemia with an apoptosis-inducing CD19-directed tyrosine kinase inhibitor. Clin Cancer Res 1999;5:3906–3913.

73. Choe S, Bennet MH, Fuji G, et al. The crystal structure of diphtheria toxin. Nature 1992;357:216–222.

74. Allured VS, Collier RJ, Carroll SF, McKay DB. Structure of exotoxin A of Pseudomonas aeruginosa at 3.0 Angstroms. Proc Natl Acad Sci USA 1986;83:1320–1324.

75. Rutenber E, Robertus JD. Structure of ricin B-chain at 2.5 Angstrom resolution. Proteins 1991;10:260–269.

76. Monzingo AF, Collins EJ, Ernst SR, Irvin JD, Robertus JD. The 2.5 Angstrom structure of pokeweed antiviral protein. J Mol Biol 1993;233:705–715.

77. Brooke JS, Cha J-H, Eidels L. Diphtheria toxin:receptor interaction: association, dissociation, and effect of pH. Biochem Biophys Res Commun 1998;248:297–302.

78. Kounnas MZ, Morris RE, Thompson MR, FitzGerald DJ, Strickland DK, Saelinger CB. The alpha2-macroglobulin receptor/low density lipoprotein receptor-related protein binds and internalizes Pseudomonas exotoxin A. J Biol Chem 1992;267:12,420–12,423.

79. Frankel AE, Burbage C, Fu T, Tagge E, Chandler J, Willingham MC. Ricin toxin contains three galactose-binding sites located in B chain subdomains 1α, 1β, and 2γ. Biochem 1996;35:14,747–14,756.

80. Lemichez E, Bomsel M, Devilliers G, et al. Membrane translocation of diphtheria toxin fragment A exploits early to late endosome trafficking machinery. Mol Microbiol 1997;23:445–457.

81. Rapak A, Falnes PO, Olsnes S. Retrograde transport of mutant ricin to the endoplasmic reticulum with subsequent translocation to cytosol. Proc Natl Acad Sci USA 1997;94:3783–3788.

82. Oh KJ, Zhan H, Cui C, Hideg K, Collier RJ, Hubbell WL. Organization of diphtheria toxin T domain in bilayers: a site-directed spin labeling study. Science 1996;273:810–812.

83. Wilson KS, Noller HF. Molecular movement inside the translational engine. Cell 1998;92:337–349.

84. Van Ness BG, Howard JB, Bodley JW. ADP-ribosylation of elongation factor 2 by diphtheria toxin. NMR spectra and proposed structures of ribosyl-diphthamide and its hydrolysis products. J Biol Chem 1980;255: 10,710–10,716.

85. Endo Y, Tsurugi K, Lambert JM. The site of action of six different ribosome-inactivating proteins from plants on eukaryotic ribosomes: the RNA N-glycosidase activity of the proteins. Biochem Biophys Res Commun 1988;150:1032–1036.

86. Kreitman RJ, Margulies I, Stetler-Stevenson M, Wang QC, FitzGerald DJ, Pastan I. Cytotoxic activity of disulfide-stabilized recombinant immunotoxin RFB4(dsFv)-PE38 (BL22) toward fresh malignant cells from patients with B-cell leukemias. Clin Cancer Res 2000;6:1476–1487.

87. Van Horssen PJ, van Oosterhout YV, Evers S, et al. Influence of cytotoxicity enhancers in combination with human serum on the activity of CD22-recombinant ricin A against B cell lines, chronic and acute lymphocytic leukemia cells. Leukemia 1999;13:241–249.

88. Kreitman RJ, Chaudhary VK, Kozak RW, FitzGerald DJP, Waldmann TA, Pastan I. Recombinant toxins containing the variable domains of the anti-Tac monoclonal antibody to the interleukin-2 receptor kill malignant cells from patients with chronic lymphocytic leukemia. Blood 1992;80:2344–2352.

89. Kreitman RJ, Pastan I. Recombinant single-chain immunotoxins against T and B cell leukemias. Leuk Lymph 1994;13:1–10.

90. Re GG, Waters C, Poisson L, Willingham MC, Sugamura K, Frankel AE. Interleukin-2 (IL-2) receptor expression and sensitivity to diphtheria fusion toxin DAB389IL-2 in cultured hematopoietic cells. Cancer Res 1996;56: 2590–2595.

91. Waters CA, Bach PA, Snider CE, et al. Interleukin 2 receptor-targeted cytotoxicity. Receptor binding requirements for entry of a diphtheria toxin-related interleukin 2 fusion protein into cells. Eur J Immunol 1990;20:785–791.

92. Sweeney EB, Foss FM, Murphy JR, vanderSpek JC. Interleukin 7 (IL-7) receptor-specific cell killing by DAB389IL-7: a novel agent for the elimination of IL-7 receptor positive cells. Bioconjugate Chem 1998;9:201–207.

93. Faguet GB, Agee JF. Four ricin chain A-based immunotoxins directed against the common chronic lymphocytic leukemia antigen: in vitro characterization. Blood 1993;82:536–543.

94. Lambert JM, Goldmacher VS, Collinson AR, Nadler LM, Blattler WA. An immunotoxin prepared with blocked ricin: a natural plant toxin adapted for therapeutic use. Cancer Res 1991;51:6236–6242.

95. Uckun FM, Evans WE, Forsyth CJ, et al. Biotherapy of B-cell precursor leukemia by targeting genistein to CD19-associated tyrosine kinases. Science 1995;267:886–891.

96. Van Horssen PJ, Oosterhout YVJM, Evers S, et al. Influence of cytotoxicity enhancers in combination with human serum on the activity of CD22-recombinant ricin A against B cell lines, chronic and acute lymphocytic leukemia cells. Leukemia 1999;13:241–249.

97. Bolognesi A, Tazzari PL, Olivieri F, et al. Evaluation of immunotoxins containing single-chain ribosome-inactivating proteins and an anti-CD22 monoclonal antibody (OM124): in vitro and in vivo studies. Br J Haematol 1998;101:179–188.

98. Hertler AA, Schlossman DM, Borowitz MJ, Blythman HE, Casellas P, Frankel AE. An anti-CD5 immunotoxin for chronic lymphocytic leukemia: enhancement of cytotoxicity with human serum albumin-monensin. Int J Cancer 1989;43:215–219.

99. Hertler AA, Schlossman DM, Borowitz MJ, et al. A phase I study of T101-ricin A chain immunotoxin in refractory chronic lymphocytic leukemia. J Biol Resp Mod 1988;7:97–113.

100. Grossbard ML, Lambert JM, Goldmacher VS, et al. Anti-B4-blocked ricin: a phase I trial of 7-day continuous infusion in patients with B-cell neoplasms. J Clin Oncol 1993;11:726–737.

101. Grossbard ML, Freedman AS, Ritz J, et al. Serotherapy of B-cell neoplasms with anti-B4-blocked ricin: a phase I trial of daily bolus infusion. Blood 1992;79:576–585.

102. LeMaistre CF, Meneghetti C, Rosenblum M, et al. Phase I trial of an interleukin-2 (IL-2) fusion toxin (DAB486IL-2) in hematologic malignancies expressing the IL-2 receptor. Blood 1992;79:2547–2554.

103. LeMaistre CF, Rosenblum MG, Reuben JM, et al. Therapeutic effects of genetically engineered Toxin (DAB486IL-2) in patients with chronic lymphocytic leukaemia. Lancet 1991;337:1124–1125.

104. LeMaistre CF, Craig FE, Meneghetti C, et al. Phase I trial of a 90-minute infusion of the fusion toxin DAB486IL-2 in hematologic cancers. Cancer Research 1993;53:3930–3934.

105. Kreitman RJ, Wilson WH, White JD, et al. Phase I trial of recombinant immunotoxin anti-Tac (Fv)-PE38 (LMB-2) in patients with hematologic malignancies. J Clin Oncol 2000;18:1622–1636.

106. Kreitman RJ, Wilson WH, Stetler-Stevenson M, et al. High complete remission rate in chemotherapy-refractory classic or variant hairy cell leukemia induced by the anti-CD22 recombinant immunotoxin RFB4 (dsFv)-PE38 (BL22). Blood 2000;96(suppl 1):577a.

107. Chaudhary VK, FitzGerald DJ, Pastan I. A proper amino terminus of diphtheria toxin is important for cytotoxicity. Biochem Biophys Res Commun 1991;180:545–551.

108. Kreitman RJ, Pastan I. Importance of the glutamate residue of KDEL in increasing the cytotoxicity of Pseudomonas exotoxin derivatives and for increased binding to the KDEL receptor. Biochem J 1995;307:29–37.

109. Hessler JL, Kreitman RJ. An early step in Pseudomonas exotoxin action is removal of terminal lysine residue, which allows binding to the KDEL receptor. Biochemistry 1997;36:14,577–14,582.

110. Keppler-Hafkemeyer A, Kreitman RJ, Pastan I. Apoptosis induced by immunotoxins used in the treatment of hematologic malignancies. Intl J Cancer 2000;87:86–94.

17 New Treatment Strategies in Chronic Lymphocytic Leukemia

Upendra P. Hegde, MD
and Wyndham H. Wilson, MD, PhD

1. INTRODUCTION

In recent years, the focus of drug discovery has moved from identifying classical cytotoxic agents to finding molecules that target specific pathways involved in signal transduction, apoptosis, and differentiation, to name a few. These efforts have been greatly aided by insights into the structure of proteins and the ability to design specific inhibitors using small molecules or monoclonal antibodies. Indeed, the development of designer molecules such as STI-571 for chronic myeloid leukemia provides an important proof of principle, and supports the application of this strategy to other diseases such as chronic lymphocytic leukemia (CLL). In many respects, CLL represents an ideal disease for the development of targeted therapies because the availability of tumor cells allows the application of powerful techniques such as cDNA microarray and proteomics, which are rapidly providing insights into pathobiology and new therapeutic targets. These developments have ushered in a new era of hope that this chronic disease may be cured in our lifetime.

2. PATHOBIOLOGY AND DRUG DEVELOPMENT IN CLL

B-CLL tumor progression results from an imbalance in tumor cell division and cell death, which arises from decreased cell death (apoptosis) and/or increased cell division (cell cycle). For the leukemic population, this is clinically measured by the lymphocyte doubling time and reflects the relevant impact of these regulatory mechanisms on the clinical outcome. The cell death and division pathways contain multiple targets for the development of mechanistically based therapies.

2.1. Apoptosis Cell Death Pathways

A prominent biological characteristic of B-cell (B)-CLL is the dysregulation of apoptosis, resulting in a survival advantage over their normal counterparts, and a gradual accumulation of the malignant B-cell clone *(1)*. Although the initiating genetic event(s) are unclear, advances in understanding the core machinery of apoptosis and attendant signal transduction pathways are revealing strategies to overcome apoptosis resistance. Assays for apoptotic pathways have been developed and can be used to screen candidate agents for mechanism of action, as well as adopted

From: *Contemporary Hematology*
Chronic Lymphocytic Leukemia: Molecular Genetics, Biology, Diagnosis, and Management
Edited by: G. B. Faguet © Humana Press Inc., Totowa, NJ

for high-throughput screens to identify new agents. Two main pathways for apoptosis, termed the intrinsic (innate pathway) and extrinsic pathways, have been identified (Fig. 1). In the extrinsic pathway, signals from stimulated death receptors on the cell surface activate caspases, which function as the ultimate effectors and lead to the biochemical and morphological changes of apoptosis. In contrast, the intrinsic pathway is activated by endogenous molecules and is dependent on mitochondrial release of cytochrome c into the cytosol, which in turn activates terminal caspases and cellular death.

The BCL-2 family of proteins plays a central role in regulation of the intrinsic pathway, where their relative balance at the mitochondria determines cell survival or apoptosis. At least 20 members of the BCL-2 family have been identified in mammalian species to date, including proteins with anti-apoptotic effects (such as BCL-2, Bcl-X_L, Bcl-W, Mcl-1, Boo/Diva, and Al/Bff-1) and others (such as Bax, Bcl-X_s, Bad, Hrk, Bim, Bik, Blk, APR/Noxa, and Bcl-G_s), which have pro-apoptotic properties. Functionally, the BCL-2 proteins determine the structural integrity of the mitochondrial membranes, endoplasmic reticulum, and nuclear envelope, thereby regulating the release of cytochrome c. The Bax protein promotes apoptosis by blocking the inhibitory activity of BCL-2 as well as by directly targeting mitochondrial membrane and inducing release of caspase activating proteins. Clinical responses to chemotherapy and radiation therapy are affected by defects in Bax, because DNA-damaging agents elicit a cell stress response that promotes apoptosis. Such responses may be mediated through induction of p53, which in turn binds to the Bax gene product and directs its transcription. Thus mutations that inactivate Bax can contribute to poor responses to anticancer agents. The increased survival of B-CLL lymphocytes has been partially ascribed to constitutive expression of BCL-2 (2). Moreover, high levels of BCL-2 protein or high ratios of BCL-2/Bax have been associated with more aggressive behavior of B-CLL, including progressive disease, chemotherapy resistance and decreased survival (3,4).

The Bim protein may play a role in resistance to the vinca alkaloids through its association with microtubules. The Bim isoforms are sequestered in microtubules, and their disruption allows Bim to translocate to the surface of mitochondria, bind BCL-2/Bcl-X_L and other related anti-apoptotic proteins, and trigger cytochrome c release and apoptosis (Fig. 1). Another potentially relevant pathway in CLL involves the apoptotic protease activating factor I (APAF-1) protein, which, when activated by cytochrome c, activates caspase-9 and produces apoptosis (5) (Fig. 1). Recent data indicate that expression of Apaf-1 may be variable in CLL, suggesting that differences in Apaf-1 levels may affect the sensitivity of CLL to apoptosis (6). B-CLL has been reported to be profoundly resistant to Fas-induced apoptosis, suggesting that defects in the Fas pathway may also contribute to chemotherapy resistance (7).

The nuclear factor-κB (NF-κB) transcription factor plays an important role in apoptosis and has been linked to CLL. Normally, NF-κB is sequestered and bound to IκB (inhibitor of kappa B) and cannot enter the nucleus to increase expression of anti-apoptotic genes like BCL-2 and IAP's (inhibitor of apoptotic proteins; Fig. 1). In response to a death stimulus, tumor necrosis factor (TNF) family receptors can trigger NF-κB activation through interaction with TNF-associated factor (TRAF) family proteins, which phosphorylate IκB. Thus, a negative feedback mechanism has been demonstrated resulting from TNF-α signaling in which NF-κB activation suppresses the signals for cell death (8). Interestingly, increased TRAF levels are found in 50% of untreated and 80% of previously treated B-CLL (9). Elevated levels of NF-κB are found in CLL, possibly related to stimulation of CD40, a TNF family receptor, by the CD40 ligand, which is found on 15–30% of B-CLL cells (10,11).

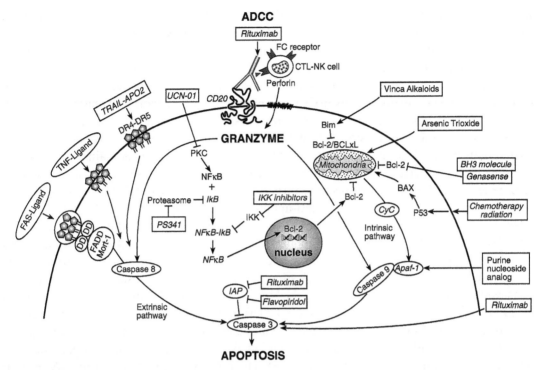

Fig. 1. Potential apoptotic mechanisms of drug (shown in boxes) actions are summarized. The extrinsic and intrinsic apoptosis pathways leading to the activation of effector cysteine proteases (caspases), ultimately leading to apoptosis, are summarized. Also depicted is the antigen-dependent cellular cytotoxicity (ADCC) pathway for rituximab. Arrows (→) represent positive regulation and bars (⊥) represent negative regulation. *See* text for details. Apaf-1, apoptotic protease-activating factor-1; APO2, apolopoprotein 2; Cyc, cytochrome C; FADD, Fas-associated death domain (Mort-1); CTL, cytotoxic T-lymphocytic; IAP, inhibitor of apoptotic protein; IKK, inhibitor of kappa B kinase; NF-kB, nuclear factor-kB; NK, natural killer (cell); PKC, protein kinase C; TNF, tumor necrosis factor; TRAIL, TNF-related apoptosis-inducing ligand.

The signal transducer and activator of transcription (STAT) proteins play a central role in mediating the response of hematopoietic cells to a diverse spectrum of cytokines. STAT proteins link cytokine receptor stimulation to gene transcription by acting as both cytosolic messengers and nuclear transcription factors. STAT proteins are activated through phosphorylation by JANUS kinase (JAK) kinases and other tyrosine kinases, and form dimers, which translocate to the nucleus and modulate gene expression. The serine residues of STAT proteins may also be phosphorylated and amplify the transcriptional activation mediated by tyrosine phosphorylation. In a recent study, inappropriate STAT-1 and STAT-3 serine phosphorylation was found in 23 patients with CLL, whereas none was found in normal control patients, suggesting that STAT proteins are involved in the pathobiology of CLL *(12)*. Therapeutically, fludarabine administration in CLL patients depletes STAT-1 protein and mRNA, but not other STAT proteins, suggesting that the STAT signaling pathway is an attractive target for the development of specific inhibitors *(13)*.

Apoptosis is an important if not principal mechanism of CLL cell death following effective therapeutic interventions, suggesting that these pathways are attractive targets for drug development (Fig. 1). BCL-2, which appears to play a central role in the survival of CLL cells through inhibition of apoptosis, may be inhibited through a variety of strategies, some of which have entered clinical trials. A promising approach involves antisense oligonucleotides, which are complementary DNA strands that bind BCL-2 mRNA, prevent protein translation, and decrease mRNA degradation *(14)*. Clinically, Genasense®, a BCL-2 antisense oligonucleotide (Fig. 1), has shown promising activity in CLL and is currently in a randomized phase III trial with fludarabine and cyclophosphamide. Using X-ray crystallographic and nuclear magnetic resonance analysis, the three-dimensional structure of BCL-2 and its homologs have been modeled to create small-molecule drugs that dock in the binding pocket of the BH3 domain (Fig. 1), which is responsible for dimerization, and inhibit its activity *(15)*. It may also be possible to inhibit BCL-2 gene expression through drugs such as flavopiridol (Fig. 1), a protein kinase inhibitor that variably downregulates the levels of the anti-apoptotic proteins BCL-2 and Mcl-1, while having little effect on the expression of pro-apoptotic proteins such as Bax and Bak *(16)*.

The TNF family ligand TNF-related apoptosis-inducing ligand (TRAIL), which binds and induces apoptosis through the death receptors DR4 and DR5, will soon enter clinical trial *(17,18)* (Fig. 1). Antibodies to CD40L, which block stimulation of CD40 and subsequent NF-κB activation, as well as small-molecule inhibitors of the NF-κB-activating IκB kinases (IKK)α and IKKβ (Fig. 1), are under development. In vitro, the CD20 monoclonal antibody rituximab activates apoptosis through the intrinsic pathway and downregulates IAPs (Fig. 1) and the anti-apoptotic Mcl-1 protein. Clinically, rituximab displays synergy with cytotoxic agents, potentially through its unique action on the apoptotic pathways *(19)*. The potential significance of the dATP/ATP binding site on Apaf-1 as a target for development of small-molecule inhibitors is suggested by the finding that purine analogs, such as fludarabine, can increase the catalytic efficiency of Apaf-1 by as much as 50-fold *(5)*.

2.2. Cell Cycle Pathways

The cell cycle consists of a set of highly ordered events that result in cell division and duplication. Multiple extracellular signals induce cells to traverse the cell cycle, through transcription of molecules, which serve as sensors to guide the cell's entry into various phases of cell cycle and division (Fig. 2). A central step in the G_1/S transition is the phosphorylation and inactivation of the retinoblastoma gene product (Rb), a tumor suppressor gene product, which results in the release of the E2F1 transcription factor and activation of E2F-responsive genes, such as cyclin E and thymidine kinase, necessary for progression to S phase. Rb phosphorylation occurs by activation of serine/threonine kinases that form complexes with cyclins and are known as cyclin-dependent kinases (CDKs). In turn, CDKs are regulated through a stoichiometric combination with small inhibitory proteins called cyclin-dependent kinase inhibitors (CDKIS), of which two families have been identified: the INK4 (inhibitor of CDK4) family of proteins (p16, p15, p18, and p19) and the KIP (kinase inhibitor protein) family of proteins (p21, p27, and p57) *(20)*, (Fig. 2). Tumors often have aberrations in the Rb pathway, resulting in hyperactivation of CDKs, through mechanisms such as amplification and/or overexpression of positive cofactors (e.g., cyclins/cdks), or downregulation of endogenous CDKIs or mutation of the Rb product. Understanding the structure and dynamics of cell cycle regulatory molecules opens the door for the development of small molecules directly targeted to the catalytic CDK subunit, or the direct manipulation of CDK activity through targeting molecules in the upstream and downstream pathways (Fig. 2). An immediate opportunity is the rational design of small-molecule CDK inhibitors that specifically interact with the ATP binding site *(21,22)*.

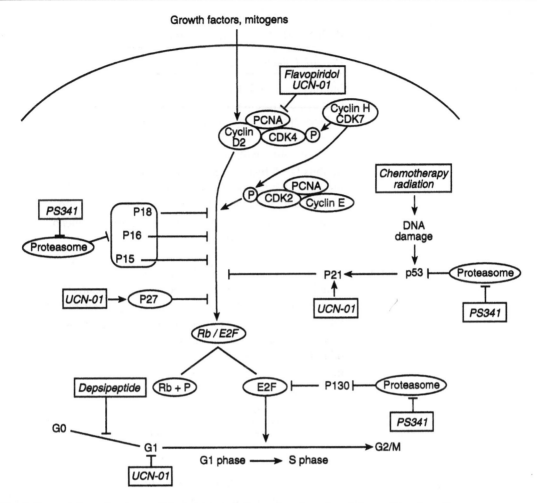

Fig. 2. Potential mechanisms of drug (shown in boxes) actions involving cell cycle pathways are summarized. Arrows (→) represent positive regulation and bars (⊥) represent negative regulation. *See* text for details. CDK, cyclin-dependent kinase; PCNA, proliferating cell nuclear antigen.

3. NOVEL THERAPEUTIC AGENTS

3.1. Agents With Novel Targets

3.1.1. FLAVOPIRIDOL

A semisynthetic flavonoid derived from rohitukine, flavopiridol is an alkaloid isolated from a plant indigenous to India. Initial studies showed that this agent could induce cell cycle arrest either in G_1 by cdk2 inhibition or in G_2/M by cdk1 inhibition. Various studies utilizing purified CDKs showed that flavopiridol inhibits cdks-1, -2, and -4 in a competitive manner through the ATP binding pocket (Fig. 2 and Table 1). A potentially important action of flavopiridol is the inhibition of cyclin D1, an oncogene that is overexpressed in mantle cell lymphoma. In vitro studies by Byrd et al. *(23)* in B-CLL demonstrated that flavopiridol can directly induce apoptosis independent of the BCL-2 and p53 pathways, suggesting that it may be active in lymphomas

Table 1
Drugs With Novel Mechanisms of Action

Agent	Potential mechanisms of action
Flavopiridol	Inhibits cyclin D1, CDK1, -2, -4 Cell cycle arrest in G1 or G2 phase of cell cycle Induces apoptosis by caspase 3 activation Downregulates BCL-2 and Mcl-1 Potential anti-angiogenesis
Depsipeptide	Inhibits DNA histone deactylase enzyme Inhibits cell cycle progression in G_0–G_1 Induces apoptosis through effects on BCL-2/Bax ratio
Bryostatin 1	Induces differentiation of CLL cells to hairy cell phenotype Inhibits protein kinase C Induces apoptosis
UCN-01 (7 hydroxy-staurosporine)	Nonspecific protein kinase C inhibitor Inhibits CDK and induces G_1 and G_2 cell cycle arrest Synergistic effects with purine analogs (e.g., fludarabine)
PS-341	Inhibits degradation of proteins important in cell cycle progression such as cyclin A, B, D, E, and CDKIs Inhibits NF-κB activation
Genasense	Reduces BCL-2 and its inhibition on apoptosis
Arsenic trioxide	Inhibits tumor proliferation and induces apoptosis Inhibits NF-κB through inhibition of IκB kinase

CDK, cyclin-dependent kinase; CDKI, CDK inhibitor; NF-κB, nuclear factor-κB.

that harbor these potential pathways of resistance. Others have suggested that flavopiridol-induced apoptosis in CLL cells is associated with early activation of the MAP kinase family [MEK, p38, c-Jun-N-terminal kinase (JNK)], which may lead to caspase activation, whereas studies by Byrd et al. (23) suggest direct activation of caspase 3. Melillo et al. (24) demonstrated anti-angiogenic properties of flavopiridol in in vitro studies. Thus far, flavopiridol administered as a continuous infusion has not shown significant clinical activity in lymphoid malignancies, but pharmacokinetic studies indicate that suboptimal concentrations of free drug are achieved owing to high protein binding. Based on this observation, new studies are under way using a short bolus schedule followed by a 4-h infusion, which is expected to provide higher target concentration of this drug in humans.

3.1.2. UCN-01

UCN-01 (7-hydroxy-staurosporine) is a potent inhibitor of Ca^{2+} and phospholipid-dependent protein kinase C (PKC), an important regulator of signal transduction. However, the inhibitory effects of staurosporine are nonspecific and have similar potencies for other protein kinases. Additional screening revealed that the 7-hydroxy analog of staurosporine, UCN-01 was a potent inhibitor of PKC (Fig. 1), and, importantly, its inhibitory effects were more selective (25), (Table 1). Whether additional protein kinases are targets for the drug is a matter of ongoing research, with recent studies indicating that the drug can inhibit cell cycle progression in conjunction with inhibition or altered activation of CDKs. More recent studies in leukemic T-cell lines have demonstrated irreversible inhibition of cell growth after 24 h of exposure, as well as evidence of internucleosomal DNA fragmentation consistent with induction of apoptosis after as little as 3–12 h of exposure. These observations correlated with apparent activation of cdk-1 and -2, and suggest that targets in addition to PKC must be considered. UCN-01 has demonstrated cytotoxic effects in various cell lines and antitumor activity against murine tumors and human tumor xenografts in vivo. Other molecules targeted by UCN-01 include various cdks, leading to abrogation of G2 and S phases of cell cycle (23). Kitada et al. (26) showed that UCN-01 enhances apoptosis in vitro by inhibition of the anti-apoptotic molecules Mcl-1 and X-linked inactivator of apoptosis (XIAP). Other groups have shown inhibitory effects on the DNA repair mechanisms in normal and CLL lymphocytes exposed to ultraviolet (UV) light or 4-hydroxy-cyclophosphamide in vitro (27). UCN-01 is currently in clinical development, primarily as a chemotherapy-sensitizing agent. Of note, as a single agent, UCN-01 produced a durable complete remission in a patient with a refractory anaplastic T-cell lymphoma and induced a complete remission with chemotherapy in a refractory large B-cell lymphoma. Combination studies of UCN-01 with fludarabine and other agents are ongoing.

3.1.3. Bryostatin

Bryostatin is a natural product isolated from the marine bryozoan *Bugula neritina* that targets PKC, initially stimulating PKC activity in the cell membrane, followed by inhibitory effects. Of potential clinical interest is the in vitro observation that it can induce differentiation of refractory B-CLL cells to a hairy cell phenotype, rendering them susceptible to 2-chlorodeoxyadenosine (28) (Table 1). A phase I study in humans identified a maximum tolerated dose of 120 µg/kg over 72 h, with a dose-limiting toxicity of generalized myalgia, headache, and fatigue as other common side effects. An in vitro assay for total PKC evaluation in patient peripheral blood mononuclear cells demonstrated activation within the first 2 h followed by downregulation, which was maintained for the duration of the infusion (29).

A phase II trial of bryostatin 1 in patients with relapsed low-grade lymphomas and CLL observed one complete and two partial remissions in 25 patients. Patients who progressed while receiving bryostatin 1 alone participated in a feasibility study by receiving vincristine administered immediately after infusion of bryostatin. Nine patients received sequential treatment with bryostatin 1 and vincristine. Phenotypic analysis by flow cytometry of the peripheral blood revealed a hairy cell phenotype in two of four CLL patients (28).

3.1.4. Depsipeptide

Depsipeptide, a bicyclic peptide produced by *Chromobacterium violaceum*, was first identified by Ueda et al. (30) through screening natural products for antitumor activity in myc expressing tumor cells. Mechanistically, depsipeptide inhibits cell cycle progression at the G_0–G_1 interface, (Fig. 2) and blocks p21 protein signal transduction, although it is not known whether if these actions explain its cytotoxic activity. Cell cycle arrest possibly occurs through inhibition of the ras-signal transduction pathway, and in vitro depsipeptide induces reversion of ras-transformed tumor cells to a normal morphology and regulates c-myc mRNA. One recent report also suggested that this agent might act via inhibition of the DNA histone deacetylase enzyme (31) (Table 1). In vitro, CLL cells demonstrate sensitivity to depsipeptide, through apoptosis, indicating it should be tested in this disease. Initial phase I trial pharmacokinetics demonstrated that plasma concentrations of this agent exceed those that cause both in vitro histone acetylation and favorable alterations in the bcl-2/bax ratio and also induce apoptosis in human CLL cells. Phase II studies in lymphoid malignancies are currently under way.

3.1.5. PROTEASOME INHIBITORS

Proteasome inhibitors, such as PS-341 are attractive targets for therapeutic intervention because of the importance of the ubiquitin proteasome pathways in the degradation and regulation of protein action (Table 1). The proteasome has numerous protein targets, such as p53, p21, and p27, and plays a key role in a broad array of cellular processes including cell cycle regulation, cell death, gene expression, and NF-κB activation *(32)* (Fig. 1). Dipeptide boronic acid analogs have been developed that inhibit the chymotryptic activity of the proteasome, with effects on tumor cell growth and apoptosis. PS-341 represents a class of novel proteasome inhibitors, which selectively inhibit the proteasome with a K_i of 6 nM and have a wide range of activity against multiple tumor cell lines. Phase I trials indicate that the drug is relatively nontoxic when administered iv twice weekly for 4 out of 6 wk at doses ranging from 0.5 to 1.25 mg/m^2. Various toxicities have been observed, including fatigue, nausea, vomiting, fever, and thrombocytopenia. Investigators have noted a direct correlation between the PS-341 dose and percent proteasome inhibition, and the biologic activity is reliably measured by inhibition of 20S proteasome activity in peripheral mononuclear cells. There is increasing evidence that proteasome inhibitors may have a potential role in the therapy of patients with CLL. Proteasome inhibition has been shown to induce apoptosis of CLL lymphocytes without affecting normal lymphocytes and can sensitize chemo- and radio-resistant CLL cells to apoptosis.

3.1.6. ARSENIC TRIOXIDE

Interest in arsenic trioxide (As_2O_3); (Table 1) has increased because of its activity in acute promyelocytic leukemia (APL), in which it has induced a high proportion of complete remissions in relapsed patients. Biologically, arsenic has been shown to inhibit tumor proliferation and induce apoptosis and to decrease or inhibit BCL-2 expression. Kapahi et al. *(33)* showed that arsenic is a potent inhibitor of NF-κB and IKBB activation. The limited clinical experience in B-CLL suggests that there may be some activity worth further study.

3.2. Monoclonal Antibodies

CLL cells express a number of antigens that are promising targets for monoclonal-based therapy (Table 2). Development of monoclonal antibodies has been largely accomplished by the empiric method of immunizing mice against human tumor cells and screening the hybridomas for antibodies of interest. Because murine antibodies have a short half-life and induce a human anti-mouse antibody (HAMA) immune response, they are usually chimeric or humanized when used as therapeutic reagents. Presently, several monoclonal antibodies have received Food and Drug Administration (FDA) approval and are used in CLL, including rituximab and alemtuzumab.

Monoclonal antibodies may be engineered to combine the antibody with a toxin (immunotoxins) or a radioactive isotope (radioimmunoconjugates) or may contain a second specificity (bispecific antibodies) (Table 2). For example, it is possible to conjugate an antibody with specificity to B-cell lymphomas with an antibody against CD3, which binds to and activates normal T-cells, in order to enhance T-cell-mediated lysis of the lymphoma cell. One such example of a bispecific antibody contains anti-CD3 and anti-CD19 specificity. Monoclonal antibodies raised against the immunoglobulin idiotype on a B-cell lymphoma represents another therapeutic strategy, which was first reported in 1982 by Levy et al. *(34)*. More recently, idiotype vaccines used to induce a polyclonal host antibody response against the malignant clone have shown promise as an effective treatment for minimal residual disease in follicular lymphomas.

3.2.1. RITUXIMAB

The first monoclonal antibody to receive FDA approval was rituximab. It is a chimeric monoclonal antibody directed against the normal CD20 antigen, which is found on over 95% of B-cell malignancies including most B-CLLs (Table 2). Rituximab has multiple potential mechanisms of cytotoxicity including antibody dependent cellular cytotoxicity (ADCC; Fig. 1), complement-dependent cytotoxicity (CDC), and direct induction of apoptosis, although which of these are the clinically important pathways is unclear *(35)*. Increasingly evident are the synergistic effects of rituximab and chemotherapy, suggesting that it sensitizes lymphoma cells to the apoptotic effects of chemotherapy by directly acting on tumor cells *(19)*. Although approved for indolent lymphomas, rituximab has gained increasing use in B-CLL. The initial experience with rituximab in B-CLL revealed a low response rate of approximately 13%, but more recent studies using either higher doses or more frequent dosing have reported response rates as high as 40–50% *(36)*. Based on in vitro studies showing synergistic effects of chemotherapy and rituximab *(37)*, rituximab is being clinically combined with agents like fludarabine and combinations such as cyclophosphamide, hydroxydaunomycin, vincristine, and prednisone (CHOP) *(38)*. In one study, rituximab and fludarabine produced an overall response rate of 93% (80% complete response and 13% partial response), in 30 patients with follicular non-Hodgkin's lymphoma. This combination was fairly well tolerated and had a median duration of response of 14 mo (range: 4–26+ mo); with 24 of 28 patients had ongoing responses. Similar response rates have been reported with CHOP plus rituximab combinations, and the long-term results are awaited.

3.2.2. ALEMTUZUMAB

Alemtuzumab (Campath) is a humanized monoclonal antibody targeted against the CD52 antigen present on the surface of normal neutrophils and lymphocytes as well as most B- and T-cell lymphomas (Table 2). CD52 is expressed at reasonable levels and does not modulate with antibody binding, making it a good target for unconjugated monoclonal antibodies. Mechanistically, alemtuzumab can induce tumor cell death through ADCC and CDC. Clinical activity has been demonstrated in patients with low-grade lymphomas and CLL, including patients with purine analog-refractory disease. In refractory CLL, response rates from 33 to 59% have been described, with higher response rates in untreated CLL patients *(39)*. The side effects of most concern are from acute infusion reactions and depletion of normal neutrophils and T-cells. Opportunistic infections are a serious side effect, particularly in patients who have received purine analogs, and have resulted in patient deaths.

3.2.3. APOLIZUMAB

Apolizumab is a humanized monoclonal antibody against the 1D10 antigen, a variant of the HLA-DR β-chain (Table 2), which is neither shed nor downmodulated on antibody binding. The 1D10 antigen is present on normal human cells, including dendritic cells, macrophages, and some activated T-cells, and is expressed in 50–70% of lymphomas and leukemias. Apolizumab is capable of mediating ADCC, CDC, and apoptosis of target cells that express the 1D10 antigen *(40)*. Apolizumab is being investigated for the treatment of B-cell malignancies including B-CLL. In a phase I study of weekly apolizumab, 4 of 8 patients with follicular center cell lymphomas achieved complete ($n = 1$, unconfirmed by bone marrow biopsy) or partial ($n = 3$) responses. Notably, all responses occurred on or beyond d 100, suggesting an immunological mechanism of action. In contrast, there was no activity in patients with more aggressive histolo-

Table 2
Monoclonal Antibody-Based Drugs

Target antigen and primary cell type	Function	Unlabeled	Radioisotope-based	Toxin-based
CD19: B cells	Activation	B4 (murine)	None	B-4 (ricin)
CD20: B cells	Proliferation/ differentiation	Rituximab (chimeric)	^{131}Iodine-tositumomab ^{90}Yttrium-ibritumomab tiuxetan	None
CD22: B cells	Activation	Epratuzumab (humanized) LL2 (murine)	LL2 ^{131}Iodine, LL2 ^{90}Yttrium	BL-22 (Pseudomonas)
CD52: B- and T-cells	Unknown	Alemtuzumab (humanized)	None	None
1D10 HLA-DR β-chain: B-cells	Activation	Apolizumab (humanized)	None	None
Lym-1 HLA-DR10: B-cells	Activation	None	^{131}Iodine ^{67}Copper	None
Tac (CD25 α-subunit): B- and T-cells	Activation	Zenapax (humanized)	None	LMB-2 (Pseudomonas)

gies *(41)*. Apolizumab is also being investigated in combination with rituximab and using more frequent dosing schedules.

3.2.4. EPRATUZUMAB

Epratuzumab is a humanized IgG1 monoclonal antibody directed against the CD22 antigen present on normal B-cells and B-cell lymphomas, with a distribution comparable to that of CD20, although the antigen density may be more variable. The CD22 antigen is a B-lymphocyte-restricted adhesion molecule of the immunoglobulin superfamily that plays a role in B-cell activation and interaction with T-cells (Table 2). It is initially expressed in the cytoplasm of pro-B and pre-B cells and occurs in mature B-cells that are IgD-positive. Initial phase I and phase II trials with this agent showed no dose-limiting toxicity with doses of 120–1000 mg/m^2/wk for four treatments *(42)* Partial depletion of B-cells was observed in some patients, with no change in hematological parameters, blood chemistries, and serum immunoglobulins. Detectable antibodies were detected in the serum 3–4 mo after completion of therapy and immunogenicity appeared to be rare. Epratuzumab is currently under evaluation in patients with rituximab-refractory indolent lymphomas and in combination with rituximab in follicular lymphomas. Radiolabeled versions of the Fab' fragment of murine antibody to CD22 (LL2) have been evaluated for lymphoma staging and radioimmunotherapy of lymphomas. Recently, a humanized, complementary determining region-grafted version of LL2 (hLL2) was generated and has shown similar pharmacokinetic and dosimetric properties to its murine counterpart. This agent has shown efficacy at low doses of administered radioactivity with acceptable toxicity.

3.2.5. IMMUNOTOXINS

Immunotoxins have been engineered using a variety of antigens and toxin combinations (Table 2). Traditionally, immunotoxins have been developed from the intact monoclonal antibody or its deglycosylated form or the Fab fragment, with conjugation to either ricin A chain or *Pseudomonas* exotoxin. Recently, bioengineered immunotoxins incorporating a single-chain Fv fragment, consisting of the antibody-variable region fused to a 38-dk truncated form of *Pseudomonas* exotoxin A (PE38), have been made. One such immunotoxin, LMB-2, targets the Tac antigen (α-subunit of CD25). In a phase I trial with a dose between 2 and 63 µg/kg, one partial response was seen among five patients with CLL. Responses were also observed in hairy cell leukemia and other lymphoma subtypes. Another immunotoxin, BL22, targets the CD22 antigen found on normal B-cells and B-cell malignancies. In a phase I study, this recombinant immunotoxin, containing an anti-CD22 variable domain (Fv) fused to truncated *Pseudomonas* exotoxin, was administered in a dose-escalation trial by iv infusion every other day for three doses each cycle. Of 16 cladarabine-refractory patients with hairy cell leukemia in this clinical trial, 11 patients achieved complete responses, 2 had partial responses, and 3 who did not respond received either a low dose or had pre-existing-toxin neutralizing antibodies *(43)*. Currently, phase I and II studies are under way to determine the optimal dose and schedule and to assess immunotoxin activity against a variety of lymphoid malignancies, including CLL. Notably, their unique spectrum of toxicities, which include vascular leak syndrome and hemolytic uremic syndrome, requires further investigation.

3.2.6. RADIOIMMUNOCONJUGATES

Radioimmunoconjugates provide monoclonal antibody-targeted delivery of radioactive particles to tumor cells (Table 2). ^{131}Iodine (^{131}I) is a commonly used radioisotope since it is readily available, relatively inexpensive, and easily conjugated to a monoclonal antibody. The γ-particles emitted by ^{131}I can be used for both imaging and therapy, but they have the drawbacks of releasing free ^{131}I and ^{131}I-tyrosine into the blood and present a potential health hazard to care givers. The β-emitter, ^{90}Yttrium (^{90}Y), has emerged as an attractive alternative to ^{131}I, based on its higher energy and longer path length, which may be more effective in tumors with larger diameters. It also has a short half-life and remains conjugated, even after endocytosis, providing a safer profile for outpatient use. However, disadvantages include its inability to image, and it is less available and more expensive. Clinically, radioimmunoconjugates have been developed with murine monoclonal antibodies against CD20 conjugated with ^{131}I [tositumomab (Bexxar®)] and ^{90}Y [ibritumomab tiuxetan Zevalin®]. Both drugs have shown responses rates in relapsed lymphoma of 65–80% *(44,45)* but are likely to be less effective and more toxic in CLL because of bone marrow involvement and the leukemic phase.

Pretargeting has been used to increase the therapeutic index of radioimmunoconjugates by taking advantage of the high binding affinity of avidin and biotin. Patients are initially treated with avidin labeled monoclonal antibody, followed 1–2 d later, after maximal binding of the monoclonal antibody to the target, by administration of yttrium-conjugated biotin. This technique may improve the specificity of radioisotope delivery to tumor cells, thus increasing the therapeutic index.

4. IMMUNE STRATEGIES

Impaired immune mechanisms are a recognized characteristic of CLL and lead to increased autoimmunity against hematological targets and increased infections late in the disease course. The cause of these defects is poorly understood, but dysregulation of the T-cell compartment may play a role. Indeed, it is possible that the altered immunity in CLL may play a permissive role in the emergence of the malignant clone during the process of lymphomagenesis *(46)*. Although investigators have recognized this factor as a potential barrier, they are developing and testing strategies to increase autoimmunity against the CLL cell. One area of active investigation is the CD40 pathway, which is involved in B-cell differentiation and activity; triggering of the CD40 pathway in germinal center B-cells results in inhibition of apoptosis, proliferation, differentiation with Ig isotype switch, and expression of activation antigens, including CD23, and Fas. In the allogeneic setting, CD40-stimulated B-CLL cells have been reported to activate CD8+ cytolytic T-cells against both untreated and CD40-stimulated B-CLL cells. When done in the autologous setting, however, the CD40-stimulated B-CLL cells could only activate CD4+ T-cells that lacked significant cytolytic activity *(47)*. Whether the absence of autologous CD8+ T-cell expansion is owing to defects in the T-cell compartment of B-CLL needs to be explored, but this possibility presents a barrier to such strategies.

Using this theory, Kato et al. *(48)* transduced B-CLL leukemic cells with an adenovirus encoding the murine CD154 antigen (CD40 ligand) and showed increased expression of the CD80 and CD86 costimulatory molecules, as well as the generation of cytotoxic T-lymphocytes against unmodified autologous B-CLL cells. Moreover, they demonstrated the activation of noninfected bystander B-CLL cells. Results of a phase I trial using this approach were recently reported by the same group. Nine intermediate or high-risk B-CLL patients received escalating doses of CD154-transduced autologous B-CLL cells. The study demonstrated activation of circulating bystander leukemia cells, as well as reductions in absolute lymphocyte counts and lymph node sizes. Based on these promising results, further studies are planned.

5. CONCLUSIONS

Although CLL remains incurable, advances in the identification and validation of targets, as well as new treatment modalities, hold significant promise. These include the identification of new targets through insights into the pathobiology of CLL, as well as identification of cell surface antigens, and extracellular cytokines and the application of immunology to the development of immune-based treatments. Not only must these new classes of agents and treatment approaches be clinically validated, but their optimal use will require extensive clinical investigation. The next 10 years promise to be an exciting time for clinical research in CLL.

REFERENCES

1. Reed JC. Molecular biology of chronic lymphocytic leukemia. Semin Oncol 1998;25:11–18.
2. Hanada M, Delia D, Aiello A, Stadtmauer E, Reed JC. Bcl-2 gene hypomethylation and high level expression in B-cell chronic lymphocytic leukemia. Blood 1993;82:1820–1828.
3. McConkey DJ, Chandra J, Wright S, et al. Apoptosis sensitivity in chronic lymphocytic leukemia is determined by endogenous endonuclease content and relative expression of BCL-2 and Bax. J Immunol 1996;156:2624–2630.
4. Pepper C, Bentley P, Hoy T. Regulation of clinical chemo-resistance by bcl-2 and bax oncoproteins in B-cell chronic lymphocytic leukemia cells. Blood 1997;89:3378–3384.
5. Genini D, Budihardjo I, Plunkett W, et al. Nucleotide requirements for the in vitro activation of the apoptosis protein activating factor-1 mediated caspase pathway. J Biol Chem 2000;275:29–34.
6. Li P, Nijhawan D, Budihardjo I, et al. Cytochrome C and ATP-dependent formation of APAF-1 caspase-9 complex initiates an apoptotic protease cascade. Cell 1997;91:479–489.
7. Rou'e G, Lancry L, Duquesne F, Salaun V, Troussard X, Sola B. Upstream mediators of the Fas apoptotic transduction pathway are defective in B-chronic lymphocytic leukemia. Leuk Res 2001;25:967–980.
8. Van Antwerp DJ, Martin SJ, Kafri T, Green DR, Verma IM. Suppression of TNF-α-induced apoptosis by NF-κB. Science 1996;274:788–789.
9. Leoni LM, Chao Q, Cottam HB, et al. Induction of an apoptotic program in cell-free extracts by 2 Chloro-2'-deoxyadenosine 5'-triphosphate and cytochrome C. Proc Natl Acad Sci USA 1998;95:9567–9571.

10. Zapata JM, Krajewska M, Krajewska S, et al. TNFR-associated factor family protein expression in normal tissues and lymphoid malignancies. J Immunol 2000;165:5084–5096.
11. Furman RR, Asgary Z, Mascarenhas JO, Schattner EJ. Modulation of NF-κb activity and apoptosis in chronic lymphocytic leukemia B cells. J Immunol 2000;164:2200–2206.
12. Frank DA, Mahajan S, Ritz J. B lymphocytes from patients with chronic lymphocytic leukemia contain signal transducer and activator of transcription (STAT)1 and STAT 3 constitutively phosphorylated on serine residues. J Clin Invest 1997;100:3140–3148.
13. Frank DA, Mahajan S, Ritz J. Fludarabine-induced immunosuppression is associated with inhibition of STAT1 signaling. Nat Med 1999;5:444–447.
14. Webb A, Cunningham D, Clarke PA, et al. Bcl-2 antisense therapy in patients with non-Hodgkin lymphoma. Lancet 1997;349:1137–1141.
15. Wang J-L, Liu D, Zhang Z-J, et al. Structure-based discovery of an organic compound that binds Bcl-2 protein and induces apoptosis of tumor cells. Proc Natl Acad Sci USA 2000;97:7124–7129.
16. Kitada S, Zapata JM, Andreeff M, Reed C. Protein kinase inhibitors flavopiridol and 7-hydroxy staurosporine down-regulate anti-apoptosis proteins in B-cell chronic lymphocytic leukemia. Blood 2000;96:393–397.
17. Ashkenazi A, Pai RC, Fong S, et al. Safety and antitumor activity of recombinant soluble Apo2 ligand. J Clin Invest 1999;104:55–162.
18. Bonavida B, Ng CP, Jazirehi A, et al. Selectivity of TRAIL-mediated apoptosis of cancer cells and synergy with drugs: the trail to non-toxic cancer therapeutics. Int J Oncol 1999;15:793–802.
19. Reed JC, Kitada S, Kim Y, Byrd J. Modulating apoptosis pathways in low-grade B-cell malignancies using biological response modifiers. Semin Oncol 2002;29:10–24.
20. Jurlander J. The cellular biology of B-cell chronic lymphocytic leukemia. Crit Rev Oncol Hematol 1998;27:29–52.
21. Ball KL, Lain S, Fahraeus R, Smythe C, Lane DP. Cell-cycle arrest and inhibition of Cdk4 activity by small peptides based on the carboxy-terminal domain of p21 WAF1. Curr Biol 1997;7:71–80.
22. Senderowicz AM, Sausville EA. Preclinical and clinical development of cyclin-dependent kinase modulators. J Natl Cancer Inst 2000;92:376–387.
23. Byrd JC, Shinn C, Waselenko JK, et al. Flavopiridol induces apoptosis in chronic lymphocytic leukemia cells via activation of caspase-3 without evidence of bcl-2 modulation or dependence on functional p53. Blood 1998;92:3804–3816.
24. Melillo G, Sausville EA, Cloud K, Lahusen T, Varesio L, Senderowitz AM. Flavopiridol, a protein kinase inhibitor, down-regulates hypoxic induction of vascular endothelial growth factor expression in human monocytes. Cancer Res 1999;59:5433–5437.
25. Saenaeve C, Kazanietz MG, Blumberg PM, et al. Differential inhibition of PKC isozymes by UCN-01, a staurosporine analog. Mol Pharmacol 1994;45:1207–1214.
26. Kitada S, Zapata JM, Andreeff M, Reed JC. Protein kinase inhibitors flavopiridol and 7-hydroxy-staurosporine down-regulate anti-apoptosis proteins in B-cell chronic lymphocytic leukemia. Blood 2000;96:393–397.
27. Yamauchi T, Keating MJ, Plunkett W. UCN-01(7-hydroxystaurosporine) inhibits DNA repair and increases cytotoxicity in normal lymphocytes and chronic lymphocytic leukemia lymphocytes. Mol Cancer Ther 2002;1:287–294.
28. Varterasian ML, Mohammad RM, Shurafa MS, et al. Phase II trial of bryostatin 1 in patients with relapsed low-grade non-Hodgkin's lymphoma and chronic lymphocytic leukemia. Clin Cancer Res 2000;6:825–828.
29. Varterasian ML, Mohammad RM, Eilender DS, et al. Phase I study of bryostatin 1 in patients with relapsed non-Hodgkin's lymphoma and chronic lymphocytic leukemia. J Clin Oncol 1998;16:56–62.
30. Ueda H, Nakajima H, Hori Y, et al. Depsipeptide: a novel antitumor bicyclic depsipeptide produced by *Chromobacterium violaceum* no. 968. Taxonomy, fermentation, isolation, physico-chemica 1, and biological properties, and antitumor activity. J Antibiotics 1994;47:301–310.
31. Nakajima H, Kim YB, Terano H, Yoshida M, Horinouchi S. FR901228, a potent antitumor antibiotic, is a novel histone deacetylase inhibitor. Exp Cell Res 1998;241:126–133.
32. Adams J, Palombella VJ, Elliott PJ. Proteasome inhibition, a new strategy in cancer treatment. Invest New Drugs 2000;18:109–121.
33. Kapahi P, Takahashi T, Natoli G, et al. Inhibition of NF-kappa B activation by arsenite through reaction with a critical cysteine in the activation loop of Ikappa B kinase. J Biol Chem 2000;275:36,062–36,066.
34. Miller RA, Maloney DG, Warnke R, et al. Treatment of B-cell lymphoma with monoclonal anti-idiotype antibody. N Engl J Med 1982;306:517–522.

35. Maloney DG, Smith B, Rose A. Rituximab: mechanism of action and resistance. Semin Oncol 2002;29(suppl 2): 2–9.

36. O'Brien SM, Kantarjian H, Thomas DA, et al. Rituximab dose-escalation trial in chronic lymphocytic leukemia. J Clin Oncol 2001;19:2165–2170.

37. Alas S, Bonavida B, Emmanouilides C. Potentiation of fludarabine cytotoxicity on non-Hodgkin's lymphoma by pentoxifylline and rituximab. Anticancer Res 2000;20:2961–2966.

38. Czuczman MS, Fallon A, Mohr A, et al. Rituximab in combination with CHOP or fludarabine in low-grade lymphoma. Semin Oncol 2002;29:36–40.

39. Osterborg A, Dyer MJ, Bunjes D, et al. Phase II multi-center study of human CD52 antibody in previously treated chronic lymphocytic leukemia, European Study Group of CAMPATH-1H treatment in chronic lymphocytic leukemia. J Clin Oncol 1997;15:1567.

40. Higaki Y, Hata D, Kanazashi S, et al. Mechanisms involved in the inhibition of growth of a human B lymphoma cell line, B104, by anti-MHC class antibodies. Immunol Cell Biol 1994;72:205–214.

41. Link BK, Wang H, Byrd JC, et al. Phase I trial of humanized 1D10 (Apolizumab) monoclonal antibody targeting class II molecules in patients with relapsed lymphoma. Proc Am Soc Clin Oncol 2000;19:24a (abstract 86).

42. Leonard JP, Link BK. Immunotherapy of non-Hodgkin's lymphoma with hLL2 (epratuzumab, an anti-CD22 monoclonal antibody) and HU1D10 (apolizumab). Semin Oncol 2002;29(suppl 2):81–86.

43. Kreitman RJ, Wilson WH, Bergeron K, et al. Efficacy of the anti-CD22 recombinant immunotoxin BL22 in chemotherapy-resistant hairy cell leukemia. N Engl J Med 2001;345:241–247.

44. Kaminski MS, Zelenetz AD, Press OW, et al. Pivotal study of Iodine I 131 Tositumomab for chemotherapy-refractory low-grade or transformed low-grade B-cell non Hodgkin's lymphomas. J Clin Oncol 2001;19:3918–3928.

45. Gordon LI, Witzig TE, Wiseman GA, et al. Yttrium 90 Ibritumomab Tiuxetan radioimmunotherapy for relapsed or refractory low-grade non-Hodgkin's lymphoma. Semin Oncol 2002;29:87–92.

46. Kipps TJ. Advances in classification and therapy of indolent B-cell malignancies. Semin Oncol 2002;29(suppl 2): 98–104.

47. Buhmann R, Nolte A, Westhaus D, Emmerich B, Hallek M. CD40-activated B-cell chronic lymphocytic leukemia cells for tumor immunotherapy: stimulation of allogeneic versus autologous T cells generates different types of effector cells. Blood 1999;93:1992–2002.

48. Kato K, Cantwell MJ, Sharma S, Kipps TJ. Gene transfer of CD40-ligand induces autologous immune recognition of chronic lymphocytic leukemia B cells. J Clin Invest 1998;101:1133–1141.

18   Gene Therapy
of Chronic Lymphocytic Leukemia

Januario E. Castro, MD and Thomas J. Kipps, MD, PhD

1. INTRODUCTION

The term *gene therapy* describes a new type of medicine mediated by the transfer of genes into somatic cells. Knowledge of viruses and how they introduce their genetic material into cells has allowed for development of virus-derived "vectors" that can infect cells and thereby introduce a selected gene(s). Through advances in molecular biology we can achieve high-level expression of the transferred genes (or *transgene*) in almost any type of mammalian cell. The transgene can direct synthesis of an intracellular, cell surface, or secreted protein(s) that complements a genetic defect or that provides for a desired phenotype. Alternatively, the transferred genetic material may mitigate expression of genes encoding unwanted or mutated proteins through "gene interference" or gene complementation. Conceivably, transfer and expression of appropriate genes could be used to correct for genetic deficiencies or allow for expression of a desired characteristic(s) by vector-infected (or *transduced*) cells. Although we have yet to realize the application of this technology in clinical practice, gene therapy arguably has tremendous potential for altering our approach to the treatment of a variety of genetic and acquired diseases, including cancer.

Chronic lymphocytic leukemia (CLL) has several features that make it amenable to gene therapy. Like many other forms of cancer, CLL results from genetic changes that affect the turnover and survival of normal B-cells, allowing for accumulation of cells descending from one clone of differentiated B-cells. Knowledge of the genes encoding proteins that contribute to the resistance of leukemia cells to programmed cell death, or *apoptosis*, has allowed for development of strategies with which to interfere with expression or function of anti-apoptotic genes. In addition, the genetic alterations and clonal distribution of unique immunoglobulin gene rearrangements in this B-cell malignancy may encode "altered-self" proteins that potentially could be recognized by the patient's immune system. Since large numbers of leukemia cells can be harvested via a relatively simple procedure (e.g., *leukapheresis*), strategies involving ex vivo gene transfer into neoplastic cells are highly feasible. This allows for in vitro evaluation of gene transfer and expression prior to reinfusion of vector-modified leukemia cells. Also, it allows for development of clinical trials that evaluate the safety and clinical response to defined numbers of transduced neoplastic cells. Relatively simple blood tests then can be used to monitor expression of the transgene(s) by the neoplastic cells in vivo, leukemia cell number, or changes in bystander cells following gene transfer. Finally, normal host cells that infiltrate

From: *Contemporary Hematology*
Chronic Lymphocytic Leukemia: Molecular Genetics, Biology, Diagnosis, and Management
Edited by: G. B. Faguet © Humana Press Inc., Totowa, NJ

the tumor are found in the blood, making such cells accessible for isolation and analysis. Thus, CLL has several features that could facilitate development of novel gene therapy approaches.

Gene therapy trials in patients with CLL are under way. Methods have been identified for effecting high-level transgene expression in CLL using virus vectors. Studies have identified means with which to alter the leukemia cell through gene transfer so as to elicit immune effector mechanisms that can contribute to leukemia cell clearance. As of August of 2002, five active clinical trials of gene therapy in CLL had been reported to the Office of Biotechnology Activities of the National Institutes of Health. These include protocols studying the effect of transducing immunomodulator genes, such as CD40 ligand (CD154) and/or interleukin-2 (IL-2), the capacity for cell marking with genes encoding neomycin phosphotransferase in the context of hematopoietic stem cell transplantation, and intramuscular injection of plasmid DNA using tumor idiotype vaccination (1). This chapter discusses the current status of gene therapy applied to CLL, recent publications, and future strategies in this field.

2. VIRUS VECTORS FOR GENE TRANSFER

2.1. Retrovirus Vectors

Retrovirus vectors are among the most popular vectors for gene transfer. They are lipid-enveloped particles containing a homodimer of linear, positive-sense, single-stranded RNA 7–11 kb in length. Because of their relatively small size, they can be manipulated easily to incorporate a gene of interest. Additionally, they produce stable and high-level transgene expression in the infected cell and its progeny.

Retrovirus vectors can be used for cell tagging with a marker gene, such as the one encoding neomycin resistance or green fluorescent protein (2,3). Such marked stem cells have been used to label transduced cells in clinical trials involving autologous stem cell transplantation, allowing for tracking of transduced cells during engraftment or clinical relapse (2,4).

The family of retroviruses includes several members that are being exploited for gene therapy. The initial evaluated types include the mammalian and avian C-type retroviruses (oncoretroviruses). More recently, spumaviruses and lentiviruses (such as HIV and other immunodeficiency viruses) have been examined for use in gene transfer. The latter, unlike other retroviruses, have the added advantage of being able to infect nondividing cells (5).

Pseudotyping can improve the range of cells that can be infected with retrovirus. Retrovirus particles can be made by cells that synthesize the envelope proteins of another virus [e.g., vesicular stomatitis virus G (VSV-G) protein] instead of the retrovirus envelope protein. Such "pseudotyped" virus particles are more resilient and better able to infect a broad range of cell types than standard retrovirus particles (6). However, CLL cells appear particularly resistant to transduction with retrovirus vectors, including vectors that are pseudotyped with VSV-G.

2.2. Adenovirus Vectors

Adenovirus vectors are also used for gene therapy. There are over 50 different human adenovirus serotypes, but current vectors are primarily derived from serotypes 2 and 5 (7). Most adenovirus vectors lack genes that are essential for virus replication, thus creating space for the insertion of a desired transgene (8). These viruses can only be grown in packaging cell lines that express the missing genes, allowing for complementation of the genetic defect.

Several qualities make adenoviruses good candidates for gene therapy. They can be produced and purified with high titers. Through the use of heterologous promoters and enhancers, they can effect high levels of transgene expression. Because the adenovirus DNA remains episomal, adenovirus vectors cannot effect insertional mutagenesis. Finally, adenovirus can infect and effect transgene expression in postmitotic nondividing cells.

Adenovirus vectors generally are not suitable for stable transgene expression. Because the virus does not integrate into the host cell's genome, it may not be retained by the daughter cells produced during cell replication. In addition, adenovirus vectors can induce antibody responses that can neutralize the ability of subsequent injections of adenovirus to infect cells in vivo. Moreover, the immune system can generate a cellular response to virus-infected cells, thereby clearing cells that express adenovirus-encoded proteins (9,10). However, this could be advantageous if the adenovirus infects tumor cells, potentially providing an adjuvant effect that could boost an otherwise weak response to tumor-associated antigens (11).

We found that adenovirus can infect CLL cells (12). The susceptibility to infection generally correlates with the relative expression of coxsackie adenovirus receptor (CAR) protein (13–15). CLL cells express low levels of CAR but can be infected by adenovirus at high multiplicity of infection (MOI). Uptake of virus appears to be mediated through interaction with integrins expressed on leukemia cells via a CAR-independent process that requires the virus to be present at a relatively high local concentration. Recognition of CAR expression is low in many human carcinomas, which has prompted development of adenovirus vectors capable of CAR-independent gene transfer (8,16,17). Such new developments may find their application in gene therapy strategies for CLL in vivo.

2.3. Adeno-Associated Viruses

Adeno-associated virus (AAV) is a human parvovirus that was initially discovered as a contaminant in adenovirus preparations. AAV requires a helper virus, such as adenovirus, to mediate a productive infection (18). There are six known human virus serotypes, of which AAV-2 is the best studied. No known human disease is associated with AAV.

AAV vectors have a number of qualities that make them highly suitable for gene therapy. AAV vectors can effect transgene expression in nondividing cells. Also, although they also can be episomal, AAV can integrate into the infected cell's genome. This provides AAV vectors with the potential for effecting long-term transgene expression, even in successive generations of daughter cells (19–21). Finally, AAV vectors generally do not induce inflammatory responses or cytotoxic immune responses against infected cells (18,22–24).

However, like adenovirus vectors, injection of free AAV can elicit neutralizing antibodies that can mitigate the ability of subsequent injections to infect cells in vivo. Also, AAV can only accept transgenes of relatively small size (<5 kb). Large-scale production and purification of this vector is problematic, and this will require the development of improved packaging cell lines and chromatographic methods for vector purification (25,26).

Another unfavorable feature is that AAV vectors apparently do not infect lymphocytes or CLL cells efficiently, making it necessary to consider ex vivo transduction strategies that use AAV vectors at high concentration. Nonetheless, AAV vectors can efficiently transfer genes encoding antigens to cells in skin or muscle, allowing for their potential use as vaccines encoding tumor-associated antigens.

2.4. Herpes Simplex Virus

Herpesviruses are promising vehicles for transferring genes into cells. Among this virus family, herpes simplex virus type 1 (HSV-1) is the most extensively studied for potential use in human gene therapy. Its genome is comprised of 152 kb of linear dsDNA containing at least 84 contiguous genes of which only 50% are essential for virus replication. For this reason, HSV-1 vectors can carry very large transgene inserts (approximately 30 kb), potentially allowing HSV-1 vectors to contain multiple transgenes that may be individually or coordinately expressed (27). After deletion of the immediate early gene region, HSV can be grown and purified in large-scale quantities without the risk of inducing replication complement virus. Such mutants have variable cytopathic effects and can enter a state of latency in non-neuronal tissues (28).

We found that CLL B-cells are highly sensitive to infection with vectors derived from replication-defective (rd)HSV-1 (29). CLL B-cells express high levels of herpesvirus entry mediator (Hve)A, but not HveC, the other known receptor for HSV-1. In contrast to B-cells of normal donors, CLL B-cells are relatively resistant to the cytopathic effects of infection by rdHSV-1 and can maintain high-level expression of the transgene for many days after infection, possibly because of the high-level expression of anti-apoptotic genes, e.g., BCL-2, by CLL cells. Consistent with this hypothesis, we found that transduction of HeLa cells with a retrovirus expression vector encoding BCL-2 rendered HeLa cells resistant to the cytopathic effects of rdHSV-1 (29).

HSV amplicon vectors represent an alternative to replication-defective recombinant genomic vectors. The amplicon is essentially a eukaryotic expression plasmid that contains the following genetic elements: (1) HSV-derived origin of DNA replication (ori) and packaging sequence ("a" sequence); (2) transcriptional unit typically driven by the HSV-1 immediate early promoter or an alternative promoter followed by an SV-40 polyadenylation site; and (3) a bacterial origin of replication and an antibiotic resistance gene for propagation in *Escherichia coli (30,31)*. Even so, amplicon plasmids are dependent on helper virus for the replication machinery and structural proteins that are necessary for packaging the amplicon-vector DNA into virus particles. Recently, helper virus-free amplicon packaging methods were developed by using complementary overlapping cosmids or bacterial artificial chromosomes (BACs) (32–34). The use of such amplicons simplifies vector construction and minimizes the potential for adverse effects caused by infection with live HSV-1.

HSV amplicons may be efficient vectors for gene therapy of CLL. Using this system, Tolba and collaborators (35) explored the effects of transduction of primary human B-cell CLL. They constructed vectors encoding CD80 (B7.1) or CD154 (CD40L) that were packaged using either a standard helper virus or a helper virus-free method. They found that helper virus-free HSV amplicon preparations were as effective as standard HSV in infecting CLL cells and in inducing high levels of transgene expression.

3. NONVIRUS VECTORS

Nonvirus vectors use different combinations of naked DNA, DNA-containing liposomes, complex polymer-based systems, and combination of lipids or peptides. In general these systems are easier to purify and to deliver (17,36). However, they generally lack the efficiency of virus vector-mediated gene delivery systems, are less predictable, and do not induce the same high level of transgene expression as that of virus-based vector systems.

3.1. DNA Vaccination

DNA plasmid expression vectors can be used for gene transfer. Generally, the transgene is placed downstream of a strong promoter, such as the heterologous cytomegalovirus promoter/

enhancer region, and upstream of a polyadenylation signal sequence, to allow for appropriate RNA processing and transport from the nucleus. Transfection of cells with such plasmid DNA can effect high-level expression of the transgene, provided the RNA has appropriate Kozak sequences for initiating effective translation of the RNA into protein *(37)*.

This technique is currently being explored as a potential strategy for treating CLL and other B-cell malignancies. For patients with B-cell tumors, the immunoglobulin idiotype expressed by the neoplastic clone provides a defined tumor-specific target antigen. However, the immunoglobulin idiotype is poorly immunogenic, especially in patients with CLL. Fusion of a gene encoding a fragment of tetanus toxin with the gene encoding the idiotype can enhance the immune response to such weak tumor-specific antigens. DNA fusion vaccines containing genes that encode immune-enhancing factors can also augment the immune response to such antigens *(38–40)*.

3.2. Oligonucleotides

Oligonucleotides (ODNs) are short stretches of synthetic DNA that can be made with the natural oxygen-containing phosphodiester backbone or a sulfur-containing phosphorothioate scaffolding. Either type of ODN can bind complementary DNA or RNA with similar efficiency. However, ODNs with phosphothioate bonds resist nuclease degradation, providing the synthetic DNA with a longer half-life than native DNA in vivo. Several other attempts have been made to improve the bioavailability and efficacy of ODNs. They include the use of lipid delivery compounds *(41)* and modifications of the ODN sequence for improved cellular uptake *(42)*.

ODNs have many uses. Aside from their use as probes or primers for the polymerase chain reaction (PCR), ODNs can be used to effect specific "gene interference" of complementary mRNA *(43)*. Such "antisense" ODNs can interfere with the processing or accelerate the degradation of the target RNA, thereby specifically mitigating expression of a selected gene. Another more recently defined use of ODNs is that of a direct stimulant of macrophages, dendritic cells, or B-cells *(44)*. We and others found that ODNs encoding sequences with cytosine followed by guanine (CpG) motifs can induce the expression of costimulatory molecules in CLL samples in vitro *(45–47)*. This effect is enhanced when the natural phosphodiester bond is replaced by a phosphorothioate backbone, thus providing at least a 10-fold increase in the ability of the ODN to activate CLL cells (J. E. Castro and T. J. Kipps, unpublished data). The mechanism(s) accounting for the direct effect of certain ODNs on such cells may involve uptake by various Toll-like receptors (TLRs) (e.g., TLR-9) that are expressed by these cells. Such immune-stimulatory ODNs may have utility for use as vaccine adjuvants.

Clinical trials using antisense ODNs in CLL are under way. CLL cells express high levels of the anti-apoptotic protein bcl-1, which can enhance the resistance of leukemia cells to chemotherapy *(48–51)*. Antisense ODNs specific for *BCL-2* mRNA can reduce CLL expression of *BCL-2* and enhance the sensitivity of treated leukemia cells to cytotoxic drugs in vitro *(49,52)*. Clinical trials testing the safety and efficacy of iv administration of the antisense *BCL-2* ODN (Genasense®) have yielded mixed results *(53)*. Six patients were treated with *BCL-2* antisense ODN administered as a continuous iv infusion for 5–7 d every 3 wk. All six patients achieved reduction of peripheral leukocytosis, and one of them had an apparent tumor lysis syndrome. Common side effects included fever, hypotension, hypoglycemia, and hemolytic anemia. The toxicity of ODN therapy in patients with CLL appeared to be greater than that observed in patients with Hodgkin's disease or solid tumors. Current studies are evaluating whether such ODNs can enhance the efficacy of chemotherapy in patients with CLL.

4. IMMUNE GENE THERAPY STRATEGIES FOR CLL

4.1. Interleukin-2

Transduction of tumor cells with the gene encoding IL-2 enables the tumor cells to secrete high levels of this T-cell stimulatory cytokine. This in turn could stimulate neighboring T-cells, producing a paracrine effect that may enhance development of antitumor immunity. Early studies in mice demonstrated that plasmacytomas transduced to express IL-2 were better able to induce antitumor immunity than nontransduced plasmacytoma cells *(54,55)*.

Recently, Takahashi and colleagues *(56)* examined whether adenovirus-encoding IL-2 (Ad-IL2) could enhance the ability of CLL cells to stimulate autologous T-cells. Although it was less effective than transduction with adenovirus encoding the ligand for CD40 (CD40L or CD154) *(57)*, transduction of CLL cells with Ad-IL2 was effective in inducing some T-cell stimulation. Furthermore, a mixture of leukemia cells transduced with Ad-IL2 with cells expressing CD154 induced greater in vitro activation of autologous T-cells against leukemia cells than could either stimulator population alone. Conceivably, co-transduction of leukemia cells with Ad-IL2 along with vectors encoding CD154 could have a greater capacity to induce autologous immune activation in vivo.

4.2. Interleukin-12

IL-12 is a heterodimeric molecule that acts as a potent stimulator of T-cells and natural killer (NK) cells. Murine lymphoma B-cells (A20) transduced with a retrovirus encoding IL-12 could induce immunity against A20 cells in syngeneic mice more efficiently than A20 cells transduced with control vectors *(58)*. Moreover, IL-12-expressing A20 cells, in contrast to control transfected A20 cells, could not form tumors upon adoptive transfer into syngeneic recipient mice *(58)*. Finally, direct injection of an adenovirus vector encoding IL-12 into solid tumors of P815 mastocytoma cells in syngeneic mice induced P815-specific T-cells that were effective in eradicating the P815 tumor in vivo *(59)*. These studies indicate that vectors encoding IL-12 may be useful for the immune gene therapy of neoplastic disease.

Vectors encoding IL-12 may be useful for treatment of patients with CLL. This is supported indirectly by studies demonstrating that the serum levels of IL-12 were significantly lower for patients with progressive disease than for those with stable disease. Such a discordance in serum cytokine levels for patients with progressive vs stable disease could not be discerned for the other cytokines measured, including tumor necrosis factor-α (TNF-α), interferon-γ (IFN-γ), IL-6, or B-cell growth factor (BCGF) *(60)*. That high levels of IL-12 are associated with stable disease suggests that IL-12 may play a role in the maintenance of stable disease. Although current studies are not sufficient to define a causal relationship, it is conceivable that treatment of CLL patients with vectors encoding IL-12 could raise the serum levels of this cytokine and possibly mitigate the tendency toward disease progression.

4.3. Tumor Necrosis Factor

TNF-α may have application in immune therapy of neoplastic disease. This cytokine is a major factor responsible for initiation of inflammatory immune responses and can induce apoptosis of some tumor cells directly. Transduction of cells to express TNF-α can inhibit development or progression of leukemia in experimental animals *(61,62)*.

CLL cells express the higher molecular weight form of the TNF receptor (CD120b). Because of this, TNF-α can stimulate CLL cells to upregulate surface expression of important immune costimulatory molecules, such as CD80 and CD54, and act synergistically with CD40 ligation to convert leukemia cells into effective antigen-presenting cells that can stimulate T-cells in autologous mixed lymphocyte reactions *(63)*. Additionally, there are reports that TNF-α can induce CLL cells to increase surface expression of other important molecules, such as CD20 *(64,65)*. Conceivably, upregulation of CD20 can enhance the therapeutic efficacy of monoclonal antibodies specific for this surface antigen in CLL (e.g., rituxamab).

The toxic effects of the soluble cytokine limit the use of TNF-α. TNF-α in the systemic circulation can cause serious toxicity, resulting in anorexia, hypotension, capillary leak syndrome, hypoxemia, hepatitis, and/or gastroenteritis *(66–68)*.

The toxicity of TNF-α can be mitigated by engineering TNF such that it cannot be released from the plasma membrane. Prior to cleavage by metalloproteinases, TNF exists as a membrane surface molecule with potent local activity on neighboring cells bearing the TNF receptor. Removal of the metalloproteinase cleavage site in TNF creates a molecule that resists cleavage, resulting in a form that has high local activity. Such constructs have been effective in the immune gene therapy of tumors in various animal models *(69,70)*. We designed a chimeric form of TNF-α that is extremely resistant to proteolysis, resulting in a membrane-stabilized form of TNF that is expressed exclusively on the cell surface *(71)*. We detected significantly higher levels of TNF on cells transfected with this membrane-stabilized form of TNF than on cells transfected with genes encoding either wild-type TNF or the TNF lacking the metalloproteinase site. However, cells transduced with the membrane-stabilized TNF produced amounts of soluble TNF that were less than 0.1% of that produced by cells transduced with vectors encoding wild-type TNF and less than less than 1% of that produced by cells expressing TNF lacking the metalloproteinase site. Coincubation of CLL cells expressing this membrane-stabilized form of TNF induced bystander CLL cells to express immune accessory molecules, such as CD80 and CD54, which are important for antigen presentation. Conceivably, transfer of the genes encoding membrane-stabilized TNF can effect high-level local concentrations of this cytokine at the sites of injection without systemic toxicity.

4.4. CD80 and CD86 (B7-1 and B7-2)

CD80 and CD86 are important immune accessory molecules that are expressed on antigen-presenting cells. CD80 and CD80 are ligands for CD28 expressed by T-cells. Coligation of CD28 and the T-cell receptor for antigen is important for inducing T-cell activation and proliferation. Phenotypic studies of human leukemia cells demonstrate that CLL cells express little or no CD80 expression and low levels of CD86 *(72)*.

Tolba and colleagues *(35)* described the use of HSV-based amplicon vectors to transduce leukemia cells to express CD80. After infection, the CLL cells that expressed this molecule were able to stimulate allogeneic T-cells in mixed lymphocyte reactions. However, in this same study, CD80-expressing CLL cells appeared to be less potent antigen-presenting cells than CLL cells that were transduced to express CD154 (the CD40 ligand; *see* just below).

4.5. CD40- Ligand (CD154)

As noted above, CLL cells express high levels of the MHC class I and II molecules required for antigen presentation but lack expression of important costimulatory molecules for T-cell activation. In addition, leukemic B-cells can downmodulate T-cell surface molecules that are required to induce expression of such molecules on antigen-presenting cells *(73)*. As a consequence, the leukemic B-cell has a tolerogenic influence on T-cells, even on those isolated from normal allogeneic donors. For any vaccine strategy to work under such conditions, it is critical to change the stealth-like phenotype of the leukemia cell to one that can stimulate T-cells to respond to leukemia-associated antigens.

A critical component to the interaction of T- and B-cells is the ligand for CD40 (CD154) *(74)*. This molecule is expressed on activated T-cells within hours after T-cell activation *(75)*, allowing activated T-cells to engage CD40 on the leukemia B-cell surface. This, along with signals derived from other members of the TNF family, triggers a cascade of events that can ultimately result in the leukemia cell expressing significantly higher levels of immune costimulatory surface accessory molecules, such as CD54 (intercellular adhesion molecule-1), CD80, and CD86. These molecules are critical for inducing a proliferative T cell response to presented antigens76,77. Moreover, these changes allow the leukemic cell to engage nonactivated autologous T-cells to respond productively to leukemia-associated antigens.

Although methods exist for inducing such changes in the leukemia cells in vitro, such methods require that the leukemia cells be cultured ex vivo for prolonged periods with foreign stimulator cells or proteins. Thus, we generated a replication-defective adenovirus that carried the gene encoding a recombinant form of CD40 ligand, designated Ad-CD154. Infection of CLL B-cells with Ad-CD154 caused dramatic changes in the leukemia cell phenotype *(57)*. Within 18 h of infection, the CLL B-cells started expressing the immune costimulatory molecules that are critical for inducing a vigorous immune response (Fig. 1). Also, factors that render the leukemia B-cells tolerogenic were downmodulated by infection with Ad-CD154. Such modified leukemia cells became highly effective stimulators in autologous mixed lymphocyte reactions and could induce generation of cytotoxic T-cells specific for autologous noninfected leukemia cells in vitro *(57)*.

5. FIRST CLINICAL STUDY OF IMMUNE GENE THERAPY FOR PATIENTS WITH CLL

Because Ad-CD154-infected CLL B-cells could induce autologous T-cells to generate cytotoxic T-cells against the patient's leukemia cells in vitro, we developed a phase I clinical trial to examine this effect in patients with CLL *(78)*. Leukemia cells were harvested by pheresis and then infected ex vivo with Ad-CD154 in a good-manufacturing practice facility. The cells were examined for expression of the CD154 and immune costimulatory molecules. After sterility testing, some of the modified leukemia cells were administered back to the same patient as a single intravenous injection given over a few minutes. This strategy allowed us to conduct a dose-escalation study, in which we could infuse defined numbers of leukemia cells that expressed defined amounts of the CD154-transgene.

Two patients in our pilot group received 3×10^8 autologous CLL cells, of which less than a few percent expressed the CD154 transgene. Although the infusion was well tolerated, the patients did not show any biological or clinical effects. Subsequently, three patients received 3×10^8 (group 1), three received 1×10^9 (group 2), and three received 3×10^{10} (group 3) autologous Ad-CD154 CLL cells. For all patients in these groups, about half of the Ad-CD154-transduced CLL cells expressed the CD154 transgene. Furthermore, unlike the cells used in the pilot patients, the modified CLL B cells for patients in groups 1–3 expressed high levels of immune costimulatory molecules resulting from high-level expression of the CD154 transgene.

The intravenous infusion of transduced cells was well tolerated. None of the patients experienced immediate toxicity or adverse events. The patients in groups 1, 2, and 3 commonly experienced flu-like symptoms. These included fever, fatigue, and anorexia, which began within

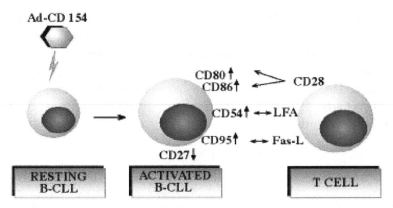

Fig. 1. Ad-CD154 activation of CLL B-cells. Leukemia B-cells are modified via transduction with an adenovirus vector encoding a recombinant CD40- ligand (Ad-CD154). This induces or enhances the expression of important immune accessory molecules, such as CD80 and CD54, which allow these cells to crosslink specific ligands on the T-cell surface that are required for T-cell activation. These accessory molecules are important in cognate intercellular immune interactions that lead to T-cell immunity. In addition, CD40 ligation downmodulates the expression of molecules, such as CD27, that can inhibit such interactions. The end result is to convert the resting leukemia cells into active antigen-presenting cells that are able to induce an immune response to leukemia-associated antigens. LFA, leukocyte factor-associated antigen.

several hours after the infusion. Less common clinical side effects included nausea, myalgia, arthralgia, and diarrhea. Laboratory abnormalities consisted primarily of minor elevations in hepatic transaminases and thrombocytopenia. Nevertheless, the clinical and laboratory abnormalities were transient and resolved within a few days after treatment. None of the patients experienced any dose-limiting toxicity.

The biological effects of this treatment were encouraging. Within 24–48 h of receiving the modified cells, virtually all the patients in groups 1, 2, and 3 had measurable increases in plasma cytokines, such as IL-12, IFN-γ, and/or IL-6. All the CLL B-cells in the blood of the treated patients started expressing low levels of immune costimulatory molecules, similar to what we had observed with the bystander effect noted in vitro. This was noted 1–2 d after treatment, when circulating Ad-CD154-infected cells could no longer be detected, and lasted for several days, if not longer. Such immune costimulatory molecules were not induced on any infected CLL B-cells that were incubated in plasma from the treated patients, indicating that a soluble factor was not responsible for this effect.

The clinical effects of this treatment were encouraging. Most of the patients in groups 1, 2, and 3 experienced acute falls in the blood leukemia cell count within the first few days after treatment. Subsequently the lymphocyte count tended to return to approximately 60% of pre-treatment levels. However, not all the blood lymphocytes that returned to such levels were CLL B-cells. In nearly all treated patients we noted significant increases in the absolute numbers of both CD4 T-cells and CD8 T-cells at 1 wk after treatment, sometimes to more than four times that of pretreatment levels. After the first week or two, many patients experienced stabilization in absolute lymphocyte counts. The CLL B-cell counts of many of the treated patients remained at or below treatment levels for several weeks, if not longer. One to two weeks after gene therapy, nearly all the treated patients experienced reductions, some significant, in lymph node size lasting for more than several weeks. Finally, several of the patients have not required additional therapy for their disease more than 2 yr after receiving gene therapy. Thus, this strategy may have activity even in patients who have advanced disease with high leukemia cell counts and diffuse adenopathy. More pronounced clinical effects are anticipated with repeat dosing, which is currently being examined in a phase II clinical study conducted at the University of California, San Diego and the Dana Farber Cancer Institute. Conceivably, we may soon experience effective gene therapy for patients with this disease.

REFERENCES

1. National Institutes of Health, Office of Biotechnology Activities. Clinical Trials in Human Gene Transfer-Recombinant and Gene Transfer, 2002, http://www4.od.nih.gov/oba/rac/clinicaltrial.htm.
2. Dunbar CE, Cottler-Fox M, O'Shaughnessy JA, et al. Retrovirally marked CD34-enriched peripheral blood and bone marrow cells contribute to long-term engraftment after autologous transplantation. Blood 1995;85:3048–3057.
3. Verhasselt B, De Smedt M, Verhelst R, Naessens E, Plum J. Retrovirally transduced CD34++ human cord blood cells generate T cells expressing high levels of the retroviral encoded green fluorescent protein marker in vitro. Blood 1998;91:431–440.
4. Stewart AK, Sutherland DR, Nanji S, et al. Engraftment of gene-marked hematopoietic progenitors in myeloma patients after transplant of autologous long-term marrow cultures. Hum Gene Ther 1999;10:1953–1964.
5. Kay MA, Glorioso JC, Naldini L. Viral vectors for gene therapy: the art of turning infectious agents into vehicles of therapeutics. Nat Med 2001;7:33–40.
6. Sharma S, Cantwell M, Kipps TJ, Friedmann T. Efficient infection of a human T-cell line and of human primary peripheral blood leukocytes with a pseudotyped retroviral vector. Proc Natl Acad Sci USA 1996;93:11,842–11,847.
7. Lukashok SA, Horwitz MS. New perspectives in adenoviruses. Curr Clin Top Infect Dis 1998;18:286–305.
8. Curiel DT. Strategies to adapt adenoviral vectors for targeted delivery. Ann NY Acad Sci 1999;886:158–171.
9. Yang Y, Ertl HC, Wilson JM. MHC class I-restricted cytotoxic T lymphocytes to viral antigens destroy hepatocytes in mice infected with E1-deleted recombinant adenoviruses. Immunity 1994;1:433–442.
10. Yang Y, Wilson JM. Clearance of adenovirus-infected hepatocytes by MHC class I-restricted CD4+ CTLs in vivo. J Immunol 1995;155:2564–2570.
11. Borgland SL, Bowen GP, Wong NC, Libermann TA, Muruve DA. Adenovirus vector-induced expression of the C-X-C chemokine IP-10 is mediated through capsid-dependent activation of NF-kappaB. J Virol 2000;74:3941–3947.
12. Cantwell MJ, Sharma S, Friedmann T, Kipps TJ. Adenovirus vector infection of chronic lymphocytic leukemia B cells. Blood 1996;88:4676–4683.
13. McDonald D, Stockwin L, Matzow T, Blair Zajdel ME, Blair GE. Coxsackie and adenovirus receptor (CAR)-dependent and major histocompatibility complex (MHC) class I-independent uptake of recombinant adenoviruses into human tumour cells. Gene Ther 1999;6:1512–1519.
14. Santis G, Legrand V, Hong SS, et al. Molecular determinants of adenovirus serotype 5 fibre binding to its cellular receptor CAR. J Gen Virol 1999;80:1519–1527.
15. Hidaka C, Milano E, Leopold PL, et al. CAR-dependent and CAR-independent pathways of adenovirus vector-mediated gene transfer and expression in human fibroblasts. J Clin Invest 1999;103:579–587.
16. Gomez-Navarro J, Curiel DT, Douglas JT. Gene therapy for cancer. Eur J Cancer 1999;35:867–885.
17. Kouraklis G. Gene therapy for cancer: from the laboratory to the patient. Dig Dis Sci 2000;45:1045–1052.
18. Muzyczka N. Use of adeno-associated virus as a general transduction vector for mammalian cells. Curr Top Microbiol Immunol 1992;158:97–129.
19. Duan D, Sharma P, Yang J, et al. Circular intermediates of recombinant adeno-associated virus have defined structural characteristics responsible for long-term episomal persistence in muscle tissue. J Virol 1998;72:8568–8577.
20. Nakai H, Iwaki Y, Kay MA, Couto LB. Isolation of recombinant adeno-associated virus vector-cellular DNA junctions from mouse liver. J Virol 1999;73:5438–5447.
21. Miao CH, Snyder RO, Schowalter DB, et al. The kinetics of rAAV integration in the liver. Nat Genet 1998;19:13–15.
22. Russell DW, Kay MA. Adeno-associated virus vectors and hematology. Blood 1999;94:864–874.
23. Monahan PE, Samulski RJ. Adeno-associated virus vectors for gene therapy: more pros than cons? Mol Med Today 2000;6:433–440.
24. Tal J. Adeno-associated virus-based vectors in gene therapy. J Biomed Sci 2000;7:279–291.
25. Clark KR, Liu X, McGrath JP, Johnson PR. Highly purified recombinant adeno-associated virus vectors are biologically active and free of detectable helper and wild-type viruses. Hum Gene Ther 1999;10:1031–1039.

26. Omori F, Messner HA, Ye C, et al. Nontargeted stable integration of recombinant adeno-associated virus into human leukemia and lymphoma cell lines as evaluated by fluorescence in situ hybridization. Hum Gene Ther 1999; 10:537–543.
27. Krisky DM, Marconi PC, Oligino TJ, et al. Development of herpes simplex virus replication-defective multigene vectors for combination gene therapy applications. Gene Ther 1998;5:1517–1530.
28. Wolfe D, Goins WF, Kaplan TJ, et al. Herpesvirus-mediated systemic delivery of nerve growth factor. Mol Ther 2001;3:61–69.
29. Eling DJ, Johnson PA, Sharma S, Tufaro F, Kipps TJ. Chronic lymphocytic leukemia B cells are highly sensitive to infection by herpes simplex virus-1 via herpesvirus-entry-mediator A. Gene Ther 2000;7:1210–1216.
30. Frenkel N, Singer O, Kwong AD. Minireview: the herpes simplex virus amplicon—a versatile defective virus vector. Gene Ther 1994;1:S40–46.
31. Spaete RR, Frenkel N. The herpes simplex virus amplicon: a new eucaryotic defective-virus cloning-amplifying vector. Cell 1982;30:295–304.
32. Fraefel C, Song S, Lim F, et al. Helper virus-free transfer of herpes simplex virus type 1 plasmid vectors into neural cells. J Virol 1996;70:7190–7197.
33. Stavropoulos TA, Strathdee CA. An enhanced packaging system for helper-dependent herpes simplex virus vectors. J Virol 1998;72:7137–7143.
34. Saeki Y, Ichikawa T, Saeki A, et al. Herpes simplex virus type 1 DNA amplified as bacterial artificial chromosome in *Escherichia coli*: rescue of replication-competent virus progeny and packaging of amplicon vectors. Hum Gene Ther 1998;9:2787–2794.
35. Tolba KA, Bowers WJ, Hilchey SP, et al. Development of herpes simplex virus-1 amplicon-based immunotherapy for chronic lymphocytic leukemia. Blood 2001;98:287–295.
36. Han S, Mahato RI, Sung YK, Kim SW. Development of biomaterials for gene therapy. Mol Ther 2000;2:302–317.
37. Kozak M. Structural features in eukaryotic mRNAs that modulate the initiation of translation. J Biol Chem 1991; 266:19867–19870.
38. Zhu D, Rice J, Savelyeva N, Stevenson FK. DNA fusion vaccines against B-cell tumors. Trends Mol Med 2001; 7:566–572.
39. Rice J, Elliott T, Buchan S, Stevenson FK. DNA fusion vaccine designed to induce cytotoxic T cell responses against defined peptide motifs: implications for cancer vaccines. J Immunol 2001;167:1558–1565.
40. Stevenson FK, Rosenberg W. DNA vaccination: a potential weapon against infection and cancer. Vox Sang 2001; 80:12–18.
41. Uchida E, Mizuguchi H, Ishii-Watabe A, Hayakawa T. Comparison of the efficiency and safety of non-viral vector-mediated gene transfer into a wide range of human cells. Biol Pharm Bull 2002;25:891–897.
42. Dalpke AH, Zimmermann S, Albrecht I, Heeg K. Phosphodiester CpG oligonucleotides as adjuvants: polyguanosine runs enhance cellular uptake and improve immunostimulative activity of phosphodiester CpG oligonucleotides in vitro and in vivo. Immunology 2002;106:102–112.
43. Yuen AR, Sikic BI. Clinical studies of antisense therapy in cancer. Front Biosci 2000;5:D588–593.
44. Hemmi H, Takeuchi O, Kawai T, et al. A Toll-like receptor recognizes bacterial DNA. Nature 2000;408:740–745.
45. Weiner GJ. The immunobiology and clinical potential of immunostimulatory CpG oligodeoxynucleotides. J Leukoc Biol 2000;68:455–463.
46. Decker T, Schneller F, Kronschnabl M, et al. Immunostimulatory CpG-oligonucleotides induce functional high affinity IL-2 receptors on B-CLL cells: costimulation with IL-2 results in a highly immunogenic phenotype. Exp Hematol 2000;28:558–568.
47. Castro JE, Motta M, Kipps TJ. The level of cell surface expression of TLR-9 does not correlate with the degree of activation mediated by immunostimulatory DNA sequences in patients with B cell CLL. In: Proceedings of the American Society of Hematology Annual Meeting, Orlando, FL, 2001, abstract 643.
48. Marschitz I, Tinhofer I, Hittmair A, et al. Analysis of Bcl-2 protein expression in chronic lymphocytic leukemia. A comparison of three semiquantitation techniques. Am J Clin Pathol 2000;113:219–229.
49. Pepper C, Thomas A, Hoy T, Cotter F, Bentley P. Antisense-mediated suppression of Bcl-2 highlights its pivotal role in failed apoptosis in B-cell chronic lymphocytic leukaemia. Br J Haematol 1999;107:611–615.
50. Klein A, Miera O, Bauer O, Golfier S, Schriever F. Chemosensitivity of B cell chronic lymphocytic leukemia and correlated expression of proteins regulating apoptosis, cell cycle and DNA repair. Leukemia 2000;14:40–46.
51. Stoetzer OJ, Pogrebniak A, Scholz M, et al. Drug-induced apoptosis in chronic lymphocytic leukemia. Leukemia 1999;13:1873–1880.
52. Pepper C, Hooper K, Thomas A, Hoy T, Bentley P. Bcl-2 antisense oligonucleotides enhance the cytotoxicity of chlorambucil in B-cell chronic lymphocytic leukaemia cells. Leuk Lymphoma 2001;42:491–498.

53. O'Brien S, et al. Bcl-2 antisense (Genasense) as monotherepy for refractory chronic lymphocytic leukemia. In: Proceeding of the American Society of Hematology Annual Meeting, Orlando, FL, 2001.

54. Bubenik J, Zeuthen J, Bubenikova D, Simova J, Jandlova T. Gene therapy of cancer: use of IL-2 gene transfer and kinetics of local T and NK cell subsets. Anticancer Res 1993;13:1457–1460.

55. Simova J, Bubenik J, Jandlova T, Indrova M. Irradiated IL-2 gene-modified plasmacytoma vaccines are more efficient than live vaccines. Int J Oncol 1998;12:1195–1198.

56. Takahashi S, Rousseau RF, Yotnda P, et al. Autologous antileukemic immune response induced by chronic lymphocytic leukemia B cells expressing the CD40 ligand and interleukin 2 transgenes. Hum Gene Ther 2001;12: 659–670.

57. Kato K, Cantwell MJ, Sharma S, Kipps TJ. Gene transfer of CD40-ligand induces autologous immune recognition of chronic lymphocytic leukemia B cells. J Clin Invest 1998;101:1133–1141.

58. Nishimura T, Watanabe K, Yahata T, et al. The application of IL-12 to cytokine therapy and gene therapy for tumors. Ann NY Acad Sci 1996;795:375–378.

59. Fernandez NC, Levraud JP, Haddada H, Perricaudet M, Kourilsky P. High frequency of specific CD8+ T cells in the tumor and blood is associated with efficient local IL-12 gene therapy of cancer. J Immunol 1999;162:609–617.

60. Aguilar-Santelises M, Gigliotti D, Osorio LM, et al. Cytokine expression in B-CLL in relation to disease progression and in vitro activation. Med Oncol 1999;16:289–295.

61. Gautam SC, Pindolia KR, Xu YX, et al. Antileukemic activity of TNF-alpha gene therapy with myeloid progenitor cells against minimal leukemia. J Hematother 1998;7:115–125.

62. Gautam SC, Xu YX, Pindolia KR, et al. TNF-alpha gene therapy with myeloid progenitor cells lacks the toxicities of systemic TNF-alpha therapy. J Hematother 1999;8:237–245.

63. Ranheim EA, Kipps TJ. Tumor necrosis factor-alpha facilitates induction of CD80 (B7-1) and CD54 on human B cells by activated T cells: complex regulation by IL-4, IL-10, and CD40L. Cell Immunol 1995;161:226–235.

64. Sivaraman S, Venugopal P, Ranganathan R, et al. Effect of interferon-alpha on CD20 antigen expression of B-cell chronic lymphocytic leukemia. Cytokines Cell Mol Ther 2000;6:81–87.

65. Sivaraman S, Deshpande CG, Ranganathan R, et al. Tumor necrosis factor modulates CD 20 expression on cells from chronic lymphocytic leukemia: a new role for TNF alpha? Microsc Res Tech 2000;50:251–257.

66. Villani F, Galimberti M, Mazzola G, et al. Pulmonary toxicity of alpha tumor necrosis factor in patients treated by isolation perfusion. J Chemother 1995;7:452–454.

67. Krigel RL, Padavic-Shaller KA, Rudolph AA, et al. Hemorrhagic gastritis as a new dose-limiting toxicity of recombinant tumor necrosis factor. J Natl Cancer Inst 1991;83:129–131.

68. Kuei JH, Tashkin DP, Figlin RA. Pulmonary toxicity of recombinant human tumor necrosis factor. Chest 1989;96: 334–338.

69. Marr RA, Addison CL, Snider D, et al. Tumour immunotherapy using an adenoviral vector expressing a membrane-mutant of murine TNF alpha. Gene Ther 1997;4:1181–1188.

70. Marr RA, Hitt M, Gauldie J, Muller WJ, Graham FL. A p75 tumor necrosis factor receptor-specific mutant of murine tumor necrosis factor alpha expressed from an adenovirus vector induces an antitumor response with reduced toxicity. Cancer Gene Ther 1999;6:465–474.

71. Cantwell M, Kipps TJ. Infection of CLL using chimeric construcs of TNF. In: Proceedings of the IWCLL, San Diego, CA, 2002.

72. Hirano N, Takahashi T, Ohtake S, et al. Expression of costimulatory molecules in human leukemias. Leukemia 1996;10:1168–1176.

73. Cantwell MJ, Hua T, Pappas J, Kipps TJ. Acquired CD40-ligand deficiency in chronic lymphocytic leukemia. Nature Med 1997;3:984–989.

74. Ranheim EA, Kipps TJ. Activated T cells induce expression of B7/BB1 on normal or leukemic B cells through a CD40-dependent signal. J Exp Med 1993;177:925–935.

75. Van Kooten C, Banchereau J, CD40-CD40 ligand: a multifunctional receptor-ligand pair. Adv Immunol 1996; 61:1–77.

76. Lanier LL, O'Fallon S, Somoza C, et al. CD80 (B7) and CD86 (B70) provide similar costimulatory signals for T cell proliferation, cytokine production, and generation of CTL. J Immunol 1995;154:97–105.

77. Matulonis U, Dosiou C, Freeman G, et al. B7-1 is superior to B7-2 costimulation in the induction and maintenance of T cell-mediated antileukemia immunity. Further evidence that B7-1 and B7-2 are functionally distinct. J Immunol 1996;156:1126–1131.

78. Wierda WG, Cantwell MJ, Woods SJ, et al. CD40-ligand (CD154) gene therapy for chronic lymphocytic leukemia. Blood 2000;96:2917–2924.

VI | CLINICAL ASPECTS: *COMPLICATIONS*

19   Infections in Patients
With Chronic Lymphocytic Leukemia

*Gerald P. Bodey, MD, Dimitrios Kontoyiannis, MD,
and Michael J. Keating, MB, BS*

1. INTRODUCTION

Since the earliest studies of chronic lymphocytic leukemia (CLL), it has been recognized that infectious complications are a major cause of morbidity and mortality. It is critically important that physicians caring for these patients have a thorough understanding of the host deficiencies predisposing to infection associated with the disease process and its therapy as well as the pathogens associated with these deficiencies. For example, introduction of the purine analogs has caused a major change in the infectious complications of these patients. Although this discussion focuses on the infectious problems in CLL, it should be recognized that many patients enjoy years of normal life, especially during the early stages of the disease.

Because of the chronicity of CLL and differing therapeutic approaches, precise information regarding the frequency of infectious complications over long periods of observation is difficult to obtain. Both the disease process itself and its therapy affect host defenses, and the types of infection depend on specific deficiencies in host defenses. Hence, there is a wide diversity of infectious complications in populations of CLL patients. It has been estimated that as many as 80% of these patients will develop at least one severe infection during the course of their disease, and approx 60% will die of infection (*1*). It has also been estimated that there is a mean of 10 severe infectious episodes per 100 patient yr and that the 5-yr risk of developing a serious infection is about 25% (*2*). These latter figures are derived from a mixture of patients in various stages of the disease. Table 1 summarizes data on infectious complications from several studies.

Prior to the availability of effective therapy, most infections were attributed to deficiencies in immunoglobulins or occasionally to neutropenia secondary to bone marrow failure. Most of these infections involved the respiratory tract and were caused by encapsulated bacteria. In most reports *Streptococcus pneumoniae* was the predominant pathogen. The first effective therapeutic agents were alkylating agents, which were administered alone or in combination with vincristine and prednisone. Since alkylating agents are myelosuppressive, there was a shift to a predominance of Gram-negative bacillary infections associated with therapy-induced neutropenia. More recently, the discovery of the efficacy of the purine analogs, especially fludarabine, which have profound effects on cellular immunity, has led to a new spectrum of infections (*see* Subheading 2.3).

From: *Contemporary Hematology*
Chronic Lymphocytic Leukemia: Molecular Genetics, Biology, Diagnosis, and Management
Edited by: G. B. Faguet © Humana Press Inc., Totowa, NJ

Table 1
Frequency of Infection in Patients With Cancer

Author	Yr	Patient	% Infected	% Died of infection
Osgood and Seaman (41)	1952	102	29	11
Shaw et al. (24)	1960	42	60	—
Aroesty and Furth (43)	1962	61	61	56
Zippin et al. (86)	1973	839	23	7
Revol et al. (87)	1974	266	39	—
Morrison et al. (50)	2001			
Fludarabine		188	77	—
Chlorambucil		189	61	—
Combination		144	85	—

2. PATHOPHYSIOLOGY OF INFECTIONS IN CLL

Among malignant diseases, CLL and its therapy are associated with the widest variety of deficiencies in host defense mechanisms (Table 2). Defects have been identified in neutrophil number and function, humoral immunity, and cellular immunity (3). The complex interaction of the various cellular and humoral components is incompletely understood, and the relative importance of each in predisposing to infectious complications is often uncertain. Also, some studies of specific host defense deficiencies have been conducted in treated and untreated CLL patients, so it is not always clear whether the deficiency is caused by the disease process or is a consequence of its therapy.

2.1. Defects in Phagocytic Cell

Impairment in monocyte and neutrophil function have been detected in CLL patients, but these seem to have no important consequences. Neutropenia from the disease or its therapy is of overriding importance in predisposing to infection. In the absence of neutrophils, many of the defects in humoral immunity have little significance, since their function is to facilitate phagocytosis.

2.1.1. DEFECTS IN PHAGOCYTIC CELL FUNCTION

Defects in both granulocytes and monocytes have been detected in CLL patients. Deficiencies in glucuronidase, lysozyme, and myeloperoxidase but not in neutral proteases and alkaline phosphatase have been found in the neutrophils of some, but not all, CLL patients (4). Some studies have found that neutrophil function is normal in untreated patients (1). Monocytes from CLL patients have been found to be deficient in glucuronidase, lysozyme, and myeloperoxidase (4). Some patients have a scarcity of large mature monocytes. These functional abnormalities appear to be reversible if patients achieve disease remission (4). Adrenal corticosteroids are often incorporated into therapeutic regimens for CLL. If given at high doses or for prolonged periods, they interfere with the fungicidal activity of monocytes. For example, the cells are able to ingest *Aspergillus* spores but are not able to kill them in vitro (5).

Inhibitory factors directed against neutrophils have been found in the sera of some CLL patients. The phagocytic and bactericidal activity of neutrophils has been inhibited in vitro by sera from CLL patients (6). CLL cells also may release into the serum a chemotactic inhibitory factor

Table 2
Important Deficiencies in Host Defenses
in Chronic Lymphocytic Leukemia

Deficiencies associated with the disease process
    Hypogammaglobulinemia
    Neutrophil inhibitory factors
    Neutropenia
    Complement deficiencies
    Impaired antibody response
    Decreased CD4+ lymphocytes
    Skin anergy
    Decreased interferon-γ, interleukin-4 (IL-4), IL-2

Deficiencies associated with conventional chemotherapy
    Neutropenia
    Impaired macrophage function
    Lymphopenia
    Inhibition of antibody production
    Skin anergy

Deficiencies associated with purine analog chemotherapy
    Neutropenia
    Decreased CD4+ lymphocytes
    Decreased CD8+ lymphocytes
    Decreased natural killer cells
    Impaired macrophage function
    Inhibition of cytokine function

directed against neutrophils *(7)*. The presence of this factor did not correlate with the stage of disease or lymphocyte count. Infections were significantly more common among patients who had this factor than in those without it. All the infections involved the respiratory tract, and respiratory infections have been associated with impaired leukocyte migration. CLL patients with recurrent infection exhibited impaired function and chemoluminescence of neutrophils in vitro compared with CLL patients without infections (8).

2.1.2. DEFECTS IN NUMBERS OF PHAGOCYTIC CELLS

Neutropenia may be caused by replacement of the bone marrow by CLL cells, suppression by tumor products, or, most often, myelosuppressive chemotherapy. Although alkylating agents cause myelosuppression, resulting in neutropenia, most conventional regimens usually do not cause severe or prolonged neutropenia *(9)*. Although not studied in CLL patients specifically, the risk of infection is inversely related to the degree of neutropenia and is directly related to its duration *(10)*. Also, the risk of hematogenous dissemination is related to the degree of neutropenia. Neutropenia is a pre-eminent factor in predisposing to most bacterial infections and also to systemic *Candida* and mold infections. Furthermore, response to appropriate therapy, especially in fungal infections, is largely dependent on neutrophil recovery.

Purine analogs (fludarabine, cladribine, and pentostatin) can cause severe myelosuppression. During 201 courses of fludarabine, the absolute neutrophil count fell below 500 cells/µL in 22% and to less than 1000 cells/mL in 46% of courses *(11)*. In a large study comparing fludarabine alone with chlorambucil and with the combination, neutropenia occurred in 27, 19, and 43%, respectively *(12)*. Severe neutropenia (<500 cells/μL) was greater with fludarabine than with chlorambucil. In one study neutropenia occurred in about 20% of patients receiving cladribine ± prednisone, whereas it occurred more frequently in other studies *(13)*. Cladribine also causes transient monocytopenia. Severe neutropenia occurs in about 20% of patients receiving pentostatin *(14)*.

2.2. Deficiencies in Humoral Immunity

Humoral immunity has been studied extensively in CLL patients, ever since decreased immunoglobulin concentrations, associated with increased risk of infection, were discovered in these patients. Complement deficiencies have also been identified in CLL patients and may also increase susceptibility to infectious complications. Deficiencies in complement components have been reported to enhance the risk of acquiring infection in CLL patients with hypogammaglobulinemia.

2.2.1. IMMUNOGLOBULIN DEFICIENCIES

The most prominent and earliest of the immune defects identified in CLL was hypogammaglobulinemia (hypo GG) *(15)*. Although decreased IgG concentration has received the most attention, deficiencies in both serum IgA and IgM concentrations occur more frequently *(16)*. Decreased duration of survival in CLL has been related to low concentrations of IgA and IgG, but not IgM *(17)*. Decreased concentrations of IgA in patients with CLL has been associated with frequent respiratory infections, as it has in patients with primary IgA deficiency. However, associations between low concentrations of IgA and IgM and infection is less apparent than with IgG *(1)*. Also, the role of deficiencies in secretory immunoglobulins (present on mucosal surfaces) has not been determined but is probably important. Decreased concentrations of secretory IgM have been detected in CLL patients *(1)*.

As their disease progress, most CLL patients develop severe, persistent hypo GG. The frequency of hypo GG is related to the stage and duration of disease *(18)*. Once it is present, it has not reversed even when a complete remission has been achieved with conventional chemotherapy, although recent experience suggests that it may reverse following successful therapy with fludarabine. Elevated serum β_2-microglobulin concentrations correlate with rapid development of hypo GG *(19)*. Normal B-lymphocytes secrete immunoglobulins, and the low levels of immunoglobulins in CLL are attributed to decreased production by B-lymphocytes. It is unclear whether this is owing to deficiencies in the number or the function of B-lymphocytes. In vitro studies showed that leukemic B-lymphocytes failed to produce immunoglobulins in the presence of normal T-lymphocytes, but also, leukemic T-lymphocytes suppressed the secretion of immunoglobulins by normal B-lymphocytes *(20)*. This finding suggests that abnormal function of both B- and T-cells may be responsible for hypo IgG. Other studies have suggested that hypo IgG is caused by dilution of normal B-lymphocytes by the accumulation of the clonal neoplastic B-lymphocyte population and not by abnormal T-lymphocyte activity *(21)*.

Most patients are deficient in at least one IgG subclass, even some with early-stage disease *(22)*. The most significant deficiencies are in IgG3 and IgG4 *(23)*. IgG3 is a major component of the humoral response to herpes simplex, which is a common cause of viral infection in CLL patients. IgG4 is an important humoral response to parasitic infections. It has been suggested that selective deficiencies in these two IgG subclasses could be caused by abnormal cytokine production by altered T-cells.

Most studies examining the frequency and severity of infection related to serum IgG concentrations have not included homogenous populations, but rather patients with varying stages and durations of disease who have received various or no therapies. In general, patients with hypo GG have two to three times more infections than those with normal concentrations, and these infections are more likely to be serious. Shaw et al. *(24)* found that 61% of patients with hypo GG had major infections compared with 33% without hypo GG. In one large study, 50% of patients with serum IgG concentrations of greater than 7g/L had no infections during the study period compared with only 13% with IgG concentrations less than 4g/L *(25)*. In the former group, 36% of patients had a severe infection, with a mortality rate of 38%, compared with 74% frequency of severe infection in the latter group, with a mortality rate of 65%.

The ability to produce specific antibodies to antigenic stimuli may be of more prognostic significance than deficient concentrations of immunoglobulins *(26)*. Deficient antibody responses to antigenic stimuli are a well-known consequence of antitumor chemotherapy, but they may also be present in CLL patients prior to any therapy. Even CLL patients with normal IgG concentrations may have poor specific antibody responses. Deficiencies in antibody response may be owing to impaired antibody production or defects in antigen presentation. Poor secondary antibody responses have been found following diphtheria, typhoid, mumps, and influenza immunizations in untreated CLL patients *(24)*. Also, deficiencies in antibody responses to *Escherichia coli* and *S. pneumoniae* have been associated with recurrent infections. When CLL patients with no infection were compared with those with recurrent or chronic infections, no patients in the latter group had an antibody response to typhoid-paratyphoid AB vaccination, but less than 40% in the former group had an antibody response *(27)*. None of the patients with hypo GG responded to the vaccination, but some with normal concentrations also failed to respond.

2.2.2. DEFICIENCIES IN COMPLEMENT COMPONENTS

Sera from as many as 55% of CLL patients have decreased properdin activity, and a defect in properdin-dependent bacteriophage neutralization has been described *(28)*. Decreased concentrations of at least one complement component have been found in nearly 70% of CLL patients at the time of diagnosis, and the concentrations remained relatively constant for a median of nearly 1 yr thereafter *(28)*. Deficiencies in complement components correlate with the stage of disease, and most patients also have hypo GG.

In one study, some patients had deficiencies in only the early classical pathway (C1–C4), the late classical pathway (C5–C9), or the alternative pathway, whereas some had deficiencies in all three *(28)*. In some studies, the most frequently detected deficiency was component C1 *(29)*. Low concentrations of C1 and C4 have been associated with increased risk of infection, although this has not been confirmed by all studies. Sera from patients with deficiencies in these components have severely impaired bactericidal activity in vitro. Poor opsinization of *Staphylococcus aureus*, *Haemophilus influenzae*, and especially *S. pneumoniae* has been associated with defective activation of complement *(30)*.

Decreased concentrations of C3b have been found in CLL patients receiving adrenal corticosteroids, although this deficiency may be disease-related. Deficient binding of C3b to *S. pneumoniae*, *S. aureus*, and *E. coli* was found in over 50% of patients with CLL, and all of these patients had abnormal binding to at least one of these bacteria *(30)*. Sera from infected CLL patients bound less C3b than that from noninfected patients. Although it seems apparent that complement deficiencies occur in CLL patients, it must be recognized that most of the data have been derived from small numbers of patients.

2.3. Defects in Cellular Immunity

Infections associated with impaired cellular immunity such as tuberculosis, cryptococcosis, listeriosis, and herpes zoster have been reported in CLL patients even before intensive therapy was available and before techniques were available to identify specific components of cellular immunity. Prominent among these abnormalities are decreased concentrations of circulating CD4+ lymphocytes, which may occur secondary to the disease process but are a significant consequence of therapy with purine analogs.

2.3.1. Skin Anergy

Early studies demonstrated that CLL patients experience delayed rejection of skin grafts. Nearly half of patients are anergic to recall skin tests, but this may be related to antileukemic chemotherapy in some patients. Impaired delayed hypersensitivity to 2,4-dinitrochlorobenzine was detected in some CLL patients, and in vitro lymphocyte transformation to phytohemagglutinin and streptolysin O was impaired (31). There does not appear to be a correlation between anergy and the risk of infection, but it does limit the value of skin tests for diagnostic purposes, such as the use of the purified protein derivative skin test for detection of tuberculosis.

2.3.2. T-Lymphocyte Abnormalities

T-cell abnormalities detected in CLL patients include increased numbers of CD8+ lymphocytes, decreased numbers of CD4+ lymphocytes, and decreased numbers of natural killer (NK) cells. Functional defects of CD4+ lymphocytes and NK cells have also been detected and are more likely to occur with advanced disease. In one study, predictors of infection included the proportion of NK cells, IgG concentration, and CD4+/CD8+ ratio (32). Abnormal CD4+/CD8+ ratios have also been related to decreased concentrations of IgG and IgA (33).

The purine analogs, fludarabine, pentostatin, and cladribine, have been found to be effective against CLL, but they have profound effects on T-lymphocytes, especially CD4+ lymphocytes. Lymphopenia occurs rapidly during fludarabine therapy and mainly affects CD4+ lymphocytes, but CD8+ lymphocytes are also diminished. The mean CD4+ lymphocyte count at the end of therapy in one small study was less than 200 cells/μL and had recovered to only 509 cells/μL at the end of approximately 1 yr (34). The mean CD8+ lymphocyte counts were less than 600 cells/μL and less than 956 cells/μL, respectively. In a large study of fludarabine plus prednisone, the median CD4+ lymphocyte count 3 mo after onset of therapy was about 170 cells/μL and was only 150 cells/μL at 6 mo (35). Low CD4+ lymphocyte counts may persist for 1–2 yr after cessation of therapy.

Cladribine causes profound suppression of CD4+ and CD8+ lymphocytes within a few days after onset of therapy. In one study, the risk of infection was related to lymphopenia. The median lymphocyte count on d 14 after onset of therapy was 200 cells/μL among seriously infected patients compared with 900 cells/μL among noninfected patients (36). The effect of cladribine is more directed against CD8+ lymphocytes and NK cells than against CD4+ lymphocytes, but CD8+ lymphocytes recover more rapidly.

Pentostatin causes immunodeficiencies similar to those observed in severe combined immunodeficiency disorder (SCID). Pentostatin binds to adenosine deaminase; the genetic deficiency of this enzyme causes SCID. It impairs the function of B- and T-lymphocytes, responses to mitogens, antibody-dependent cellular cytotoxicity, and NK activity (37). In vitro pentostatin is more toxic to T-lymphocytes than B-lymphocytes and impairs macrophage, monocyte, and NK cell function. Lymphopenia is universal following pentostatin therapy, with suppression of both CD4+ and CD8+ lymphocytes. Low CD4+ lymphocyte counts may persist for 15–18 mo or longer (14).

Recently, it has been shown that fludarabine inhibits the cytokin-induced activation of signal transducer and activator of infection 1 (STAT-1) and STAT-1-dependent transcription in normal lymphocytes *(38)*. STAT-1 is a protein that is activated in response to many lymphocyte-activating cytokines; it is essential for cell-mediated immunity and plays a role in control of viral infections. Fludarabine also induces apoptosis in proliferating and quiescent lymphocytes.

2.3.3. OTHER ABNORMALITIES IN LYMPHOCYTE FUNCTION IN CLL

The intracellular expression of interferon-γ and interleukin-4 (IL-4) in CD4+ lymphocytes of CLL patients in vitro was found to be significantly lower than in CD4+ lymphocytes from normals *(39)*. This impairment occurs early and may worsen with progression of the disease. Production of IL-2 by T-lymphocytes is also reduced in CLL. Other abnormalities detected in CLL patients that may impact on risk of infection include increased IL-2 receptors, decreased coexpression of CD7+ by CD4+ cells, and decreased suppression of CD28+ by CD4+ and CD8+ lymphocytes. CD28+ is an important accessory molecule in creating T-cell antigenic responses *(3)*.

3. INFECTIONS ASSOCIATED WITH THERAPY OF CLL

The deficiencies associated with the disease process itself cause CLL patients to be susceptible to infectious complications. The myelosuppressive and immunosuppressive side effects of chemotherapy substantially enhance this susceptibility. Whereas most of the infections associated with earlier chemotherapeutic regimens were attributed to neutropenia, the profound and prolonged effect of purine analogs on CD4+ lymphocytes has resulted in a major shift in the spectrum of infections.

3.1. Infections in Untreated Patients

Prior to the availability of effective therapeutic regimens, most infections were attributed to deficiencies in immunoglobulin production associated with the disease process. There are few data regarding the frequency, sites, and causes of infection prior to the advent of chemotherapy. In early reports, about 15–25% of patients were infected at the time of diagnosis *(40)*. An early study of 102 patients treated with radiation reported infection in 30% of patients, and 10% died of infection *(41)*. Most of the infections were pneumonias, upper respiratory tract infections, and septicemias. These infections were caused predominantly by encapsulated bacteria, especially *S. pneumoniae* and *H. influenzae*. *S. aureus* was also a frequent pathogen in some series. Urinary tract infections were common in some series, often associated with ureteral obstruction owing to enlarged abdominal lymph nodes.

Herpesvirus infections, predominantly dermatomal herpes zoster and oral herpes simplex, accounted for about 10% of infections *(42,43)*. Other infections associated with CLL were generally identified from studies of specific infections and included tuberculosis, salmonellosis, cryptococcosis, and, rarely, pneumocystosis and progressive multifocal leukoencephalopathy. All of these infections are associated with impaired cellular immunity, indicating that hypo GG was not the sole deficiency in host defenses in nontreated and minimally treated patients.

3.2. Infections Associated With Conventional Chemotherapy

The most frequently used agents for initial therapy of CLL have been the alkylating agents chlorambucil and cyclosphosphamide, alone or in combination with prednisone ± vincristine (CVP). Alkylating agents are both myelosuppressive and immunosuppressive, but neutropenia is the single most important factor predisposing to infection in patients receiving these drugs.

With the extensive use of these regimens, Gram-negative bacilli, including Enterobacteraceae and *Pseudomonas aeruginosa*, emerged as the predominant pathogens *(40)*.

Adrenal corticosteroids (prednisone) have multiple effects on host defenses. Especially important is their effect on macrophages and monocytes. These cells are an important defense against mold infection such as aspergillosis since they ingest and kill spores. Steroids interfere with the sporicidal activity of these cells, although phagocytosis remains intact *(5)*. Steroids also interfere with neutrophil function and inhibit release of vasoactive factors, chemoattractants, and proteolytic enzymes *(44)*. Shaw et al. *(45)* randomly assigned half of a group of patients to 1 mg/kg prednisone daily for 3 mo followed by a 3-mo washout period vs the opposite sequence for the other half. During the administration of prednisone, patients experienced more frequent and more severe infections, especially infections caused by *S. aureus*.

3.3. Infections Associated With Purine Analog Therapy

The therapy of CLL has changed dramatically with the introduction of the purine analogs. Unfortunately, although these agents are highly efficacious, they are associated with substantial risks of infection even for prolonged periods after cessation of therapy. Fludarabine has been combined with prednisone, which proved to be no more effective than fludarabine alone but was associated with a higher risk of infections *(11)*. What is most impressive and probably related to reduced CD4+ lymphocyte numbers, is the increased frequency of infections that are also seen in AIDS patients such as *Pneumocystis carinii*, cytomegalovirus, herpesviruses, and *Listeria monocytogenes* infections *(46)*.

3.3.1. Infections Associated With Fludarabine Therapy

The largest amount of information on infectious complications following purine analog therapy has been obtained from CLL patients receiving fludarabine. Early studies focused on the increased frequency of *L. monocytogenes* and *P. carinii* infections *(47)*. Subsequently, a variety of infections, most of which are typically associated with defects in cellular immunity were reported, primarily as single case reports or only small series. These include infections caused by *Legionella* species, atypical *Mycobacterium* species, *Nocardia* species, and *Cryptococcus* neoformans *(46)*. Viral infections have included herpes simplex, herpes zoster, cytomegalovirus, adenoviruses, JC virus, respiratory syncytial virus, and astrovirus *(48,49)*. An association between fludarabine therapy may be spurious in some cases, since only single cases have been reported.

The largest review of infections associated with fludarabine included 402 CLL patients who received the drug alone or with prednisone *(46)*. The frequency of infection was 58% among prior treated patients vs 34% among those who had no prior therapy. More than 50% were pneumonias, and 12% were herpes zoster infections. Among the 158 patients who had CD4+ lymphocyte counts determined, herpes zoster occurred in 26%, with CD4+ lymphocyte counts of less than 50 cells/μL compared with 6% of those with CD4+ lymphocyte counts greater than 50 cells/μL. Mucocutaneous herpes simplex infection was three times more frequent in the former group. Cytomegalovirus and mycobacterial infection also occurred in patients with low CD4+ lymphocytes counts. *L. monocytogenes* and *P. carinii* infections only occurred in patients who received fludarabine plus prednisone.

Another large study examined the frequency of fever and infection among 518 previously untreated CLL patients who were randomly assigned to fludarabine, chlorambucil, or the combination *(50)*. The frequency of all types of infection was highest among those receiving the combination and lowest among those receiving chlorambucil, although the duration of follow-up was substantially shorter for the latter group. Considering only the 188 patients who received fludarabine alone, 77% experienced at least one febrile episode, and 29% developed a major infection. The most frequent sites of infection were the lower respiratory tract (14% of patients) and skin and soft tissue (7% of patients). The most frequent infections were herpes zoster, occurring in 13% of patients, followed by herpes simplex (10%), Gram-positive cocci (8%), Gram-negative bacilli (5%), *Candida* species (3%), and *P. carinii* (0.5%). Only 19% of major infections occurred when patients were neutropenic, and none of them died of infection.

In a study of fludarabine administered by continuous infusion, more than 30% of patients developed major infections; 60% were respiratory infections and more than 50% were fatal *(51)*. In a randomized study comparing fludarabine with chlorambucil with the combination in previously untreated patients, the frequency of infection was 16, 9, and 28%, respectively *(12)*. The proportions of the infections requiring hospitalization were 29, 17, and 45%, respectively.

In a study examining the long-term effects of fludarabine ± prednisone therapy, 43% of all fatalities were owing to infection *(52)*. There were 94 episodes of infection in 137 patients who achieved complete or partial remission, although the frequency was less for those in complete remission. The most common infections were sinopulmonary (41%), localized herpes zoster (20%), and urinary tract (9%) infections. There was no correlation between the CD4+ lymphocyte count at the end of therapy and risk of subsequent infection.

3.3.2. INFECTIONS ASSOCIATED WITH CLADRIBINE THERAPY

Infections during cladribine therapy may be caused by neutropenia or lymphopenia. In one study of patients with hematological malignancies, 68% of patients who developed neutropenia had fever or infection. The frequency of infection among patients with hematological malignancies almost doubled during the 6 mo following the first course of cladribine compared to the previous 6 mo *(53)*. In another study, half of the infections were caused by viruses, predominantly herpes simplex *(36)*. About 20% of cases were pneumonias and septicemias. Organisms responsible for infection included Gram-positive and Gram-negative bacteria, *L. monocytogenes*, *P. carinii*, adenoviruses, cytomegalovirus, *Candida* species, and *Aspergillus* species *(3)*. In a study of 378 CLL patients, 123 received cladribine alone and 255 received cladribine + prednisone *(13)*. Fever and infection was higher among previously treated patients (49% vs 38%) and, surprisingly, lower among those receiving prednisone (36% vs 58%). The most common site of infection was the respiratory tract, and over 20% had reactivation of herpes zoster or herpes simplex infection. There were no cases of listeriosis or pneumocystosis. Infection was responsible for 54% of deaths, predominantly owing to pneumonia and septic shock.

3.3.3. INFECTIONS ASSOCIATED WITH PENTOSTATIN THERAPY

Infection has occurred in about 25% of CLL patients receiving pentostatin at appropriate dosage schedules *(14)*. Infections occur predominantly during the first few weeks of therapy and include bacterial (especially *L. monocytogenes*), *P. carinii*, *Toxoplasma gondii*, *Candida* species, and *Aspergillus* species infections. Herpes simplex and herpes zoster infections were especially common, including several cases of disseminated zoster *(37)*. A substantial number of pneumonias occurred, associated with a high fatality rate. As many as 70% of patients were not neutropenic at the onset of their infection.

3.4. Infections Associated with Splenectomy

The spleen plays an important role in controlling infection since it is very effective in removing nonopsonized bacteria and hence serves as an important filtering system, especially for organisms against which the individual has no immunity. Splenectomy is used less frequently in the therapy of CLL than in the past, but this procedure is still performed in patients with hypersplenism or very large spleens. Asplenic patients are especially susceptible to infections caused by the encapsulated bacteria, *S. pneumoniae, H. influenzae*, and *Neisseria meningitidis*. These infections may be fulminant, resulting in death even with appropriate therapy. These patients are also susceptible to babesiosis and infections caused by *Capnocytophaga canimorus*.

4. SPECIFIC PATHOGENS ASSOCIATED WITH CLL

Because of the many deficiencies in host defense mechanisms caused by the disease process or its therapy, it is not surprising that a wide variety of pathogens have been reported in CLL. Often it is difficult to identify the specific underlying deficiency responsible for susceptibility to a particular infection. Reports of association based on a single case or only a few cases may be misleading. Obviously, in order to contract an infection, the patient must be exposed to the pathogen, and some pathogens truly associated with CLL can be contracted only in limited geographical regions. Despite these caveats, it is clear that some infections are associated with CLL.

4.1. Bacterial Infections

A substantial proportion of bacterial infections occurring in CLL patients involve the respiratory tract and are caused by *S. pneumoniae* and *H. influenzae (40)*. The propensity for these infections relates to several factors including decreased production of secretory and serum immunoglobulins, impaired complement binding to organisms, and deficiencies in neutrophils and CD4+ lymphocytes. The most common respiratory infections are acute and chronic sinusitis, otitis media, and pneumonia. In the past most pneumonias were caused by *S. pneumoniae*, but with current chemotherapeutic regimens, the spectrum of pathogens includes Gram-negative bacilli, *Nocardia* species, *Legionella* species, and *P. carinii*. In a study from the 1980s, the estimated frequency of pneumococcal bacteremia was 10.8 episodes/1000 patients *(54)*. The lung was the site of origin of 75% of cases and even when treated with appropriate antibiotics, the fatality rate was 20%. The increasing proportion of penicillin-resistant strains of *S. pneumoniae* is disconcerting and may lead to a resurgence of these infections in CLL patients. Chronic and recurrent sinusitis is a significant problem for some CLL patients.

Infection is the most common cause of neurological complications in CLL patients, most of which are caused by nonbacterial pathogens *(55)*. Bacterial meningitis is most likely to be caused by *S. pneumoniae* or *L. monocytogenes*. The latter infection has been associated with fludarabine therapy, especially when given with prednisone *(47)*. Septicemia occurs predominantly in patients with moderate to severe neutropenia, and the most common pathogens are *Pseudomonas aeruginosa, E. coli, Klebsiella* species, and *S. aureus*, the latter organism also causing skin and soft tissue infections *(40)*. Interestingly, low-grade malignant lymphocytic infiltrates of the skin have been associated with chronic *Borrelia burgdorferi* skin lesions *(56)*. Some early studies reported an association between CLL and tuberculosis. A few cases of atypical mycobacterial infection have been reported in patients receiving purine analog therapy.

4.2. Fungal Infections

The association between cryptococcosis and CLL has been recognized for many years. In a study from 1956 to 1972, the estimated occurrence of cryptococcosis among CLL patients was 24 episodes/1000 admissions, the highest among all cancers *(57)*. The most common form of infection is meningitis, but some patients have fulminant pneumonia, fungemia, disseminated infection, or skin and subcutaneous lesions.

P. carinii (now considered to be a fungus) occasionally caused pneumonia in CLL patients prior to the introduction of fludarabine therapy, but most cases of *Pneumocystis* pneumonia have occurred in patients who were treated with fludarabine plus prednisone *(46,58)*. The association of this infection with adrenocorticosteroid therapy is well recognized; hence, the role of fludarabine is less certain. Systemic *Candida* infections have been reported in patients receiving fludarabine, as well as sporadic cases of infection caused by *Aspergillus* species, *Fusarium* species, *Histoplasma capsulatum*, and *Onchocronis* species *(59)*. It is somewhat surprising that superficial *Candida* infections and *Aspergillus* sinusitis have not been reported more frequently, the former infections being associated with low CD4+ lymphocyte counts and the latter with neutropenia and adrenal corticosteroid therapy.

4.3. Viral Infections

Herpes zoster is the most common severe viral infection associated with CLL *(48)*. Less than 10% of patients experience cutaneous dissemination, and only a few develop visceral dissemination. About 20% suffer from postherpetic neuralgia, and a few develop polyradiculopathy or meningoencephalitis *(55,60)*. Herpes simplex infections of the circumoral area and oropharynx are more common than herpes zoster but are usually not as severe. A chronic indolent form of orofacial herpes simplex infection has been described in a few patients *(61)*. Slowly or rapidly progressive local or widespread lymphadenitis and, rarely, visceral dissemination may occur *(62)*. Occasional patients may develop persistent or recurrent skin lesions after herpes zoster or simplex infection that are caused by infiltration by CLL cells *(63)*.

Reactivation of Epstein-Barr virus (EBV) infection has been observed following fludarabine therapy *(64)*. EBV-transformed cells can cause a mononucleosis syndrome or clonal lymphoid malignancies. A few patients with EBV infection transformed from a low-grade to higher grade B-cell malignancy, and this virus has been implicated in the transformation of Reed-Sternberg cells in T-cell and B-cell CLL *(64)*. EBV infection may be responsible for some cases of Richter's transformation and also possibly for the development of disseminated Hodgkin's disease in CLL patients *(65,66)*. However, although CLL cells can be infected with EBV in vitro, the infection rarely gives rise to immortalized cell lines *(67)*.

Parvovirus B19 has been associated with aplastic crises in diseases in which the life span or production of red blood cells is reduced. Several CLL patients have developed severe parvovirus B19 infection manifested by a flu-like illness followed by anemia owing to pure red cell aplasia in the bone marrow *(68)*. The infection may be followed by an incapacitating polyarthritis.

Progressive multifocal leukoencephalopathy (PML) is a demyelinating disease of the brain caused by the JC virus. The disease results from reactivation of latent infection. About 80% of normal adults demonstrate JC virus antibodies by middle age. PML was first described in patients with CLL and Hodgkin's disease *(69)*. Symptoms include visual disturbances, speech defects, and mental deterioration, leading to dementia and coma. The mortality rate is 80% at 1 yr and the mean time from diagnosis to death is 4 mo. No consistently effective therapy is available, but arabinosyl cytosine may cause improvement in some patients *(69)*.

Several other viral infections have been reported sporadically in CLL patients, including reactivation of hepatitis B, lethal disseminated adenovirus infection, and astrovirus enteritis *(70)*. Cytomegalovirus infection has also been reported, generally following allogeneic bone marrow transplantation or, occasionally, purine analog therapy *(71)*.

4.4. Other Infections

Reactivation of leishmaniasis and strongyloidiasis have occurred in CLL patients more than 40 yr after the original infection *(72,73)*. Sporadic cases of toxoplasmosis have also been reported.

5. INFECTION PROPHYLAXIS

Until recently, prophylaxis of infection in CLL focused on replacement of immunoglobulins which became possible with the availability of intravenous preparations (IVIG). Although conventional chemotherapy regimens cause neutropenia, the frequency of severe infections has not been sufficient to consider antimicrobial prophylaxis. The increased risk and expanded spectrum of infections in patients receiving fludarabine has caused some physicians to suggest several prophylactic measures. It must be emphasized that no organized clinical trials of any of these prophylactic measures, other than IVIG, have been attempted.

5.1. Immunoglobulin Prophylaxis

Multiple studies have shown some reduction in infectious complications among patients with hypo IgG who received IVIG, but all the studies (including randomized trials) included less than 100 patients. In the largest trial, patients with IgG concentrations less than 50% of normal who had at least one serious infection were randomized to receive 400 mg/kg IVIG or normal saline every 3 wk for 1 yr *(74)*. Moderately severe bacterial infections were reduced by 50%, but there was no effect on the occurrence of viral and fungal infections, and the proportion of patients remaining free of infection was the same in both groups. A cost-effectiveness analysis of this study concluded that IVIG does not increase the quality or length of life and is not cost-effective *(75)*. A subset of patients from this trial then continued in a double-blind crossover study *(76)*. Serious bacterial infections were significantly less frequent in the months during which patients received IVIG and in patients whose IgG concentrations were maintained above 6.49 mg/dL.

Because of the significant cost of IVIG, several studies have examined lower dose therapy. The administration of 10 g IVIG every 3 wk eventually led to normal IgG concentrations after 11 doses *(77)*. Febrile episodes were reduced by 50%, and hospital admissions for infection were reduced from 16 to 5. In another study, 30 evaluable patients were given IVIG 300 mg/kg every 4 wk for 6 mo and then changed to no IVIG *(78)*. There were 67% of patients with no infection during the period of IVIG administration vs 30% during the period of no therapy. The number of serious infections per year was reduced by 50% during IVIG therapy. In another study, patients were randomized to IVIG 500 mg/kg every 4 wk or to 250 mg/kg every 4 wk *(79)*. There were no apparent differences in infectious complications between the two regimens. A recent study compared a higher dose with conventional replacement therapy in patients with primary hypo GG *(80)*. Patients were randomly assigned to IVIG 600 mg/kg or 300 mg/kg every 4 wk (adults) for 9 mo, and then to the alternate dosage schedule. There were a median of 2.5 infections/patient during high-dose therapy vs 3.5 during low-dose therapy. The median numbers of severe infections were 1.2 vs 1.5. Also, the median duration of respiratory infections was longer during low-dose therapy (29 vs 22 d).

There are several problems with the use of IVIG. These preparations do not correct deficiencies in IgM and IgA, which also play a role in protecting against infections. Weeks et al. *(75)* concluded that 1 quality-adjusted life-year achieved per patient costs $6 million without any increase in life expectancy. Hence, while IVIG replacement reduces the frequency of infections, it is not cost-effective and should be reserved only for selected patients who have recurrent severe bacterial infections and IgG concentrations less than 400 mg/dL. In addition, therapy with IVIG is not likely to be useful for preventing viral or fungal infections. Also, the optimum dose of IVIG has not been determined.

5.2. Immunizations

Live attenuated virus vaccines are contraindicated in patients with CLL. Vaccinations have not been successful in many patients with CLL because poor antibody responses correlate with hypo GG and advanced disease, those groups of patients who most need protection.

Immunization with the pneumococcal polysaccharide vaccine has also produced disappointing results because patients can be infected with serotypes of *S. pneumoniae* that are not incorporated in the vaccine *(81)*. Attempts at immunizing patients with influenza vaccine have resulted in poor long-term antibody responses, which could be improved in some patients by administering a second dose. Scheduling is problematic, since cancer chemotherapeutic agents can mute antibody response *(82)*.

Patients who have undergone splenectomy should receive vaccination with pneumococcal polyvalent capular polysaccharide vaccine every 3 yr. Vaccination with *H. influenzae* type B conjugated polysaccharide vaccine and yearly influenza vaccination are also recommended. Quadrivalent meningococcal vaccination should only be given in the setting of an epidemic.

5.3. Antimicrobial Prophylaxis

In recent years, ciprofloxacin has been used most extensively for prevention of bacterial infections in patients with prolonged severe neutropenia. Although it has reduced the frequency of Gram-negative bacterial infections, its use has been associated with an increase in Gram-positive infections and the emergence of resistance among Gram-negative bacilli. Also, in most studies, its use did not reduce the frequency of fever and empiric antibacterial therapy. Hence, its use should be restricted to those patients who are likely to experience severe neutropenia following chemotherapy. Outpatients at risk for pneumococcal or *Listeria* infections could be given a supply of amoxicillin-clavulanate to be initiated at the onset of fever, as should splenectomized patients *(3)*. Since serious fungal infections occur rather infrequently in CLL patients, it is difficult to justify the routine use of antifungal prophylaxis, especially since it has been associated with colonization by resistant *Candida* species.

Herpes simplex infections are painful, interfere with nutrition, and may become superinfected with bacterial pathogens. Hence, patients who receive therapy with purine analogs should be considered for prophylaxis with acyclovir or valcyclovir if they have had previous infection *(46)*. Long-term prophylaxis to prevent herpes zoster infections is probably not necessary since nearly all infection is localized to a few dermatomes.

Trimethoprim-sulfamethoxazole (TMP-SMX) has been used effectively to prevent *P. carinii* pneumonia in AIDS patients and also has activity against *L. monocytogenes*. Some physicians have suggested that CLL patients who are receiving fludarabine should be given TMP-SMX (1 double strength tablet 3 times weekly) until at least 2 mo after completion of therapy *(46,83)*. However, the frequency of this infection was only 0.5% in a large group of patients treated with fludarabine, which suggests this is not necessary *(50)*.

The use of growth factors [granulocyte and granulocyte/macrophage colony-stimulating factor (G-CSF, GM-CSF)] in patients receiving therapy resulting in severe neutropenia may be considered. In a group of patients receiving fludarabine plus G-CSF, the frequencies of neutropenia and severe neutropenia (<500 cells/µL) were 45 and 15% compared with 79 and 63%, respectively, in historical controls who received only fludarabine *(84)*. The frequency of pneumonia was 8% versus 37%, but the frequencies of other infections were similar in both groups. In a small group of CLL patients with chronic neutropenia caused by hypersplenism and autoimmune problems, GM-CSF administration substantially increased patients' neutrophil counts and improved the chemoluminescence of neutrophils in vitro *(85)*.

Some physicians have suggested that patients receiving fludarabine should avoid potential sources of *L. monocytogenes* such as unpasteurized milk and cheese, raw vegetables, and undercooked poultry or meat *(46)*. It may be wiser to stress the importance of careful cleaning of raw vegetables rather than total abstention.

6. CONCLUSIONS

Infection is a common complication in patients with CLL owing to the disease and to its therapy. The development of effective chemotherapeutic agents, such as the purine analogs, has increased the frequency and severity of those infections and has changed the spectrum of infecting organisms. Most of infections involve the respiratory tract, but a substantial number involve the central nervous system. Common bacterial pathogens include *S. pneumoniae, S. aureus, E. coli, P. aeruginosa*, and *Klebsiella* species. Cryptococcosis is the most common fungal infection and herpes simplex and herpes zoster are the most prevalent viral infections. Less common, but important, pathogens associated with purine analog therapy include *L. monocytogenes, P. carinii*, EBV, and JC virus. The only prophylactic measure that has been studied in an organized fashion is IVIG, and it should be administered only to selected patients with hypo IgG who have a history of repeated severe bacterial infections. Careful studies are needed to determine the appropriate use of other prophylactic measures.

REFERENCES

1. Morrison VA. The infectious complications of chronic lymphocytic leukemia. Semin Oncol 1998;25:98–106.
2. Molica S, Levato D, Levato L. Infections in chronic lymphocytic leukemia. Analysis of incidence as a function of length of follow-up. Haematologica 1993;78:374–377.
3. Tsiodras S, Samonis G, Keating MJ, Kontoyiannis DP. Infection and immunity in chronic lymphocytic leukemia. Mayo Clin Proc 2000;75:1039–1054.
4. Zeya HI, Keku E, Richards F II, Spurr CL. Monocyte and granulocyte defect in chronic lymphocytic leukemia. Am J Pathol 1979;95:43–53.
5. Schaffner A, Douglas H, Braude A. Selective protection against *Conidia* by mononuclear and against *Mycelia* by polymorphonuclear phagocytes in resistance to *Aspergillus*. J Clin Invest 1982;69:617–631.
6. Sbarra AJ, Shirley W, Selvaraj RJ, et al. The role of the phagocyte in host-parasite interactions. I. The phagocytic capabilities of leukocytes from lymphoproliferative disorders. Cancer Res 1964;24:1958–1968.
7. Siegbahn A, Simonsson B, Venge P. The chemokinetic inhibitory factor (CIF) in serum of CLL patients: correlation with infection propensity and disease activity. Scand J Haematol 1985;35:80–87.
8. Itälä M, Vainio O, Remes K. Functional abnormalities in granulocytes predict susceptibility to bacterial infections in chronic lymphocytic leukaemia. Eur J Haematol 1996;57:46–53.
9. Raphael B, Andersen JW, Silber R, et al. Comparison of chlorambucil and prednisone versus cyclophosphamide, vincristine, and prednisone as initial treatment for chronic lymphocytic leukemia: long-term follow-up of an Eastern Cooperative Oncology Group Randomized Clinical Trial. J Clin Oncol 1991;9:770–776.
10. Bodey GP, Buckley M, Sathe YS, Freireich EJ. Quantitative relationships between circulating leukocytes and infection in patients with acute leukemia. Ann Intern Med 1966;64:328–340.
11. Keating MJ. Fludarabine phosphate in the treatment of chronic lymphocytic leukemia. Semin Oncol 1990;17:49–62.
12. Rai KR, Peterson BL, Appelbaum FR, et al. Fludarabine compared with chlorambucil as primary therapy for chronic lymphocytic leukemia. N Engl J Med 2000;343:1750–1757.

13. Robak T, Blonski JZ, Kasznicki M, et al. Cladribine with or without prednisone in the treatment of previously treated and untreated B-cell chronic lymphocytic leukaemia—updated results of the multicentre study of 378 patients. Br J Haematol 2000;108:357–368.

14. Margolis J, Grever MR. Pentostatin (Nipent): a review of potential toxicity and its managment. Semin Oncol 2000;27:9–14.

15. Ultmann JE, Fish W, Osserman E, Gellhorn A. The clinical implications of hypogammaglobulinemia in patients with chronic lymphocytic leukemia and lymphocytic lymphosarcoma. Ann Intern Med 1959;51:501–516.

16. Montserrat E, Marques-Pereira JP, Gallart MT, et al. Bone marrow histopathologic patterns and immunologic findings in B-chronic lymphocytic leukemia. Cancer 1984;54:447–451.

17. Rozman C, Montserrat E, Vinolas N. Serum immunoglublins in B-chronic lymphocytic leukemia. Cancer 1988; 61:279–283.

18. Rai KR, Montserrat F. Prognostic factors in chronic lymphocytic leukemia. Semin Hematol 1987;24:252–256.

19. Gamm, H, Chuber C, Chapel H, Lee M, Ries F, Dicato MA. Intravenous immune globulin in chronic lymphocytic leukaemia. Clin Exp Immunol 1994;97:17–20.

20. Hersey P, Wotherspoon J, Reid G, Gunz FW. Hypogammaglobulinaemia associated with abnormalities of both B and T lymphocytes in patients with chronic lymphatic leukaemia. Clin Exp Immunol 1980;39:698–707.

21. Kurec AS, Davey DR. Impaired synthesis of immunoglobulin in patients with chronic lymphocytic leukemia. Am J Hematol 1987;25:131–142.

22. Lacombe C, Gombert J, Dreyfus B, Brizard A, Preud'Homme JS. Heterogeneity of serum IgG subclass deficiencies in B chronic lymphocytic leukemia. Clin Immunol 1999;90:128–132.

23. Copson ER, Ellis BA, Westwood NB, Majumdar G. IgG subclass levels in patients with B cell chronic lymphocytic leukaemia. Leuk Lymphoma 1994;14:471–473.

24. Shaw RK, Szwed C, Boggs DR, et al. Infection and immunity in chronic lymphocytic leukemia. Arch Intern Med 1960;106:467–478.

25. Itälä M, Helenius H, Nikoskelainen J, Remes K. Infections and serum IgG levels in patients with chronic lymphocytic leukemia. Eur J Haematol 1992;48:266–270.

26. Chapel HM, Bunch C. Mechanisms of infection in chronic lymphocytic leukemia. Semin Hematol 1987;24:291–296.

27. Miller DG, Karnofsky DA. Immunologic factors and resistance to infection in chronic lymphatic leukemia. Am J Med 1961;31:748–757.

28. Schlesinger M, Broman I, Lugassy G. The complement system is defective in chronic lymphatic leukemia patients and in their healthy relatives. Leukemia 1996;10;1509–1513

29. Fust G, Czink E, Minh D, Miszlay Z, Varga L, Hollan SR. Depressed classical complement pathway activities in chronic lymphocytic leukaemia. Clin Exp Immunol 1985;60:489–495.

30. Health ME, Cheson BD. Defective complement activity in chronic lymphocytic leukemia. Am J Hematol 1985; 19:63–73.

31. Block JB, Haines HA, Thompson WL, Neiman PE. Delayed hypersensitivity in chronic lymphocytic leukemia. J Natl Cancer Inst 1969;42:973–980.

32. Apostolopoulos A, Symeonidis A, Zoumbos N. Prognostic significance of immune function parameters in patients with chronic lymphocytic leukaemia. Eur J Haematol 1990;44:39–44.

33. Freedman AS. Immunobiology of chronic lymphocytic leukemia. Hematol Oncol Clin North Am 1990;4:405–429.

34. Wijermans PW, Gerrits WJB, Haak HL. Severe immunodeficiency in patients treated with fludarabine monophosphate. Eur J Haematol 1993;50:292–296.

35. O'Brien S, Kantarjian H, Beran M, et al. Results of fludarabine and prednisone therapy in 264 patients with chronic lymphocytic leukemia with multivariate analysis-derived prognostic model for response to treatment. Blood 1993; 82:1695–1700.

36. Betticher DC, Fey MF, von Rohr A, et al. High incidence of infections after 2-chlorodeoxyadenosine (2-CDA) therapy in patients with malignant lymphomas and chronic and acute leukaemias. Ann Oncol 1994;1:57–64

37. O'Dwyer PJ, Spiers ASD, Marsoni S. Association of severe and fatal infections and treatment with pentostatin. Cancer Treat Rep 1986;70:1117–1120.

38. Frank DA, Mahajan S, Ritz J. Fludarabine-induced immunosuppression is associated with inhibition of STAT1 signaling. Nat Med 1999;4:444–447.

39. Hill SJ, Peters SH, Ayliffe MJ, Merceica J, Bansal AS. Reduced IL-4 and interferon-gamma (INF-[gamma]) expression by CD4 T cells in patients with chronic lymphocytic leukaemia. Clin Exp Immunol 1999;117:8–11.

40. Kontoyiannis DP, Anaissie EJ, Bodey GP. Infection in chronic lymphocytic leukemia: a reappraisal. In: Cheson, BD, ed. Chronic Lymphocytic Leukemia. Marcel Dekker, New York, 1993, pp. 399–417.

41. Osgood EE, Seaman AJ. Treatment of chronic leukemias: results of therapy by titrated, regularly spaced total body irradiation phosphorus, or roentgen irradiation. JAMA 1952;150:1372–1379.

42. Twomey JJ. Infections complicating multiple myeloma and chronic lymphocytic leukemia. Arch Intern Med 1973;132:562–565.

43. Aroesty JM, Furth FW. Infection and chronic lymphocytic leukemia. A review of 61 cases. NY State J Med 1962;62:1946–1952.

44. Go CHU, Cunha BA. Infections in patients on steroids. Infect Dis Pract Clin 2000;24:61–65.

45. Shaw RK, Boggs DR, Silberman HR, Frei E III. A study of prednisone therapy in chronic lymphocytic leukemia. Blood 1961;17:182–195.

46. Anaissie EJ, Kontoyiannis DP, O'Brien S, et al. Infections in patients with chronic lymphocytic leukemia treated with fludarabine. Ann Intern Med 1998;129:559–566.

47. Anaissie E, Kontoyiannis DP, Kantarjian H, Elting L, Robertson LE, Keating M. Listeriosis in patients with chronic lymphocytic leukemia who were treated with fludarabine and prednisone. Ann Intern Med 1992;117:466–469.

48. Byrd JC, McGrail LH, Hospenthal DR, Howard RS, Dow NA, Diehl LF. Herpes virus infections occur frequently following treatment with fludarabine: results of a prospective natural history study. Br J Haematol 1999;105:445–447.

49. Coppo P, Scieux C, Ferchal F, Clauvel JP, Lassoued K. Astrovirus enteritis in a chronic lymphocytic leukemia patient treated with fludarabine monophosphate. Ann Hematol 2000;79:43–45.

50. Morrison VA, Rai KR, Bercedis L, et al. Impact of therapy with chlorambucil, fludarabine, or fludarabine plus chlorambucil on infections in patients with chronic lymphocytic leukemia: intergroup study cancer and leukemia group B 9011. J Clin Oncol 2001;19:3611–3621.

51. Puccio CA, Mittelman A, Lichtman SM, et al. A loading dose/continuous infusion schedule of fludarabine phosphate in chronic lymphocytic leukemia. J Clin Oncol 1991;9:1562–1569.

52. Keating MJ, O'Brien S, Lerner S, et al. Long-term follow-up of patients with chronic lymphocytic leukemia (CLL) receiving fludarabine regimens as initial therapy. Blood 1998;92:1165–1171.

53. Van Den Neste E, Delannoy A, Vandercam B, et al. Infectious complications after 2-chlorodeoxyadenosine therapy. Eur J Haematol 1996;56:235–240.

54. Chou MY, Brown AE, Blevins A, Armstrong D. Severe pneumococcal infection in patients with neoplastic disease. Cancer 1983;51:1546–1550.

55. Bower JA, Hammack JE, McDonnell SK, Tefferi A. The neurologic complications of B-cell chronic lymphocytic leukemia. Neurology 1997;48:407–412.

56. Goodlad JR, Davidson MM, Hollowood K, et al. Primary cutaneous B-cell lymphoma and *Borrelia burgdorferi* infection in patients from the highlands of Scotland. Am J Surg Pathol 2000;24:1279–1285.

57. Kaplan MH, Rosen PP, Armstrong D. Cryptococcosis in a cancer hospital. Clinical and pathological correlates in forty-six patients. Cancer 1977;39:2265–2274.

58. Bastion Y, Coiffier B, Tigaud JD, Espinouse D, Bryon PA. *Pneumocystis* pneumonia in a patient treated with fludarabine for chronic lymphocytic leukaemia. Eur J Cancer 1991;27:671.

59. Bowyer JD, Johnson EM, Horn EH, Gregson RMC. *Ochroconis gallopava* endophthalmitis in fludarabine treated chronic lymphocytic leukaemia [Letters to the Editor]. Br J Ophthalmol 2000;84:117.

60. Hughes BA, Kimmel DW, Aksamit AJ. Herpes zoster-associated meningoencephalitis in patients with systemic cancer. Mayo Clin Proc 1993;68:652–655.

61. Barrett AP. Chronic indolent orofacial herpes simplex virus infection in chronic leukemia: a report of three cases. Oral Surg Oral Med Oral Pathol 1988;66:387–390.

62. Higgins JPT, Warnke RA. Herpes lymphadenitis in association with chronic lymphocytic leukemia. Cancer 1999;86:1210–1215.

63. Cerroni L, Zenahlik P, Kerl H. Specific cutaneous infiltrates of B-cell chronic lymphocytic leukemia arising at the site of herpes zoster and herpes simplex scars. Cancer 1995;76:26–31.

64. Lazzarino M, Orlandi E, Baldanti F, et al. The immunosuppression and potential for EBV reactivation of fludarabine combined with cyclophosphamide and dexamethasone in patients with lymphoproliferative disorders. Br J Haematol 1999;107:877–882.

65. Ansell SM, Li CY, Lloyd RV, Phyliky RL. Epstein-Barr virus infection in Richter's transformation. Am J Hematol 1999;60:99–104.

66. Quintallia-Martinez L, Fend F, Monguel LR, et al. Peripheral T-cell lymphoma with Reed-Sternberg-like cells of B-cell phenotype and genotype associated with Epstein-Barr virus infection. Am J Surg Pathol 1999;23:1233–1240.

67. Doyle MB, Catovsky D, Crawford DH. Infection of leukemia B lymphocytes by Epstein Barr virus. Leukemia 1993;7:1858–1864.

68. Hitchins R, Sloots TP. Another parvovirus B19 infection of a chronic lymphatic leukaemia patient. Aust NZ J Med 1993;23:217–218.
69. Berger JR, Concha M. Progressive multifocal leukoencephalopathy: the evolution of a disease once considered rare. J NeuroVirol 1995;1:5–18.
70. Ljungman P, Ehrnst A, Bjorkstrand B, et al. Lethal disseminated adenovirus type 1 infection in a patient with chronic lymphocytic leukemia. Scand J Infect Dis 1990;22:601–605.
71. Schilling PJ, Vadhan-Raj S. Concurrent cytomegalovirus and pneumocystis pneumonia after fludarabine therapy for chronic lymphocytic leukemia. N Engl J Med 1990;323:833–834.
72. Jewell AP, Giles FJ. Cutaneous manifestation of leishmaniasis 40 years after exposure in a patient with chronic lymphocytic leukaemia. Leuk Lymphoma 1996;21:347–249.
73. Wilkinson R, Leen CLS. Chronic lymphocytic leukaemia and overt presentation of underlying *Strongyloides stercoralis* infection [Letters to the Editor]. J Infect 1993;27:99–100.
74. Cooperative Group for the Study of Immunoglobulin in Chronic Lymphocytic Leukemia. Intravenous immunoglobulin for the prevention of infection in chronic lymphocytic leukemia. A randomized, controlled clinical trial. N Engl J Med 1988;319:902–907.
75. Weeks JC, Tierney MR, Weinstein MC. Cost effectiveness of prophylactic intravenous immune globulin in chronic lymphocytic leukemia. N Engl J Med 1991;325:81–86.
76. Griffiths H, Brennan V, Lea J, Bunch C, Lee M, Chapel H. Crossover study of immunoglobulin replacement therapy in patients with low-grade B-cell tumors. Blood 1989;73:366–368.
77. Jurlander J, Hartmann GC, Hansen MM. Treatment of hypogammaglobulinaemia in chronic lymphocytic leukaemia by low-dose intravenous gammaglobulin. Eur J Haematol 1994;53:114–118.
78. Molica S, Musto P, Chiurazzi J, et al. Prophylaxis against infections with low-dose intravenous immunoglobulins (IVIG) in chronic lymphocytic leukemia. Results of a crossover study. Haematology 1996;81:121–126.
79. Chapel H, Dicato M, Gamm H, et al. Immunoglobulin replacement in patients with chronic lymphocytic leukaemia: a comparison of two dose regimens. Br J Haematol 1994;88:209–212.
80. Eijkhout HW, van der Meer JWM,, Kallenberg CGM, et al. The effect of two different dosages of intravenous immunoglobulin on the incidence of recurrent infections in patients with primary hypogammaglobulinemia. Ann Intern Med 2001;135:165–174.
81. Shapiro ED, Berg AT, Austrian R, et al. The protective efficacy of polyvalent pneumococcal polysaccharide vaccine. N Engl J Med 1991;325:1453–1460.
82. Gribabis DA, Panayiotidis P, Boussiotis VA, Hannoun C, Pangalis GA. Influenza virus vaccine in B-cell chronic lymphocytic leukaemia patients. Acta Haematol 1994;91:115–118.
83. Sudhoff T, Arning M, Schneider W. Prophylactic strategies to meet infectious complications in fludarabine-treated CLL. Leukemia 1997;11:S38–S41.
84. O'Brien S, Kantarjian H, Beran M, et al. Fludarabine and granulocyte colony-stimulating factor (G-CSF) in patients with chronic lymphocytic leukemia. Leukemia 1997;11:1631–1635.
85. Itälä M, Pelliniemi TT, Remes K, Vanhatalo S, Vainio O. Long-term treatment with GM-CSF in patients with chronic lymphocytic leukemia and recurrent neutropenic infections. Leuk Lymphoma 1998;32:165–174.
86. Zippin C, Culter SJ, Reeves WJ Jr, Lum D. Survival in chronic lymphocytic leukemia. Blood 1973;42:367–376.
87. Revol L, Cressel R, Bryon PA, Coeur P, Gentilhomme O. Leucime lymphoide chronique. Enc Med Chir Paris Sang 1974;1303 B 20.

20 Autoimmune and Hypersplenic Cytopenias

Terry Hamblin, MB, DM

1. INTRODUCTION

Perhaps the most important observation concerning chronic lymphocytic leukemia (CLL) made in the 20th century was the assertion by Rai in America *(1)* and Binet in France *(2)* that anemia or thrombocytopenia carries a grave prognosis. Although neither of these authors' scoring system demands it, it is axiomatic that for this to be true, the cytopenia must be the consequence of bone marrow suppression. As it happens, there are two other important reasons for cytopenias in CLL: autoimmunity and hypersplenism. Neither of these causes necessarily carries the same dire consequences.

2. AUTOIMMUNITY

2.1. History

The pioneering work of Winifred Ashby *(3)* established a technique to determine the life span of red blood cells. Transfusion of compatible but serologically distinct red cells allowed them to be tracked by differential agglutination. In nine patients with CLL, Berlin *(4)* used this technique to demonstrate a shortened red cell survival, even though only one had a reticulocytosis. This was probably the first demonstration that the anemia of CLL might be hemolytic in nature.

According to Ehrlich and Morgenroth *(5)* the body should not make an antibody that destroys its own tissues, yet within 3 yr Donath and Lansteiner *(6)* had described an antibody that did precisely that. Four years later, Fernand Widal *(7)* was the first to recognize acquired hemolytic anemia caused by red cell agglutination. It was another 30 yr before Dameshek and Schwartz *(8)* realized the importance of "hemolysins" in the commonest type of acquired hemolytic anemia, although it was not clear what these "hemolysins" were until the development of the direct antiglobulin test (DAT) by Robin Coombs *(9)* and its application to hemolytic anemia *(10)*.

In a series of 58 consecutive patients with CLL, Wasserman et al. *(11)* found hemolytic anemia to be present in 9; 5 out of 7 tested had a positive Coombs' test. Thereafter a number of studies suggested that autoimmune hemolytic anemia (AIHA) occurs at some time in the course of CLL in between 10 and 26% of cases *(11–16)*.

Thrombocytopenia used to be "idiopathic" until Harrington and his colleagues *(17)* demonstrated that the plasma of patients with chronic idiopathic thrombocytopenic purpura (ITP) transfused into a normal recipient (himself) would produce thrombocytopenia. Shulman et al. *(18)* showed that this plasma factor was present in the 7S γ-globulin fraction and was absorbed

From: *Contemporary Hematology*
Chronic Lymphocytic Leukemia: Molecular Genetics, Biology, Diagnosis, and Management
Edited by: G. B. Faguet © Humana Press Inc., Totowa, NJ

by human platelets. Hence, for a new generation of hematologists, ITP stands for immune thrombocytopenic purpura.

Thrombocytopenia is, of course, quite common in CLL. Minot and Buckman (19) found it in half their patients at presentation and in virtually all those whose white count rose above 175 × 10^9/L. Most of these cases were because of bone marrow infiltration or hypersplenism. Harrington and Arimura (20) reported seven cases of autoimmune thrombocytopenia occurring in CLL, and Ebbe et al. (21) reported five more. However, because of the unsatisfactory nature of platelet antibody tests, the true prevalence of immune thrombocytopenia in CLL is unknown. Increase in bone marrow megakaryocytes remains the surest touchstone, but in a marrow full of small lymphocytes they may be difficult to estimate.

Immune neutropenia (22) and pure red cell aplasia (23) have both also been reported to complicate CLL. It is natural, therefore, to suggest that autoimmunity is generally more common in CLL. Several other immunologically mediated diseases, including Sjøgren's syndrome (24), nephrotic syndrome (25), bullous pemphigoid (26), and Graves' disease (27) have been reported in association with CLL, and reviews by Miller (28) and Dameshek (29) have also mentioned systemic lupus erythematosus, rheumatoid arthritis, ulcerative colitis, allergic vasculitis, and pernicious anemia.

2.2. The CD5-Positive B-Cell

A commonly advanced hypothesis to explain these findings is the suggestion that CLL is derived from a CD5-positive B-cell of separate lineage akin to the Ly-1 (CD5) B-cell of mice. This subset, which is particularly enriched in the peritoneal cavity, comprises 5% of circulating B-cells in mice but is markedly expanded in strains such as NZB and MeV, which are prone to autoimmunity (30–33). The link between CD5 and autoimmunity appears as an important buttress supporting unifying theories of CLL (34). The hypothesis gains extra weight with the observation that in both mice and human the germline configuration of many immunoglobulin V_H gene products of CD5 positive B-cells tends to favor weak reactions with autoantigens (35–37).

It was therefore an important observation that the autoimmunity associated with CLL is largely confined to antibodies against mature blood cells (38). Thus, although Hamblin et al. (38) found that 22% of 195 patients with CLL had autoantibodies detectable in their sera, they observed that autoantibodies are found quite commonly in an elderly population. In an age- and gender-matched control population, tissue-specific autoantibodies were detected by immunofluorescence in 21.5%.

If the autoimmunity associated with CLL is so specific, the theory that it is a product of the CD5-ness of the B-cells begins to collapse. Also, against it is the fact that CD5-positive B-cells are not augmented in other strains of mice prone to autoimmunity (39), whereas Xid mice have a similar incidence of autoimmunity as other strains, yet they have no CD5-positive B-cells (40).

In fact, in both mice and human the germline configuration of many V_H gene products tends to favor weak reactions with autoantigens irrespective of whether they are carried by CD5-positive or -negative B-cells (41–43). Hybridomas made from fusing CD5-negative lymphoma cells with nonsecreting murine myeloma cells also secrete autoantibodies (44). The reactivity of 30% of monoclonal IgMs found in patient sera is with only four specificities: rheumatoid factor, cold agglutinins, polyreactivity, and myelin-associated glycoproteins (45).

CD5-negative B-cells express CD5 when stimulated with phorbol ester (46). It is most likely that the expression of CD5 by CLL B-cells represents a state of partial activation rather than their derivation from a separate lineage.

2.3. Prevalence

2.3.1. AUTOIMMUNE HEMOLYTIC ANEMIA

The precise prevalence of AIHA in CLL is disputed. The highest reported prevalence is 35% *(47)*, whereas only 1.8% of patients entered into the French Cooperative Group CLL1980 and CLL1985 trials had a positive antiglobulin test at diagnosis *(48)*. The prevalence is closely related to stage and progression. In stable stage A disease, Hamblin et al. *(38)* found a prevalence of 2.9% compared with 10.5% in stage B and C disease and 18.2% in progressive stage A disease. More patients have a positive Coombs' test than have hemolytic anemia. However, it is clear that CLL is a disease in which disordered control of autoreactivity is a hallmark. Indeed, the commonest known cause of AIHA is CLL. Engelfriet et al. *(49)* found that 14% of his large series of patients with AIHA also had CLL

2.3.2. IMMUNE THROMBOCYTOPENIA

A prevalence of 2%, as suggested by Ebbe et al. *(21)* and confirmed by both Hamblin et al. *(38)* and Dührsen et al. *(50)*, is based on three series each with small numbers of cases. The diagnosis of ITP in CLL requires isolated thrombocytopenia, normal or increased bone marrow megakaryocytes with an excess of early forms, increased mean platelet volume and platelet distribution width, and the detection of platelet antibodies in the serum or on the platelet membrane. However, platelet antibody tests are unreliable. Hegde et al. *(51)* found increased levels of platelet-associated IgG in 3/10 CLL patients with thrombocytopenia and in 1/10 nonthrombocytopenic patients. Kuznetsov et al. *(52)* found antibodies in the serum using an enzyme-linked immunosorbent assay (ELISA) technique in 7/54 thrombocytopenic patients with CLL and platelet-bound antibodies by radioimmunoassay in 21/27. Although these assays are probably oversensitive, they stress the disordered autoreactivity characteristic of the condition. About one-third of patients with ITP secondary to CLL also have a positive direct antiglobulin test, a much higher rate than for primary ITP *(53)*.

2.3.3. AUTOIMMUNE NEUTROPENIA AND PURE RED CELL APLASIA

Confusion has arisen because of the clearly established relationship between large granular lymphocytic (LGL) leukemia *(54)* and both neutropenia and pure red cell aplasia (PRCA) *(55)*. The cytopenias appear to be mediated by a direct action of the leukemic T-cells. Until fairly recently this condition masqueraded under the name of T-CLL.

Whether antibody-mediated neutropenia occurs in CLL is still moot, but higher numbers of CD3+, CD8+, and CD57+ cells have been reported in those patients with true CLL who were neutropenic than in those who were not *(56)*. These authors also demonstrated that CD8+ cells from neutropenic patients exerted a greater suppressive effect on colony-forming units-granulocyte/macrophage (CFU-GM) colony growth than similar cells from non-neutropenic patients *(56)*. Another more recent hypothesis implicates the secretion of high levels of Fas ligand as a cause of the neutropenia that is sometimes seen in B-CLL *(57)*.

It is probable that the PRCA sometimes accompanying CLL is also T-cell-mediated. In 1986 a review by Chikkappa et al. *(58)* identified 23 cases of PRCA associated with CLL, and in the subsequent 12 yr a further 5 cases were recognized *(53)*. This is clearly a rare complication of CLL with a prevalence nothing like the 6% suggested by Chikkappa et al. *(58)*.

2.4. Pathogenesis of Autoimmunity in CLL

2.4.1. AUTOANTIBODIES SECRETED BY THE TUMOR

2.4.1.1. Warm Antibodies. The most obvious explanation for autoimmune disease in CLL would be that the autoantibodies were the product of the tumor. I am constantly surprised by the many eminent immunologists who believe this to be so. The CLL cell does secrete immunoglobulin. Stevenson et al. *(59)* demonstrated secretion of small amounts of idiotypic IgM by CLL cells using a highly sensitive radioimmunoassay. The immunoglobulin secreted by CLL cells is often autoreactive. Stimulation by phorbol ester induced the CLL cells from 12/14 patients to secrete IgM that reacted with a variety of autoantigens, including the Fc portion of IgG, both single- and double-stranded DNA, histones, cardiolipin, and cytoskeletal proteins *(60)*. Similar polyreactive antibodies have been described by Sthoeger et al. *(61)*, who demonstrated that the antibodies were of the same light chain types as the surface IgM of the CLL cells and therefore not the product of contaminating normal B-cells. They also demonstrated the production of IgG autoantibodies from CLL cells expressing surface IgG.

However, it is important not to read too much into these experiments. Beaume et al. *(62)*, who found monoclonal immunoglobulins in the sera of 80% of patients with CLL using a highly sensitive immunoblotting technique, were disappointed to find that the light chain type was the same as that of the surface immunoglobulin in only half the cases. Monoclonal immunoglobulins in the sera of patients with CLL may not necessarily be derived from the tumor.

Most workers agree that the red-cell autoantibodies found on the cells and in the sera in CLL-associated AIHA are detectable with both anti-κ and anti-λ antisera and therefore the product of residual normal B-cells and not of the tumor. In a landmark early case, Sikora et al. *(63)* demonstrated that the monoclonal IgM rescued from CLL cells was not responsible for a concurrent warm antibody AIHA. In contrast, and contrary to accepted wisdom, Sthoeger et al. *(64)* reported two cases of CLL in which it was claimed that immunoglobulin eluted from direct antiglobulin-positive red cells reacted with anti-κ but not anti-λ antibodies. In addition, the CLL cells produced in culture a monoclonal IgM that reacted with red cells, although more strongly at 4°C than at 37°C.

2.4.1.2. Cold Agglutination Syndrome. Occasionally, the AIHA accompanying CLL is caused by cold-reacting rather than warm-reacting antibodies. Cold agglutination syndrome is the best understood disease in which the antibody activity of a monoclonal protein is responsible for clinical manifestations. An essential reagent for unraveling the molecular nature of cold agglutinins was a rat monoclonal antibody, 9G4, raised against the surface IgM of a B-cell lymphoma. This antibody recognized a shared idiotypic determinant on all anti-I or anti-i cold agglutinins *(65)*. Tumor cells from patients with cold agglutination syndrome were immortalized with Epstein-Barr virus. The immunoglobulin V_H genes of these 9G4-positive lines were sequenced and found to use the V_{4-34} gene exclusively *(66,67)*. The antibody continued to react with the V_{4-34} gene product whether the V_H gene was in germline configuration or showed evidence of somatic mutation.

Neither complementarity determining region (CDR) 3 nor light chain sequences were required for binding either to 9G4 or to red cells. Other V_H4 family genes did not react with the anti-idiotype or with red cells in the cold. There are three sections of V_{4-34} that are distinct from other V_H gene segments: the framework region (FR) 1, CDR1, and the first amino acids of CDR2. Recombinant mutants with changed sequences in all these areas demonstrated that the 9G4 idiotope is determined by the motif AVY at amino acid positions 23–25 in FR1 *(68)*.

Binding to the I or i antigens also requires FR1 of V_{4-34}, but other parts of the V_H gene are permissive for binding and determine specificity *(69)*. Anti-I antibodies use VκIII light chains almost exclusively, whereas anti-i antibodies make use of a much broader array of κ and λ light chains *(70)*.

Cold agglutination syndrome is rare in CLL. Among 78 patients with persistent cold agglutinins reported by Crisp and Pruzanski in 1982 *(71)*, only 6 had CLL, and since the diagnostic criteria for CLL were not as stringent in 1982, doubt must exist whether these diagnoses were correct. In retrospect, the single case of CLL with cold agglutination syndrome reported by us *(38)* had a spillover lymphoma. The same may be true of the single case report from Feizi et al. *(72)*. A more recent case was also CD5-negative *(73)*. In this case also the heavy chain gene used by the surface immunoglobulin was DP54 and not V_{4-34}, an indication that the cold agglutinin was not the product of the tumor. We have recently seen a patient with long-standing cold agglutination syndrome who developed definite CLL during his last illness. The tumor made use of the V_{4-34} gene. None of the 11 other patients of CLL who made use of the V_{4-34} gene in our series developed cold agglutination syndrome *(74)*.

There is therefore little evidence to suggest that immunoglobulin produced by the malignant B-cells is responsible for autoimmune phenomena in CLL. A number of paraneoplastic conditions associated with B-cell lymphomas have been attributed to just such a cause; chief among them are acquired angioedema *(75)* and glomerulonephritis *(76,77)*. However, lymphomas more proficient at secreting immunoglobulin are responsible for the larger proportion of such disorders.

2.4.2. THE V GENE HYPOTHESIS

Notwithstanding the lack of direct involvement of the idiotypic immunoglobulin in the autoimmune process, Efremov and co-workers *(78)* produced a startlingly different hypothesis for the pathogenesis of AIHA in CLL. They suggested that AIHA was particularly associated with the use by the tumor of the V_H genes DP10 and DP50 (modern nomenclature V_{1-69} and V_{3-33}), the D segment gene DXP4 (modern nomenclature D3-3), and J_H6. Such a combination of genes would code for a particularly shaped antibody-combining site on the surface of the CLL cells, which, it was hypothesized, would engender an immune attack on red cells, perhaps by invoking idiotype networks in an unspecified way.

Only 12 cases of AIHA were included in the study, 5 using V_{1-69} and 4 using V_{3-33}, neither being used in 12 controls. It is likely that because of small numbers, this apparent association was a chance finding despite the statistics. In two rather larger but unpublished studies *(79,80)* comprising 40 patients with AIHA, only 7 (17.5%) with AIHA used the V_{1-69} gene, close to the usage in 166 controls. Similarly, there was no excess use of V_{3-33} or D3-3. AIHA in CLL is associated with progressive disease. Since the use of V_{1-69} is also associated with progressive disease *(74)*, it is likely that this is a case of guilt by association.

2.4.3. AUTOIMMUNITY TRIGGERED BY TREATMENT

More than 30 yr ago, William Dameshek *(81)* suggested that hemolysis might be triggered by treatment of CLL with X-rays or alkylating agents. Only two such case reports have subsequently appeared in the literature *(82,83)*, and among 37 hemolytic episodes in his large series of patients Hansen found only 5 in which treatment with X-rays or alkylating agents had been given in the previous 2 mo *(84)*. However, since the introduction of fludarabine, reports of treatment-induced hemolysis have become commonplace *(85)*.

Fludarabine-triggered AIHA was first reported in a letter in 1992 *(86)*. Some doubt remained about the association, since the group at M.D. Anderson, with the most experience in the world of the new drug, believed that the 5 patients they had seen with AIHA among 112 patients treated with fludarabine represented the natural prevalence of AIHA in CLL *(87)*. Among patients with pre-existing AIHA, four deteriorated after fludarabine treatment, but four experienced a remission of both CLL and AIHA.

An abstract from the 1994 American Society of Clinical Oncology meeting *(88)* reported a further case and stated that the association had been reported to the Food and Drug Administration on 30 occasions. In 1995, Myint et al. *(89)* reported that of 52 heavily pretreated patients 12 developed AIHA after between 2 and 6 courses of fludarabine. Since then, many reports involving over 100 cases have confirmed the association *(85,90)*. It is important to emphasize that this phenomenon does not represent an allergic reaction to fludarabine, rather, it is an indication of the profound degree of disordered immunity that may occur in CLL, especially in end-stage disease. Fludarabine is an extremely effective drug in CLL, but it is also highly immunosuppressive; so much so that it regularly forms part of the immunosuppressive regimens used for non-myeloablative stem cell transplants. In fact, only about 2% of patients with CLL treated for the first time with fludarabine develop AIHA, probably no more than those treated with other drugs *(91)*. This compares with about 5% of patients who have received some previous treatment and more than 20% of heavily pretreated patients *(85)*.

Fludarabine may also trigger autoimmune thrombocytopenia. This was first reported by Montillo et al. *(92)*, and more than 25 cases have since entered the literature *(85,93)*. In addition, there are reports of one possible case of immune neutropenia *(94)* and three cases of PRCA *(87,95,96)*. The other purine analogs, cladribine and pentostatin, which are equally immunosuppressive, are also capable of triggering autoimmune complications *(85)*, as can the immunosuppressive monoclonal antibody Campath 1H *(85)*.

Although our working hypothesis has been that autoimmunity in CLL is directed against the formed elements of the blood, it appears that a restricted range of other autoimmune conditions can be triggered by fludarabine in CLL. There are two reports of glomerulonephritis associated with antineutrophil cytoplasmic antibodies (ANCAs), one of which followed treatment with fludarabine *(97,98)*. Even more striking has been a rush of reports of paraneoplastic pemphigus. Five cases have been reported following treatment of CLL with fludarabine *(99–101)*.

Blistering skin diseases have been associated with CLL since 1910 *(102,103)*. At that time the autoimmune nature of these diseases was not appreciated, and there was confusion over whether pemphigus vulgaris or bullous pemphigoid was associated with CLL *(26,104)*. This conundrum was solved when Anhalt et al. *(105)* described paraneoplastic pemphigus. The clinical features were painful erosions of the oropharynx, severe pseudomembranous conjunctivitis, pruritic, polymorphous cutaneous lesions including confluent erythema with skin denudation, and papules on the trunk and extremities forming target lesions with central blistering. Histologically, three elements were observed: suprabasilar intraepithelial acantholysis, necrosis of individual keratinocytes, and vacuolar interface change. Immunofluorescence studies revealed the presence in the serum of antibodies that reacted with the intracellular spaces, such as is seen in pemphigus vulgaris, but direct immunofluorescence studies of the skin also demonstrated complement deposition along the basement membrane typical of bullous pemphigoid.

Although it is rare, paraneoplastic pemphigus is a discrete autoimmune blistering skin disease with characteristic clinical features, a pathognomonic pattern of antibody specificity, and an association with lymphoid tumors. It may occur in an array of lymphoid tumors, and especially in Castleman's disease, but about 30% of cases occur in CLL *(106)*.

Some general conclusions can be drawn from these observations. Most cases of post-fludarabine autoimmunity have occurred in patients who have been heavily pretreated, usually with alkylating agents. Hemolysis or thrombocytopenia is severe, difficult to treat, and often fatal. If control is achieved, then re-exposure to any of the purine analogs or even alkylating agents retriggers the complication in an even more virulent form. Although it is commonest in CLL autoimmunity, it may also be induced in other low-grade lymphoproliferative diseases.

2.4.4. THE T-CELL HYPOTHESIS

The suppression of CD4+ T-cells following fludarabine treatment reaches levels as low as those seen in AIDS *(107)*. We have previously suggested that autoimmunity in CLL is caused by loss of T-cell regulatory control of autoreactive T-cells *(89)*. Recent understanding of T-suppressor cells supports this hypothesis.

There is accumulating evidence that T-cell-mediated control of self-reactive T-cells contributes to the maintenance of immunological self-tolerance and that its alteration can cause autoimmune disease. A regulatory T-cell subpopulation expressing CD4 and CD25 has been identified. In normal naive animals, these cells prevent autoimmune disease in vivo and, upon antigenic stimulation, suppress the activation/proliferation of other T-cells in vitro. These CD25+/CD4+ regulatory T-cells, which are naturally anergic and suppressive, appear to be produced by the normal thymus as a functionally distinct subpopulation of T-cells. They play critical roles not only in preventing autoimmunity but also in controlling tumor immunity and transplantation tolerance *(108)*.

Mice thymectomized on the third day of life develop a wide spectrum of organ-specific autoimmune diseases. Reconstitution of these mice with CD4+/CD25+ T-cells from normal mice prevents the development of disease. These cells can also prevent the transfer of disease by autoantigen-specific cloned T-cells derived from neonatally thymectomized mice. Elimination of CD4+/CD25+ T-cells, which constitute 5–10% of peripheral CD4+ T-cells, leads to spontaneous development of various autoimmune diseases *(109)*. They suppress autoreactive T-cells by specifically inhibiting the production of IL-2, an action remarkably like that of cyclosporin *(110)*. This subset of T-cells is highly susceptible to killing with chemotherapeutic agents compared with the CD4+/CD25– subset.

Most of the animal models of autoimmune disease refer to T-cell-mediated, organ-specific autoimmunity. It should not be imagined that this is irrelevant to the production of autoantibodies. Using gene expression profiling, Bystry et al. *(111)* demonstrated that activation of B-cells and professional antigen-presenting cells (APCs) induced the expression of common chemokines. Among these, CCL4 was the most potent chemoattractant of the CD4+/CD25+ T-cell population. Depletion of either regulatory T-cells or CCL4 resulted in a deregulated humoral response, which culminated in the production of autoantibodies. This suggested that the recruitment of regulatory T-cells to B-cells and APCs by CCL4 plays a central role in the normal initiation of T-cell and humoral responses and that failure to do this leads to autoimmune activation.

The CD4+/CD25+ subset has been detected in humans, and appears to have the same function as in mice *(112)*. Scrivener et al. *(113)* have reported a marked reduction in the number of T-cells expressing CD25 in CLL.

2.5. Treatment of Autoimmunity in CLL

Treatment of the autoimmune complications of CLL is not guided by good data. In general, the same treatments have been applied as when the disease occurs spontaneously. However, some treatments are less appropriate, and there is also the question of whether and how to treat the CLL itself. The possibility that the immunosuppression caused by the disease or its treatment has triggered the autoimmunity has to be weighed against the prospect that treating the disease will eliminate the complication.

2.5.1. Autoimmune Hemolytic Anemia

There are no controlled trials of treatment for AIHA secondary to CLL. Autoimmune destruction of blood cells in CLL is frequently vigorous, especially when triggered by purine analogs. Some patients have died because of the mistaken belief that, because the immune process will also destroy transfused red cells, transfusion is of no value. On the contrary, the transfusion of red cells is often vital. It is also important to replenish folic acid. The type of specific treatment used is guided by what has been established for idiopathic AIHA.

2.5.1.1. Corticosteroids and Cytotoxic Drugs. Most patients will respond to the standard treatment for acute hemolysis of prednisolone 1 mg/kg for 10–14 d *(114)*, reducing slowly over the next 3 mo. The usual steroid side effects should be looked for, and, especially in immunodeficient patients, prophylaxis against fungal infections should be given. There are multiple modes of action of steroids including decreased lymphocyte proliferation, decreased interleukin-2 (IL-2) production, decreased T-cell activation and T-helper function, impaired natural killer (NK) function, monocyte maturation and handling of antigen by macrophages, and deficient macrophage chemotaxis *(115)*.

Since most cases occur in progressive CLL, it would be usual to treat the CLL also, either with chlorambucil or fludarabine, but this carries a risk. In patients in which the AIHA has been triggered by fludarabine, further exposure to purine analogs or even to alkylating agents. may be hazardous.

2.5.1.2. Splenectomy. Only four of a series of 113 splenectomies for AIHA were for hemolysis secondary to CLL *(116)*. The well-known hazards of splenectomy are certainly increased in frail, elderly, immunodeficient patients. Laparoscopic splenectomy extends the possibility of operation to a less healthy population. Patients with AIHA with IgG alone and no complement components on their red cells respond better *(117)*. Before elective splenectomy, vaccination against pneumococcus is recommended, and some groups also recommend long-term prophylactic penicillin or the equivalent.

2.5.1.3. Intravenous Immunoglobulin. Of 73 cases of AIHA treated with intravenous immunoglobulin in the literature *(118)*, 40% responded to doses of 0.4 g/kg/d for 5 d. Only 18 of the 73 also had CLL. In these, although reduction in the size of lymph nodes and spleen was also noted, response was transient, lasting only 3–4 wk.

2.5.1.4. Cyclosporin. Cyclosporin is used in AIHA when other modalities have failed. Since treatment of AIHA complicating CLL is often unsuccessful, cyclosporin has been used most frequently in this situation *(119)*. The dose is 5–8 mg/kg/d, tapering to a maintenance dose of about 3 mg/kg/d. We aim to keep the blood level at about 100 µg/L. In a series from the M.D. Anderson Cancer Center, 63% of patients with AIHA complicating CLL responded to cyclosporin 300 mg/d with an increase in Hb of more than 3 g/dL *(120)*.

2.5.1.5. Other Treatments. In patients too sick for splenectomy, especially when the spleen is very large, splenic irradiation may be substituted *(121)*. Danazol may have a role in steroid sparing, although its use in CLL is unreported. Plasma exchange has been successful in a few reports of idiopathic AIHA, but there are no reports in cases secondary to CLL *(53)*. Immunoadsorption onto a column containing protein A is sometimes used as an adjunct to plasma exchange. At least one patient has been successfully treated in this way *(122)*. The infusion of vincristine-loaded platelets to inactivate macrophages has been successful in one patient whose

CLL-related AIHA was unresponsive to other modes of treatment *(123)*. Rituximab has produced responses in AIHA caused by both warm *(124,125)* and cold (126, 127) reacting antibodies. It was very effective in a patient with cold agglutinins associated with a CD20-positive, low-grade non-Hodgkin's lymphoma *(128)*, and it has some activity in CLL *(129)*, but there have so far been no reports of its use in AIHA associated with CLL. Similarly, although there have been no reports of the use of Campath 1H in the treatment of AIHA associated with CLL, it has a beneficial effect in patients with refractory AIHA *(130)*.

2.5.2. AUTOIMMUNE THROMBOCYTOPENIA

There are no reported clinical trials of therapy in CLL-associated ITP, and it is wise to follow the Clinical Guidelines of the American Society of Hematology *(131)* for the treatment of ITP and treat the CLL independently as required. These recommend that asymptomatic thrombocytopenia should only be treated when the platelet count is less than 30×10^9/L. Hospitalization should be confined to patients with mucous membrane or other severe bleeding. Conventional-dose oral prednisolone is the treatment of choice for those who need any treatment, (those with severe bleeding or a platelet count less than 30×10^9/L).

Prednisolone should be given in the same dose as for AIHA, and those patients failing to respond should be treated with intravenous immunoglobulin 0.4 g/kg/d for 5 d. A higher response rate than for AIHA, should be expected. Splenectomy is also more effective than in AIHA with response rates of over 70% in patients unresponsive to steroids *(132)*. Other treatments that work in AIHA may also be tried, but of special value in ITP is bolus or slow infusions of vincristine at a dose of 1 mg iv weekly × 6 *(133)*.

ITP complicating CLL may cause intractable bleeding and be a medical emergency. In this circumstance, intravenous immunoglobulin followed immediately by platelet transfusion *(134)* or methylprednisolone 1 g/d iv × 3 followed by platelet transfusion may be effective. Alternatively, tranexamic acid is worth trying. In refractory cases Campath 1H may be effective *(130)*.

2.5.3. PURE RED CELL APLASIA

On the basis of literature reports of 41 treatments in 33 patients, Diehl and Ketchum *(53)* recommend instituting treatment to control the CLL since this will be necessary to achieve long-term remission of the PRCA. At the same time the PRCA may be treated with prednisolone 1 mg/kg/d. If it is unresponsive, then cyclosporin should be added. The reticulocyte count should increase within 2–3 wk and the hemoglobin should normalize in 1–2 mo. At this point the steroid dose can be reduced and stopped. Cyclosporin should be continued for 6–7 mo and then gradually withdrawn. Campath 1H may be effective in unresponsive cases *(130)*.

2.5.4. MANAGEMENT OF POST-FLUDARABINE AUTOIMMUNITY

The severity of hemolysis or thrombocytopenia following fludarabine is often extreme, and it may be fatal. It is important not to stint on transfusions of red cells or platelets. Immunosuppression is a hazard in these patients, and further immunosuppressive treatment will intensify the risk of infection. When treatment with steroids fails, most patients should be started on cyclosporin, even though intravenous immunoglobulin and splenectomy may still be tried.

A special risk is the retriggering of autoimmunity by re-exposure to purine analogs and even chlorambucil may retrigger the complication *(135)*. However it is possible to reintroduce fludarabine while the patient is maintained on cyclosporin *(120)*. Whether it is safe to use purine analogs in patients with a positive Coombs' test or evidence of pre-existing AIHA is difficult to answer. Some patients have had an exacerbation of their hemolysis or thrombocytopenia when treated this way, but both fludarabine and cladribine have been used successfully in these circumstances *(136,137)*. Our current advice is to introduce purine analogs under the cover of cyclosporin with careful regard to renal function.

3. THE ROLE OF THE SPLEEN

3.1. The Concept of Hypersplenism

Galen called the spleen the "organ of mystery," and in the 19th century both Banti and Gretsel believed that the spleen could exert harmful effects by the exaggeration of its normal function *(138)*. Chauffard coined the term hypersplenism in 1907 *(138)*, but it was made popular by Dameshek 40 yr later *(139)*. The term defined a condition associating splenomegaly with pancytopenia. A debate ensued between Dameshek and Doan. Dameshek held that the spleen exerted an influence on the bone marrow, inhibiting the production of blood cells, whereas Doan's position was that the pancytopenia was caused by the sequestration and destruction of cells in the spleen. After a demonstration in his own laboratory that transfused platelets failed to emerge in the splenic vein, Dameshek conceded defeat, "Well, it looks as though Charley Doan is right" *(140)*.

The anemia of hypersplenism has two causes. There is an expansion of the total plasma volume as well as a pooling of red cells. In very large spleens, up to 40% of red cells may be sequestered there *(141,142)*. The neutropenia of hypersplenism is usually only moderate and asymptomatic. It is caused by an increase in the marginated pool, some of which may be located within the spleen *(143,144)*. On the other hand, the thrombocytopenia of hypersplenism is caused by splenic pooling *(144,145)*. In massively enlarged spleens, up to 90% of platelets can be sequestered there. Nevertheless, the splenic transit time for platelets remains normal at about 10 min, and the splenic platelets remain part of the exchangeable pool *(145)*.

3.2. Hypersplenism in CLL

The importance of hypersplenism in CLL lies in distinguishing it from other causes of cytopenias. There is no doubt that massive splenomegaly may occur in CLL, and there are circumstances in which splenectomy rather than chemotherapy is the treatment of choice. It can be difficult to distinguish hypersplenism from true stage C disease, but clues for diagnosis include moderate or massive splenomegaly, nondiffuse marrow infiltration, and mild, nonprogressive cytopenias.

4. CONCLUSIONS

Anemia, thrombocytopenia, and neutropenia are important features of CLL and usually herald a poor prognosis since their usual cause is bone marrow suppression by infiltrating lymphocytes. Although neither the Binet nor the Rai scoring system specifies it, cytopenias with other causes do not necessarily have such dire consequences. The two most important other causes are autoimmunity and hypersplenism.

Autoimmune hemolytic anemia and thrombocytopenia are relatively common complications of CLL, usually, but not exclusively, occurring in progressive disease. Autoimmune neutropenia and pure red cell aplasia are much rarer and may have a different etiology. Both anemia and thrombocytopenia are usually caused by circulating autoantibodies that are not secreted by the tumor cells but are the product of residual normal B-cells.

Recent reports of an increased number of autoimmune complications following treatment with the purine analogs have led to the suggestion that disturbances of T-cell function are the cause of autoimmunity in CLL. There has been a fresh awakening of interest in suppressor T-cells, and a subpopulation marking with CD4 and CD25 is thought to have a regulatory action over autoreactive T-cells that is lost in autoimmune disease.

Treatment of autoimmune complications of CLL is often difficult, as the diseases are often aggressive and unresponsive, and the patient is often immunosuppressed and susceptible to infection. Cyclosporin is often the most useful drug.

Hypersplenism often accompanies an enlarged spleen in CLL. The cytopenias are usually not severe, and their chief importance is that they allow recognition of when splenectomy rather than chemotherapy is the treatment of choice.

REFERENCES

1. Rai KR, Sawitsky A. Cronkite ER, et al. Clinical staging of chronic lymphocytic leukemia. Blood 1975;46:219–234.
2. Binet, J-L, Leporier M, Dighiero G, et al. A clinical staging system for chronic lymphocytic leukemia. Cancer 1977;40:855–864.
3. Ashby W. Determination of the length of life of transfused blood corpuscles in man. J Exp Med 1919;29:267–281.
4. Berlin R. Red cell survival studies in normal and leukaemic subjects; latent hemolytic syndrome in leukaemia with splenomegaly—nature of anemia in leukaemia—effect of splenomegaly. Acta Med Scand 1951;139 (suppl 252):1–141.
5. Ehrlich P, Morgenroth J. Ueber Hämolysine. V. Berlin Klin Wschr 1901;38:251.
6. Donath J, Landsteiner K. Ueber paroxysmale Hämoglobinurie. Münchenr Medzin Wochenschr, 1904;51:1590–1593.
7. Widal F, Abrami P, Brulé M. Les ictères d'origine hémolytique. Arch Mal Coeur 1908;1:193–231.
8. Dameshek W, Schwartz SO. Hemolysins as the cause of clinical and experimental hemolytic anemias. With particular reference to the nature of spherocytosis and increased fragility. Am J Med Sci 1938;196:769–792.
9. Coombs RRA, Mourant AE, Race RR. A new test for the detection of weak and "incomplete" Rh agglutinins. Br J Exp Pathol 1945;26:255–266.
10. Boorman KE, Dodd BE, Loutit JF. Hemolytic icterus (acholuric jaundice) congenital and acquired. Lancet 1946; i:812–814.
11. Wasserman LR, Stats D, Schwartz L, Fudenberg H. Symptomatic and hemopathic hemolytic anemia. Am J Med 1955;18:961–989.
12. Pisciotta AV, Hirschboeck JS. Therapeutic considerations in chronic lymphocytic leukemia. Arch Int Med 1957;99:334–335.
13. Beickert A. Die hämolytische Verlausform der chronischen lymphatischen Leukämie. Munchen Med Woschenschr 1959;101:2067–2072.
14. Dameshek W, Schwartz RS. Leukemia and auto-immunization. Some possible relationships. Blood 1959; 14:1151–1158.
15. Troup SB, Swisher SN, Young LE. The anemia of leukemia. Am J Med 1960;28:751–763.
16. Videbæk AA. Auto-immune hemolytic anemia in some malignant systemic diseases. Acta Med Scand 1962;171:463–476.
17. Harrington J, Minnich V, Hollingsworth JW, Moore CV. Demonstration of a thrombocytopenic factor in the blood of patients with thrombocytopenic purpura. J Lab Clin Med 1951;38:1–10.
18. Shulman NR, Marder VJ, Weinrach RS. Similarities between known anti-platelet antibodies and the factor responsible for thrombocytopenia in idiopathic purpura: physiologic serologic and isotopic studies. Ann NY Acad Sci 1965;124:499.
19. Minot GR, Buckman TE. The blood platelets in the leukemias. Am J Med Sci 1925;169:477–485.
20. Harrington WJ, Arimura G. Immune reactions of platelets. In: Johnson SA, Monto RW, Rebuck JW, Horn RC, eds. Blood Platelets. Little, Brown, Boston, 1961.
21. Ebbe S, Wittels B, Dameshek W. Autoimmune thrombocytopenic purpura ("ITP type") with chronic lymphocytic leukemia. Blood 1962;19:23–27.
22. Killman S-Å. Auto-aggressive leukocyte agglutinins in leukaemia and chronic leukopenia. Acta Med Scand 1959;163:207–222.
23. Abeloff MD, Waterbury MD. Pure red cell aplasia and chronic lymphocytic leukemia. Arch Intern Med 1974;134:721–724.

24. Lehner-Netsch G, Barry A, Delage JM. Leukemias and autoimmune diseases: Sjøgren's syndrome and hemolytic anemia associated with chronic lymphocytic anemia. Can Med Assoc J 1969;100:1151–1154.

25. Dathan JRE, Heyworth MF, MacIver AG. Nephtotic syndrome in chronic lymphocytic leukaemia. BMJ 1974; 3:655–657.

26. Cuni LJ, Grünwald H, Rosner F. Bullous pemphigoid in chronic lymphocytic leukemia with the demonstration of anti-basement membrane antibodies. Am J Med 1974;57:987–992.

27. Haubenstock A, Zalusky R. Autoimmune hyperthyroidism and thrombocytopenia in a patient with chronic lymphocytic leukemia. Am J Hematol 1985;19:281–283.

28. Miller DG. Patterns of immunological deficiency in lymphomas and leukemias. Ann Intern Med 1962;57:703–715.

29. Dameshek W. Chronic lymphocytic leukemia—an accumulative disease of immunologically incompetent lymphocytes. Blood 1967;24:566–584.

30. Manohar V, Brown E, Leiserson WM, Chused TM. Expression of Ly-1 by a subset of B-lymphocytes. J Immunol 1982;129:532–538.

31. Hayakawa K, Hardy RR, Parks DR, Herzenberg LA. The Ly-1 B cell subpopulation in normal, immunodefective and autoimmune mice. J Exp Med 1983;157:202–218.

32. Herzenberg LA, Stall AM, Lalor PA, et al. The Ly1-B cell lineage. Immunol Rev 1986;93:81–102.

33. Hayakawa K, Hardy RR, Herzenberg LA. Peritoneal Ly1-B-cells: genetic control, autoantibody production, increased lambda light chain expression. Eur J Immunol 1986;16:450–456.

34. Caligaris-Cappio F. B-chronic lymphocytic leukemia: a malignancy of anti-self B-cells. Blood 1996;87:2615–2620.

35. Holmberg D, Forsgren S, Ivars F, Coutinho A. Reactions among IgM antibodies derived from normal neonatal mice. Eur J Immunol 1984;14:435–440.

36. Lymberi P, Dighiero G, Ternyck T, Avrameas S. A high incidence of cross reactive idiotypes among murine natural autoantibodies. Eur J Immunol 1985;5:702–707.

37. Kearney JF, Vakil M. Idiotype directed interactions during ontogeny play a major role in the establishment of the adult B cell repertoire. Immunol Rev 1986;94:39–62.

38. Hamblin TJ, Oscier DG, Young BJ. Autoimmunity in chronic lymphocytic leukaemia. J Clin Pathol 1986;39:713–716.

39. Dighiero G. Relevance of murine models in elucidating the origin of B-CLL lymphocytes and related immune associated phenomena. Semin Hematol 1987;24:240–251.

40. Dighiero G, Poncet P, Rouyre S, Mazie JC. Newborn Xid mice carry the genetic information for the production of natural autoantibodies. J Immunol 1986;136:4000–4005.

41. Holmberg D, Forsgren S, Ivars F, Coutinho A. Reactions among IgM antibodies derived from normal neonatal mice. Eur J Immunol 1984;14:435–440.

42. Lymberi P, Dighiero G, Ternyck T, Avrameas S. A high incidence of cross reactive idiotypes among murine natural autoantibodies. Eur J Immunol 1985;5:702–707.

43. Kearney JF, Vakil M. Idiotype directed interactions during ontogeny play a major role in the establishment of the adult B cell repertoire. Immunol Rev 1986;94:39–62.

44. Dighiero G, Hart S, Lim A, Borche L, Levy R, Miller RA. Autoantibody activity of immunoglobulins isolated from B cell follicular lymphomas. Blood 1991;78:581–585.

45. Dellagi K, Brouet JC, Danon F. Cross reacting idiotypic antigens among monoclonal immunoglobulin M from patients with Waldenström's macroglobulinemia and polyneuropathy. J Clin Invest 1979;64:1530–1539.

46. Miller RA, Gralow J. The induction of Leu-1 antigen expression in human malignant and normal B-cells by phorbolmyristic acetate (PMA). J Immunol 1984;133:3408–3412.

47. Bergsagel DE. The chronic leukemias: a review of disease manifestations and the aims of therapy. Can Med Assoc J 1967;96:1615–1620.

48. Dighiero G. Hypogammaglobulinemia and disordered immunity in CLL. In: Cheson BD, ed. Chronic Lymphocytic Leukemia: Scientific Advances and Clinical Developments. Marcel Dekker, New York, 1993, pp. 167–180.

49. Engelfriet CP, Overbeeke MAM, von dem Borne AEGK. AIHA. Semin Hematol 1992;29:3–12.

50. Dührsen U, Augener W, Zwingers T, Brittinger G. Spectrum and frequency of autoimmune derangements in lymphoproliferative disorders: analysis of 637 cases and comparison with myeloproliferative diseases. Br J Haematol 1987;67:235–239.

51. Hegde UM, Williams K, Devereux S, et al. Platelet associated IgG and immune thrombocytopenia in lymphoproliferative and autoimmune disorders. Clin Lab Haematol 1983;5:9–15.

52. Kuznetsov AI, Idel'son LI, Ivanov AL, Mazurov AV. Antithrombocyte antibodies in the serum and on the surface of the thrombocytes in patients with chronic lymphoproliferative diseases. Ter Arkh 1991;63:26–30.

53. Diehl LF, Ketchum LH. Autoimmune disease and chronic lymphocytic leukemia: AIHA, pure red cell aplasia and autoimmune thrombocytopenia. Semin Hematol 1998;25:80–97.

54. Loughran TP, Kardin ME, Starkebaum G, et al. Leukemia of large granular lymphocytes: association with clonal chromosomal abnormalities and autoimmune neutropenia, thrombocytopenia, and hemolytic anemia. Ann Intern Med 1985;102:169–175.

55. Lacy MQ, Kurtin PJ, Tefferi A. Pure red cell aplasia: association with large granular lymphocytic leukemia and the prognostic value of cytogenetic abnormalities. Blood 1996;87:3000–3006.

56. Katrinakis G, Kyriakou D, Alexandrakis M, Sakellariou D, Foudoulakis A, Eliopoulos GD. Evidence for involvement of activated CD8+/HLA-DR+ cells in the pathogenesis of neutropenia in patients with B-cell chronic lymphocytic leukaemia. Eur J Haematol 1995;55:33–41.

57. Lamy T, Loughran TP. Current concepts: large granular lymphocyte leukaemia. Blood Rev 1999;13:230–240.

58. Chikkappa G, Zarrabi MH, Tsan MF. Pure red cell aplasia in patients with chronic lymphocytic leukemia. Medicine (Baltimore) 1986;65:339–351.

59. Stevenson FK, Hamblin TJ, Stevenson GT, Tutt A. Extracellular idiotypic immunoglobulin arising from human leukemia B-lymphocytes. J Exp Med 1980;152:1484–1496.

60. Broker BM, Klajman A, Youinou P, et al. Chronic lymphocytic leukemia (CLL) cells secrete multispecific autoantibodies. J Autoimmune 1988;1:469–481.

61. Sthoeger ZM, Wakai M, Tse DB, et al. Production of autoantibodies by CD5-expressing B-lymphocytes from patients with chronic lymphocytic leukemia. J Exp Med 1989;169:255–268.

62. Beaume A, Brizard A, Dreyfus B, Preud'homme JL. High incidence of serum monoclonal Igs detected by a sensitive immunoblotting technique in B-cell chronic lymphocytic leukemia. Blood 1994;84:1216–1219.

63. Sikora K, Kirkorian J, Levy R. Monoclonal immunoglobulin rescued from a patient with chronic lymphocytic leukemia and AIHA. Blood 1979;54:513–518.

64. Sthoeger ZM, Stoeger D, Shtalrid M, et al. Mechanism of AIHA in chronic lymphocytic leukemia. Am J Hematol 1993;43:259–264.

65. Stevenson FK, Wrightham M, Glennie MJ, et al. Antibodies to shared idiotypes as agents for analysis and therapy for human B cell tumours. Blood 1986;68:430–436.

66. Pascual V, Victor K, Lelsz D, et al. Nucleotide sequence analysis of the V regions of two IgM cold agglutinins. Evidence that the V_H4-21 gene segment is responsible for the major cross-reactive idiotype. J Immunol 1991; 146:4385–4391.

67. Pascual V, Victor K, Spellerberg M, Hamblin TJ, Stevenson FK, Capra JD. VH restriction among human cold agglutinins: the VH4-21 gene segment is required to encode anti-I and anti-i specificities. J Immunol 1992; 149:2337–2344.

68. Potter KN, Li Y, Pascuel V, et al. Molecular characterization of a cross-reactive idiotope on human immunoglobulins utilizing the V_H4-21 gene segment. J Exp Med 1993;178:1419–1428.

69. Li Y, Spellerberg M, Stevenson FK, Capra JD, Potter KN. The I binding specificity of V_H4-34 (V_H4-21) encoded antibodies is determined by both V_H framework region 1 and complementarity determining region 3. J Mol Biol 1996;256:577–589.

70. Silberstein LE, Jefferies LC, Goldman J, et al. Variable region gene analysis of pathologic human autoantibodies related to the i and I red blood cell antigens. Blood 1991;78:2372–2388.

71. Crisp D, Pruzanski W. B-cell neoplasms with homogeneous cold-reacting antibodies (cold agglutinins). Am J Med 1982;72:915–922.

72. Feizi T, Wernet P, Kunkel HG, Douglas SD. Lymphocytes forming red cell rosettes in the cold in patients with chronic cold agglutinin disease. Blood 1973;42:753–762.

73. Ishida F, Saito H, Kitano K, Kiyosawa K. Cold agglutinin disease by auto-i blood type antibody associated with B cell chronic lymphocytic leukemia. Int J Hematol 1998;67:69–73.

74. Hamblin TJ, Davis Z, Gardiner A, Oscier DG, Stevenson GT. Unmutated Ig V_H genes are associated with a more aggressive form of chronic lymphocytic leukemia. Blood 1999;94:1848–1854.

75. He S, Tsang S, North J, Chohan N, Sim RB, Whaley K. Epitope mapping of C1 inhibitor autoantibodies from patients with acquired C1 inhibitor deficiency. J Immunol 1996;156:2009–2013.

76. Gouet D, Marechaud R, Touchard G, Abadie JC, Pourrat O, Sudre Y. Nephrotic syndrome associated with chronic lymphocytic leukaemia. Nouv Presse Med 1982;11:3047–3049.

77. Moulin B, Ronco PM, Mougenot B, Francois A, Fillastre JP, Mignon F. Glomerulonephritis in chronic lymphocytic leukaemia and related B cell lymphomas. Kidney Int 1992;42:127–135.

78. Efremov DG, Ivanovski M, Siljanovski N, et al. Restricted immunoglobulin V_H regopn repertoire in chronic lymphocytic leukemia patients with AIHA. Blood 1996;87:3869–3876.
79. Bessudo A, Chen A, Rassenti LZ, Savin A, Kipps TJ. AIHA in patients with chronic lymphocytic leukemia apparently is not associated with leukemia cell expression of Ig V_H 1-69 (51p1) genes. Blood 1997;90(suppl 1): 209b, abstract 3672.
80. Hamblin TJ, Davies Z, Oscier D, Stevenson F. In chronic lymphocytic leukaemia (CLL) AIHA (AIHA) is not related to any particular immunoglobulin V gene usage. Br J Haematol 1999;105(suppl 1):88.
81. Lewis FB, Schwarz RS, Damashek W. X-irradiation and alkylating agents as possible trigger mechanisms in autoimmune complications of malignant lymphoproliferative diseases. Clin Exp Immunol 1966;1:3–11.
82. Catovsky D, Foa R. B-cell chronic lymphocytic leukaemia. In: Catovsky D, Foa R, eds. The Lymphoid Leukaemias. Butterworths, London, 1990, pp. 73–112.
83. Thompson-Moya L, Martin T, Heuft HG, Neubaur A, Herrmann R. Allergic reaction with immune hemolytic anemia arising from chlorambucil. Am J Hematol 1989;32:230–231.
84. Hansen MM. Chronic lymphocytic leukaemia: clinical studies based on 189 cases followed for a long time. Scand J Haematol 1973;18(suppl 1):1–282.
85. Hamblin TJ. Autoimmune disease and its management in chronic lymphocytic leukemia. In: Cheson BD, ed. Chronic Lymphocytic Leukemia: Scientific Advances and Clinical Developments. Marcel Dekker, New York, 2001, pp. 435–458.
86. Bastion Y, Coiffier B, Dumontet C, Espinouse D, Bryon PA. Severe AIHA in two patients treated with fludarabine for chronic lymphocytic leukemia. Ann Oncol 1992;3:171–172
87. Di Raimondo F, Guistolisi R, Caccio;a E, et al. AIHA in chronic lymphocytic leukemia patients treated with fludarabine. Leuk Lymphoma 1993;11:63–68.
88. Byrd JC, Weiss RB, Kweeder SL, Deihl LF. Fludarabine therapy with lymphoid malignancies is associated AIHA. Proc ASCO 1994;13:304a.
89. Myint H, Copplestone JA, Orchard J, et al. Fludarabine-related AIHA in patients with chronic lymphocytic leukaemia. Br J Haematol 1995;91:341–344.
90. Leporier M, Chevret S, Cazin B, et al. Randomized comparison of fludarabine, CAP, and ChOP in 938 previously untreated stage B and C chronic lymphocytic leukemia patients. Blood 2001;98:2319–2315.
91. Mauro FR, Foa R, Cerretti R, et al. Autoimmune haemolytic anemia in chronic lymphocytic leukemia: clinical, therapeutic, and prognostic features. Blood 2000;95:2786–1792.
92. Montillo M, Tedeschi A, Leoni P. Recurrence of autoimmune thrombocytopenia after treatment with fludarabine in a patient with chronic lymphocytic leukemia. Leuk Lymphoma 1994;15:187–188.
93. Churn M, Clough V. Autoimmune thrombocytopenia associated with the first cycle of fludarabine therapy in the treatment of relapsed non-Hodgkin'd lymphoma. Clin Radiol 2001;13:273–275.
94. Stern SC, Shah S, Costello C. Probable autoimmune neutropenia induced by fludarabine treatment for chronic lymphocytic leukaemia. Br J Haematol 1999;106:836–837.
95. Antich Rojas J, Balaguer H, Cladera A. Selective aplasia of the red-cell series after fludarabine administration in a patient with chronic B-cell lymphatic leukemia. Sangre (Barc) 1997;42:254–256.
96. Leporier M, Reman O, Troussard X. Pure red cell aplasia with fludarabine for chronic lymphocytic leukemia. Lancet 1993;342:555.
97. Tisler A, Pierratos A, Lipton JH. Crescentic glomerulonephritis associated with p-ANCA positivity in fludarabine-treated chronic lymphocytic leukemia. Nephrol Dial Transplant 1996;11:2306–2308.
98. Dussol B, Brunet P, Vacher-Coponat H, Bouabdallah R, Chetaille P, Berland Y. Crescentic glomerulonephritis with antineutrophil cytoplasmic antibodies associated with chronic lymphocytic leukaemia. Nephrol Dial Transplant 1997;12:785–786.
99. Bazarbachi A, Bachelez H, Dehen L, Delmer A, Zittoun R, Dubertret L. Lethal paraneoplastic pemphigus following treatment of chronic lymphocytic leukemia with fludarabine. Ann Oncol 1995;6:730–731.
100. Braess J, Reich K, Willert S, et al. Mucocutaneous autoimmune syndrome following fludarabine therapy for low-grade non-Hodgkin's lymphoma of B-cell type (B-NHL). Ann Hematol 1997;75:227–230.
101. Gooplu C, Littlewood TJ, Frith P, et al. Paraneoplastic pemphigus—an association with fludarabine. Br J Dermatol 2001;144:1102-1104.
102. Oppenheim M. Verhandlungen Der Weiner dermatologischen Gesellschaft. Arch Dermatol Syphiligr 1910; 101:379–382.
103. Sachs O. Ueber pemphigoide Hauteruption in einem Falle von Lymphatischer Leukaemie. Wien Klin Wochenschr 1921;34:317.

104. Laskaris GC, Papavasilou SS, Bovopoulou OD, Nicolis GD. Association of oral pemphigus with chronic lymphocytic leukemia. Oral Surg Oral Med Oral Pathol 1980;50:244–249.
105. Anhalt GJ, Kim SC, Stanley JR, et al. Paraneoplastic pemphigus. An autoimmune mucocutaneous disease associated with neoplasia. N Engl J Med 1990;323:1729–1735.
106. Anhalt GJ, Nousari HC. Paraneoplastic autoimmune syndromes. In: Rose NR, Mackay IR, eds. The Autoimmune Diseases. 3rd ed. Academic Press, San Diego, 1998, pp. 795–804.
107. Boldt DH, Van Hoff DD, Kuhn JG, Hersh M. Effect on human peripheral lymphocytes of the in vivo administration of 9-β-D-arabinofuranosyl-5'-monophosphate (NSC312887) a new purine antimetabolite. Cancer Res 1984;44:4661–4666.
108. Sakaguchi S, Sakaguchi N, Shimizu J, et al. Immunologic tolerance maintained by CD25+ CD4+ regulatory T-cells: their common role in controlling autoimmunity, tumor immunity, and transplantation tolerance. Immunol Rev 2001;182:18–32.
109. Shevach EM, McHugh RS, Piccirillo CA, Thornton AM. Control of T-cell activation by CD4+ CD25+ suppressor T-cells. Immunol Rev 2001;182:58–67.
110. Thornton AM, Shevach EM. CD4+ CD25+ immunoregulatory T-cells suppress polyclonal T cell activation by inhibiting interleukin 2 production. J Exp Med 1998;188:287–296.
111. Bystry RS, Aluvihare V, Welch KA, Kallikourdis M, Betz AG. B-cells and professional APCs recruit regulatory T-cells via CCL4. Nat Immunol 2001;2:1126–1132.
112. Ng WF, Duggan PJ, Ponchel F, et al. Human CD4(+)CD25(+) cells: a naturally occurring population of regulatory T-cells. Blood 2001;98:2736–2744.
113. Scrivener S, Kaminski ER, Demaine A, Prentice AG. Analysis of the expression of critical activation/interaction markers on peripheral blood T-cells in B-cell chronic lymphocytic leukaemia: evidence of immune dysregulation. Br J Haematol 2001;112:959–964.
114. Dameshek W, Komninos ZP. The present status of treatment of AIHA with ACTH and cortisone. Blood 1956; 11:648–664.
115. Collins PW, Newland AC. Treatment modalities of autoimmune blood disorders. Semin Hematol 1992;29: 64–74.
116. Coon WW. Splenectomy in the treatment of hemolytic anemia. Arch Surg 1985;120:625–628.
117. Dacie JV. Autoimmune hemolytic anemia. Arch Intern Med 1975; 135:1293–1300.
118. Flores G, Cunningham-Rundles C, Newland AC, Bussel J. Efficacy of intravenous immunoglobulin in the treatment of AIHA: results in 73 patients. Am J Hematol 1993;44:237–242.
119. Ruess-Borst MA, Waller HD, Muller CA. Successful treatment of steroid resistant hemolysis in chronic lymphocytic leukemia with cyclosporin A. Am J Hematol 1994;9:357–359.
120. Cortes J, O'Brien S, Loscertales J, et al. Cyclosporin A for the treatment of cytopenia associated with chronic lymphocytic leukemia. Cancer 2001;92:2016–2022.
121. Guinet MJ, Liew KH, Quong GG, Cooper IA. A study of splenic irradiation in chronic lymphocytic leukemia. Int J Rad Oncol Biol Phys 1989;16:225–229.
122. Esa EC, Ray PK, Swami VK, et al. Specific immunoadsorption of IgG antibody in a patient with chronic lymphocytic leukemia and AIHA. Am J Med 1981;71:1035–1040.
123. Sigler E, Shtalrid M, Goland S, Stoeger ZM, Berrebi A. Intractable acute AIHA in B-cell chronic lymphocytic leukemia successfully treated with vincristine loaded platelet infusion. Am J Hematol 1995;50:313–315.
124. Ahrens N, Kingreen D, Seltsam A, Salama A. Treatment of refractory autoimmune haemolytic anaemia with anti-CD20 (rituximab). Br J Haematol 2001;114:241–242.
125. Zecca M, De Stefano P, Nobili B, Locatelli F. Anti-CD20 monoclonal antibody for the treatment of severe, immune-mediated pore red cell aplasia and haemolytic anemia. Blood 2001;97:3995–3997.
126. Laylos N, Van Den Neste E, Jost E, Deneys V, Schieff JM, Ferrant A. Remission of severe cold agglutinin disease after rituximab therapy. Leukemia 2001;15:187–188.
127. Zaja F, Russo D, Fuga G, et al. Rituximab in a case of cold agglutinin disease. Br J Haematol 2001;114: 232–233.
128. Bauduer F. Rituximab: a very efficient therapy in cold agglutinins and refractory autoimmune haemolytic anaemia associated with CD20-positive, low-grade non-Hodgkin's lymphoma. Br J Haematol 2001;112:1085–1090.
129. Huhn D, von Schilling C, Wilhelm M, et al. Rituximab therapy in patients with B-cell chronic lymphocytic leukemia. Blood 2001;98:1326–1331.
130. Willis F, Marsh JCW, Bevan DH, et al. Effect of treatment with Campath-1H in patients with autoimmune cytopenias. Br J Haematol 2001;114:891–898.

131. The American Society of Hematology ITP Practice Guideline Panel. Diagnosis and treatment of idiopathic thrombocytopenic purpura: recommendations of the American Society of Hematology. Ann Intern Med 1997; 126:319–326.
132. McMillan R. Therapy for adults with refractory chronic immune thrombocytopenic purpura. Ann Intern Med 1997;126:307–314.
133. Ahn YS, Harrington WJ, Mylvagnam R, Allen LM, Pall LM. Slow infusion of vinca alkaloids in the treatment of idiopathic thrombocytopenic purpura. Ann Intern Med 1984;100:192–196.
134. Baumann MA, Menitove JE, Aster RH, Anderson T. Urgent treatment of idiopathic thrombocytopenic purpura with single dose gammaglobulin infusion followed by platelet transfusion. Ann Intern Med 1986;104:808–809.
135. Orchard J, Bolam S, Myint H, Oscier DG, Hamblin TJ. In patients with lymphoid tumours recovering from the autoimmune complications of fludarabine, relapse may be triggered by conventional chemotherapy. Br J Haematol 1998;102:1112–1113.
136. Montillo M, Tedeschi A, O'Brien S, Lerner S, Morra E, Keating MJ. Autoimmune phenomena against hemato-poietic cells and myelosuppression in CLL treated with fludarabine-including regimens as front-line therapy. InL Proceedings of the IWCLL VIII Workshop on CLL, 1999, p. 54, abstract P091.
137. Tosti S, Caruso R, D'Adamo F, et al. Severe AIHA in a patient with chronic lymphocytic leukemia responsive to fludarabine responsive treatment. Ann Hematol 1992;65:238–239.
138. Wintrobe MM. Clinical Hematology, 7th ed. Lea & Febiger, Philadelphia, 1974, p. 1317.
139. Crosby WM. The spleen. In:Wintrobe MM, ed. Blood, Pure and Eloquent. McGraw Hill, New York, 1980, pp. 96–138.
140. Dameshek W, Estren S. Hypersplenism. Med Clin North Am 1950;34:1271–1292.
141. Blendis LM, Banks DC, Ramboer C, Williams R. Spleen blood flow and splanchnic haemodynamics in blood dyscrasia and other splenomegalies. Clin Sci 1970;38:73–84.
142. Bowdler AJ. Splenomegaly and hypersplenism. Clin Haematol 1983;12:467–488.
143. Brubaker LH, Johnson CA. Correlation of splenomegaly and abnormal neutrophil pooling (margination). J Lab Clin Med 1978;92:508–515.
144. Schaffner A, Augustiny N, Otto RC, Fehr J. The hypersplenic spleen. A contractile reservoir of granulocytes and platelets. Arch Intern Med 1985;145:651–654.
145. Aster RH. Pooling of platelets in the spleen: role in the pathogenesis of "hypersplenic" thrombocytopenia. J Clin Invest 1966;45:645–657.

21

Clonal Evolution and Second Malignancies in B-CLL

Guy B. Faguet, MD

1. INTRODUCTION

Chronic lymphocytic leukemia (CLL) is a malignancy of B-lymphocytes characterized by accumulation of neoplastic cells with low proliferative capacity but a disrupted apoptotic pathway that hampers programmed cell death, resulting in their prolonged life span *(1,2)*. As a consequence, many patients afflicted by CLL follow an indolent or slowly progressive course often, requiring no treatment *(3)*. Because of this slow course and because CLL primarily affects the elderly [mean age at diagnosis, 60–65 *(4)*] most patients die with rather than of the disease or its complications. Indeed, many CLL patients with early-stage disease [Rai low risk *(5)* or Binet stage A *(6)*] have a normal life span *(7)*. However, in a substantial number of patients, survival is shortened by the multifaceted pathological impact of progressive disease *(8,9)* or its treatment *(10)* and (to a much lesser extent) by clonal evolution to a more aggressive disease *(11)* or the development of second malignancies *(12–16)*. This chapter examines the most recent literature on CLL clonal evolution, especially Richter's syndrome, and reviews Surveillance, Epidemiology, and End Results (SEER) data in order to quantify the risk for and types of second malignancies suffered by patients with CLL.

2. RICHTER'S SYNDROME

Hematological malignancies develop as second cancers in CLL with some frequency and include diffuse large cell lymphoma (DLCL), Hodgkin's disease (HD), and multiple myeloma (MM), with relative incidences of 3, 0.5, and 0.1, respectively. Of these, an aggressive and rapidly fatal form of DLCL described by Richter in 1928 is the best known second malignancy associated with CLL *(17)*. The term Richter's syndrome was coined by Lortholary et al. *(18)*, who reported four additional cases exhibiting the clinical and pathological syndrome. It includes the emergence of an aggressive DLCL occurring in a patient with pre-existing CLL, severe constitutional symptoms, and swift disease progression resulting in rapid clinical deterioration and death within 1 yr of onset. Given its low incidence, most reports on RS are anecdotal or are limited to only a few patients, and some have included rapidly progressive DLCL arising from low-grade lymphoproliferative disorders other than CLL *(19,20)*. This review focuses on RS supervening in CLL, highlighting differences that relate to the primary underlying disorder, if other than CLL, especially when addressing its clonal origin.

From: *Contemporary Hematology*
Chronic Lymphocytic Leukemia: Molecular Genetics, Biology, Diagnosis, and Management
Edited by: G. B. Faguet © Humana Press Inc., Totowa, NJ

2.1. Clinical Profile

The largest series (39 cases) addressing RS emerged from a retrospective analysis of the M.D. Anderson Cancer Center computerized database of 1374 CLL cases diagnosed between 1972 and 1992 *(21)*. The authors included in their definition of RS cases of immunoblastic non-Hodgkin's lymphomas. The median interval between the initial diagnosis and the onset of RS was approximately 4 yr. Salient presenting features included male predominance (62%), progressive lymphadenopathy (64%), systemic symptoms (59%), and extranodal involvement (41%), mainly pleura and central nervous system, and increased levels of lactic dehydrogenase (82%). Several observations made by the authors merit emphasis, as they have major clinical and pathogenic relevance: whereas nearly half of the patients had stage III/IV CLL at the onset of RS, 25% were in a complete remission induced by a fludarabine-based regimen. Likewise, whereas 82% of patients had been treated for CLL prior to the onset of RS, 8% had not. Thus, neither disease stage nor successful treatment, including that with fludarabine monophosphate, seemed to affect the risk for CLL patients to develop RS. Alternatively, three or more cytogenetic abnormalities were detected in 9 of the 11 RS patients who exhibited abnormal karyotypes, confirming previous reports that complex clonal chromosomal abnormalities increase the risk for RS *(22)*. Finally, of the 33 patients (85%) who were treated for RS (32 with systemic chemotherapy, including 9 who received adjuvant radiation therapy, and 1 with radiotherapy alone), 10 achieved a complete remission. However, only three survived longer than 1 yr, and the group's median survival was 5 mo from the onset of RS, exposing the inability of our current therapeutic modalities to reverse or control this disorder's relentless progression and rapid demise.

An earlier series from Paris *(19)* had reported 25 cases of RS, identified by the authors as "histiocytic lymphoma in 23 cases and Hodgkin's disease in 2 cases": 19 arose from CLL, 4 from Waldenström's macroglobulinemia, and 2 from small cell lymphoma (SCL). The time interval to the diagnosis of RS was 49 mo and the median survival was 4 mo even though complete remissions were achieved in six, four of whom had localized disease. An additional relatively large series of nine RS patients *(23)* mirrored the M.D. Anderson Cancer Center and Paris reports with respect to clinical features, time interval to RS, and a dismal median survival.

As described above, most cases of RS occur some time after the primary clonal disease has been recognized and usually treated. However, in addition to this "classic" presentation, a "variant" form of RS is said to occur when RS is diagnosed concomitantly with a previously unrecognized low-grade lymphoproliferative disease *(19,24)*. From a clinical standpoint, these cases appear indistinguishable from the classic type, except for a higher response rate (50% complete remission) reported by one group *(24)*. Hodgkin's disease supervening in patients with CLL has been referred to as HD variant of RS, whereas it should more appropriately be viewed as a second malignancy. According to the M.D. Anderson Cancer Center CLL group *(25)*, these patients present with a histological profile indistinguishable from *de novo* HD, with a median time to HD diagnosis of 45 mo. However, unlike patients with *de novo* HD, they exhibit a poor response to chemotherapy (25%), and a short median survival (12 mo).

2.2. Karyotype Profile

The scarcity of RS cases has precluded an adequate assessment of the cytogenetic abnormalities associated with this condition, as most reports over the years have been anecdotal and were limited to karyotype banding. The largest series on RS included either no karyotype data *(19)* or data from cytogenetic analysis performed only during the CLL phase of the disease *(21,26)*. Additionally, interpretation of published data is hampered by uncertainties regarding the cellular origin, whether CLL or RS, of the metaphases studied. A report of chromosomal abnormalities in a series of 6 RS cases, plus a review of 10 additional RS cases from the literature *(27)*, made the following observations:

1. No specific chromosomal abnormalities were present in RS.
2. Abnormalities were complex, as is frequently seen in advanced or progressive CLL, and instability was frequent.
3. Chromosomes 14 and 11 were the most frequently involved, with band 14q32 rearrangement noted in 8 of 16 RS cases and t(11;14)(q13;q32) in 2.
4. Trisomy 12, frequently observed in CLL, was reported in only 2 of 16 RS cases, and deletion involving 13q14 was not observed in RS.
5. Two patients had structural rearrangements of 12q with t(5;12)(q21-q22;q23-q24).

The fact that 4 of the 16 cases had not received chemotherapy prior to the cytogenetic study suggests an inherent disease-associated rather than treatment-induced genomic instability.

Newer molecular karyotype techniques have been used with increasing frequency and success in recent years. These include polymerase chain reaction (PCR) and fluorescence *in situ* hybridization (FISH) *(28)* to highlight preselected marker chromosomes, comparative genomic hybridization (CGH) *(29)*, which allows a comprehensive mapping of chromosomal gains and losses without any preknowledge of affected chromosomal regions, in a single experiment, and spectral karyotyping *(30)*, a technique that uses multiple painting probes hybridized on metaphase chromosomes and identifies each chromosome by a unique spectral signature, enhancing detection of rearrangements and subtle translocations.

Of these, CGH alone or in combination with standard chromosome banding or with RNA or DNA probing techniques has anecdotally uncovered gains in C-MYC oncogene copies in six different chromosomes in a patient with RS *(31)*, as well as a mutation of *p53* exon 7, in addition to a 17p deletion with a potentially pathogenic role in another RS case *(32)*. However, a recent CGH analysis of CLL patients studied at diagnosis (*n* = 30), at the time of disease progression (*n* = 7), and at transformation to RS (*n* = 4), plus six RS patients with no prior cytogenetics study, is the largest and most informative assessment of cytogenetics abnormalities associated with progressive CLL *(33)*. Overall, DNA imbalances were observed in 22 (70%) CLL patients at diagnosis, with the most common imbalances being gains in chromosome 12 (30%), losses in chromosome 13 (17%), and losses of 17p (17%), 8p, 11q, and 14q (7% each). All patients who progressed to a more advanced clinical stage of CLL or to RS had abnormal initial CGH profiles. Sixty percent of patients with progressive CLL exhibited additional imbalances, and 89% of RS patients had gains (*n* = 28) and losses (*n* = 12). The most common imbalances in these latter patients included gains in chromosome 12 (33%), and 11q (22%) and losses of 8p, 17p (44% each) and 9 (33%). Deletions of 17p were associated with *p53* gene mutations and greater additional chromosomal imbalances than cases with normal chromosome 17. In contrast, no relationship was demonstrated between 9p deletions and p16[ink] (located at 9p12) gene alterations. The authors concluded that chromosomal imbalances might increase during progression of CLL and transformation to RS and that genetic alterations detected by CGH in the CLL phase might have prognostic significance.

2.3. Clonal Origin

CLL and DLCL cells are morphologically distinct: the former resemble mature lymphocytes, and the latter are generally larger and immature looking. However, immature lymphoid cells can be found in nonprogressive, uncomplicated CLL and are not in themselves diagnostic of RS. In

RS, DLCL cells predominate, especially in biopsy specimens of rapidly enlarging lymph nodes, or they can be found admixed with CLL cells, particularly in extranodal tissues biopsied to assess clinical deterioration without apparent CLL progression. Given the common lymphoid origin of CLL and DLCL the question is whether DLCL in RS represents a *de novo* malignancy or an evolution or a true "transformation" of the CLL clone. Until recently, our ability to distinguish between these two possibilities was hampered by the low incidence of RS and by the low discriminant power of techniques used for that purpose. More recent methods have included cytogenetics analysis, immune techniques such as immunophenotypic and immunohistochemical analysis of cellular antigens, and molecular techniques including southern blotting and PCR to facilitate gene probing *(34)*.

Based on concordance of immunoglobulin isotype and idiotypes, immunoglobulin gene rearrangement, and cytogenetics of lymphoid malignancies arising from CLL reported in the English literature, it has been suggested that approximately half of RS cases occur as a result of the evolution of the CLL clone, whereas the other half represents *de novo* malignancies unrelated to the CLL clone *(35)*. Alternatively, an analysis of 37 cases of RS arising from CLL in a single institution studied by Southern blot and cytogenetics analyses revealed that 28 cases of RS (75.7%) appeared to have evolved from the CLL clone, whereas in 9 cases (24.3%) the two malignancies seemed to have distinct origins *(36)*.

One of the earliest tools used in attempts to distinguish *de novo* from evolutional clones was the analysis of cell surface antigens via immunophenotype or immunohistochemistry. However, because most cases of CLL and DLCL express cell surface $\mu\kappa$, isotype identity by both clones is probable on statistical grounds alone regardless of the origin of the DLCL clone. Likewise, isotype disparity can occur as a result of isotype switch, an occurrence that, in addition to having no diagnostic value, is biologically and prognostically inconsequential. For example, a progressive $\mu/\delta\kappa$ to $\mu\lambda$ to $\gamma\lambda$ switch was documented through 12 immunophenotype assays of peripheral blood performed over a 3-yr period in one of the author's stage II CLL patients who died 1 yr later of progressive disease. Likewise, in a case of RS in which DLCL cells failed to express the μ heavy-chain phenotype present on CLL cells, Southern blotting revealed identical κ light-chain rearrangements on CLL and DLCL cells and a post-rearrangement deletion of the μ gene in the DLCL cells, confirming a common precursor cell for both malignancies *(37)*.

Similarly, numerous authors have demonstrated a common clonal origin for DLCL and CLL despite different surface immunoglobulins. In one such report the CLL cells expressed $\mu\lambda$ surface immunoglobulins whereas DLCL cells showed $\mu\kappa$ *(38)*. However, both clones demonstrated identical rearrangements for the immunoglobulin heavy chain and surface markers (CD5, CD19, and CD20). In another case report studied via immunophenotype, cytogenetics, and molecular studies, the CLL cells expressed λ, whereas DLCL cells showed κ surface light chains. However, both exhibited trisomy 12 and identical heavy chain rearrangements in the *Bam*HI and *Eco*RI digests, although the *Hin*dIII and *Pst*I digests were different, suggesting to the authors a common clonal origin *(39)*. Similar conclusions were reached in a case of RS by comparing the nucleotide sequences of the heavy chain genes of the two clones by PCR *(40)*. Alternatively, in a case of RS in which CLL cells expressed the $\mu\lambda$ phenotype but DLCL cells did not, Southern blot analysis of the J_H region of the heavy- and light-chain genes revealed a different heavy-chain gene rearrangement for CLL and DLCL cells and a light-chain rearrangement only for CLL cells *(41)*.

In an analysis of the complementarity determining region 3 (CDR3) of the primary CLL/SLL and the secondary DLCL of three cases of RS, one case revealed an identical heavy-chain rearrangement pattern of both clones by Southern blotting. In the remaining two cases in which the rearrangement patterns were different, one showed a nonidentical sequence and the other an identical sequence *(42)*. The authors concluded that analysis of the oligonucleotide sequence of the CDR3 region including the V_HDJ_H gene rearrangements, rather than Southern blotting, is useful to establish whether the CLL and DLCL clones are identical.

Finally, clonal evolution from low- to high-grade lymphoma may involve distinct pathways depending on the cellular origin and the type of progenitor B-cell tumor. This suggestion derives from longitudinal analysis of immunoglobulin gene sequence expressed in a case each of CLL, SCL, and follicular lymphoma that transformed to DLCL *(43)*. Whereas neither the CLL, SCL, nor their DLCL transformants exhibited clonogenic shift or acquired mutations in the V_HDJ_H gene segments, as confirmed by specific and sensitive PCR-single strand polymorphism analysis, follicular lymphoma cells exhibited a high degree of intraclonal divergent V_HDJ_H gene sequences but unique sequences in the DLCL cells, suggesting that a new neoplastic clonotypic variant gave rise to the DLCL clone and that this more aggressive clone had lost its capacity to undergo mutation in the immunoglobulin gene. In a recent report, six cases of digestive RS supervening in CLL patients were studied by immunohistochemical analysis in paired samples of CLL and DLCL specimens (*n* = 6) and by PCR for immunoglobulin heavy-chain gene rearrangements (*n* = 4) *(44)*. Similar rearrangements demonstrated by PCR in the paired CLL and DLCL specimens from two patients were confirmed by sequence analysis. In two additional cases one of the two bands observed in CLL was lost in the DLCL specimen, suggesting allelic loss, and in one case different rearrangement patterns were observed in the CLL and DLCL specimens.

Finally, cytogenetic studies of a clinically deteriorating patient with CLL with concomitant blasts in blood, bone marrow, and ascitic fluid revealed karyotypic evolution with trisomy 7 and del(17p) in ascitic blasts, in addition to the t(11;14) previously observed in the CLL cells *(32)*. FISH confirmed trisomy 7, and PCR-single-strand polymorphism and direct sequence analysis revealed a mutation of *p53* exon 7, in addition to 17p deletion. The authors concluded that the latter might have played a role in the development of RS.

2.4. Management

At present the management of RS is unsatisfactory. Most successfully treated patients have received conventional chemotherapy appropriate for the treatment of DLCL, such as cyclophosphamide, Adriamycin, vincristine, and prednisone (CHOP) or the equivalent. Anecdotal reports of treatment results are skewed toward success, and only three series have been published from which to assess treatment success rates and patient outcomes. In the first one, published in 1981 *(19)*, of the 19 cases of RS that received treatment, 6 (including 4 with localized disease) achieved a complete remission that at the time of the publication had lasted for 15–17 mo, whereas the group's overall median survival was only 4 mo. Treatment consisted of chemotherapy alone (15 patients) and chemotherapy plus irradiation (4 patients).

The other series was published in 1998 by the CLL group at the M.D. Anderson Cancer Center *(26)*. Given their extensive involvement with fludarabine in the treatment of CLL, the authors conducted a pilot study comparing two fludarabine-based regimens [fludarabine plus cytosine arabinoside, and platinum (PFA) or cyclophosphamide (CFA)] in 12 patients with RS. The rationale for these drug combinations was multiple and included the efficacy of fludarabine in CLL, its ability to enhance the intracellular conversion of cytosine arabinoside to its triphosphatated active metabolite by CLL cells, its ability to inhibit DNA repair, its ability to enhance formation and retention of platinum/DNA crosslinks in certain cell lines, and the activity of the platinum/cytosine arabinoside in non-Hodgkin's lymphoma. Of the 12 RS patients accrued to the study, 3 had previously responded to fludarabine, 3 had no exposure, and 6 were refractory to this drug. Of the 11 evaluable patients, 2 achieved a complete remission, 3 had a partial response, 5 had refractory or progressive disease, and 1 died during treatment. Their median survival was 17 mo.

More recently, the same group reported their experience *(45)* with a salvage regimen designed for poor-prognosis non-Hodgkin's lymphoma *(46)* consisting of fractionated cyclophosphamide, vincristine, liposomal daunorubicin, and dexamethasone (hyperCVXD). Twenty-nine patients with RS patients arising from CLL (26 patients), non-Hodgkin's lymphoma (2 patients), and prolymphocytic leukemia (1 patient) were given a total of 95 cycles of hyperCVXD. Six patients (20%) died while receiving treatment, and toxicity included grade 4 granulocytopenia in all 95 cycles (100%), fever in 23 (24%), associated with pneumonia in 15 (16%) and sepsis in 8 (8%), and neuropathy in 5 (5%). Thrombocytopenia greater than 50% of pretreatment levels occurred in 79% of first cycles and overt bleeding in 4% of all cycles. Eleven patients (38%) achieved a complete remission; four of them relapsed within 1 yr, and one patient had a partial response. The overall survival was 10 mo: 19 mo for patients who experienced complete remission and 3 mo for those who did not.

Thus, experience to date shows that even the most aggressive chemotherapy regimen achieved only modest gains in survival rates despite unacceptably high mortality and toxicity. This confirms the view that RS, like most malignancies, is refractory to cytotoxic chemotherapy. It also suggests that progress in the management of RS, and of most malignancies, is not likely to result from new cytotoxic drugs or new combinations thereof, but from translating our ever increasing knowledge of the genetic defects responsible for cancer development and progression into molecularly targeted therapies focused on preventing, reverting, or controlling the aberrant genetics pathways responsible for RS, whether resulting from CLL clonal transformation or emerging as a *de novo* second malignancy. Until such target-specific therapeutic approaches are designed and implemented, the prognosis of RS, under the cell-kill paradigm *(47)*, will remain dismal.

3. SECOND MALIGNANCIES

CLL has long been known to be associated with an increased risk for second malignancies *(15,17,48)*. A recent report, based on 16,367 patients with CLL registered in the SEER program of the National Cancer Institute between 1973 and 1996, represents the largest study to date addressing this issue *(48)*. The mean patient follow-up was 5.2 yr, representing 84,667 person-years of follow-up data. Follow-up end points were the dates of diagnosis of a second cancer, death, or the study cutoff (December 31, 1996). Second cancers, which excluded lymphoid malignancies, occurred in 1820 patients for an observed/expected (O/E) ratio of 1.20 (with a 95% confidence interval of 1.15–1.26). The risk of second malignancies remained relatively constant between less than 1 yr (O/E ratio of 1.25) and over 10 yr (O/E ratio of 1.16) from diagnosis of CLL. Although scant data were available regarding the treatment patients had received over the follow-up period, no differences were observed between treated and untreated patients. Likewise, a similar O/E ratio for second malignancies was recorded before and after 1990, when chlorambucil and other alkylators were progressively replaced by nucleoside analogs, especially fludarabine monophosphate, perceived by many to be the drug of choice for the treatment of CLL *(49)*, suggesting a quantitatively equivalent or absent carcinogenic role for these two classes of cancer drugs when they are administered to patients with CLL. However, a recent Cancer and Leukemia Group B (CALGB) study *(50)* comparing chlorambucil (C), fludarabine monophosphate (F), and a combination of both (C + F) in 544 previously untreated B-CLL patients identified six patients

(1.2%) who developed myelodysplastic syndrome (three patients or 0.6%), acute myelocytic leukemia (two patients or 0.4%), or myelodysplastic syndrome evolving into acute myelocytic leukemia (one patient or 0.2%),after a median follow up of 4.2 yr. They included 5 patients (or 3.5%) of 142 patients who were treated with C + F, and 1 patient (or 0.5%) of 188 who received F alone. Patients who received C alone did not experience such complications, prompting the authors to warn of the possible carcinogenic potential of alkylator-purine analog combination therapies.

A significantly increased risk was found in the SEER study for Kaposi's sarcoma (O/E ratio, 5.09), malignant melanoma (O/E ratio, 3.18), laryngeal carcinoma (O/E ratio, 1.72), and lung cancer (O/E ratio, 1.66). It is noteworthy that although the risk of Kaposi's sarcoma was increased in men and women, the latter exhibited more than a ninefold greater risk for this type of sarcoma than men (O/E ratio, 19.13 vs 2.06). Additionally, gender-specific risks for second malignancies were observed: men exhibited an increased risk of brain cancers, particularly glioblastoma (O/E ratio, 1.91), and women demonstrated increased risk for stomach (O/E ratio, 1.76) and bladder (O/E ratio, 1.52) cancers.

As suggested by the authors, possible mechanisms to explain the increased risk of specific second malignancies suffered by patients with CLL include the immunodeficiency associated with this disease (48,51–53), the carcinogenic role of drugs used for its treatment (54), the possibility that the carcinogenic effects of sunlight and tobacco are enhanced by chemotherapy and immunodeficiency (55,56), and the likely effect of increased medical surveillance in patients with CLL compared with the general population. Of these, immunodeficiency is most frequently invoked as a contributing factor for second malignancies developing in a variety of conditions linked only by an immunodeficiency background whether induced by drugs (54–56), viruses (57–60), or congenital defects (59,61,62). However, in this setting the most frequent second cancer is non-Hodgkin's lymphoma, a second tumor infrequently associated with CLL.

The role of chlorambucil, the drug most widely used in the treatment of CLL until recently, is less convincing. Indeed, acute myelocytic leukemia, a second malignancy that affects nearly one in four patients with polythemia rubra vera treated with chlorambucil (63,64), is conspicuously absent in CLL patients treated in the long term with the same drug. Moreover, the fact that comparable O/E rates and similar types of second cancers occurred during the pre- and post-1990 periods, when chlorambucil and fludarabine prevailed, respectively, as the drug of choice for CLL, suggests that neither plays a significant carcinogenic role in the development of second cancers.

Finally, closer medical scrutiny would be expected to uncover more cases of the types of cancers associated with the highest incidence in the general population, rather than the ones observed. Although longevity is not discussed in the article, it is evident that it is a prerequisite for the full expression of genomic instability underlying second malignancies. Indeed, the risk of developing second malignancies appears to be greater for patients whose primary tumors or immunodeficient conditions are compatible with prolonged survival, as in the case of CLL, HIV infection (58), kidney transplant (57), and Hodgkin's disease (65,66), although in the latter second malignancies are more clearly therapy-related: acute myelocytic leukemia associated primarily with chemotherapy and solid tumors linked to radiation therapy. Taken together, these observations suggest the existence of complex and largely unknown multifactorial endogenous and exogenous factors underlying the heightened risk and the type of second malignancies associated with CLL and other malignant and nonmalignant conditions.

REFERENCES

1. Lin CW, Manshouri T, Jilani I, et al. Proliferation and apoptosis in acute and chronic leukemias and myelodysplastic syndrome. Leuk Res 2002;26:551–559.

2. Oliveira GB, Pereira FG, Metze K, Lorand-Metze I. Spontaneous apoptosis in chronic lymphocytic leukemia and its relationship to clinical and cell kinetic parameters. Cytometry 2001;46(6):329–335.

3. Faguet GB, Agee JF, Marti GE. Clone emergence and evolution in chronic lymphocytic leukemia: Characterization of clinical, laboratory, and immunophenotypic profiles of 25 patients. Leuk Lymphoma 1992;6:345–356.

4. Faguet GB. Chronic lymphocytic leukemia: An updated review J Clin Oncol 1994;12(9):1974–1990.

5. Rai KR, Han T. Prognostic factors and clinical staging in chronic lymphocytic leukemia. Hematol Oncol Clin North Am 1990;4:447–456.

6. Binet JL, Auquier A, Dighiero G, et al. A new prognostic classification of chronic lymphocytic leukemia derived from multivariate survival analysis. Cancer 1981;48:198–207.

7. Montserrat E, Vinolas N, Reverter JC, Rozman C. Natural history of chronic lymphocytic leukemia: On the progression and prognosis of early stages. Nouv Rev Fr Hematol 1988;30:459–461.

8. Tsiodras S, Samonis G, Keating MJ, Kontoyiannis DP. Infection and immunity in chronic lymphocytic leukemia. Mayo Clin Proc 2000;75:1039–1054.

9. Fairley GH, Scott RB. Hypogammaglobulinemia in chronic lymphocytic leukemia. BMJ 1961;2:290–294.

10. Morrison VA, Rai KR, Peterson BL, et al. Impact of therapy with chlorambucil, Fludarabine, or Fludarabine plus chlorambucil on infections in patients with chronic lymphocytic leukemia: Intergroup Study of Cancer and Leukemia Group B9011. J Clin Oncol 2001;19:3611–3621.

11. Long JC, Aisenberg AC. Richter's syndrome: a terminal complication of chronic lymphocytic leukemia with distinct clinical pathologic features. Am J Clin Pathol 1975;63:7786–7795.

12. Kjeldberg CR, Marty J. Prolymphocytic transformation of chronic lymphocytic leukemia. Cancer 1981;48: 2447–2457.

13. Frenkel EP, Ligler FS, Graham MS, Hernandez JA, Kettman JR Jr, Smith RG. Acute lymphocytic leukemia transformation of chronic lymphocytic leukemia: substantiation by flow cytometry. Am J Hematol 1981;10:391–398.

14. Brouet JC, Fermand JP, Laurent G, et al. The association of chronic lymphocytic leukemia and multiple myeloma: a study of eleven patients. Br J Haematol 1985;59:55–66.

15. Greene MH, Hover RN, Fraumeni JF Jr. Second cancers in patients with chronic lymphocytic leukemia—a possible immunologic mechanism. J Natl Cancer Inst 1978;61:337–340.

16. Travis LB, Curtis RE, Hankey BF, Fraumeni JF Jr. Second cancers in patients with chronic lymphocytic leukemia. Natl Cancer Inst 1992;84:1422–1427.

17. Richter MN. Generalized reticular cell sarcoma of lymph nodes associated with lymphocytic leukemia. Am J Pathol 1928;4:285–292.

18. Lortholary P, Boiron M, Ripault P, et al. Leucemie lymphoide chronique secondairement associee a une reticulopathie maligne, syndrome de Richter. Nouv Rev Fr Hemat 1964;78:621–644.

19. Harousseau JL, Flandrin G, Tricot G, et al. Malignant lymphoma supervening in chronic lymphocytic leukemia and related disorders. Richter's syndrome: a study of 25 cases. Cancer 1981;48:1302–1308.

20. Nakamura N, Kuze T, Hashimoto Y, et al. Analysis of the immunoglobulin heavy chain gene of secondary diffuse large B-cell lymphoma that subsequently developed in four cases with B-cell chronic lymphocytic leukemia or lymphoplasmacytoid lymphoma (Richter syndrome). Pathol Intl 2000;50:636–643.

21. Robertson LE, Pugh W, O'Brien S, et al. Richter's syndrome: a report on 39 patients. J Clin Oncol 1993;11: 1985–1989.

22. Han T, Henderson ES, Emrich LJ, Sandberg AA. Prognostic significance of karyotypic abnormalities in B cell chronic lymphocytic leukemia: an update. Semin Hematol 1987;24:257–263.

23. Foucar K, Rydell RE. Richter's syndrome in chronic lymphocytic leukemia. Cancer 1980;46:116–134.

24. Han T, Henderson ES, Emrich LJ, Sandberg AA. Richter syndrome with emphasis on large-cell non-Hodgkin's lymphoma in previously unrecognized subclinical chronic lymphocytic leukemia. Neoplasma 1997;44:63–68.

25. Fayad L, Roberson LA, O'Brien S, et al. Hodgkin's disease variant of Richter's syndrome: experience at a single institution. Leuk Lymphoma 1996;23:333–337.

26. Giles FJ, O'Brien S, Keatin MJ. Chronic lymphocytic leukemia in (Richter's) transformation. Semin Oncol 1998;25:117–125.

27. Hebert J, Jonveaux P, d'Agay MF, Berger R. Cytogenetic studies in patients with Richter's syndrome. Cancer Genet Cytogenet 1994;73:65–68.

28. Sanderg AA, Chen Z. FISH analysis. In: Faguet GB, ed. Hematologic Malignancies: Methods and Techniques. Humana, Totowa, NJ, 2001, pp. 19–42.

29. Baudis M, Bentz M. Comparative genomic hybridization for the analysis of leukemias and lymphomas. In: Faguet GB, ed. Hematologic Malignancies: Methods and Techniques. Humana, Totowa, NJ, 2001, pp. 43–64.

30. Hildgenfeld E, Padilla-Nash H, Haas OA, Serve H, Schrock E, Ried T. Spectral karyotype (SKY) of hematologis malignancies. In: Faguet GB, ed. Hematologic Malignancies: Methods and Techniques. Humana, Totowa, NJ, 2001, pp. 65–69.
31. Arranz E, Martinez B, Richart A, et al. Increased C-MYC oncogene copy number detected with combined modified comparative genomic hybridization and FISH analysis in a Richter syndrome case with complex karyotype. Cancer Genet Cytogenet 1998;106:80–83.
32. Cuneo A, De Angeli C, Roberti MG, et al. Richter's syndrome in a case of atypical chronic lymphocytic leukemia with the (11;14)(q13;132): role for a p53 exon 7 gene mutation. Br J Haematol 1996;92:375–381.
33. Bea S, Lopez-Guillermo A, Ribas M, et al. Genetic imbalances in progressed B-cell chronic lymphocytic leukemia and transformed large-cell lymphoma (Richter's syndroem). Am J Pathol 2002;161:957–968.
34. Faguet GB, ed. Hematologic Malignancies: Methods and Techniques. Humana, Totowa, NJ, 2001.
35. Foon KA, Thiruvengadam R, Saven A, Bernstein ZP, Gale RP. Genetic relatedness of lymphoid malignancies. Transformation of chronic lymphocytic leukemia as a model. Ann Intern Med 1993;119:63–73.
36. Besudo A, Kipps TJ. Origin of high-grade lymphomas in Richter's syndrome. Leuk Lymphoma 1995;18:367–372.
37. Schots R, Dehou MF, Jochmans K, et al. Southern blot analysis in a case of Richter's syndrome. Evidence for a postarrangement heavy chain gene deletion associated with the altered phenotype. Am J Clin Pathol 1991;95:571–577.
38. Miyamura K, Osada H, Yamauchi T, et al. Origin of neoplastic B-cells with different immunoglobulins light chains in a patient with Richter's syndrome. Cancer 1990;66:14–144.
39. Nakamine H, Masih AS, Sanger WG, et al. Richter's syndrome with different immunoglobulins light chain types. Molecular and cytogenetic features indicate a common clonal origin. Am J Clin Pathol 1992;97:656–663.
40. Cherepakhin V, Baird SM, Meisenholder GW, Kipps TJ. Common clonal origin of chronic lymphocytic leukemia and high grade lymphoma in Richter's syndrome. Blood 1993;82:3141–3147.
41. Ostrowski M, Minden M, Wang C, Bailey D. Immunophenotypic and gene probe analysis of a cased of Richter's syndrome. Am J Clin Pathol 1989;91:215–221.
42. Matolcsy A, Inghirami G, Knowles DM. Molecular genetic demonstration of the diverse evolution of Richter's syndrome (chronic lymphocytic leukemia and subsequent large cell lymphoma). Blood 1994;83:1363–1372.
43. Matolcsy A, Schattner EJ, Knowles DM, Casali P. Clonal evolution of B cells in transformation from low- to high-grade lymphoma. Eur J Immunol 1999;29:1253–1264.
44. Parrens M, Sawan B, Dubus P, et al. Primary digestive Richter's syndrome. Mod Pathol 2001;14:452–457.
45. Dabaja BS, O'Brien SM, Kantarjian HM, et al. Fractionated cyclophosphamide, Vincristine, liposomal daunorubicin (daunoXome), and dexamethasone (hyperCVXD) regimen in Richter's syndrome. Leuk Lymphoma 2001;42:329–337.
46. McBride NC, Cavenagh JD, Ward MC, et al. Liposomal daunorubicin (DaunoXome) in combination with cyclophosphamide, Vincristine and prednisosne (COP-X) as salvage therapy for poor-prognosis non-Hodgkin's lymphoma. Leuk Lymphoma 2001;42:89–98,2001.
47. Schipper H. Treating cancer: is kill cure? Ann Acad Med Singapore 1994;23:382–386.
48. Hisada M, Biggar RJ, Greene MH, Fraumeni JF, Travis LB. Solid tumors after chronic lymphocytic leukemia. Blood 2001;98:1979–1981.
49. Cheson BD. Recent advances in the treatment of chronic lymphocytic leukemia. Oncology 1990;4:71–84.
50. Morrison VA, Rai KR, Peterson B, et al. Therapy-related myeloid leukemias are observed in patients with chronic lymphocytic leukemia after treatment with fludarabine and chlorambucil: results of an intergroup study, Cancer and Leukemia Group B 9011. J Clin Oncol 2002;20:3878–3884.
51. Faguet GB. Mechanisms of lymphocyte activation: the role of suppressor cells in the proliferative responses of chronic lymphocytic leukemia lymphocytes. J Clin Invest 1979;63:67–74.
52. Bartik MM, Welker D, Kay NE. Impairments in immune function in B cell chronic lymphocytic leukemia. Semin Oncol 1998;25:27–33.
53. Linet MS, Cartwright RA. The leukemias. In: Schottenfeld D, Fraumeni JF, eds. Cancer Epidemiology and Prevention, 2nd ed. Oxford University Press, New York, 1996, pp. 841–892.
54. Travis LB, Curtis RE, Glimelius B, et al. Bladder and kidney cancer following cyclophosphamide therapy for non-Hodgkin's lymphoma. J Natl Cancer Inst 1995;87:524–530,.
55. Hoover R. Effects of drugs—Immunosuppression. In: Hiatt HH, Watson JD, Winsten JA, eds. Origins of Human Cancer. Book A. Incidence of Cancer in Humans. Cold Spring Harbor Laboratory Press, Cold Spring Harbor, NY, 1977, pp. 369–379.

56. Swerdlow AJ, Schoemaker MJ, Allerton R, et al. Lung cancer after Hodgkin's disease: a nested case-control study of the relation to treatment. J Clin Oncol 2001;19:1610–1618.

57. Hanto DW, Frizzera G, Gajl-Peczalska KJ, et al. Epstein-Barr virus-induced B-cell lymphoma after renal transplantation: acyclovir therapy and transition from polyclonal to monoclonal B-cell proliferation. N Engl J Med 1982;306:913–918.

58. Ziegler JL, Beckstead JA, Volberding PA, et al. Non-Hodgkin's lymphoma in 90 homosexual men: Relation to generalized lymphadenopathy and the acquired immunodeficiency syndrome. N Engl J Med 1984;311:565–570.

59. Beral V, Newton R. Overview of the epidemiology of immunodeficiency-associated cancers. J Natl Cancer Inst Monogr 1998;23:1–6.

60. Boshoff C, Weiss R. AIDS-related malignancies. Natl Rev Cancer 2002;2:373–382.

61. Mueller BU, Pizzo PA. Cancer in children with primary or secondary immunodeficiencies. J Pediatr 1995;126:1–10.

62. Gatti RA, Good RA. Occurrence of malignancy in immunodeficiency diseases. A literature review. Cancer 1971;28:89–98.

63. Berk PD, Goldberg JD, Silverstein MN, et al. Increased incidence of acute leukemia in polycythemia vera associated with chlorambucil therapy. N Engl J Med 1981;304:441–447.

64. Polycythemia Vera Study Group minutes, 1987.

65. Cellai E, Magrini SM, Masala G, et al. The risk of second malignant tumors and its consequences for the overall survival of Hodgkin's disease patients and for the choice of their treatment at presentation: analysis of a series of 1524 cases consecutively treated at the Florence University Hospital. Int J Radiat Oncol Biol Phys 2001;49:1327–1337.

66. van Leeuwen FE, Klokman WJ, Veer MB, et al. Long-term risk of second malignancy in survivors of Hodgkin's disease treated during adolescence or young adulthood. J Clin Oncol 2000;18:487–497.

VII | FAMILIAL AND JUVENILE CHRONIC LYMPHOCYTIC LEUKEMIA

22   Inherited Predisposition to Chronic Lymphocytic Leukemia

Martin R. Yuille, PhD, Daniel Catovsky, MD, DSc and Richard S. Houlston, MD, PhD

1. INTRODUCTION

B-cell chronic lymphocytic leukemia (CLL) and other associated B-cell lymphoproliferative disorders (LPDs; i.e., lymphomas and Hodgkin's disease) have not been thought of until recently as having an inherited genetic component. By contrast, it has long been recognized that a small number of acute leukemia cases occur at a higher frequency in individuals with genetic disease, such as Down syndrome and other constitutional chromosome anomalies as well as some mendelian cancer syndromes (e.g., Li-Fraumeni syndrome).

There is now, however, increasing evidence strongly implicating inherited genetic factors in a subset of CLL patients. Identification of CLL predisposition genes should be useful for diagnosis and could also serve as a model for CLL tumorigenesis.

2. EVIDENCE FOR A GENETIC PREDISPOSITION TO CLL

2.1. Epidemiological Studies

Four case-control and three cohort studies have systematically examined the risk of CLL and other LPDs in relatives of patients. Table 1 summarizes the characteristics of each of the studies and the estimates of the familial risks obtained. All the studies found that risk of leukemia or lymphocytic leukemia was elevated in relatives. The study reported by Gunz et al. in 1975 *(1)* was based on a survey of 909 families ascertained through leukemia cases. Giles et al. *(2)* made no distinction between types of LPD in their analysis of the family histories of cases diagnosed between 1972 and 1980 in Tasmania. In 1994, Goldgar et al. *(3)* systematically analyzed the clustering of malignancy at 28 distinct sites using the Utah population database. Relatives of lymphocytic leukemia cases were at a sixfold increased risk of the same hematological malignancy. The risk of LPD in relatives reported in the three cohort studies was comparable to that observed in the four case-control studies. Although none of these studies has systematically estimated familial risks by specific leukemia type, it is likely that the familial risk reflects an increased risk of CLL since acute lymphoblastic leukemia—the primary potential confounding diagnosis—does not display an increased sibling risk *(4)*.

A number of inherited susceptibility genes cause cancer at several sites. Therefore any excess of cancer at sites other than CLL in relatives may reflect in part the pleiotropic effects of an

From: *Contemporary Hematology*
Chronic Lymphocytic Leukemia: Molecular Genetics, Biology, Diagnosis, and Management
Edited by: G. B. Faguet © Humana Press Inc., Totowa, NJ

Table 1
Familial Risks of CLL and other LPDs

Study	Diagnosis in index case	Relative	Observed (no.)	Expected (no.)	Risk (%) (95% CI)
Cohort studies					
Giles et al. (2)	LPD	LPD in first-degree relatives	35	10.3	3.4 (2.4–4.7)
Gunz et al. (1)	Leukemia	Leukemia in first-degree relatives	16	6.61	2.4 (1.9–3.9)
Goldgar et al. (3)	Lymphocytic leukemia	Lymphocytic leukemia in first-degree relatives	18	3.6	5.7 (2.6–10.0)
Case-control studies					
Cartwright et al. (45)	CLL	Lymphocytic leukemia in blood relatives	5/330	2/559	4.3 (0.9–19.5)
Linet et al. (46)	CLL	Leukemia in parents and siblings	25/342	10/342	2.6 (1.2–5.5)
Pottern et al. (47)	CLL	Leukemia in parents and siblings	13/237	30/1207	2.3 (1.2–4.4)
Radovanovic et al. (48)	CLL	Leukemia in first- and second-degree relatives	7/130	0/130	—

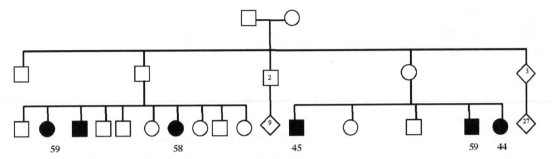

Fig. 1. Chronic lymphocytic leukemia (CLL) in one family. CLL was not recorded in the first two generations, which is consistent with incomplete penetrance. Solid symbols, diagnosis of CLL. (Adapted from ref. *59.*)

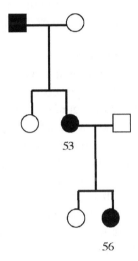

Fig. 2. Chronic lymphocytic leukemia recorded in one family. (Adapted from ref. *54.*)

inherited predisposition gene. In addition to a possible relationship between CLL and other B-cell LPDs, a relationship between lymphocytic leukemia and granulocytic leukemia and rectal cancer was observed in the study reported by Goldgar et al. *(3).*

2.2. Survey of Published Familial Cases

There is strong evidence from literature reports over eight decades that multiple cases of CLL do occur in families. Two of these are illustrated in Figs. 1 and 2. Both are consistent explicitly or implicitly with vertical transmission of an autosomal trait over three generations. In Fig. 1, the absence of recorded CLL in the first two generations is consistent with incomplete penetrance.

Although early reports on familial CLL were published before B-cells had been described, most of the diagnoses are likely to be accurate. This is because the characteristic morphology of CLL B-lymphocytes makes diagnosis clinically robust. Reports in the literature describe over 80 pedigrees that show clustering of CLL and sometimes other LPDs. Some of these studies have been reviewed *(5,6),* and we have recently reported 14 families *(7).* It has often been suggested that even very striking familial clusters of common malignancies might be ascribed to ascertainment bias. This is, however, a statistical fallacy. For example, Table 2 identifies reports of 24 families with three or more affected individuals, nine of which were ascertained by the authors, yet a family with three affected sibs would be expected to occur by chance about every 1000 yr.

A few reports of relatively large kindreds clearly show vertical transmission of CLL and other LPDs, suggesting that predisposition to CLL and other LPDs is caused by the inheritance of a dominantly acting gene (or genes) with incomplete penetrance and pleiotropic effects. Although most of the families reported are nuclear rather than multigenerational, it is conceivable that many family members may have subclinical disease, as CLL generally has an indolent course. Such a notion is supported by the observation that in some of the families reported, apparently unaffected family members had a persistent lymphocytosis (8).

It is relatively difficult to determine the proportion of CLL cases that have a family history of the disease because in a good number of patients the disease goes undetected. However, in our recent systematic survey of CLL, 6% of patients reported a family history of CLL and another 5% a family history of a LPD (7).

Published CLL pedigrees appear to be characterized by an earlier onset than sporadic forms of the disease, suggesting a more aggressive clonal expansion. One intriguing feature seen in the expression of CLL in many of the families reported is anticipation, the phenomenon of earlier onset and more severe phenotype in successive generations (9–13). This phenomenon is observed in other mendelian diseases in which it is known to have a specific molecular basis. Anticipation in familial CLL may have a similar basis, although other possibilities exist, such as the cohort effect in relation to viral or other environmental exposures, which act as risk factors.

Anticipation has been described for a range of neurological conditions and been shown to arise from a single gene defect (14). In these disorders anticipation is a function of the instability of certain repetitive sequences—usually trinucleotide motifs—in the disease gene. Although there is a normal range of variation in repeat number, in affected families the repeat number increases in the germline from generation to generation. At a certain threshold, this expansion begins to give rise to phenotypic effects through its deleterious effects on gene function. Further expansion occurs in the next generation, resulting in earlier onset and greater severity of the disease phenotype. It is premature to speculate on whether such a mechanism is operative in CLL families. Other possible mechanistic bases for anticipation have been proposed (15). The mutation might become more severe between generations by a persistent shared environmental factor (rather than intrinsic instability). An epigenetic effect—perhaps involving DNA methylation or gene conversion—that, instead of being eliminated, is fixed in the genome during subsequent meiosis might lead to an accumulation of defects during following generations. In families in which only two affected generations are detected, a shared transient environmental factor cannot be excluded.

3. MOLECULAR GENETICS OF FAMILIAL CLL

Molecular studies of neoplastic disease have shown that multiple genetic alterations are an essential feature of the tumorigenic process. These alterations involve two broad classes of genes: tumor suppressor genes—whose products normally directly inhibit neoplastic development by negatively regulating growth and differentiation—and oncogenes that positively contribute to the neoplastic transformation when activated. Inactivation of tumor suppressor genes coupled with activation of oncogenes leads to malignancy. Genetic alterations involved in the transformation of normal cells to the malignant state can be both inherited in the germline and arise somatically in the tissue in which the cancer arises.

Table 2

Published Familial Cases of Chronic Lymphocytic Leukemia

Reference	Affected family members	Additional information
Guasch, 1954 *(5)*	Sibs, M, M	
	Parent F, offspring M	
	Sibs M, M	
	Sibs M, M, M, F	
	Sibs M, M, M	
	Sibs M, M	
	Sibs M, M	
	Sibs M, M	
	Sibs M, M, F	
	Parent F, offspring F	
	MZ twins M, M	
	Parent M, offspring M	
	Parent M, offspring M	
	Sibs M, M	
Brem and Morton, 1955 *(49)*	Sibs M, M	Sib M LK
Videbaek, 1958 *(50)*	Uncle, nephew	
Hudson and Wilson, 1960 *(51)*	Sibs M, M	
	Sibs M, M	
Gunz et al, 1962 *(52)*		
Fitzgerald and Hamer *(53)*	Sibs F, M, M	
Furbetta and Solinas, 1963 *(54)*	Grandparent M, parent F, offspring F	
Wisniewski and Weinrich, 1966 *(55)*	Parent M, offspring M	
Rigby et al., 1966 *(56)*	2 half-sibs	
Ardizzone et al., 1968 *(57)*	Sibs M, M	
Magaraggia and Vettori, 1968 *(58)*	Sibs M, M	
McPhedran et al., 1969 *(59)*	Sibs F, M, F, cousins F, M, M	
Fraumeni et al., *(60)*; Blattner et al., 1969 *(61)*	Sibs F, M, M	
Gunz and Veale, 1969 *(62)*	Sibs M, F	
	Sibs M, M	Sib CGL
Undritz et al., 1971 *(63)*	Sibs M, M, M, F	
Potolosky et al., 1971 *(64)*	Sibs F, F	Sib LY, sib LY, sib acute LK
Schweitzer et al., 1973 *(65)*	Sibs F, M, M, F, F	
Blattner et al. *(66)*; Neuland et al. *(67)*; Shen et al. *(68)*; Caporaso et al., 1975 *(69)*	Parent M, offspring M, M, F, F	
Gunz et al., 1975 *(70)*	3 first degree; 3 others	
Petzholdt et al., 1976 *(71)*	Sibs M, M, M	
Fazekas et al., 1978 *(72)*	Sibs, M, M, M	
Branda et al., 1978 *(73)*	Parent F; offspring M	

(continued)

Table 2 (continued)

Reference	Affected family members	Additional information
Conley et al., 1980 *(74)*	Sibs F, F	
	Sibs M, M	
	Nephew , maternal aunt;	
	Nephew M; great-aunt	
Alfinito et al., 1982 *(75)*	Sibs F, F	
Vanni and Deambrogio, 1983 *(76)*	Sibs F, F	
Brok-Simoni et al., *(77)*; Hakim et al., 1987 *(78)*	MZ twins F, F, sib F	
Eriksson and Bergstrom, 1987 *(79)*	Sibs M, M	
	Sibs M, F	
	Sibs M, F	
	MZ twins M	
	Parent M, offspring M	
	Parent M, offspring M	
Shah et al., 1992 *(80)*	Sibs F, M, F	
Cuttner, 1993 *(81)*	Sibs M, M	
	Parent M, offspring M	
	MZ twins M, M	Sib M NHL
Fernhout et al., 1997 *(82)*	Sibs F, F, F, F	
Yuille et al., 2000 *(7)*	Parent M, offspring M, pat cousin F	
	Parent F, offspring M	
	Parent F, offspring M	
	Parent F, offspring F	
	Parent M, offspring M	
	Parent F, offspring M	
	Sibs M, F	
	Sibs M, M	
	Parent M, offspring M	
	Parent F; offspring M	
	Parent F, offspring F	Nephew NHL
	Sibs M, M	
	Parent F, offspring M	Sib F LK
	Parent M, offspring M	Offspring F LK
		Offspring M HL

CGL, chronic granulocytic leukemia; HL, Hodgkin's lymphoma; LK, leukemia; LY, lymphoma; NHL, non-Hodgkin's leukemia; MZ, monozygotic.

The genetics of CLL are conceivably similar to that of breast and colon cancers, in which a subset of the disease occurs in individuals who possess in their germline one or more of the causal genetic alterations required for the neoplastic transformation. In most cases, these genes are altered at the tissue level by random errors in cellular processes. According to the multistep model of carcinogenesis, development of the full neoplastic phenotype in both inherited and noninherited forms of CLL depends on multiple genetic alterations.

3.1. Ataxia Telangiectasia Gene and Risk of CLL

The genetic basis of CLL is largely unknown. Probably for technical reasons, cytogenetic abnormalities appear to be less frequent in CLL than in many other hematological malignancies although the use of techniques such as *in situ* hybridization, comparative genomic hybridization, and others has significantly increased the proportion of cases with cytogenetic abnormalities *(16)*. A number of chromosome breakage syndromes have been known for many years to be associated with an increased risk of leukemia *(17)* including the recessive disease ataxia telangiectasia (AT). AT maps to chromosome 11q23 *(18)*. AT patients have an increased risk of lymphomas and leukemias, and AT heterozygotes may have a significantly increased risk of breast cancer *(19,20)*. CLL has also been reported in AT families *(21)*, suggesting that AT heterozygotes may be at an increased risk. In a retrospective study of the cancer incidence in 110 AT families, the risk of hematological and lymphoid malignancies was increased in blood relatives of AT patients, and CLL accounted for all but one of the leukemias seen in adult blood relatives. However, these observations did not attain statistical significance. It has been demonstrated that the *ATM* gene is mutant in approx 20% of samples from CLL patients and that some patients have germline mutations *(22–25)*. The *ATM* gene specifies a 12-kb mRNA encoding an approx 350-kDa pattern *(26)*. The 3' end of the gene has some homology to phosphinositide 3-kinases and to *Streptomyces cerevisiae* TEL1, which controls telomere length and maintenance of genome integrity *(27)*. Homozygous germline mutations in *ATM* are associated with radio-sensitivity and genomic instability: the mutation rate is increased, double-strand breaks are mis-repaired, there is a high frequency of cytogenetic rearrangements, and homologous recombination is increased and error-prone. AT cells also show defects in cell cycle checkpoints. These defects underlie a model *(28)* in which the Atm protein functions to survey the genome for radiation damage.

This and the prevalence of leukemia in relatives of patients with AT led a number of researchers to question whether germline *ATM* mutations were involved in familial cases of CLL. Stankovic et al. *(22)* observed two germline *ATM* mutations in 32 (6.3%) cases of CLL [$p = 0.04$; 95% confidence interval (CI): 1–21%]. We assessed the role of *ATM* in familial CLL through a linkage analysis of 28 families *(29)*. The observed distribution of sharing of *ATM* haplotypes between affected individuals did not lend support to the notion that *ATM* is involved in familial CLL. However, our study was not sufficiently large to preclude that *ATM* might account for up to a twofold sibling relative risk. Multigenerational families are characteristic of highly penetrant susceptibility genes: it is therefore conceivable that genes conferring susceptibility to CLL are associated with more modest risks. Assuming that approx 6% of CLL is caused by *ATM (22)*, mutations in this gene should only confer a sibling relative risk of 1.1. *ATM* therefore represents a credible candidate predisposition locus for CLL, but more evidence is needed.

To resolve this question, we subjected 29 CLL families to a mutational analysis of the *ATM* gene (unpublished data). Truncating *ATM* mutations, including a known AT mutation, were detected in 2/61 cases, but the mutations did not co-segregate with CLL. Three new *ATM* missense mutations were detected, but no significant or compelling evidence suggested that they contributed to the genotypic risk of CLL. Common *ATM* missense mutations were not over-represented in familial CLL.

Based on this observation, there is no evidence to implicate *ATM* as a CLL predisposition gene ($p = 0.12$). Furthermore, when these data are combined with those of Stankovic et al. *(22)*, there is no overwhelmingly significant evidence of over-representation of truncating *ATM* mutations in CLL ($p = 0.08$). Although nonconservative amino acid changes in *ATM* were detected, the frequency of these collectively in the population is high, and in the absence of functional assays it is difficult to assign pathogenic status to any specific variant. However, the absence of cosegregation of mutations in families strongly implies that the nonconservative mutations confer at best only small genotypic risks.

3.2. Relationship Between the HLA and Risk of CLL

The established relationship between HLA and Hodgkin's lymphoma, another B-cell disorder, and the association between autoimmune disease and CLL raise the possibility that genes within the MHC region may be determinants of CLL susceptibility. Hodgkin's lymphoma shows strong linkage to HLA *(30,31)*. The underlying basis of linkage is not through a common haplotype, but it appears that certain HLA-DPB1 alleles may affect susceptibility and resistance to specific subtypes of Hodgkin's lymphoma *(32,33)*. Patients with CLL frequently share common HLA haplotypes with relatives who have autoimmune disease. Leukemic cells from most CLL cases are CD5+ B-lymphocytes, and these B-cells are implicated in autoimmunity. Hence, genetic determinants leading to CD5+ B-cell proliferation or differentiation are likely to be involved in both B-CLL and autoimmune disease. The notion of a relationship between CLL and autoimmune disease is supported by animal studies using congenic New Zealand mouse strains *(34,35)*. In Hodgkin's disease the allele sharing probabilities between affected siblings suggests that the HLA locus is likely to explain a twofold sibling relative risk with more than half of all cases arising in susceptible individuals. There is no evidence such a situation exists with respect to familial CLL. In the linkage study reported by Bevan et al. *(36)*, there was no evidence for linkage in an analysis of 27 families. However, the 95% CI for the estimate of the sibling relative risk ascribable to the HLA did not preclude that variation within HLA or the MHC is a determinant of CLL susceptibility in some instances.

3.3. Other Candidate CLL Predisposition Genes

Linkage of Hodgkin's disease to the pseudoautosomal region of the genome has recently been proposed by Horwitz and Wiernik *(37)* on the basis of an excess of sex concordance among affected siblings. The common lineage of Hodgkin's disease and CLL prompted us to examine whether familial CLL also shows pseudoautosomal linkage. An analysis of published CLL families shows that the frequency of sex-concordant sib pairs is skewed beyond random expectation; however, it is impossible to preclude publication bias, and so the implicated pseudoautosomal linkage in CLL is questionable *(38)*.

In a number of mendelian diseases anticipation has been shown to be indicative of a dynamic mutation mechanism involving expansion of triplet repeat motifs *(39)*. If the genetic basis of familial CLL involves a similar mechanism, this offers a novel method of identifying a predisposition locus for the disease since specialized methods exist specifically for cloning genes associated with such expansions *(40)*.

3.4. CLL Families Show Homogeneity for IgV Mutational Status

CLL was traditionally viewed as a homogenous disease. However, evidence is accumulating that the disease is heterogeneous, from both the clinical and laboratory perspectives. One laboratory phenotype that distinguishes CLL subsets is IgV mutation status. This distinguishes between cases with unmutated IgV (associated with "naïve" pregerminal center cells) and cases with IgV mutations (associated with "memory" postgerminal center cells). IgV mutation status is associated with differing prognoses *(41,42)*.

Table 3
IgV Mutational Status in CLL Families[a]

IgV mutation status, familial phenotype	Pritsch et al. (43)	Sakai et al. (44)	Combined
N/N	1	5	6
N/Mut	2	2	4
Mut/Mut	11	6	17

[a]IgV mutational status is shown for affected sibs of two sets of published families. All affected sibs are treated in pairs. N, no IgV hypermutation; Mut, IgV hypermutation detected.

This IgV phenotype may offer an attractive means of delineating CLL families in any linkage analysis. Pritsch et al. (43) reported the IgV mutation status of 25 affected individuals from 12 CLL families. In one pair of affecteds, both individuals had no mutations; in two pairs one individual had a mutation; in eight pairs both had mutations; and in one kindred of three affecteds all had mutations. Sakai et al. (44) reported the IgV mutation status of 23 affected individuals from 11 CLL families. In five pairs of affecteds, both individuals had no mutations; in two pairs one individual had a mutation; in three pairs both had mutations; and in one sibship of three affecteds all had mutations.

Using the data from these studies, it is possible to assess whether there is intrafamilial concordance. Table 3 shows the number of concordant and discordant pairs in each of these studies. To assess the significance formally, we compared the observed distribution with the random distribution predicted on the basis of the observed prevalence of the mutated phenotype.

Although the distribution of phenotypes in the families reported by Pritsch et al. (43) is not significantly different from that expected, the distribution in the families reported by Sakai et al. (44) shows a clear deviation. When data from the two studies are combined, the concordance is significant within families ($\chi^2 = 11.2$, 1 df, $p < 0.001$). Studies have shown that between 20 and 50% of all CLL cases have mutations in IgV (41,42). The frequency of these mutations in familial forms of the disease is significantly higher [assuming a mutation frequency of 50%, significance levels are <0.001 in Pritsch et al. (43) and 0.04 in Sakai et al. (44)]. These observations strongly suggest that determining IgV status will be helpful in subgroup analyses of linkage data and future meta-analyses.

4. CONCLUSIONS

CLL has not until recently been thought of as having an inherited basis. However, there is increasing evidence that a subset of cases is caused by an inherited predisposition. The evidence at present is largely indirect. However, it appears that some familial forms of the disease have a more aggressive phenotype, which may warrant more attentive clinical management than sporadic forms of the disease.

Identification of the genes involved in inherited forms of CLL should provide insights into the pathogenesis of CLL in general. At present there is no convincing evidence that any specific gene acts as a susceptibility locus, and identification of these genes for CLL awaits future linkage studies. In these studies, the power to detect linkage using any set of families depends critically on the degree of heterogeneity. With a threefold increase in risk of CLL in relatives of affected individuals, 57 affected sibling pairs (ASPs) are required to detect linkage (defined as a LOD score of 3.0) under homogeneity. However, if two genes (dominantly acting with equal effect) are involved, then approx 250 ASPs will be required. Subcategorization of a disease provides a powerful strategy to mitigate the impact of heterogeneity on linkage. The observation of concordance of IgV hypermutation status within families strongly suggests that determining IgV status will be helpful in subgroup analyses of linkage data and future meta-analyses.

ACKNOWLEDGMENTS

The authors' work is supported by the Leukemia Research Fund.

REFERENCES

1. Gunz FW, Gunz JP, Veale AM Chapman CJ, Houston IB. Familial leukemia: a study of 909 families. Scand J Haematol 1975;15:117–131.
2. Giles GG, Lickiss JN, Baikie MJ, Lowenthal RM, Panton J J. Myeloproliferative and lymphoproliferative disorders in Tasmania, 1972–80: occupational and familial aspects. Natl Cancer Inst 1984;72:1233–1240.
3. Goldgar DE, Easton DF, Cannon-Albright LA, Skolnick MH. Systematic population-based assessment of cancer risk in first-degree relatives of cancer probands. J Natl Cancer Inst 1994;86:1600–1608.
4. Miller RW. Deaths from childhood leukemia and solid tumours among twins and other sibs in the United States, 1960-67. J Natl Cancer Inst 1971;46:203–209.
5. Guasch J. Heredité des leucémies. Sang 1954;25:384–421.
6. Conley CL, Misiti J, Laster AJ. Genetic factors predisposing to chronic lymphocytic leukemia and to autoimmune disease. Medicine 1980;5:323–334.
7. Yuille MR, Matutes E, Marossy A, Hilditch B, Catovsky D, Houlston RS. Familial chronic lymphocytic leukemia: a survey and review of published studies. Br J Haematol 2000;109:794–799.
8. Thiersch JB. Aspects of leuchaemia: a leuchaemic family in South Australia. Proc R Aust Coll Phys 1947;2:35–38.
9. Penrose LS. The problem of anticipation in pedigrees of dystrophica myotonica. Ann Eugenics 1949;14:124–132.
10. Yuille MR, Houlston RS, Catovsky D. Anticipation in familial chronic lymphocytic leukemia families. Leukemia 1998;12(11):1696–1698.
11. Horwitz M, Goode EL, Jarvik GP. Anticipation in familial leukemia. Am J Hum Genet 1996;59:990–998.
12. Goldin LR, Sgambati M, Marti GE, Fontaine L, Ishibe N, Caporaso N. Anticipation in familial chronic lymphocytic leukemia Am J Hum Genet 1999;65:265–269.
13. Pritsch O, Troussard X, Magnac C, et al. VH gene usage by family members affected with chronic lymphocytic leukemia. Br J Haematol 1999;107:616–624.
14. Ashley CT, Warren ST. Trinucleotide repeat expansion and human disease. Ann Rev Genet 1995;29:703–728.
15. Howeler CJ, Busch HFM, Geraedts JPM, Niermeijer MF, Staal A. Anticipation in myotonic dystrophy: fact or fiction? Brain 1989;112:779–797.
16. Wierda WG, Kipps TJ. Chronic lymphocytic leukemia. Curr Opin Hematol. 1999;6:253–261.
17. German J. Chromosome-breakage syndromes: different genes, different treatments, different cancers. Basic Life Sci 1980;15:429–439.
18. Gatti RA, Berkel I, Boder E, et al. Localization of an ataxia-telangiectasia gene to chromosome 11q22-23. Nature 1988;336:577–578.
19. Taylor AMR, Metcalfe JA, Thick J, Mak Y-F. Leukemia and lymphoma in ataxia telangiectasia. Blood 1996;87:423–428.
20. Athma P, Rappaport R, Swift M. Molecular genotyping shows that ataxia-telangiectasia heterozygotes are predisposed to breast cancer. Cancer Genet Cytogenet 1996;92:130–134.
21. Swift M, Reitnauer PJ, Morrell D, Chase CL. Breast and other cancers in families with ataxia-telangiectasia. N Engl J Med 1987;316:1289–1294.
22. Stankovic T, Weber P, Stewart G, et al. Inactivation of ataxia telangiectasia mutated gene in B-cell chronic lymphocytic leukemia. Lancet 1999;353:26–29.
23. Schaffner C, Stilgenbauer S, Rappold GA, Dohner H, Lichter P. Somatic *ATM* mutations indicate a pathogenic role of *ATM* in B-cell chronic lymphocytic leukemia. Blood 1999;94:748–753.
24. Bullrich F, Rasio D, Kitada S, et al. ATM mutations in B-cell chronic lymphocytic leukemia. Cancer Res 1999; 59:24–27.
25. Starostik P, Manshouri T, O'Brien S, et al. Deficiency of the *ATM* protein expression defines an aggressive subgroup of B-cell chronic lymphocytic leukemia. Cancer Res 1998;58:4552–4557.

26. Savitsky K, Sfez S, Tagle DA, et al. The complete sequence of the coding region of the *ATM* gene reveals similarity to cell cycle regulators in different species Hum Mol Genet 1995;4:2025–2032.
27. Savitsky K, Bar-Shira A, Gilad S, et al. A single ataxia-telangiectasia gene with a product similar to PI-3 kinase. Science 1995;268:1749–1752.
28. Meyn MS. Ataxia-telangiectasia, cancer and the pathobiology of the ATM gene. Clin Genet 1999;55:289–304.
29. Bevan S, Catovsky D, Marossy A, et al. Linkage analysis for ATM in familial chronic lymphocytic leukemia. Leukemia 1999;13:1497–1500.
30. Klitz W, Aldrich CL, Fildes N, Horning SJ, Begovich AB. Localization of predisposition to Hodgkin disease in the HLA class II region. Am J Hum Genet 1994;54:497.
31. Risch N. Assessing the role of HLA-linked and unlinked determinants of disease. Am J Hum Genet 1987;40:1–14.
32. Klitz W, Aldrich CL, Fildes N, Horning SJ, Begovich AB. Localization of predisposition to Hodgkin disease in the HLA class II region. Am J Hum Genet 1994;54:497–505.
33. Taylor GM, Gokhale DA, Crowther D, et al. Further investigation of the role of HLA-DPB1 in adult Hodgkin's disease (HD) suggests an influence on susceptibility to different HD subtypes. Br J Cancer 1999;80:1405–1411.
34. Hirose S, Hamano Y, Shirai T. Genetic factors predisposing to B-CLL and to autoimmune disease in spontaneous murine model. Leukemia 1997;11(suppl 3):267–270.
35. Okada T, Takiura F, Tokushige K, et al. Major histocompatibility complex controls clonal proliferation of CD5+ B cells in H-2-congenic New Zealand mice: a model for B cell chronic lymphocytic leukemia and autoimmune disease. Eur J Immunol 1991;21:2743–2748.
36. Bevan S, Catovsky D, Matutes E, et al. Linkage analysis for MHC related genetic susceptibility in familial chronic lymphocytic leukemia. Blood 2000;96:3982–3984.
37. Horwitz M, Wiernik PH. Pseudoautosomal linkage of Hodgkin disease. Am J Hum Genet 1999;65:1413–1422.
38. Yuille MR, Catovsky D, Houlston RS. Pseudoautosomal linkage in chronic lymphocytic leukemia. Br J Haematol 2000;109:899–900.
39. Ashley CT, Warren ST. Trinucleotide repeat expansion and human disease. Annu Rev Genet 1995;29:703–728.
40. Koob MD, Benzow KA, Bird TD, et al. Rapid cloning of expanded trinucleotide repeat sequences from genomic DNA. Nat Genet 1998;18:72–75.
41. Oscier DG, Thompsett A, Zhu D, Stevenson FK. Differential rates of somatic hypermutation in V(H) genes among subsets of chronic lymphocytic leukemia defined by chromosomal abnormalities. Blood 1997;89:4153–4160.
42. Fais F, Ghiotto F, Hashimoto S, et al. Chronic lymphocytic leukemia B cells express restricted sets of mutated and unmutated antigen receptors. J Clin Invest 1998;102:1515–254.
43. Pritsch O, Troussard X, Magnac C, et al. VH gene usage by family members affected with chronic lymphocytic leukemia. Br J Haematol 1999;107:616–624.
44. Sakai A, Marti GE, Caporaso N, et al. Analysis of expressed immunoglobulin heavy chain genes in familial B-CLL. Blood 2000;95:1413–1419.
45. Cartwright RA, Bernard SM, Bird CC, et al. Chronic lymphocytic leukemia: case-control epidemiological study in Yorkshire. Br J Cancer 1987;56:79–82.
46. Linet MS, Van Natta ML, Brookmeyer R, et al. Familial cancer history and chronic lymphocytic leukemia. A case-control study. Am J Epidemiol 1989;130:655–664.
47. Pottern LM, Linet M, Blair A, et al. Familial cancers associated with subtypes of leukamia and non-hodgkin's lymphoma. Leukemia Res 1991;15:305–314.
48. Radovanovic Z, Markovic-Denic L, Jakovic S. Cancer mortality of family members of patients with chronic lymphocytic leukemia. Eur J Epidemiol 1994;10:211–213.
49. Brem TH, Morton ME. Defective serum gamma globulin formation. Ann Intern Med 1955;43:465–479.
50. Videbaek A. Familial leukemia. Acta Pathol Microbiol Scand 1958;44:372.
51. Hudson RP, Wilson SJ. Hypogammaglobulinemia and chronic lymphatic leukemia. Cancer 1960;13:200–204.
52. Gunz FW, Fitzgerald PH, Adams A. An abnormal chromosome in chronic lymphocytic leukemia. BMJ 1962;2:1097.
53. Fitzgerald PH, Hamer JW. Third case of chronic lymphocytic leukemia in a carrier of the inherited Ch1 chromosome. BMJ 1969;3:752.
54. Furbetta D, Solinas P. Hereditary chronic lymphatic leukemia. Proc Sec Intern Congr Hum Genet 1961;2:1078–1079.
55. Wisniewski D, Weinreich J. Lymphatische leukamie bei Vater und Sohn. Blut 1966;12:241–244.
56. Rigby PG, Rosenlof RC, Pratt PI, Lemon HM. Leukemia and lymphoma. JAMA 1966;197:95–100.
57. Ardizzone G, Rossi-Ferrini PL, Montali E, Matassi L. Anomalia chromosomica Ch1 in una famiglia con due casi di leukemia linfatica cronica. Rev Crit Clin Med 1968;68:1102.

58. Magaraggia L, Vettori G. Leucemia linfatica cronica familiare associata ad epitelioma cutaneo. Fracastoro 1968;61:269–273.

59. McPhedran P, Heath CW, Lee J. Patterns of familial leukemia: 10 cases of leukemia in two inter-related families. Cancer 1969;24:403–407.

60. Fraumeni JF, Vogel CL, DeVita VT. Familial chronic lymphocytic leukemia. Ann Intern Med 1969;71:279–284.

61. Blattner WA, Dean JH, Fraumeni JF. Familial lymphoproliferative malignancy: clinical and laboratory follow-up. Ann Intern Med 1979;90:943–944.

62. Gunz FW, Veale AMO. Leukemia in close relatives—accident or predisposition? J Natl Cancer Inst 1969;42:517–524.

63. Undritz E, Schnyder F. Vier Geschwister mit chronischer lymphatischer leukamie im Wallis. Scweiz Med Wochenschr 1971;101:1779–1780.

64. Potolosky AI, Heath CW, Buckley CE, Rowlands DT. Lymphoreticular malignancies and immunologic abnormalities in a sibship. Am J Med 1971;50:42–48.

65. Schweitzer M, Melief CMJ, Ploem JE. Chronic lymphocytic leukemia in five siblings. Scand J Haematol 1973; 11:97–105.

66. Blattner WA, Strober W, Muchmore AV, Blaese R, Broder S, Fraumeni J. Familial chronic lymphocytic leukemia. Immunologic and cellular charcaterisation. Ann Intern Med 1976;84:554–557.

67. Neuland CY, Blattner WA, Mann DL, Fraser MC, Tsai, Strong DM. Familial chronic lymphocytic leukemia. J Natl Cancer Inst 1983;71:1143–1150.

68. Shen A, Humphries C, Tucker P, Blattner F. Human heavy-chain variable region gene family nonrandomly rearranged in familial chronic lymphocytic leukemia. Proc Natl Acad Sci USA 1987;84:8563–8567.

69. Caporaso NE, Whitehouse J, Bertin P, et al. A 20-year clinical and laboratory study of familial B-chronic lymphocytic leukemia in a single kindred. Leuk Lymphoma 1991;3:331–342.

70. Gunz FW, Gunz JP, Veale AMO, Chapman CJ, Houston IB. Familial leukemia: a study of 909 families. Scand J Haematol 1975;15:117–131.

71. Petzholdt R, Hartwich G, Demmler K. Familiar-gehauftes Auftreten der chronischen lymphatischen Leukamie. Med Klin 1976;71:2123–2126.

72. Fazekas VT, Bach K, Toth S, Bodor F. Familiares Vorkommen von chronischer lympatischer leukamie. HLA-antigen und zytogenetische Untersuchungen. Wien Med Wochenschr 1978;9:262–264.

73. Branda RF, Ackerman SK, Handwerger BS, Howe RB, Douglas SD. Lymphocyte studies in familial chronic lymphatic leukemia. Am J Med 1978;64:508–514.

74. Conley CL, Misiti J, Laster AJ. Genetic factors predisposing to chronic lymphocytic leukemia and to autoimmune disease. Medicine 1980;5:323–334.

75. Alfinito F, Formisano S, Rotoli B. Familial leukemia: uncommon type of chronic lymphocytic leukemia in two sisters. Haematologica 1982;67:406–410.

76. Vanni M, Deambrogio P. Riscontro in due membri della stressa di leucemia linfatica chronica. Min Med 1983; 74:443–446.

77. Brok-Simoni F, Rechavi G, Katzir N, Ben-Bassat I. Chronic lymphocytic leukemia in twin sisters: monozygous but not identical. Lancet 1987;1:329–330.

78. Hakim I, Brok-Simoni F, Grossman Z, et al. CLL in three sisters: preferred usage of specific IG gene segments. Eur J Cancer 1993;29A(suppl 6):S38.

79. Eriksson M, Bergstrom I. Familial malignant blood disease in the county of Jamtland, Sweden. Eur J Haematol 1987;38:241–245.

80. Shah AR, Maeda K, Deegan MJ, Roth MS, Schnitzer B. A clinicopathologic study of familial chronic lymphocytic leukemia. Am J Clin Pathol 1992;97:184–188.

81. Cuttner J. Increased incidence of hematological malignancies in first-degree relatives of patients with chronic lymphocytic leukemia. Cancer Invest 1992;10:103–109.

82. Fernhout F, Dinkelaar RB, Hagemeijer A, Groeneveld K, van Kammen E, van Dongen JJ. Four aged siblings with B cell chronic lymphocytic leukemia. Leukemia 1997;11:2060–2065.

23 Young Patients With Chronic Lymphocytic Leukemia

Francesca R. Mauro, MD and Robin Foa, MD, PhD

1. INTRODUCTION

Chronic lymphocytic leukemia (CLL) is the most common leukemia in the Western world. In view of the mean age of CLL patients at presentation, the frequently indolent clinical course, and the overall restricted treatment options, for many years there has been only somewhat limited interest in this disease, and management has been largely conservative. However, the overall scenario and approach has changed significantly during the last few years, for the following reasons: (1) the progressive and constant increase in the "biological" age of CLL patients; (2) the availability of new drugs, namely, the purine analogs, which have a marked antileukemic action in CLL; (3) the knowledge that transplantation may have a role and may impact on this disease; (4) the evidence that monoclonal antibodies (MAbs) may be utilized in CLL; and (5) the progressive recognition of biological features that have prognostic implications.

Taken together, these realities are such that more aggressive, debulking approaches have been utilized for subgroups of patients with CLL. In this setting, particularly in light of the broader therapeutic armamentarium available today for the management of CLL patients, the issue of age has become of primary relevance. Although CLL has always been considered a disease of the elderly, with a median age at presentation of approx 65 yr, it should be recalled that about 20% of patients are younger than 55 yr at the time of diagnosis. In the last decade, retrospective studies (mainly multicentric) have focused attention on patients 50–55 yr old or younger (1–9). These studies have aimed at analyzing whether CLL in younger patients showed different features than CLL affecting older individuals. In an attempt to identify a hypothetically different clinical pattern of disease presentation, the clinical characteristics at diagnosis of the two age groups have been compared. In addition, the prognostic relevance for survival of some traditional clinical factors has been tested, and in some studies the outcome of young patients after first-line and advanced-line therapy has been also analyzed (9,10). The overall poor survival observed in young CLL patients requiring therapy justifies the general agreement that young patients deserve potentially curative therapeutic efforts. Two important questions then arise: which young patients should be treated and what kind of treatment should be recommended? In the present chapter we discuss different epidemiological, biological, clinical, and therapeutic features that pertain to young CLL patients.

From: *Contemporary Hematology*
Chronic Lymphocytic Leukemia: Molecular Genetics, Biology, Diagnosis, and Management
Edited by: G. B. Faguet © Humana Press Inc., Totowa, NJ

2. EPIDEMIOLOGY AND CLINICAL CHARACTERISTICS AT DIAGNOSIS OF YOUNG PATIENTS

As mentioned, CLL is the most common leukemia type among the elderly, with a median age at presentation of 65 yr. The disease is extremely rare before the third decade of life and increases after the fourth decade exponentially until the seventh decade *(11)*. The increased practice of periodic blood examinations has also increased the observation of CLL cases at an earlier stage of the disease and, possibly, at a younger age *(12,13)*. Within our series of 1011 CLL patients managed during the 1984–1994 period at our institution, we have observed a progressively increasing number of newly diagnosed CLL cases matched by a constant rate of about 20% per year of young patients (55 yr old or younger) (Figs. 1 and 2). Eleven percent of these patients were 50 yr old, and 9% were between 50 and 55 yr old; 9% were between 40 and 50 yr, and only 1.5% were younger than 40 yr. In their series, Bennett et al. *(2)* and Molica et al. *(7)* reported that 7–12% of CLL patients were younger than 50 yr.

As previously described *(3–7,9)*, in our series younger and older patients showed at diagnosis a similar distribution of different clinical features: stage, lymphocyte count, bone marrow histology, lymphocyte doubling time (LDT), and active disease (AD). The only unexplained difference between the two age groups in our series and also in the series described by Montserrat et al. *(3)* was a significantly higher male/female ratio in the younger group that could be partly caused by a hypothetical protective endocrine effect in young female subjects (Fig. 2).

3. DIFFERENTIAL DIAGNOSIS

It is becoming more evident that a sizable proportion of CD5-positive B-cell chronic lymphoproliferative disorders may indeed not be represented by true CLL. Thus, the heterogeneity always recorded in the clinical course of CLL cases may, at least in part, be attributed by an inadequate diagnostic workup. Although it is important at all ages, a correct etiopathogenetic definition appears to be essential in younger patients. In particular, a differential diagnosis must be made between CLL and non-Hodgkin's lymphoma (NHL) in the leukemic phase. A correct diagnosis must be based on an adequate morphological and immunophenotypic workup *(14–18)*. On morphological grounds, the presence of atypical lymphoid cells suggests NHL in leukemic phase. An accurate immunophenotypic analysis is essential for the differential diagnosis. In addition to CD5 positivity, CLL is characterized by weak surface Ig (sIg) expression, CD23 positivity, and frequent CD22 negativity. The sIg expression level should be quantified. Despite CD5 positivity, in the presence of high sIg expression, CD23 negativity, and CD22 positivity, further investigations should be performed. A lymph node biopsy in the presence of lymphadenopathy, or otherwise a bone biopsy with an accurate immunohistochemical workup, should be performed. It should be stressed that a diagnosis of NHL can be often made on the basis of a bone biopsy *(19)*. In our opinion, the importance of the differential diagnosis in CD5-positive lymphoproliferative disorders between CLL and NHL with a leukemic presentation has so far been understated. The practical implications are readily apparent in light of the different management techniques required.

4. SURVIVAL AND PROGNOSTIC FACTORS

A 5-yr relative survival rate of 78.8% (observed expected survival compared withy the same age control population) was recorded by the Surveillance, Epidemiology, and End Results (SEER)

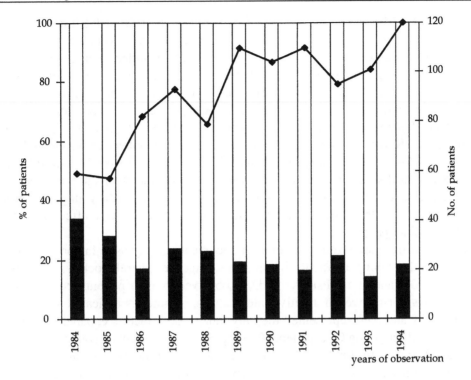

Fig. 1. CLL cases recorded during the 1984–1994 period and proportion of younger and older patients observed per year. Black bars, 55 yr old or younger; open bars, 55 yr or older; solid black line, no. of patients.

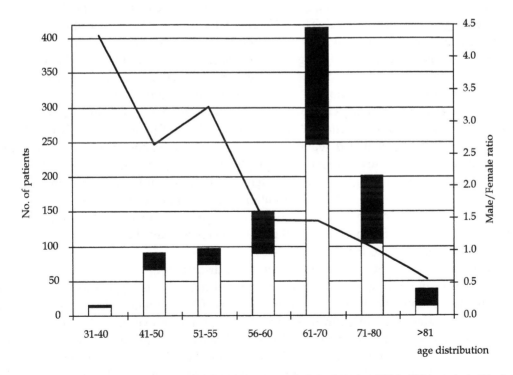

Fig. 2. Gender and age distribution of CLL cases recorded during the 1984–1994 period. Black bars, women; open bars, men; solid black line, no. of patients.

program registry for CLL patients younger than 65 yr during the 1989–1985 time period *(20)*. In our series, the overall median survival probability for patients 55 yr or younger was 10 yr, in line with the range of median survival values for young patients included in other series *(3–6,8,9)*. Paradoxically, young age did not represent a survival advantage, since both younger and older patients showed a similar survival probability. The 10-yr survival probability for young and old CLL patients was significantly lower compared with the expected survival probability for the age- and sex-matched Italian population: 55 yr or younger, controls 96.2% vs CLL 45.3%; older than 55 yr, controls 81.7% vs CLL 54.8%. When the relative survival rates were calculated, younger patients showed a lower relative survival rate than older patients (47% vs 67%). In addition to the greater impact of the disease on survival in the younger than in the older age group, deaths from causes directly related to CLL progression were significantly greater in the younger age group *(9)*. These findings indicate that a diagnosis of CLL implies a more adverse effect on survival in younger than in older people.

Several authors have analyzed whether well-documented prognostic factors have the same impact on survival of younger patients. In our series, stage, peripheral blood lymphocytes, marrow histology, LDT, and clinical signs of AD, as observed in older patients, correlated significantly with survival. However, in multivariate analysis, parameters indicative of early disease progression (LDT and AD) represented the only independent factors capable of significantly predicting survival for young CLL patients *(9)* (Fig. 3). Forty percent of young patients with an extremely good prognostic likelihood could be identified within stage A: 94% of them were projected long-term survivors at 12 yr from diagnosis without treatment *(9)* (Fig. 4).

The different outcome of CLL patients has recently been better defined by the exciting identification of biological features, such as the presence of certain cytogenetic abnormalities and the mutational pattern of the IgV_H genes *(21–23)*, which have had a high predictive value for disease progression and survival. The different patterns of genomic aberrations, i.e., 17p deletion, 11q deletion, 12q trisomy, and 13q deletion as a single aberration, are observed in approx 80% of cases using molecular genetic techniques *(21)*. The pattern of cytogenetic aberrations appears to be related to clinical features at CLL presentation, to the time of disease progression, and to survival probability. Preliminary results of a new prospective study performed by the German CLL Study Group in stage A patients revealed the presence of genomic aberrations with unfavorable prognostic value in approx 15% of patients *(13)*. Two different CLL variants have been identified according to the mutational status of the IgV genes. The pregerminal variant originates from naive B-lymphocytes, shows no IgV gene mutation, and is characterized by a poor prognosis. The postgerminal variant originates from memory B-lymphocytes, shows IgV gene somatic hypermutations and is characterized by a better outcome *(22–25)*. Cytogenetic aberrations with unfavorable prognostic effects, such as 17p and 11q deletion, as well as a CD38 expression level greater than 30%, have been found in CLL cases characterized by nonmutated IgV genes *(23–25)*.

In a series of CLL patients with long-lasting stable disease without treatment for 10–23 yr observed at our institution, we documented a number of features that appear to correlate with indolent disease: an immunophenotypic profile of classic CLL, a mutated IgV gene status, the absence of *p53* aberrations, a very low incidence of poor-prognosis cytogenetic abnormalities, a lack of CD38 expression, and a normal CD4/CD8 T-cell subset distribution (ms. in preparation).

To our knowledge, no study has yet specifically focused on the distribution and prognostic significance of such biological markers within the younger age group of CLL patients. Ideally, an integrated clinical-biological prognostic assessment at CLL presentation should be offered to

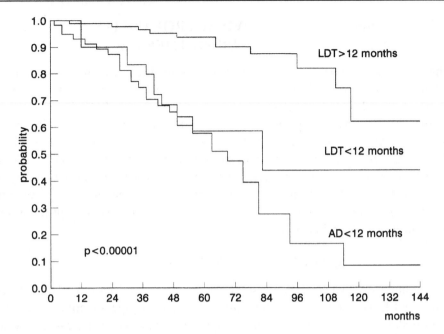

Fig. 3. Survival of young CLL patients according to lymphocyte doubling time (LDT) or presence of active disease (AD).

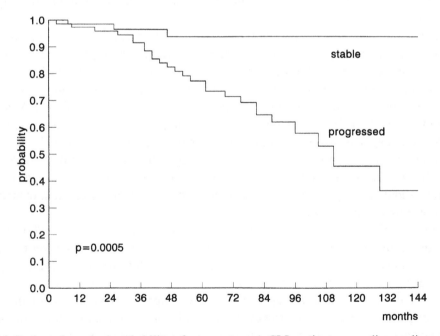

Fig. 4. Projected survival probability of young stage A CLL patients according to disease status.

all patients, particularly to the younger ones, since it may prove of primary relevance in predicting a stable or a progressive outcome and may thus be important to plan the most adequate therapeutic management, particularly for stage A patients.

5. RESPONSE AND SURVIVAL PROBABILITY
OF PATIENTS REQUIRING THERAPY

Young age has a favorable impact on the possibility of achieving a response to conventional therapy (26,27). In our series, 60% of younger CLL patients required treatment, and the overall response rate (complete and partial responses) to first-line therapy was 86%. Despite the high response rate to first-line therapy, young patients showed a median survival probability from the start of therapy of only 5 yr. Patients receiving second-line therapy had lower response and lower survival rates: only 32% responses and a median survival probability of 28 mo (9). The poor outcome of young CLL patients requiring advanced treatment has also been reported by Seymour et al. (10), who identified (in fludarabine-refractory patients and in patients relapsing from a fludarabine-induced remission) a subset of young CLL patients with very poor prognosis who showed a median survival probability of less than 18 mo.

6. TREATMENT OPTIONS

It is important to emphasize that younger age should not be considered per se a sufficient reason to treat every young CLL patient early after diagnosis. The same therapeutic policy is at present recommended for both younger and older patients: stage A patients should be treated only at the time of disease progression, whereas advanced stage patients require treatment earlier. This is in agreement with the observation of a lack of survival advantage for early treatment of all stage A CLL patients reported in the past (26) and recently confirmed in a large randomized study by Dighiero et al. (27).

In our series, over half of stage A patients had disease progression and required treatment after a median time of 23 mo from diagnosis, and the remaining approx 40% represented a group of young patients with an extremely good prognostic likelihood: 94% of them were projected long-term survivors at 12 yr from diagnosis without treatment (9) (Fig. 4). As mentioned above, biological markers—such as cytogenetic abnormalities, the mutational pattern of the IgV genes, and the degree and level of CD38 expression (22–25)—could provide helpful prognostic information to determine at diagnosis stage A patients who will have stable or progressive disease. The early identification of stage A patients who will show progressive disease could be useful to design an early therapeutic intervention for such patients, particularly in the younger age group. Controlled studies should attempt to evaluate the potential benefit of early treatment of stage A patients with poor prognostic biological markers.

It should be recalled that at the present time CLL is still incurable by conventional therapies and that the disease itself represents the main cause of death for younger patients. Over time, the profile of survival curves of CLL patients has not been modified by the different chemotherapeutic approaches, because chemotherapy is not curative.

In CLL patients, the first goal of therapy should be to improve survival expectancy and quality of life for patients of all ages. However, although for elderly patients a traditional conservative management is a realistic and reasonable strategy, for younger patients this approach may prove unsatisfactory. Thus, there is general agreement that young patients with advanced or progressive disease deserve curative therapeutic efforts. Once the decision to treat is made, the question of which treatment to use arises. The availability of highly active drugs such as purine analogs, the recent utilization of monoclonal antibodies, and the increasing use of autologous stem cell transplantation procedures have improved the quality and duration of remissions. Thus, different therapeutic options are now available, in an attempt to obtain a profound cytoreduction of the leukemic clone, better quality remissions, and, in some cases, molecular remissions. Considering their poor prognosis, there is a consensus that young CLL patients with good performance status and advanced disease should be included in randomized trials in which the potential benefit of possibly eradicative programs is investigated.

Young CLL patients may be treated more aggressively for several reasons: (1) the median survival probability of younger patients after conventional first-line therapy is only 5 yr and is only 2 yr or less after second-line therapy *(9,10)*; (2) CLL, or its complications, is responsible for 98% of deaths in young patients *(9)*; (3) young patients may tolerate high-dose therapy better, and the currently available supportive care measures have significantly decreased the morbidity and mortality related to transplantation procedures; thus, the age limit for transplantation has increased during the last decade; and (4) at the present time, a correlation between quality of responses and survival has not been clearly demonstrated *(29)*. However, the achievement of better quality responses may translate into a longer treatment-free duration, better outcome after transplantation *(13)*, and, ultimately, longer relapse-free survival duration *(30,31)*.

At the present time, there are no indications for a specific treatment modality to be implemented in young CLL patients, since the best treatment strategy has not yet been identified. However, there is a agreement that the treatment goal is achievement of better quality complete responses with the greatest possible leukemia debulking since the response duration is inversely related to the amount of residual disease. Thus, controlled trials with purine analogs in association with synergistic drugs (combined or followed by monoclonal antibodies, or autologous or allogeneic stem cell transplantation) are currently under investigation. Potentially, all treatment modalities may be combined in a therapeutic strategy directed toward maximum reduction of the leukemic clone.

In younger patients there is an agreement that a fludarabine-containing protocol should be used as initial therapy, since this regimen has effected a higher response rate and a longer response duration compared with alkylating agents *(32)*. For patients of any age, a complete response rate of approx 30% after fludarabine ± prednisone as initial therapy is to be expected *(32)*, with a median response duration of approx 3 yr. O'Brien et al. *(33)* reported a similar rate of complete using the fludarabine and cyclophosphamide combination regimen; these responses were of better quality, since residual disease detected by flow cytometry was very low and the remission duration seemed to be prolonged.

In patients achieving a response to front-line therapy, current clinical trials are evaluating the role of postremission treatment (such as monoclonal antibodies or autologous transplantation) aimed at further reducing residual disease and improving duration of response. The possibility of obtaining complete responses with very little residual disease after combined fludarabine schedules has allowed a broader utilization of autologous stem cell transplantation procedures. Although transplantation procedures are currently under extensive investigation, data are still insufficient to establish their potential benefit. This is not surprising, considering that about 30% of patients show active disease that requires treatment, that about 30% are 60 yr or younger, and that an intensive treatment procedure such as a stem cell transplantation can probably be considered only for 10% or fewer of CLL patients with an adequate performance status *(34)*. The transplant-related mortality of approx 10% should be weighed when the autograft option is considered. Furthermore, the absence of a plateau in the disease-free survival curves suggests that autotransplantation does not cure CLL *(13)*. However, in the subset of good-prognosis patients, the survival duration after autologous transplant is likely to be improved. Retrospective data suggest that the sensitivity of CLL is a key factor for predicting the outcome after transplant. Patients with sensitive disease (who have a complete remission before autograft, with less bone marrow lymphocyte infiltration and less heavy pretreatment and in an earlier phase of the disease) in fact have a better outcome, with sustained disease control *(35–39)*.

The option of allogeneic bone marrow transplantation is limited by the small number of eligible patients and by the consistent transplant-related mortality rate, which ranges between 25 and 50%. However, it should be noted that after allogeneic stem cell transplantation, responses have been observed in some refractory patients, and a survival plateau of 40–60% can be reached. These findings suggest the occurrence of a graft-vs-CLL effect after allogeneic stem cell transplantation *(13)*. Allogeneic stem cell transplantations in which nonmyeloablative and more immunosuppressive conditioning regimens are employed may represent a noneradicating therapeutic approach in which both the stem cell engraftment and the graft-vs-CLL effect are preserved. Preliminary results of this alternative allogeneic transplantation, which may be potentially curative with less transplanted-related toxicity, are promising *(40,41)*. This approach, which could be offered to a larger number of patients, needs to be investigated further in the setting of controlled studies.

Since the main objective of therapy should be the prolongation of survival, the potential morbidity and mortality of intensive therapies needs to be carefully weighed in patients with associated risks of poor compliance to intensive treatments: heavily and pretreated CLL patients, refractory patients, patients with recurrent infections, and bad performance status. Despite the (relatively) young age, this subset of patients has a significant risk of poor outcome after both autologous and allogeneic transplantation and may have a better benefit in terms of quality of life and survival duration by a conservative approach.

Given the extremely poor survival of patients refractory to purine analogs, new drugs and experimental treatment approaches should be considered in this subset of patients. Young patients refractory to chemotherapy are the best candidates for investigational treatments and should be enrolled in experimental trials.

7. COMPLICATIONS

7.1. Infections

Infections represent the major cause of morbidity and of mortality of CLL patients. In our series, we observed the same rate of fatal infections in young and old CLL patients *(9)*. Heavily treated patients and refractory patients, particularly if they are treated with purine analogs, are subgroups with an increased risk of developing infections *(42,43)*. In young CLL patients receiving intensive treatment, the risk of infectious complications should be always considered. Adequate supportive management, including prophylaxis against herpesviruses, fungi, and *Pneumocystis carinii* and the use of granulocyte colony-stimulating factor in the presence of neutropenia may reduce the occurrence of fatal infections that could have an adverse impact on the outcome of patients treated with curative intent *(44,45)*.

7.2. Second Primary Cancers and Richter's Syndrome

The association of a second primary malignancy with CLL is well known. Epidemiological studies were carried out on large series of CLL patients enrolled in tumor registries participating in the National Cancer Institute Surveillance, Epidemiology, and End Results program. CLL patients were found to have a significantly increased risk, constant over time, of developing second cancers, with an overall observed/expected ratio of 1.2 *(46,47)*. In our series, we recorded an overall incidence of 8.3% with a nonstatistically different rate of second primary cancers in the old and young age groups of *(9)*. The rate of second cancers did not appear to be influenced by therapy. This finding suggests that the disease-related immunodeficiency state of CLL that most likely predisposes to the development of second malignancies is independent of treatment and age. The simultaneous occurrence of a leukemia of the elderly and of a second cancer at a younger age strongly suggests that some patients may have an increased risk of developing a tumor early because of individual predisposing factors.

The incidence of Richter's syndrome in CLL patients recorded in our series *(9)* and reported by Robertson et al. *(48)* and by Morrison et al. *(49)* ranges between 1 and 2.8%. No predictive risk factors for the occurrence of Richter's syndrome have been identified so far. In the Cancer and Leukemia Group B study *(47)*, age did not have a predictive effect on the occurrence of Richter's syndrome. In our series, younger patients showed a Richter's syndrome rate fivefold higher than that of older patients. However, it should be recalled that the rate of lymphomas in the older age group is possibly underestimated, since very old patients with advanced and unresponsive disease are not always surgically biopsied, for ethical reasons. Most of Richter's syndrome occur as a consequence of a clonal transformation from the original CLL cells; a small proportion of cases may occur as a consequence of an immunosuppressive state.

Since younger patients are usually treated with purine analogs, an important point to analyze is whether the immunosuppression caused by purine analogs therapy may facilitate the occurrence of both second cancers and Richter's syndrome. An absence of a relationship between fludarabine and 2-chlorodeoxyadenosine (2-CDA) therapy and a higher occurrence of Richter's syndrome has been reported by Robertson et al. *(48)*, whereas other authors *(50)* have reported a higher risk of Richter's syndrome in patients receiving fludarabine. In a large study reported by Cheson et al. *(51)*, the rate of second malignancies in CLL patients treated with fludarabine was not increased compared with those never treated with purine analogs. However, the value of these findings is limited by two factors: the immunosuppressive state related to CLL itself and the short patient follow-up.

No information is yet available about the rate of Richter's syndrome and second malignancies occurring after autologous and allogeneic stem cell transplantation.

8. ETHICAL AND EMOTIONAL ASPECTS

Physicians should recall that a diagnosis of CLL can have a devastating effect on the pateint's quality of life, independently of age, clinical stage, and the therapy requirements. A leukemia diagnosis at a relatively young age may cause worries about the future course of the disease, the need for therapy, the potential complications, the ability to face professional and familial engagements, and, most of all, the risk of premature death. This is particularly so in light of the progressive increase in mean life expectancy. Patients with a diagnosis of CLL need to be helped to accept their new reality, which is related to the diagnosis of a chronic but incurable disease. Adequate and detailed information should be given to the patients and their families. Because of the high heterogeneity of this form of leukemia, each patient will have his or her own clinical picture, which depends on the stage and clinical activity of the disease.

The nature of the disease, the different clinical profiles and patterns of outcome, and the need for therapy or only clinical observation should be explained clearly. Providing detailed information is paramount for an optimal clinical management of patients and for preserving a good quality of life. Patients with early disease are usually encouraged not to modify their usual life style; in approx one-fourth of patients, life duration of cases, may be similar to that of nonaffected individuals of the same age and sex. However, patients with early-stage disease should also be informed about the possibility of disease progression, which in about half of cases justifies periodic clinical assessment. A normal social and family life should also be recommended for patients requiring therapy. Because of the chronic course of the disease, it is usually not hard for the physician to arrange a treatment strategy compatible with an active life style.

If therapy is required, the treatment strategy should be clearly explained. In particular, patients need to know their life expectancy and be given clear information about the potential objectives and risks of intensive therapies. The physician's clear explanations can form the basis of participation in clinical trials, which should be encouraged. However, in the treatment choice, managing physicians should also take into account the expectations of the patient. A good physician-patient relationship is essential both for the emotional needs of patients and as the basis for an optimal therapeutic management with patient cooperation.

Some specific points need to be discussed clearly. Many patients are afraid they will transmit the leukemia to their partner or family members. They need to be reassured that CLL is not infectious or transmissible. Younger patients also need to know that birth control should be practiced during chemotherapy because of the potential effects of purine analogs and intensive chemotherapy on the fetus. Information on the substantial risk of transient or permanent infertility after chemotherapy should also be given. Thus, patients aware of the life expectancy related to the diagnosis of CLL who wish to procreate should be informed about procedures to circumvent sterility. Only anecdotial cases concerning pregnancy during CLL have been reported *(52)*. Thus, relatively limited information on the risks for the child and for the affected patient is available.

The uncertainty and the inability to plan long-term projects following the diagnosis of CLL may induce a different pattern of psychological responses, such as denial, anxiety, despair, and depression. A pre-existing quiescent psychological distress may be activated by anxiety and depression *(53)*. Patients who are potentially at risk of psychological distress should be identified and considered for psychological support and/or treatment, which may considerably improve their quality of life and compliance with diagnostic and therapeutic procedures.

9. CONCLUSIONS

Patients younger than 55 yr, defined as "young" patients, represent about one-third of all CLL patients and have no major distinctive presenting clinical features compared with older patients. Although the two age groups display similar clinical features and overall survival, the disease itself appears to have a more adverse effect on the expected survival of younger individuals.

About 40% of young patients have long-lasting stable disease requiring no treatment, with a very good prognosis that may not differ from that of the age-matched normal population. For this category, any form of therapeutic intervention would be inappropriate. On the other hand, 60% of young CLL patients have progressive disease, with a relatively short median survival probability of 5 yr following conventional therapy. The possibility of identifying features associated with disease stability or progression at diagnosis or early during clinical follow-up is of primary relevance, in order not to administer unnecessary treatment to patients with favorable features and, vice versa, to implement as early as possible potential eradicative strategies in the presence of adverse prognostic features. Current advances in knowledge are such that nowadays all young CLL patients should probably undergo an extensive biological workup. The recently documented high prognostic relevance for CLL progression of cytogenetic markers, *p53* mutations, the mutational pattern of the IgV$_H$ genes, and CD38 expression represents an exciting improvement that may help to explain the clinical heterogeneity of CLL. Further studies are needed to understand the biological pathways of CLL and their potential therapeutic applications. Better prognostic information could be very useful, for better early definition (at CLL diagnosis) of young patients with a poor prognostic profile and an increased risk of progression.

Younger patients can benefit from more aggressive treatment strategies aimed at obtaining a true eradication of the disease. Younger patients refractory to therapy are also the best candidates for evaluating the activity of new drugs. The poor prognosis shown by younger CLL patients with active disease should be taken into account, and the inclusion of these patients in controlled trials investigating the potential benefits of such potentially eradicative programs and the activity of new treatment approaches needs to be encouraged.

ACKNOWLEDGMENTS

This work was partly supported by the Associazione Italiana per la Ricerca sul Cancro (AIRC), Milan, and by the Ministero dell'Istruzione, dell'Università e della Ricerca (MIUR), Rome, Italy.

REFERENCES

1. Spier CM, Kjeldsberg CR, Head DR, Di Fiore KC, Tudor B. Chronic lymphocytic leukemia in young adults. Am J Clin Pathol 1985;84:675–678.
2. Bennett JM, Raphael B, Oken MM, Rubin P, Silber R. The prognosis of chronic lymphocytic leukemia under age 50 years. Nouv Rev Fr Hematol 1988;30:411–412.
3. Montserrat E, Gomis F, Vallespi T, et al Presenting features and prognosis of chronic lymphocytic leukemia in younger adults. Blood 1991;78:1545–1551.
4. Pangalis GA, Reverter JC, Boussiotis VA, Montserrat E. Chronic lymphocytic leukemia in younger adults: preliminary results of a study based on 454 patients. IWCLL/Working Group. Leuk Lymphoma 1991;5:175–181.
5. De Rossi G, Mandelli F, Covelli A, et al. Chronic lymphocytic leukemia (CLL) in younger adults: a retrospective study of 133 cases. Hematol Oncol 1989;7:127–131.
6. Dhodapkar M, Tefferi A, Su J, Phyliky RL. Prognostic features and survival in young adults with early/intermediate chronic lymphocytic leukemia (B-CLL): a single institution study. Leukemia 1993;7:1232–1235.
7. Molica S, Brugiatelli M, Callea V, et al. Comparison of younger versus older B-cell chronic lymphocytic leukaemia patients for clinical presentation and prognosis. A retrospective study of 53 cases. Eur J Haematol 1994;52: 216–221.
8. De Lima M, O'Brien S, Lerner S, Keating MJ. Chronic lymphocytic leukemia in the young patient. Semin Oncol 1998;25:107–116.
9. Mauro FR, Foa R, Giannarelli D, et al. Clinical characteristics and outcome of "young" chronic lymphocytic leucemia patients: a single institution study of 204 cases. Blood 1999;94:448–454.
10. Seymour JF, Robertson LE, O'Brien S, Lerner S, Keating MJ. Survival of young patients with chronic lymphocytic leukemia failing fludarabine therapy: a basis for the use of myeloablative therapies. Leuk Lymphoma 1995;18:493–496.
11. Sgambati MT, Linet MS, Devesa SS. Chronic lymphocytic leukemia. Epidemiological, familial, and genetic aspects. In: Cheson BD, ed. Chronic Lymphoid Leukemias. 2nd ed. Marcel Dekker, New York, 2001, pp. 33–62.
12. Diehl LF, Karnell LH, Menck HR. The National Cancer data base on age, gender, treatment, and outcomes of patients with chronic lymphocytic leukemia. Cancer 1999;86:2684–2692.
13. Rai RR, Dohner H, Keating MJ, Montserrat E. Chronic lymphocytic leukemia: case-based session. Hematology (Am Soc Hematol Educ Program) 2001:140–156.
14. Bennett JM, Catovsky D, Daniel MT, et al. The French-American-British (FAB) Cooperative Group. Proposals for the classification of chronic (mature) B and T lymphoid leukaemias. J Clin Pathol 1989;42:567–584.
15. Catovsky D, Foa R. The Lymphoid Leukaemias. Butterworths, London, 1990.
16. Criel A, Verhoef G, Vlietinck R, et al. Further characterization of morphologically defined typical and atypical CLL: a clinical, immunophenotypic, cytogenetic and prognostic study on 390 cases. Br J Haematol 1997;97:383–391.

17. Matutes E, Owusu-Ankomah K, Morilla R, et al. The immunological profile of B-cell disorders and proposal of a scoring system for the diagnosis of CLL. Leukemia 1994;8:1640–1645.

18. Moreau EJ, Matutes E, A'Hern RP, et al. Improvement of the chronic lymphocytic leukemia scoring system with the monoclonal antibody SN8 (CD79b). Am J Clin Pathol 1997;108:378–382.

19. Pezzella F, Munson PJ, Miller KD, Goldstone AH, Gatter KC. The diagnosis of low B-cell neoplasm in bone marrow trephines. Br J Haematol 2000;108:369–376.

20. Ries LAG, Kosary CL, Hankley BF, Miller BA, Clegg LX, Edwards BK. SEER Cancer Statistics Review, 1973–1996. NIH Publication No. 99-2789. National Cancer Institute, Bethesda, MD, 1999, pp. 262–283.

21. Döhner H, Stilgenbauer S, Benner A, et al. Genomic aberrations and survival in chronic lymphocytic leukemia. N Engl J Med 2000;343:1910–1916.

22. Hamblin TJ, Davis Z, Gardiner A, Oscier DG, Stevenson FK. Unmutated Ig V_H genes are associated with a more aggressive form of chronic lymphocytic leukemia. Blood 1999;94:1848–1854.

23. Damle JN, Wasil T, Fais F, et al. IgV gene mutation status and CD38 expression as novel prognostic indicators in chronic lymphocytic leukemia. Blood 1999;94:1840–1847.

24. Kröber A, Seiler T, Leupolt E, Döhner H, Stilgenbauer S. IgV$_H$ mutated and unmutated B-CLL tumors show distinct genetic aberration patterns. Blood 2000; 96(Suppl 1):835a.

25. Hamblin TJ, Orchard JA, Ibbotson RE, et al. CD38 expression and immunoglobulin variable region mutation are independent prognostic variables in chronic lymphocytic leukemia, but CD38 expression may vary during the course of the disease. Blood 2002;99:1023–1029.

26. Montserrat E, Vinolas N, Reverter JC, Rozman C. Natural history of chronic lymphocytic leukemia: on the progression and prognosis of early stages. Nouv Rev Fr Hematol 1998;30:359–361.

27. Catovsky D, Richards S, Fooks J, Hamblin TJ. CLL trials in the United Kingdom: MRC trial 1, 2 and 3. Leuk Lymphoma 1991;5(suppl 14):105.

28. Dighiero G, Maloum K, Desablens B, et al. for The French Cooperative Group on Chronic Lymphocytic Leukemia. Chlorambucil in indolent chronic lymphocytic leukemia. N Engl J Med 1998;338:1506–1514.

29. CLL Trialist' Collaborative Group. Chemotherapeutic options in chronic lymphocytic leukemia: a meta-analysis of the randomized trials. J Natl Cancer Inst 1999;91:861–868.

30. Keating MJ, O'Brien S, Kantarjian H, et al Long-term follow-up of patients with chronic lymphocytic leukemia treated with fludarabine as a single agent. Blood 1993;81:2878.

31. The French Cooperative Group on CLL, Johnson S, Smith AG, Loffler H, et al. Multicentre prospective randomised trial of fludarabine versus cyclophosphamide, doxorubicin and prednisone (CAP) for treatment of advanced-stage chronic lymphocytic leukaemia. Lancet 1996;347:1432–1438.

32. Rai KR, Peterson BL, Appelbaum FR, et al. Fludarabine compared with chlorambucil as primary therapy for chronic lymphocytic leukemia. N Engl J Med 2000;343:1750–1757.

33. O'Brien SM, Kantarjian HM, Cortes J, et al. Results of the fludarabine and cyclophosphamide combination regimen in chronic lymphocytic leukemia. J Clin Oncol 2001;19:1414–1420.

34. Montserrat E. Developing risk-adapted treatment strategies for chronic lymphocytic leukemia. In: Cheson BD, ed. Chronic Lymphoid Leukemias, 2nd ed. Marcel Dekker, New York, 2001, pp. 377–392.

35. Montserrat E, Esteve J, Schmitz N, et al. Autologous stem-cell transplantation (ASCT) for chronic lymphocytic leukemia (CLL): results in 107 patients. Blood 1999;94(suppl 1):397a.

36. Dreger P, von Neuhoff N, Sonnen R, et al: Efficacy and prognostic implications of early autologous stem cell transplantation for poor-risk chronic lymphocytic leukemia. Blood 2000;96(suppl 1):483.

37. Horowitz MM, Montserrat E, Sobocinski K, et al. for the Chronic Leukemia Working Committee, International Bone Marrow Transplant Registry (IBMTR) and the Autologous Blood and Marrow Transplant Registry (ABMTR). Hematopoietic stem-cell transplantation (SCT) for chronic lymphocytic leukemia (CLL). Blood 2000; 96(suppl 1):522a

38. Esteve J, Villamor N, Colomer D, et al. Stem cell transplantation for chronic lymphocytic leukemia: different outcome after autologous and allogeneic transplantation and correlation with minimal residual disease. Leukemia 2001;15:445–451.

39. Dreger P, van Biezen A, Brand R, et al Outcome after autologous stem cell transplantation for CLL: a prognostic factor analysis from the EBMT database. Hematol J 2001;1(suppl 1):219a.

40. Khouri I, Keating M, Körbling M, et al. Transplant-lite: induction of graft-versus-malignancy using fludarabine-based nonablative chemotherapy and allogeneic blood progenitor cell transplantation as treatment for lymphoid malignancies. J Clin Oncol 1998;16:2817–2824.

41. Khouri I, Munsell M, Zajzi S, et al. Comparable survival for nonablative and ablative allogeneic transplantation for chronic lymphocytic leukemia (CLL): the case for early intervention. Blood 2000;96(suppl 1):205a.
42. Anaissie EJ, Kontoyiannis DP, O'Brien S, Kantarjian H, Robertson L, Keating MJ. Infections in patients with chronic lymphocytic leukemia treated with fludarabine. Ann Int Med 1998;129:559–566.
43. Morrison VA, Rai KR, Peterson BL, et al. Impact of therapy with chlorambucil, fludarabine, or fludarabine plus chlorambucil on infections in patients with chronic lymphocytic leukemia: Intergroup Study Cancer and Leukemia Group B 9011. J Clin Oncol 2001;19:3611–3621.
44. Sudhoff T, Arning M, Schneider W. Prophylactic strategies to meet infectious complications in fludarabine-treated CLL. Leukemia 1997;11(suppl 2):S38–41.
45. O'Brien S, Kantarjian H, Beran M, et al. Fludarabine and granulocyte colony-stimulating factor (G-CSF) in patients with chronic lymphocytic leukemia. Leukemia 1997;11:1631–1635.
46. Travis LB, Curtis RE, Hankey BF, Fraumeni JF Jr. Second cancers in patients with chronic lymphocytic leukemia. J Natl Cancer Inst 1992;84:1422–1142.
47. Hisada M, Biggar RJ, Greene MH, Fraumeni JF Jr, Travis LB. Solid tumors after chronic lymphocytic leukemia. Blood 2001;98:1979–1981.
48. Robertson LE, Pugh W, O'Brien S, et al. Richter's syndrome: a report on 39 patients. J Clin Oncol 1993;11:1985.
49. Morrison VA, Rai KR, Peterson BL, et al. Transformation to Richter's syndrome or to prolymphocytic leukemia (PLL) and other second hematologic malignancies in patients with chronic lymphocytic leukemia (CLL): an Intergroup Study (CALGB 9011). Blood 1999;94:539a.
50. Desablens B, Garidi R, Fernandes J, et al. Does fludarabine increase the risk of Richter's syndrome (RS) among chronic lymphocytic leucemia? Haematologica 1999;84:259.
51. Cheson BD, Vena DA, Barret J, Freidlin B. Second malignancies as a consequence of nucleoside analog therapy for chronic lymphocytic leukemias. J Clin Oncol 1999;17:2454–2460.
52. Welsh TM, Thompson J, Lim S. Chronic lymphocytic leukemia in pregnancy. Leukemia 2000;14:1155.
53. Saifollahi J, Rouhani M, Roth AJ, Holland JC. Psychological aspects of chronic lymphocytic leukemias. In: Cheson BD, ed. Chronic Lymphoid Leukemias. 2nd ed. Marcel Dekker, New York, 2001, pp. 593–608.

Index

Lightning Source UK Ltd.
Milton Keynes UK
UKHW05n1921220218
318321UK00004B/31/P